Illustrated Handbook
of
NURSING
CARE

SPRINGHOUSE CORPORATION
SPRINGHOUSE, PENNSYLVANIA

STAFF

Senior Publisher
Matthew Cahill

Art Director
John Hubbard

Clinical Manager
Judith Schilling McCann, RN, MSN

Senior Editor
H. Nancy Holmes

Project Manager
Judith A. Lewis

Clinical Editors
Beverly Ann Tscheschlog, RN (clinical project manager); Collette Bishop Hendler, RN, CCRN; Marybeth Morrell, RN, CCRN; Clare M. Brabson, RN, BSN

Copy Editors
Cynthia C. Breuninger (manager), Karen C. Comerford, Stacey A. Follin, Brenna H. Mayer

Designers
Arlene Putterman (associate art director), Matie Patterson (assistant art director), Stephanie Peters (book designer), Donald G. Knauss (project manager), Joe Clark, Jeff Sklarow

Typography
Diane Paluba (manager), Joyce Rossi Biletz, Phyllis Marron, Valerie Rosenberger

Manufacturing
Deborah Meiris (director), Pat Dorshaw (manager), T.A. Landis, Otto Mezei

Editorial Assistants
Beverly Lane, Mary Madden

Production Coordinator
Margaret Rastiello

Indexer
Dorothy Hoffman

CONTENTS

CONTRIBUTORS AND CONSULTANTS

Linda S. Baas, RN, PhD, CCRN
Assistant Professor
University of Cincinnati (Ohio)
College of Nursing and Health

Heather Boyd-Monk, SRN, BSN, CRNO
Assistant Director of Nursing for
Ophthalmic Education Programs
Wills Eye Hospital
Philadelphia

Susan J. Brown-Wagner, RN, MSN, CRNP, AOCN
Administrative Director, Oncology
Initiative
Anne Arundel Medical Center
Annapolis, Md.

Kathleen C. Byington, RN, MSN, CS
Pediatric Clinical Nurse Specialist,
Case Manager
Vanderbilt University
Nashville, Tenn.

Claire Campbell, RN, MSN, CFNP
Family Nurse Practitioner
Health South Medical Center
Dallas

Janice T. Chussil, RN,C, MSN, ANP
Dermatology Nurse Practitioner
Dermatology Associates
Portland, Ore.

Jacqueline Crocetti, RN,C, MSN, CRNP
Nursing Professor
Northampton Community College
Bethlehem, Pa.

Jane Curnow, RN,C, MSN, CNA
Director, Physician Affiliations
Mercy Hospital of Philadelphia

Robin Donohoe Dennison, RN, MSN, CCRN, CS
Critical Care Consultant
Lexington, Ky.

Harriet W. Ferguson, RN,C, MSN, EdD
Associate Professor
Temple University
Philadelphia

Janine Fiesta, JD, BSN
Vice President
Lehigh Valley Hospital
Allentown, Pa.

Margaret A. Fitzgerald, RN-CS, MS, CFNP
Family Nurse Practitioner
Greater Lawrence (Mass.) Family
Health Center

Marilyn A. Folcik, RN, MPH, ONC
Assistant Director, Department of
Surgery
Hartford (Conn.) Hospital

Ellie Z. Franges, RN, MSN, CNRN, CCRN
Director, Neuroscience Services
Sacred Heart Hospital
Allentown, Pa.

Karen Alyce Graf, RN, BSN, CURN
Urology Nurse Coordinator
New York University Medical Center
Rusk Institute of Rehabilitation
Medicine

Peg Gray-Vickrey, RN,C, DNS
Associate Professor
Florida Gulf Coast University
Fort Myers, Fla.

Linda B. Haas, RN, PhC, CDE
Endocrinology Clinical Nurse
Specialist
VA Pugent Sound Health Care System
Seattle (Wash.) Division

**Janet C. Ross Kerr, RN, BScN, MS,
PhD**
Professor, Faculty of Nursing
University of Alberta (Can.)
Edmonton

Margaret Massoni, RN, MS, CS
Assistant Professor
City University of New York
The College of Staten Island

Paula L. Rich, RN, MSN
Consultant
Professional Nursing Development
Mountaintop, Pa.

**Judith M. Saunders, RN, DNSc,
FAAN**
Assistant Professsor
Department of Nursing
University of Southern California
Los Angeles

**Regina Shannon-Bodnar, RN, MS,
MSN, OCN**
Director of Patient Care Services
Hospice of Baltimore
Towson, Md.

Sharon Valente, RN,CS, PhD, FAAN
Assistant Professor
Clinical Specialist in Mental Health
Department of Nursing
University of Southern California
Los Angeles

FOREWORD

Understanding health care trends helps provide nurses with direction for managing clinical practice. Two of these trends—the rising cost of health care and increased mortality from emerging and resistant diseases—present challenges that nurses must meet. Other challenges facing nurses are the management of advancements in technology and changes in health care delivery. Telematics, the process of communications and information storage and retrieval technologies, will become an even more integral part of the nurse's role.

Shifts to community-based settings for nursing practice affect competency and quality of the nurse's role in practice. Outcome-driven, multidisciplinary plans of care are being developed in health care facilities nationwide to decrease cost and increase the quality of care. Nurses have a primary role on multidiscliplinary care teams and a direct involvement in cross-training skills and expansion of skills for health care personnel, regardless of practice site.

The answer for nurses

To help you meet these nursing challenges, you'll find that the *Illustrated Handbook of Nursing Care* will serve as one of the best resources available. Along with nursing theory, this quick-reference handbook includes up-to-date professional issues that encompass the evolutionary process of the discipline of nursing. It explores legal and ethical issues in nursing practice and emphasizes the nurse's growing accountability. Another important focus is the nurse's central role in health promotion.

Body-system chapters include assessment components, nursing diagnoses, and pertinent disorders. You'll find causes, assessment findings, nursing interventions, treatment, and evaluation. What's more, you'll find chapters that detail nursing care for patients with special needs. The chapter on geriatric care demystifies the aging process. Pediatric care includes the principles of growth and development along with environmental influences, assessment of systems, and treatment modalities. The psychiatric care chapter includes the latest diagnostic and treatment information for the common disorders described.

This comprehensive, easy to carry book has an impressive format. It includes hundreds of illustrations and charts as well as a 16-page anatomic atlas in full color.

One of the most exciting components of the *Illustrated Handbook of Nursing Care,* among the many other features, are the graphic logos to help you find specific information:

• *Critical thinking* — problem-solving techniques using analytic and prioritization skills
• *Focus on caring* — clinical skills or techniques that enhance comfort and care
• *Charting tips* — charting tips and sample documentation entries
• *Clinical paths* — model clinical pathways on selected common disorders
• *Alternative therapy* — samples of nontraditional treatments.

In addition to the color atlas, you'll find an appendix with Internet sites for nurses.

This cutting-edge reference should help any nurse become a truly effective professional.

Bonnie L. Saucier, PhD, RN
Associate Dean, Undergraduate
Nursing Program
University of Texas Health Science
Center
San Antonio

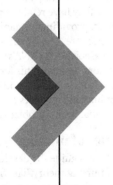

Part 1

PROFESSIONAL ISSUES

1

NURSING PRACTICE

Optimistic about the role that nursing will play in the health care system of the 21st century, the profession has, for the first time in its history, given clear expression to its own principles and ideals by advancing nursing's own health agenda. Comprehensive health care reform is well underway, and nurses are positioned to assume a major role in solving the problems of cost, access, and quality of health care. Nurses have gained a foothold in national, regional, and local public-policy arenas. The demand for health care reform has created a favorable climate for promoting nursing's themes and messages.

The profession has a reputation for successfully delivering high-quality, cost-effective care. In fact, a recent survey of public attitudes toward health care and nurses revealed that the public admires nurses and that most people are willing to have more of their care delivered by nurses.

What is nursing?

Florence Nightingale once wrote that the profession aims "to put the patient in the best condition for nature to act upon him." Although definitions of nursing have changed over time, they have retained a common focus: providing humanistic and holistic care. The American Nurses' Association's (ANA's) definition of nursing shares this focus: "Nursing is the diagnosis and treatment of human responses to actual and potential health problems."

Theories of nursing

Three themes guide the development of nursing theory. The first considers the principles and laws that govern life processes, well-being, and the optimal functioning of people, sick or well. The second looks at patterns of human behavior in interaction with the environment in critical life situations. The third concerns the processes by which positive changes in health status can be brought about. (See *Comparing nursing theories,* pages 4 to 7.)

NURSING EDUCATION

Until recently, registered nurses (RNs) were commonly employed with little regard to their differing educational backgrounds. Increasingly, however, nursing roles and expectations are becoming more closely linked to education and abilities.

This direct connection between education and particular levels of responsibility and salary offers several advantages. For employers, making this connection clarifies entry-level job requirements and encourages equitable pay differentiation. Health care consumers benefit from knowing the educational preparation and experience of each nurse and the services that nurse is prepared to provide. Finally, prospective nursing students gain a clearer idea of how time and money invested in one educational path may translate into future earnings potential and career mobility.

Higher education and career advancement

A broad range of innovative educational programs available today makes it easier than ever for an RN to seek an advanced degree. For example, an experienced RN seeking a bachelor of science in nursing (BSN) may qualify for admission to one of the advanced-placement tracks now offered by many undergraduate nursing programs. There are also BSN programs designed exclusively for RNs as well as articulated associate degree in nursing (ADN) and BSN programs. Some nursing schools also provide competency-based programs for RNs who are unable to attend an accredited school. More recently, accelerated programs leading to both BSN and master of science in nursing (MSN) degrees have been established for RNs as well as students with a prior college degree. More recently, some schools have begun to offer advanced practice programs — such as nurse-midwife, nurse-anesthetist, or family nurse practitioner. These types of nursing practices require certification, for example, advanced nurse practitioner (ANP) or advanced registered nurse practitioner (ARNP). The requirements for certification can vary from state to state. For many RNs, tuition reimbursement from employers defrays the cost of returning to school.

How valuable is an advanced degree? Holding formal credentials helps nurses advance up the career ladders that many health care facilities have established. In addition, advanced degrees open the door to increased compensation, key roles on institutional committees, and higher status within the organization. In most facilities, an advanced degree is a prerequisite for the leading clinical and administrative positions. (See *Higher education: Passport to career advancement,* page 8.)

Comparing nursing theories

Nursing theories differ in their assumptions about patients and health, the
goals of nursing, and the methodologies for research and practice. Taken
together, they help define nursing's domain. A nursing theory is expressed as

Model	Definition of nursing	Purpose of nursing
Nightingale	• A profession for women that seeks to discover and use nature's laws governing health to serve humanity	• To put the person in the best condition for nature to restore or preserve health • To prevent or cure disease and injury
Henderson	• A profession that assists the individual, sick or well, in activities contributing to health or recovery	• To carry out the 14 components of nursing care
Levine	• A human interaction incorporating scientific principles into the nursing process	• To provide individualized holistic care • To support each person's adaptations.
Orem	• A human service designed to overcome limitations in health-related self-care	• To make judgments responding to a person's need for self-care to sustain life and health
Roy	• Analysis and action related to the care of an ill or potentially ill person	• To manipulate stimuli within a prescribed process of nursing assessment and intervention
Neuman	• A profession concerned with the variables that affect the person's response to stressors	• To reduce a person's encounter with stressors • To mitigate the effect of stressors

a conceptual model, which usually includes a definition of nursing, statement of nursing purpose, and definitions of *person*, *health*, and *environment*. This chart describes eight models.

Definition of person	Definition of health	Definition of environment
• A being composed of physical, intellectual, and metaphysical attributes and potentials	• To be free of disease and able to use one's own powers to the fullest	• External elements that affect the healthy or sick person
• A biological being with inseparable mind and body	• To be able to function independently (using the 14 components of nursing care as a guide)	• Not clearly defined, but can act on a person in a positive or negative way
• A complex individual who interacts with internal and external environments and adapts to change	• A pattern of adaptive change • To be whole	• Internally, the person's physiology • Externally, the perceptual, operational, and conceptual components
• An integral whole that functions biologically, symbolically, and socially	• A state of wholeness or integrity of the individual, his or her parts, and modes of functioning	• A subcomponent of the person; together, they compose an integrated system related to self-care
• A biopsychosocial being in constant interaction with a changing environment • An open, adaptive system	• Part of the health-illness continuum, a continuous line representing states or degrees of health or illness that a person might experience at a given time	• All conditions, circumstances, and influences surrounding and affecting the development of an organism or group of organisms
• A physiologic, psychological, sociocultural, and developmental being • Must be viewed as a whole	• A state of wellness or illness determined by physiologic, psychological, sociocultural, and developmental variables that are relative and in a state of flux	• Internally, the state of the person in terms of physiologic, psychological, sociocultural, and developmental variables • Externally, all is outside the person

(continued)

Comparing nursing theories (continued)

Model	Definition of nursing	Purpose of nursing
King	• Human interaction between nurse and client	• To exchange information with the patient and take action together to attain mutually set goals
Rogers	• A learned profession that promotes and maintains health and cares for and rehabilitates the sick and disabled	• To promote harmonious interaction between the environment and person

NURSING'S EMERGING ROLE

Profound changes in hospital care and a new emphasis on alternative health care settings have altered the nature of nursing practice. As patients become older and hospital stays become shorter, long-term care facilities are increasingly common alternatives to a prolonged hospital stay. Furthermore, as health care delivery shifts from the hospital to the community, the demand for highly skilled nurses in out-of-hospital settings increases. This trend gives nurses more career options than ever before.

Independent care

By delivering primary health care to individuals and families in convenient, familiar places, nurses promote health and prevent disease. Health education, screening, immunizations, well-child care, and prenatal care are being provided by licensed nurse practitioners in the community. Nurses educate consumers and promote healthful lifestyles.

Hospital nursing

Patients come to a hospital needing skilled clinical observation and intervention. Depending on the complexity of the health problem, patients and their families may also require teaching, counseling, coordination of services, development of

Definition of person	Definition of health	Definition of environment
• An open system with permeable boundaries that permit the exchange of matter, energy, and information with the environment	• Dynamic adjustment to stressors in the internal and external environment • Makes optimal use of resources to achieve maximum potential for daily living	• An open system with permeable boundaries that permit the exchange of matter, energy, and information with human beings
• A four-dimensional energy field identified by pattern and organization and manifesting characteristics and behaviors that differ from those of its parts and that can't be predicted from knowledge of the parts	• A value word broadly defined by cultures and individuals to describe behaviors considered to be of high or low value	• A four-dimensional energy field identified by pattern and organization and encompassing all that exists outside any given human field

community support systems, and help in coping with health-related lifestyle changes.

Staff nurses, primary nurses, and clinical nurse specialists must now deliver vital services under complex conditions. Not only are patients older, more acutely ill, and hospitalized for shorter stays, but technological advances make today's medical-surgical units look like yesterday's intensive care units. Because patients commonly move through a number of units, the nurse's traditional relationship with patients and their families is jeopardized.

Case management
To counter the trend toward fragmented, depersonalized nursing care, some hospitals are turning to case management, which gives a single nurse-manager the opportunity to provide continuous, comprehensive care. A case manager may schedule preadmission interviews and tests, coordinate care in all hospital units, visit the patient after discharge, and continue to manage care during subsequent hospitalizations.

Telematics
Telematics refers to communications and information storage and retrieval technologies (such as computers and video recorders). As these technologies become more important, nurses must consider their ethical, social, and economic ramifica-

Higher education: Passport to career advancement

Having an advanced degree in nursing gives you a competitive edge in career advancement. The rewards include greater responsibility, compensation, and professional status. The outline below describes the basic features that characterize four nursing degrees — the associate degree in nursing (ADN), the bachelor of science in nursing (BSN) degree, the master of science in nursing (MSN) degree, and the doctor of philosophy in nursing (PhD) and doctor of nursing science (DNSc) degrees.

ADN
• Minimum education requirement for beginning associate nurses
• Prepares nurses to fulfill technical nursing functions
• Obtained at 2-year community and junior colleges

BSN
• Minimum education requirement for beginning professional nurses
• Emphasis on nursing process to prepare graduate nurses who are "advanced beginners"
• Obtained at 4-year colleges and universities

MSN
• Increasingly, the minimum education requirement for advanced clinical positions such as clinical nurse specialist and administrative roles such as head nurse
• Prerequisite bachelor's degree in nursing or another field
• Obtained at colleges and universities, through generic programs

(range from 1 calendar year to 2 academic years in length) or accelerated BSN-MSN programs

PhD or DNSc
• Preparation for a lifetime of intellectual inquiry.
• Research doctorate leading to careers in university teaching and public policy and leadership roles in research and practice settings
• Clinical, applied, or professional doctorate building on clinical specialization to prepare advanced practitioners, applied researchers, clinical faculty, and public policy analysts
• Prerequisite MSN; though some programs accept students with a BSN
• Obtained through doctoral programs offered at colleges of nursing (*Note:* BSN and MSN programs are accredited by the National League for Nursing in the United States, whereas doctoral programs are not. In Canada, accreditation of graduate programs in nursing has not been initiated.)

tions. More nursing schools now encourage this critical thinking.

Families and ancillary personnel
In the future, health care services in the hospital and other settings will increasingly rely on family members, certified health care assistants, and nursing aides. While nurses will still be accountable for the care of patients and their families, they'll need to delegate more activities.

Along with using ancillary personnel comes increased accountability for your nursing judgments, decisions, and actions — and for those of others. This legal responsibility rests with the professional nurse.

Long-term nursing care

As the number of elderly and chronically ill patients increases, so do opportunities to provide long-term nursing care. Negative images associated with caring for these populations have kept many nurses from considering this career option. Currently only about 7% of all RNs work in long-term care facilities, where the nursing shortage has become critical. Gradually, a more enlightened public and profession are recognizing the importance of long-term care. Nursing schools teach about the health of older adults and the care of the chronically ill. This education now receives higher priority because of the complexities involved in caring for this growing group of health care consumers.

Community nursing

Continuity of care between the hospital and the community is one of the most important issues confronting nurses. Patients' health care needs are more complex because they're discharged earlier. Nurses need "high-tech" skills to manage seriously ill patients in the home.

Because patients and their families assist in complex home care, community-based nurses also need effective interpersonal, counseling,

and management skills to coordinate services from myriad community resources.

The need for intensive home nursing services has diverted resources away from health promotion and prevention. However, growing public awareness of health promotion should increase the support community health nurses receive for preventive practice such as immunization. Nurses can tackle teenage pregnancy, substance abuse, the spread of acquired immunodeficiency syndrome, and malnourishment.

NURSING PROCESS

One of the most significant advances in nursing has been the development and acceptance of the nursing process. This problem-solving approach provides a systematic method of determining the patient's health problems, devising a plan of care to address those problems, implementing the plan, and evaluating the plan's effectiveness.

The nursing process offers several important advantages:
• The patient's specific health problems, not the disease, become the focus of health care. This emphasis promotes the patient's participation and encourages his independence and compliance — factors important to a positive outcome.
• Identifying a patient's health problems improves communication by providing nurses, who care for the patient, with a common list of recognized problems.

• The nursing process provides a consistent and orderly professional structure. It promotes accountability for nursing activities based on evaluation and, in so doing, leads to quality assurance.

Evolution of the nursing process

The nursing process emerged during the 1960s as the concept of team health care came into wider practice and nurses were increasingly called upon to define the problems they solve. However, its origins can be traced to World War II, when sophisticated technology, medical advances, and a growing need for nurses began to change both the profession and the concept of nursing.

In its early stages, the nursing process consisted of four distinct but interrelated phases: assessment, planning, intervention, and evaluation. Within the past 20 years, a fifth phase has emerged: nursing diagnosis. Several events promoted the acceptance of nursing diagnosis:

• The ANA, in its publication *Standards of Nursing Practice,* mentioned nursing diagnosis as a separate and definable act performed by the RN.

• Several states passed nurse practice acts that listed diagnosis as part of a nurse's legal responsibility.

• In an effort to define a taxonomy, the North American Nursing Diagnosis Association (NANDA) began meeting biennially in 1973.

Currently, there is interest in developing a nursing diagnosis language for international use on a computer-based patient record. In the future, vocabulary will be developed as well as taxonomies and coding, which will facilitate easy retrieval and meet the multicultural needs of nurses throughout the world.

Five phases

The five phases of the nursing process are dynamic and flexible. They include assessment, nursing diagnosis, planning, intervention, and evaluation.

Assessment

Assessment involves continuous data collection used to identify a patient's actual and potential health needs. According to ANA guidelines, data should accurately reflect the patient's life experiences and patterns of living. To accomplish this, you must assume an objective and nonjudgmental approach when gathering data. You can obtain data through a nursing history, a physical examination, and a review of pertinent laboratory and medical information.

Nursing diagnosis

After clustering significant assessment data and analyzing the pattern, your next step is to label the patient's actual and potential health problems. NANDA has developed a taxonomic scheme to help you identify and formulate nursing diagnoses. This system helps you organize the basic nursing data you've obtained during your initial assessment. You'll identify the patient's problem, write a diagnostic statement, and validate the diagnosis. You'll probably establish several nursing diagnoses for each patient. (See *NANDA taxonomic structure*, pages 12 to 14.)

Maslow's hierarchy of needs is one way of prioritizing human needs based on the idea that lower-level, physiologic needs must be met before higher-level, abstract needs. (See *Maslow's hierarchy of needs*, page 15.)

Nursing plan of care

After you establish the nursing diagnoses, you'll develop a written plan of care. Designed to help you deliver quality patient care, the plan consists of two parts: *patient outcomes*, or expected outcomes, that describe behaviors or results to be achieved within a specified time and *nursing interventions* needed to achieve these outcomes.

Intervention

The actions you take to carry out the plan of care and the subsequent documentation compose the fourth phase of the nursing process: intervention.

Continue to monitor the patient after you implement the plan of care to gauge the effectiveness of interventions and adjust them as the patient's condition changes. Expect to review, revise, and update the entire plan of care regularly, according to institutional policy. Keep in mind that the plan of care usually forms a permanent part of the patient's medical record. Documentation of outcomes achieved should be reflected in the plan.

Evaluation

After enough time has elapsed for the plan of care to bring about desired changes, you're ready for the final step in the nursing process: evaluation. During evaluation, you decide if the interventions have enabled the patient to achieve the desired outcomes.

CLINICAL PATHWAYS

In many areas, clinical pathways are gradually replacing plans of care and are a current method for recording patient outcomes. They encourage health care workers to join together to form plans of care for patient care that reflect all of the patient's needs.

Clinical pathways are multidisciplinary guidelines for patient care. A clinical pathway is a documentation tool for nurses as well as other health care providers. It provides the sequences of multidisciplinary interventions that incorporate education, consultation, discharge planning, medications, nutrition, diagnostics, activities, treatments, and therapeutics. The goal of a clinical pathway is to achieve realistic, expected outcomes for the patient and his family. It should promote a professional and collaborative goal for care and practice as well as assure continuity of care. It should also guarantee appropriate use of resources, which will reduce costs and hospital length of stay while also providing the framework for quality improvement.

Clinical pathways were originally developed to guide the care of acutely ill patients during their hospitaliza-

(Text continues on page 15.)

NANDA taxonomic structure

The North American Nursing Diagnosis Association (NANDA) endorsed its first nursing diagnosis taxonomic structure, NANDA Taxonomy I, in 1986. Revised in 1989, this taxonomy is organized around nine human response patterns and constitutes the currently accepted classification system for 1997–1998.

Pattern 1. Exchanging: A human response pattern involving mutual giving and receiving

1.1.2.1	Altered nutrition: More than body requirements
1.1.2.2	Altered nutrition: Less than body requirements
1.1.2.3	Altered nutrition: Potential for more than body requirements
1.2.1.1.	Risk for infection
1.2.2.1	Risk for altered body temperature
1.1.2.2	Hypothermia
1.1.2.3	Hyperthermia
1.2.2.4	Ineffective thermoregulation
1.2.3.1	Dysreflexia
1.3.1.1	Constipation
1.3.1.1.1	Perceived constipation
1.3.1.1.2	Colonic constipation
1.3.1.2	Diarrhea
1.3.1.3	Bowel incontinence
1.3.2	Altered urinary elimination
1.3.2.1.1	Stress incontinence
1.3.2.1.2	Reflex incontinence
1.3.2.1.3	Urge incontinence
1.3.2.1.4	Functional incontinence
1.3.2.1.5	Total incontinence
1.3.2.2	Urinary retention
1.4.1.1	Altered (specify type) tissue perfusion (renal, cerebral, cardiopulmonary, gastrointestinal, peripheral)
1.4.1.2.1	Fluid volume excess
1.4.1.2.2.1	Fluid volume deficit
1.4.1.2.2.2	Risk for fluid volume deficit
1.4.2.1	Decreased cardiac output
1.5.1.1	Impaired gas exchange
1.5.1.2	Ineffective airway clearance
1.5.1.3	Ineffective breathing pattern
1.5.1.3.1	Inability to sustain spontaneous ventilation
1.5.1.3.2	Dysfunctional ventilatory wheezing response
1.6.1	Risk for injury
1.6.1.1	Risk for suffocation
1.6.1.2	Risk for poisoning
1.6.1.3	Risk for trauma
1.6.1.4	Risk for aspiration
1.6.1.5	Risk for disuse syndrome
1.6.2	Altered protection
1.6.2.1	Impaired tissue integrity
1.6.2.1.1	Altered oral mucous membrane
1.6.2.1.2.1	Impaired skin integrity
1.6.2.1.2.2	Risk for impaired skin integrity

Pattern 2. Communicating: A human response pattern involving sending messages

2.1.1.1	Impaired verbal communication

NANDA taxonomic structure *(continued)*

Pattern 3. Relating: A human response pattern involving establishing bonds

3.1.1	Impaired social interaction
3.1.2	Social isolation
3.1.3	Risk for loneliness
3.2.1	Altered role performance
3.2.1.1.1	Altered parenting
3.2.1.1.2	Risk for altered parenting
3.2.1.1.2.1	Risk for altered parent/infant/child attachment
3.2.1.2.1	Sexual dysfunction
3.2.2	Altered family processes
3.2.2.1	Caregiver role strain
3.2.2.2	Risk for caregiver role strain
3.2.2.3.1	Altered family process: Alcoholism
3.2.3.1	Parental role conflict
3.3	Altered sexuality patterns

Pattern 4. Valuing: A human response pattern involving the assigning of relative worth

4.1.1	Spiritual distress (distress of the human spirit)
4.2	Potential for enhanced spiritual well-being

Pattern 5. Choosing: A human response pattern involving the selection of alternatives

5.1.1.1	Ineffective individual coping
5.1.1.1.1	Impaired adjustment
5.1.1.1.2	Defensive coping
5.1.1.1.3	Ineffective denial
5.1.2.1.1	Ineffective family coping: Disabling
5.1.2.1.2	Ineffective family coping: Compromised
5.1.2.2	Family coping: Potential for growth
5.1.3.1	Potential for enhanced community coping
5.1.3.2	Ineffective community coping
5.2.1	Ineffective management of therapeutic regimen (individual)
5.2.1.1	Noncompliance (specify)
5.2.2	Ineffective management of therapeutic regimen: Families
5.2.3	Ineffective management of therapeutic regimen: Community
5.2.4	Effective management of therapeutic regimen: Individual
5.3.1.1	Decisional conflict (specify)
5.4	Health-seeking behaviors (specify)

Pattern 6. Moving: A human response pattern involving activity

6.1.1.1	Impaired physical mobility
6.1.1.1.1	Risk for peripheral neurovascular dysfunction
6.1.1.1.2	Risk for perioperative positioning injury
6.1.1.2	Activity intolerance
6.1.1.2.1	Fatigue
6.1.1.3	Risk for activity intolerance
6.2.1	Sleep pattern disturbance

(continued)

NANDA taxonomic structure *(continued)*

6.3.1.1	Diversional activity deficit
6.4.1.1	Impaired home mainte-nance management
6.4.2	Altered health mainte-nance
6.5.1	Feeding self-care deficit
6.5.1.1	Impaired swallowing
6.5.1.2	Ineffective breastfeed-ing
6.5.1.2.1	Interrupted breastfeed-ing
6.5.1.3	Effective breastfeeding
6.5.1.4	Ineffective infant feed-ing pattern
6.5.2	Bathing/hygiene self-care deficit
6.5.3	Dressing/grooming self-care deficit
6.5.4	Toileting self-care deficit
6.6	Altered growth and development
6.7	Relocation stress syn-drome
6.8.1	Risk for disorganized infant behavior
6.8.2	Disorganized infant behavior
6.8.3	Potential for enhanced organized infant behav-ior

Pattern 7. Perceiving: A human response pattern involving the reception of information

7.1.1	Body image distur-bance
7.1.2	Self-esteem distur-bance
7.1.2.1	Chronic low self-esteem
7.1.2.2	Situational low self-esteem
7.1.3	Personal identity distur-bance
7.2	Sensory/perceptual alterations (specify — visual, auditory, kines-thetic, gustatory, tactile, olfactory)
7.2.1.1	Unilateral neglect
7.3.1	Hopelessness
7.3.2	Powerlessness

Pattern 8. Knowing: A human response pattern involving the meaning associated with information

8.1.1	Knowledge deficit (specify)
8.2.1	Impaired environmental interpretation syndrome
8.2.2	Acute confusion
8.2.3	Chronic confusion
8.3	Altered thought processes
8.3.1	Impaired memory

Pattern 9. Feeling: A human response pattern involving the subjective awareness of information

9.1.1	Pain
9.1.1.1	Chronic pain
9.2.1.1	Dysfunctional grieving
9.2.1.2	Anticipatory grieving
9.2.2	Risk for violence: Self-directed or directed at others
9.2.2.1	Risk for self-mutilation
9.2.3	Post-trauma response
9.2.3.1	Rape-trauma syndrome
9.2.3.1.1	Rape-trauma syndrome: Compound reaction
9.2.3.1.2	Rape-trauma syndrome: Silent reaction
9.3.1	Anxiety
9.3.2	Fear

Maslow's hierarchy of needs

Maslow's hierarchy of needs, diagrammed below, is a system of classifying human needs based on the idea that a person's physiologic needs must be met before more abstract needs can be addressed. By considering these different levels of need when trying to understand and resolve your patient's problems, you'll be better able to provide more holistic care.

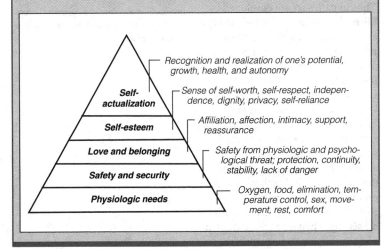

Recognition and realization of one's potential, growth, health, and autonomy

Self-actualization

Sense of self-worth, self-respect, independence, dignity, privacy, self-reliance

Self-esteem

Affiliation, affection, intimacy, support, reassurance

Love and belonging

Safety from physiologic and psychological threat; protection, continuity, stability, lack of danger

Safety and security

Oxygen, food, elimination, temperature control, sex, movement, rest, comfort

Physiologic needs

tion. They are now being developed to manage patients in other settings: home care patients, those in long-term care settings, and outpatients.

Clinical pathways are also referred to as clinical paths, anticipated recovery plans, multidisciplinary action plans, action plans, and multidisciplinary plans. Originally, they were developed by a member of a health care team for specific diagnoses, usually high-risk, high-volume, and high-cost cases.

How are expected outcomes achieved?

Clinical pathways are outcome-driven. Patients are expected to achieve stated outcomes at specific times or phases of recovery. If the expected outcome is achieved, the patient is encouraged to move forward to the next expected outcome and to do so within a specific time frame. If the patient doesn't achieve the expected outcome, a variance is documented in the clinical pathway.

A variance in the pathway is recorded as either a provider, system, or patient variance. A provider variance is related to the experience of the health care provider. A system variance can be the unavailability of a certain diagnostic procedure. An unexpected change in the patient's condition is regarded as a patient variance. When the reason for the variance is established, new interventions are proposed and implemented.

How are clinical pathways developed?

Clinical pathways are developed by the health care agencies and are very specific to that agency. Literature reviews, chart reviews, expert opinion, and insurance reimbursement information on the specific case is used to develop the pathway. Usually, high-cost, high-volume, and high-risk cases are investigated. A multidisciplinary team is formed, composed of individuals from all areas of the health care team who develop the clinical pathway based on the information gathered. The clinical pathway is piloted in a clinical setting. Then it's revised as often as necessary depending upon the variances encountered, until it best meets the needs of the patient in the practice setting.

REFERENCES AND READINGS

Carpiento, L. *Nursing Diagnosis: Application to Clinical Practice,* 6th ed. Philadelphia: J.B. Lippincott Co., 1996.

Chang, B., and Hirsch, M. "Nursing Diagnosis Research: Computer Aided Research," *Nursing Diagnosis* 5(1):6-13, January-March 1994.

Dobrynz, J. "Components of Written Diagnostic Statements," *Nursing Diagnosis* 6(1):29-36, January-March 1995.

Fitzpatrick, J. and Zanotte, R. "Nursing Diagnoses Internationally," *Nursing Diagnosis* 6(1):42-43, January-March 1995.

Kozier, B., et al. *Fundamentals of Nursing: Concepts, Process, and Practice,* 5th ed. New York: Addison-Wesley Publishing Co., 1995.

NANDA. *Nursing Diagnosis: Definitions and Classification.* Philadelphia: North American Nursing Diagnosis Association, 1997-1998.

Sparks, S., et al. *Nursing Diagnosis Pocket Manual.* Springhouse, Pa.: Springhouse Corp., 1996.

2

LEGAL ISSUES IN NURSING PRACTICE

Growing professional recognition for nurses has brought with it growing legal accountability. And with this growing accountability has come concern about malpractice and other legal issues. This chapter will help you understand malpractice and recognize and avoid malpractice pitfalls, including those encountered in specialty areas. The chapter also describes another type of lawsuit nurses sometimes must defend against: intentional torts. What's more, the chapter includes a discussion of your legal rights and responsibilities and measures to protect your license.

MALPRACTICE

Our legal system's view of malpractice evolved from negligence law and the premise, basic to all law, that an individual is responsible for the consequences of his own acts. For nurses, malpractice refers to the failure to follow a reasonable, professional standard of care that results in injury to a patient.

A malpractice action seeks to compensate a person for an injury he received because of a health care provider's negligence. This compensation usually includes medical expenses, lost salary, and a certain sum for pain and suffering. Some cases also seek compensation for emotional damages. Most health care facilities and insurance companies will try to work out a fair settlement with the patient if they determine that malpractice has occurred. However, if the patient isn't satisfied with the offer, he may pursue his claim through legal action.

Filing a complaint

The patient's attorney will evaluate a potential malpractice case by asking the health care facility for pertinent medical records.

If the attorney decides that a claim is appropriate, he drafts a complaint describing in legal terms what the injured party, or plaintiff, will try to prove. He files the complaint and serves a copy to the defendants, who have a set number of days in which to respond.

Gathering evidence

After the complaint has been served, the discovery period begins. During discovery, the parties gather evidence and learn the facts of the case. Another purpose of discovery is to encourage a settlement, when appropriate. In complex cases, the discovery period may last several years.

Once the case reaches trial, the plaintiff, the defendants, family members, and witnesses to the patient's care may testify. Expert witnesses will testify to explain professional standards of care. You may be called as a witness to provide your firsthand knowledge of the case or as an expert witness to provide your professional opinion.

Proving malpractice

The plaintiff must establish duty, breach of duty, causation, and damages to prove malpractice.

Duty

Duty refers to the relationship between the health care provider and the patient. For nurses, courts have determined that this relationship can develop easily, even through a single telephone conversation. Therefore, no matter where you practice nursing, you must give advice prudently.

Breach of duty

Breach of duty against a nurse can be a difficult determination because her responsibilities commonly overlap those of other health care providers, particularly doctors. A key question is how would a reasonable nurse have acted in the same or similar circumstances.

Nurses, for instance, are responsible for continually assessing patients, and failing to do so can constitute breach of duty.

Even if you do recognize that a patient's condition has worsened and you notify the doctor, you may not have fulfilled your legal duty. If the patient's situation is an emergency and the doctor doesn't respond or responds in an obviously negligent manner, legal precedent has held that you have a duty to proceed further, including notifying your nursing manager.

Causation

Even if the plaintiff establishes a breach of duty, he must prove that the breach caused his injury. Causation is the most difficult factor to prove.

Because causation is so difficult to prove, courts sometimes resort to a theory called *res ipsa loquitur* to satisfy the requirement of proof. *Res ipsa loquitur* means that the plaintiff can prove negligence through circumstantial evidence. When using this theory, the plaintiff must prove that the injury wouldn't have occurred unless someone had been negligent, that the defendant exclusively controlled whatever caused the injury, and that no action of the plaintiff caused the injury.

Defending a malpractice claim

An attorney's request for a patient's medical records may signal to the health care facility that a patient is considering a suit. However, the risk manager may have already been aware of that possibility because of a previously filed incident report. (See *Importance of incident reports.*)

If not already done, the risk manager will review the patient's records and investigate the case. She will also notify the facility's insurance carrier as well as the health care providers involved. If you learn you're a potential defendant, you may review the records, but you shouldn't make any changes. Altered medical records may injure the credibility of the defendant in the eyes of the jurors and result in an additional award of punitive damages.

Once the plaintiff files suit, the defense lawyers will assert that the nurse's care met professional standards or that, even if it didn't, it didn't cause the injury.

Contributory negligence

Contributory or comparative negligence means that the patient may have contributed to his injury. For instance, he may have left the facility against medical advice, failed to return for follow-up care, refused to follow instructions, or tampered with traction or other equipment. However, to apply this defense, the

Importance of incident reports

Health care facility standards vary for incident reports, also called event reports, occurrence reports, or situation reports. One common definition of an incident is any occurrence not consistent with the facility's routine operation or patient care. Incident reports highlight areas of potential liability for the risk manager. Always chart the facts of an incident if they're pertinent to the patient's clinical condition. However, because they are a management tool, don't refer to incident reports in the patient's chart. Typically, if the risk manager feels that an incident is serious and may involve a liability claim, the insurance carrier is notified and then the business office will be notified to cancel all or part of the patient's bill. Most states don't view cancelling a patient's bill as an admission of liability, and it can help satisfy an angry patient or family.

A patient representative may visit the patient and his family to hear their description of the incident. Findings are then reported to the doctor, facility administrator, and risk manager. In the meantime, the risk manager reviews the patient's medical record for accurate and complete documentation.

Even if the incident isn't serious, the risk manager's report can be useful for statistical studies that identify repetitive incidents and consequent need for change.

Good Samaritan laws

Good Samaritan laws are state laws that encourage health care professionals to care for accident victims at the scene without fear of a lawsuit. Such statutes usually don't apply to the care the patient receives in a hospital. Although the laws differ by state, most Good Samaritan laws specifically include nurses. To be protected by the law, you should not charge the patient for your services. Although health care professionals often fear being held liable for their patient care in such emergencies, it has not happened in any state.

defendant must show that the plaintiff could understand the consequences of his actions. This may prove especially difficult because the plaintiff was ill and may have been in pain, making it difficult for him to exercise reasonable judgment. You should always document the patient's actions in the medical record, especially if they are examples of noncompliant behavior.

Statute of limitations

Another defense is the statute of limitations, which defines the time allowed for a plaintiff to file a lawsuit. This span varies by state and may begin from the date the injury occurred or the date the patient discovered what happened. Because the patient may not immediately discover the injury or its full extent, courts tend to be lenient in applying the statute of limitations. In nearly all states, the statute of limitations

for minors is longer than that for adults. In some states, it doesn't begin until the minor reaches the age of maturity.

If someone has tried to keep the patient from learning what happened, then the statute of limitations may not bar the claim. If the doctor, or even the health care facility, simply keeps silent, the court may view that as fraudulent concealment. Honesty *is* the best policy.

The nurse as defendant

Until recently, the law didn't recognize nurses as independent health care providers, and nurses were rarely named as malpractice defendants. Instead, the courts typically held either the facility or the doctor accountable for the nurse's acts. Today, however, an increasing number of medical malpractice cases include nurses as defendants. While this may seem unsettling, it actually reflects the evolving independence of the professional nurse and recognition of nursing as a profession with its own standards and accountability. (See *Good Samaritan laws.*)

The primary defendant in a malpractice case is usually the person accused of harming the patient. Because nurses provide direct patient care, many of them become primary defendants. With the increasing number of unlicensed health care providers, it's important for the nurse to know that these individuals are also held accountable for their own actions. Also, many patients realize when a nurse makes a mistake during a procedure. In fact, many malpractice cases involve common procedures. For instance, nurses have been held liable for activities such as failing to catheterize a patient properly, failing to give an enema properly, and damaging a nerve with an injection.

The level of your accountability depends upon your job description and your facility's policies as well as customary practices.

Malpractice suits usually involve joint or shared liability, which means the case has more than one defendant. The case may name the entire health care team — for example, an operating room team that fails to respond appropriately when a patient has an adverse reaction to an anesthetic.

Employer's responsibility

While you're responsible for your own actions, your employer will also share in the responsibility under the principle of vicarious liability, or *respondeat superior.*

As managed care organizations evolve, corporate liability judgments have addressed accountability issues. Under the doctrine of corporate accountability, health care facilities may be liable for situations involving staffing, equipment, security, environmental safety, and the acts of attending doctors who aren't employed by the facility. As a nurse, this doctrine directly affects you, as you're the one most likely to become aware of these problems. When you do notice a problem and clearly can't correct it, you must tell someone with more authority about it. If your manager can't correct a problem such as being short staffed,

then she must tell her superior. In some cases, the problem may have to be brought before upper management or the facility's board of directors. (See *Short staffing: Who's responsible?* page 22.)

Many nurses become frustrated by a lack of response to their complaints, and they stop reporting the problem. That's a mistake. Tell your manager each time the problem arises, not just once. After all, you may be held liable if an injury occurs because of an unreported problem.

Always document repetitive, serious problems in writing. If your facility has a management reporting system, use it. If not, simply describe the problem, giving particular attention to its effects on patient care, on a plain sheet of paper. Sign and date the report, and submit it to your superior (remember to keep a copy, so that you can document that you communicated the problem). In addition, you may want to use your facility's risk management or quality assurance system to report problems. (For more information, see *How continuous quality improvement and risk management differ,* page 23.)

INTENTIONAL TORTS

While most lawsuits against nurses involve negligence, others involve intentional torts, which are infringements on the patient's basic civil rights. A tort is a civil wrong punishable by monetary compensation.

Intentional torts include assault and battery, defamation of charac-

Short staffing: Who's responsible?

Short staffing is a chronic problem for many health care facilities and can significantly affect patient care. Many nurses express concern over their risk of liability when faced with a short-staffing situation. As long as you exercise reasonable professional judgment, establish priorities, and communicate problems to nursing management, you can defend a claim based on short staffing.

The facility's responsibility

Health care facilities have a legal duty to provide the level of staffing needed to care safely for patients and may be held liable for any injuries that occur because of short staffing. However, to satisfy your legal duty, you must communicate the problem to someone in a position to solve it.

In one case, a neonate suffocated in the hospital's nursery. The parents claimed that their baby died because of the hospital's short staffing and because of the nurses' negligence. On the day of the incident, 3 nurses — 2 staff nurses and a charge nurse — were caring for 18 neonates in 3 rooms. For 30 minutes, all 3 nurses were occupied in the nursery's first 2 rooms. When a nurse checked on the third room, she found 1 neonate lying face down and not breathing. The neonate's pediatrician testified that the incident probably wouldn't have happened if a nurse had been in the room at all times, as required by hospital policy. The charge nurse testified that the unit was understaffed, and another witness testified that the hospital had been repeatedly warned of a chronic staffing shortage in the nursery. The court issued a directed verdict in favor of the 2 staff nurses, and the jury found in favor of the charge nurse but against the hospital.

The nurse's responsibility

Keep in mind, though, that a nurse working in a short-staffed situation may still be liable for making an inappropriate professional judgment.

In *Horton v. Niagara Falls Memorial Medical Center (1976),* someone discovered a patient standing on his balcony asking for a ladder. The doctor then requested that the patient be watched closely and placed in a Posey belt and cloth wristlets. The charge nurse telephoned the patient's wife at home and asked her to come to the hospital and watch her husband.

The wife said that she would ask her mother, who lived closer to the hospital, to come and that her mother could be there in 10 minutes. She then asked the charge nurse to watch her husband until her mother arrived. The charge nurse responded that that would be impossible. During the 10-minute lapse in supervision, the patient fell from the balcony and died.

The court decided that the charge nurse had been negligent and that the hospital was liable for the nurse's negligence under the theory of *respondeat superior.* The court noted that another nurse could have watched the patient until the mother-in-law arrived. The court also noted that the charge nurse had allowed an aide to take a supper break.

ter, breach of confidentiality, misrepresentation or fraud, and false imprisonment. To prove an intentional tort, the plaintiff doesn't have to have been injured and doesn't have to prove duty, breach of duty, causation, or damages. The significance of the infringement determines the amount of compensation. Standard malpractice or liability insurance policies may not cover intentional torts. (See *Intentional torts*, page 24.)

RESPONSIBILITIES AND RIGHTS

Knowing your legal responsibilities can help you avoid malpractice claims. Knowing your rights and your patient's rights can guide you when confronting difficult decisions about your work and your colleagues.

Documentation

The medical record plays a vital role in most lawsuits involving nurses. If the medical record shows that the patient received reasonable care, it may prevent a lawsuit. On the other hand, if the record is poorly documented, a patient may sue and win even though he may have actually received reasonable care. The nurses' notes are usually the key to this evaluation.

Its legal role aside, the medical record is a historic document that can influence the patient's medical care. With that in mind, chart everything that is clinically significant. A good rule is to err on the side of overdocumentation.

How continuous quality improvement and risk management differ

Although continuous quality improvement and risk management are related, they don't serve the same purpose. Continuous quality improvement evaluates the facilty's role in delivering health care services, while risk management focuses on legal standards and the patient's perception of the health care services he has received.

Risk management also evaluates a situation according to what the law *requires* the facility to do. Continuous quality improvement often applies a higher standard, analogous to an ethical standard. Continuous quality improvement refers to the quality of care the facility would like to provide for its patients, rather than what the law requires it to provide.

To protect yourself in the event of a malpractice claim, document the care you give precisely. For example, always note the site of an injection; you could be held liable for an alleged injury from an injection given by someone else.

Just as you should never chart medications given by someone else, never document an action performed by someone else. If nursing assistants participate in direct patient care, they should chart those activities on the medical record. Remember that all health care providers are accountable for their

Intentional torts

Intentional torts are infringements against the patient's basic civil rights. Below are some examples of intentional torts a nurse may commit.

Assault and battery

An actionable battery occurs, for instance, when a surgeon performs an operation without the patient's consent. An alert, oriented adult has the right to refuse any aspect of treatment. If you have a competent adult patient held down while you administer an injection or if you force a patient to take an oral medication, then you have committed an intentional tort.

Defamation of character

Injuring someone's reputation through false and malicious statements is termed defamation of character. Written defamation is called *libel;* verbal defamation, *slander.* In some states, the defendant doesn't have to prove specific financial injury if the slanderous statement alleges a contagious or venereal disease, alleges a crime of moral turpitude, or affects a person's profession, trade, or business.

Breach of confidentiality

Typically, you shouldn't disclose confidential information about a patient to a third party who doesn't need to know. Confidential information includes the patient's medical record. In some instances, however, you may have a legal duty to disclose confidential information such as in cases of suspected child abuse.

Fraud

If a doctor misleads a patient to conceal a mistake made during treatment, the doctor, and even the hospital, may be sued for fraud. Remaining silent may also constitute fraudulent concealment.

False imprisonment

False imprisonment occurs when a person's freedom of movement is restricted. Although most actions for false imprisonment involve psychiatric patients, others have involved patients who were improperly physically restrained or who weren't permitted to leave the facility but should have been.

own actions, whether they're professionals or nonprofessionals.

At the end of every shift, take time to make sure that your charting is clear, legible, and reflects the patient care. If you encounter a patient care problem that you can't handle, ask your manager for help and chart that you did so. Tell your manager what you charted so that

she can respond on the medical record.

Verbal and telephone orders

Most health care facilities have specific policies — usually written to comply with state regulations — regarding verbal orders. Many facilities require doctors to sign verbal orders within 24 hours to authenticate them, although the nurse will have already carried out the order in most cases. Although verbal orders aren't illegal, they do increase the risk of an error, as the nurse may misunderstand what the doctor has said. That situation is quite difficult to defend in court.

A colleague's incompetence

Nurses are responsible for helping patients receive adequate and safe care. If a nurse fails to identify a situation in which reasonable standards of care have been violated, the nurse and any other participating health care professional may be liable.

An even more difficult problem arises when the doctor doesn't respond to a patient's complaint or only responds in a perfunctory manner. Again, if the lack of response results in poor patient care, you're legally obligated to advise facility administrators.

Employee rights

You have legal rights just as any other employee does. An employer may not discriminate against you on the basis of race, sex, age, religion, or nationality. What's more, you have certain other rights related to your legal obligation as a nurse. For example, a nurse can't be fired for refusing to perform a legally unauthorized activity.

Whistle-blowing

Some states have laws to protect employees who publicly disclose perceived wrongdoing by their employer, which is called whistle-blowing. These laws hold that whistle-blowing may be in the public interest.

Before deciding to take an issue outside your place of employment, consider whether you have enough evidence to warrant action. To make a serious accusation, you must have enough documentation to be fair and to maintain your credibility. Also consider whether you've used all channels within your place of employment, including the risk management and quality assurance departments and the facility's administration.

Right to refuse a work assignment

As a general rule, nurses can't refuse patient care assignments. However, if you feel that you aren't qualified to perform a particular assignment, document your concerns in writing and submit the note to your manager. Emphasize your belief that you might harm the patient if you accept the assignment. If your manager still insists that you accept the assignment because no alternative exists, then accept the assignment.

Under most circumstances, you aren't allowed to refuse an assignment because of ethical or personal beliefs. However, many states allow nurses to refuse to participate in abortions and even sterilization procedures. No court has upheld a nurse's right to refuse to care for a patient with acquired immunodeficiency syndrome.

Patient rights

The patient also has rights, including the right to informed consent, the right to refuse treatment, and the right to control access to his records.

Informed consent

All competent adults have the right to make decisions about their own health care. To make an informed decision, the patient must have sufficient information, such as the nature of the procedure and its benefits, alternatives, and risks. Obtaining an informed consent is clearly the doctor's legal duty, not the nurse's.

The consent form documents that the patient has received an explanation of the procedure and that he has had an opportunity to ask questions. However, if the nurse accepts responsibility for obtaining the patient's consent, then she may make herself liable for what normally would not be her responsibility.

If the patient isn't competent, his next-of-kin (as determined by state laws) must assume responsibility for giving consent. A person's next-of-kin is usually his spouse; if he has no spouse, his next-of-kin would be his adult children, followed by his parents, and then his siblings. The doctor needs the consent of only one of the responsible parties.

In emergencies, the law doesn't require an informed consent, although it's always preferable to obtain one if time allows. Also, always notify the doctor if the patient has decided not to have the procedure. The patient has a right to revoke his consent at any time before the procedure.

Refusal of treatment

Competent adults also have a right to refuse treatment, even if the treatment is lifesaving — in which case the patient must clearly understand that his refusal could cause his death.

This same legal principle applies when a patient refuses care because of religious or personal beliefs. However, the courts occasionally limit this right, such as in cases where blood transfusions are necessary or when the patient is pregnant and the decision affects the fetus' life. Also, parents can't impose their religious beliefs on their children when those beliefs could cause the child's death.

The courts usually follow the patient's wishes when the patient is competent and clearly understands the results of his decision. If the patient is unconscious or incompetent, the family assumes responsibility for expressing the patient's wishes, which he may have documented through an advance directive, such as a living will or a durable power of attorney. A living will is a document, legally binding in most states, that allows an incapacitated patient to refuse life-sustaining treatment in certain circumstances. In states where living wills aren't legally binding, they still indicate the patient's wishes.

The durable power of attorney allows the patient to give another person the power to make medical decisions for him if he cannot make his own. The durable power of attorney is also legally binding in many states. Some states utilize a proxy consent document, which is a combination of these two.

Patient access to records

While records are the health care facility's physical property, their content belongs to the patient. If someone requests a copy of his record, the patient must sign a statement authorizing release. State law or facility policy usually gives patients the right to review their own records, even while still in the facility.

PROTECTING YOUR LICENSE

A state's nurse practice act establishes the standards for licensure as a registered nurse, defines the nurse's scope of practice, and defines the grounds for disciplinary action. Each state legislature establishes an agency such as a board of nursing examiners to enforce its nurse practice act. After investigating, if the state board decides to consider disciplinary action it must notify the nurse of the charges and the time and place of a hearing.

Grounds for disciplinary action

While the reasons for disciplinary action differ among states, usual categories include fraud and deceit, criminal acts, substance abuse, mental or professional incompetence, and unprofessional conduct.

According to the American Nurses' Association's Model Act, fraud and deceit includes falsification of patient records or repeated negligence in documentation. Practicing nursing without a license also constitutes a basis for disciplinary action. Furthermore, in some states, a nurse who knows that another person is practicing without a license but doesn't report the infraction can have her license revoked.

Nurses commonly become concerned about the possibility of losing their licenses when their health care facility asks them to take on new responsibilities. However, such action is rare because most nurse practice acts have considerable flexibility. While some nurses wish their state's act contained more specific direction and guidance, the act's flexibility offers the advantage of allowing the profession to develop its own standards.

However, a third party, such as a doctor or health care facility, can't insist that you take on responsibility that the state hasn't authorized. If a facility is requiring its nursing staff to delegate activities previously performed by professional nurses to unlicensed individuals, the nursing management should determine the scope, limits, and appropriateness of the delegated activities so that state licensure requirements are observed. If you take on an unauthorized activity at another party's insistence, that third party can't protect you from losing your license.

If a health care facility requires you to accept questionable duties, ask the facility to contact the state board of nursing — or contact it yourself — to clarify whether your license is in jeopardy. Also ask if the facility's insurance company covers the activity. Usually, if the facility specifically authorizes or requires you to perform the activity, you'd be acting "within the scope of your employment," and the facility's insurance would cover you.

LEGAL ISSUES FOR CANADIAN NURSES

In Canada, the roots of the legal system in nine of the provinces originate in English common law. In Quebec, however, the legal system derives from Roman civil law, the basis of which is enacted law.

Although liability for negligence applies to nurses, legal actions against nurses tend to be rare because juries are uncommon in civil trials, which usually lowers monetary awards to the plaintiff. What's more, in most provinces, lawyers aren't permitted to charge contingency fees (a percentage of the damages awarded the plaintiff).

Canadian nurses, of course, bear responsibility for the results of their actions and should carry liability insurance. In most provinces, liability insurance is usually obtained as part of the licensure and registration fee and is offered through the Canadian Nurses Protective Association.

REFERENCES AND READINGS

Hall J.K. *Nursing Ethics and Law.* Philadelphia: W.B. Saunders Company, 1996.

Fiesta, J. J. *20 Legal Pitfalls for Nurses to Avoid.* Albany, N.Y.: Delmar Publishers, 1994.

Moniz, D. "The Clock Stops Ticking on Potential Lawsuits, Eventually," *RN* 58(7):57, July 1995.

Nurse's Legal Handbook, 3rd ed. Springhouse, Pa.: Springhouse Corp., 1996.

Prent, Nancy J. *Nurses and the Law: A Guide to Principles and Applications.* Philadelphia: W.B. Saunders Company, 1997.

Tammello, A.D. "Are You Responsible for the Doctor 'Covering' for You?" *Reagan Report on Medical Law* 28(6):4, June 1995.

Part 2

CLINICAL PRACTICE

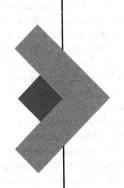

3

HEALTH PROMOTION

Research shows that poor health practices contribute to a wide range of illnesses, a shortened life span, and spiraling health care costs. In contrast, good health practices have the opposite effect: fewer illnesses, a longer life span, and lower health care costs. What's more, good health practices can benefit most people no matter when they're begun. Of course, the earlier in life they're begun, the less they have to overcome. But, fortunately, later is better than never.

What is health promotion?

Health promotion is teaching good health practices and finding ways to help people correct their poor health practices. It's something you'll do in a variety of settings in your clinic or hospital, in your patient's home, and even at a community meeting.

But what specifically should you teach? The report *Healthy People 2000: National Health Promotion and Prevention of Disease* sets forth comprehensive health goals for the nation with the aim of reducing mortality and morbidity in all ages. These guidelines set a national agenda to prevent unnecessary disease and disability by establishing goals that increase the span of a healthy life, reduce health disparities, and increase the access of preventive health care to all Americans. These guidelines are focused around 20 health objectives. (For a complete list of the goals, see *Goals for promoting health.*)

These health objectives are divided into three categories: health protection, health prevention, and health promotion. While nurses can be involved in all these activities, the focus of this chapter is health promotion.

Health promotion strategies are linked to lifestyle choices that affect health status. These include level of physical activity and fitness, nutrition, mental health and disorders, and violent and abusive behaviors. Nurses can promote health by teaching patients to increase physi-

Goals for promoting health

The list below designates the specific objectives that the U.S. Department of Health and Human Services has indicated to be the focus of health promotion priority.

- Reduce tobacco use.
- Reduce alcohol and other abuse.
- Improve nutrition.
- Increase physical activity and fitness.
- Improve mental health and prevent mental illness.
- Reduce violent and abusive behavior.
- Increase access to family planning services.
- Promote health education and community-based health programs.
- Improve environmental public safety.
- Improve occupational health and safety.
- Prevent and control unintentional injuries.

- Improve oral health.
- Improve food and drug safety.
- Increase clinical preventive health services.
- Prevent and control human immunodeficiency virus infection and acquired immunodeficiency syndrome.
- Prevent and control sexually transmitted diseases.
- Immunize against and control infectious diseases.
- Improve maternal and infant health.
- Prevent, detect, and control hypertension, heart disease, and stroke.
- Prevent, detect, and control diabetes and other disabling conditions.

Source: U.S. Department of Health and Human Services. *Healthy People 2000: National Health Promotion and Disease Prevention Objectives*. Boston: Jones & Bartlett Pubs., Inc., 1996.

cal activity, improve nutrition and reduce the abuse of alcohol, tobacco, and other drugs. The goals outlined in *Healthy People 2000* should direct your teaching.

This chapter is organized by age group: infants, children, adolescents, adults, and older adults.

INFANT HEALTH PROMOTION

How a woman cares for herself during pregnancy directly affects the health of her unborn infant. Two

factors especially can jeopardize the infant's health: low birth weight (LBW) and birth defects. LBW infants are more likely to develop complications and are less likely to survive.

Prenatal care

Your teaching will highlight ways that early and ongoing prenatal care promotes the birth of a healthy infant. During the first prenatal visit, you'll help obtain a thorough patient history including a genetic history, a physical examination, and laboratory tests. Screening should also be done for inherited disorders such as Tay-Sachs disease and Down syndrome. The doctor will probably order measurement of alpha-fetoprotein levels to detect fetal neural tube defects, such as spina bifida or anencephaly.

Focus your teaching efforts on prenatal nutrition and exercise and the adverse effects of cigarette smoking, alcohol, caffeine, and drugs on the fetus. Additionally, you'll want to teach the patient how to avoid exposure to certain infectious and toxic agents associated with birth defects.

Childbirth education

You will also want to educate the parents about birth practices and birth choices. For example, they may opt to forego routine administration of analgesics and anesthetics during labor. Or they may question whether the traditional hospital delivery room is the best birth setting. Suggest that the patient and her coach attend childbirth education classes. Equally important is making certain that your patient is properly taught how to detect — and correctly respond to — complications of pregnancy or labor and delivery. For example, explain that any bleeding from the vagina should be evaluated promptly.

After your patient delivers, your teaching will focus on nutrition, exercise, breast- or bottle-feeding as well as infant care, such as feeding and safety. For instance, remind the patient and her partner always to use an infant car seat, beginning with the infant's trip home from the hospital.

Growth and development

As the infant develops, your teaching centers around the child's growth and development. Teach parents about physical and emotional growth and development by describing developmental milestones at different ages. Stress that infants develop at their own pace and that parents shouldn't compare their infant with anyone else's or worry if he doesn't progress "by the book."

For all infants, stress the importance of following the immunization schedule recommended by their doctor or nurse practitioner.

Special problems

When an infant is born with a disease or a birth defect, your teaching becomes more difficult. If the infant has been identified as positive for human immunodeficiency virus (HIV) infection, explain to the parents the precautions required to prevent exposure to infections. Although some who are HIV positive may never develop acquired immunodeficiency syndrome (AIDS), they will have severe medical and developmental problems. Stress the need for reevaluating developmental skills every 6 months.

Parents of infants with other disorders, such as cerebral palsy, cystic fibrosis, and Down syndrome, also need intensive teaching. Discuss causes, symptoms, prognosis, and special care problems. Tell them about support groups and special services and resources. Explain the purpose of health care visits, and answer their questions — they'll probably have many.

CHILD HEALTH PROMOTION

Perhaps more than any other stage of life, childhood has a profound impact on health. During this period, a child acquires habits that can produce lifelong benefits or ill effects. To promote healthful habits, help parents teach children the importance of taking care of themselves. Explain to parents that children should have regular screening for preventable diseases. Provide counseling about injury prevention, and give parents the information they need about sound nutrition, exercise, drug avoidance, and dental health. Emphasize the need for reducing violence, and managing common health concerns, such as obesity, asthma, hypertension, stress, and behavioral disorders. Remind parents that their efforts now can help establish healthful habits that won't collapse under the peer pressures of adolescence.

Maintaining health and safety

Because accidents account for almost half of all fatalities in childhood, you'll need to emphasize such safety measures as consistent use of seat belts and precautions to prevent burns and poisoning. Your teaching must also stress nutrition, to enhance growth and development, and the importance of timely immunization against infectious diseases. (See *Schedule for childhood immunizations*, page 34.)

Even a young child can experience stress, which may cause depression and jeopardize his psychological well-being. Stress also raises blood pressure and increases susceptibility to certain illnesses such as ulcers. To minimize these effects, your teaching must emphasize how to cope with stress effectively and, better yet, how to prevent it. Teach them that exercise helps prevent stress, while enhancing strength, cardiac fitness, agility, and balance.

ADOLESCENT HEALTH PROMOTION

The adolescent years can be trying for both a teenager and his family. As he passes from childhood into adulthood, a teenager develops his own set of values and sense of identity, chiefly by testing and experimenting. Little by little, he pulls away from the family and asserts his independence. He has a strong desire to belong to his peer group. He's also overly self-conscious about his appearance, largely because he's maturing sexually.

The dramatic physical and psychological changes of adolescence can certainly affect a teenager's health. As a result, to promote health in adolescence, you'll need to teach about such health problems as poor nutrition, teenage pregnancy, and alcohol and drug abuse.

Addressing teenage sexuality

Each year more than half a million American teenagers give birth, commonly to an infant whose conception wasn't planned. Still other

Schedule for childhood immunizations

Before immunizing a child, ask the parents about contraindications, such as:
• an anaphylactic reaction to a vaccine, vaccine constituent, neomycin, streptomycin, eggs, baker's yeast, or gelatin
• pregnancy
• moderate or severe illness with or without fever
• encephalopathy within 7 days of previous diphtheria/tetanus/pertussis (DTP/DTaP) shot
• infection with human immunodeficiency virus or known altered immunodeficiency

Inform the parents about the risks and benefits of the immunization and provide vaccine information pamphlets. After immunization, tell the parents to watch for and report any reactions other than local swelling and pain or mild temperature elevation. Give them the child's immunization record. Explain that the American Academy of Pediatrics recommends that childhood immunizations follow this schedule.

Age	Immunization
1 day to 2 months	Hepatitis #1
1 month to 4 months	Hepatitis #2
2 months	First dose: DTP vaccine, poliovirus vaccine (oral [OPV] or inactivated [IPV]), *Haemophilus influenzae* B (HIB) vaccine
4 months	Second dose: DTP, OPV or IPV, HIB
6 months	Third dose: DTP, HIB
6 months to 18 months	Hepatitis #3, OPV or IPV
12 months to 15 months	Measles, mumps, rubella (MMR) #1, HIB #4
12 months to 18 months	DTP booster (DTaP at 15 months or older), Varicella vaccine
4 years to 6 years	DTP or DTaP booster, OPV or IPV booster, MMR #2, Tetanus booster every 10 years

teenagers choose to have an abortion, rather than carry an unwanted fetus. To help prevent an unwanted pregnancy, you'll need to provide basic information about how conception occurs and, most important, information about ways to prevent it, including contraception and abstinence. You'll also need to teach them about safe sex practices and proper care during pregnancy. (See "Prenatal care," pages 31 and

Danger signs of teenage suicide

More than likely, you've read or heard about cases in which a teenage boy or girl commits suicide. Sometimes, young lovers or friends even commit suicide together. Do these adolescents give any warning signs of their intentions? Quite commonly, they do. You should be aware of these signs — and teach parents how to recognize them.

Consider the possibility of a suicide attempt if an adolescent:
• talks frequently about death or about the futility of life
• exhibits dramatic mood changes
• appears sad or downcast or expresses feelings of hopelessness
• shows loss of interest in his friends or previous activities
• becomes increasingly withdrawn or spends more and more time alone

• begins having trouble at school or receiving poorer grades than usual
• exhibits behavioral changes that suggest alcohol or drug abuse
• starts giving away his favorite possessions
• seems unusually apathetic about the future.

Supporting the parents
Teach parents never to take any behavior for granted, and encourage them to follow their instincts. If they think something is wrong with their son or daughter, they're probably right. They shouldn't try to rationalize or deny any behavior. If they suspect a problem, tell them to seek professional help. Also stress the need to maintain communication with their child.

32, and "Sexually transmitted diseases," page 37.)

Preventing self-inflicted injuries

You'll need to provide information about how to prevent motor vehicle accidents, drug and alcohol abuse, and suicide. Point out that drug- and alcohol-related motor vehicle accidents are the leading cause of teenage deaths.

Suicide, the third leading cause of death among teenagers, is usually accomplished by self-inflicted gunshot wounds, drug overdose, or carbon monoxide poisoning by automobile exhaust fumes. Suggest that parents keep guns and medicine

properly secured. Be aware that most teenagers who successfully commit suicide have made previous attempts. What's more, a suicidal teenager will typically give warning signs of his intentions. (See *Danger signs of teenage suicide*.)

ADULT HEALTH PROMOTION

The leading causes of death in adults between ages 25 and 64 are heart disease, cancer, and cerebrovascular accident (CVA). Although some of these problems stem from genetic predisposition, many are linked to unhealthy habits, such as overeating, smoking, lack of exercise, and alcohol and drug abuse. Your teaching can help an adult recognize and correct these habits to help ensure a longer and healthier life.

Your goals include promoting good nutrition, combating inactivity, teaching how to avoid safety risks and how to detect early signs of illness — especially cancer, myocardial infarction (MI), and CVA.

Nutrition and exercise

To promote health in adulthood, you'll need to cover such topics as preventing poor nutrition and combating inactivity. Explain that exercise improves circulation and helps the heart and lungs function more efficiently. By helping the body metabolize carbohydrates and fats, exercise may reduce the risk of atherosclerosis. It can also increase stamina, improve stress management, and improve the quality of sleep. However, exercise can aggravate hidden or existing health problems and heighten the risk of injuries. So instruct the patient to seek medical advice before starting an exercise program if he:
• has diagnosed heart disease or a heart murmur or has had an MI
• feels pain or pressure in the chest, neck, shoulder, or arm during or after exercise
• feels faint or has dizzy spells
• experiences extreme breathlessness after mild exertion
• is hypertensive or hasn't had a recent blood pressure check
• has bone or joint problems such as arthritis
• is a male older than age 45 or a female older than age 50 who isn't used to vigorous exercise

• has a family history of coronary artery disease
• has any other medical condition such as diabetes.

Refer the patient to the American Heart Association for brochures that teach how to start an exercise program, choose enjoyable exercises, and prevent injury.

Smoking cessation

Cigarette smoking remains the largest single cause of preventable illness and premature death. Smokers risk developing heart disease, CVA, chronic lung disease, and cancer of the lung or other organs. For women, smoking during pregnancy may account for low birth weight, preterm delivery, and 10% of all infant deaths. In addition, smokers have a 70% greater chance of premature death than nonsmokers.

To encourage your patient to kick the habit, discuss the health hazards for the smoker and others affected by secondhand smoke. Advise the smoker to ask his doctor about the use of nicotine-resin-complex gum or nicotine patches to help him quit smoking. Support groups can also be helpful.

Substance abuse counseling

You will also need to teach your adult patient about substance abuse. Screen your patient for signs of substance abuse — especially alcohol abuse. Referral to a community help and support group such as Alcoholics Anonymous can be helpful.

Stress and coping skills

Reducing stress and teaching coping skills are another important health promotion objective. Occasional stress during adulthood is normal and helps an individual rise to challenges. However, chronic or overwhelming stress can tax a person's coping ability, which can eventually lead to alcohol or drug abuse, mental illness, depression, hypertension, or GI upset. Teaching your patients coping skills will help them reduce or better manage their stress, preventing stress-induced illness.

Sexually transmitted diseases

Each year, sexually transmitted diseases (STDs) strike millions of people, most of them between the ages of 15 and 30. AIDS is perhaps the most widely known STD. Intimate sexual contact (heterosexual and homosexual) remains the most common mode of HIV transmission. Because AIDS is fatal, prevention is key. Unsafe sexual practices dramatically increase the risk of HIV infection for all patients.

To help prevent and control STDs, teach the patient that each type of STD results from a different organism. Point out that more than one STD may occur at any given time. Recommend limiting sexual contacts, avoiding infected partners, and urinating and cleaning the genitals right after intercourse. Urge an infected patient to inform sexual partners so they can seek treatment. Explain safer sex practices to the adolescent in a nonjudgmental way.

Point out that unsafe sex — even once — can cause HIV infection. (See *Guide to safer sexual practices*, page 38.)

Discussing HIV testing is a high-level skill requiring detailed knowledge of risks and benefits. Refer the patient for appropriate HIV counseling.

Domestic violence

Domestic violence is the single largest cause of injury to women in the United States. Women seek medical treatment for injuries inflicted by current or former partners. Don't overlook spousal abuse. Males, though not as commonly as females, can be victims of abuse. Same-sex partners can also fall victim to abuse.

Nurses can identify victims by routine screening with direct questions during history taking. Counsel patients who have been abused about available resources and referrals.

Early signs and symptoms of illness

Teach adults about early signs and symptoms of illness — especially breast, cervical, testicular, prostatic, and lung cancer as well as MI and CVA. This will help ensure prompt treatment, which can be lifesaving.

One in eight women will develop breast cancer if she lives to age 85. Emphasize to your patient the importance of early detection through monthly breast self-examination and mammography. (See

Guide to safer sexual practices

Abstinence is the safest activity. Next safest is a stable, monogamous relationship with another uninfected person. (*Both* partners must be monogamous.) Sexual relations with anyone whose human immunodeficiency virus status is unknown or positive are risky.

Safe activities
• Massage or body rubbing (*without* genital contact)
• Hugging
• Dry kissing
• Phone sex
• Solo masturbation
• Unshared sex toys
• Mutual masturbation

Activities that have some risks (because condoms might break, tear, or slip)
• Vaginal sex with condom
• Anal sex with condom
• Oral sex with condom or dental dam

High-risk sexual behaviors
• Anal sex without a condom
• Vaginal sex without a condom
• Unprotected vaginal intercourse during menstruation
• Contact with semen
• Anal-oral contact ("rimming")
• Penetration of the anus with the fist ("fisting")
• Sharing sex toys (for example, dildos) without condoms or proper cleaning

Teaching about breast self-examination.)

Thanks to the Papanicolaou (Pap) test and regular gynecologic checkups, deaths from cervical cancer have fallen by more than 70% over the past 45 years. Annual Pap tests are recommended for all women ages 20 to 85, with more frequent testing if previous abnormal tests have been noted. Also instruct your female patients to watch for warning signs of uterine cancer, such as unusual bleeding or discharge, and to seek medical attention if such signs develop.

Describe the warning signs and symptoms of lung cancer, including a persistent cough, blood-streaked sputum, and chest pain. Unfortunately, lung cancer is typically advanced by the time it causes signs and symptoms. As a result, focus your teaching on high-risk groups: smokers, especially if they've had the habit for more than 20 years, and adults exposed to asbestos or other industrial contaminants.

Inform the patient that the American Cancer Society recommends these tests for early detection of colorectal cancer: a digital rectal examination performed annually after age 40, a fecal occult blood test performed annually after age 50, and a proctosigmoidoscopy performed every 3 to 5 years after age 50 following two negative annual examinations. Also teach him the warning signs of colorectal cancer: rectal bleeding, bloody stool, or a change in bowel habits.

Testicular cancer usually strikes men between ages 20 and 35. To

Teaching about breast self-examination

Teach your patients to conduct their own monthly self-examination. If your patient hasn't reached menopause, the best time for this examination is immediately after her menstrual period.

Standing before a mirror
1. Have the patient undress to the waist and stand in front of a mirror, with her arms at her sides. She should observe her breasts for any change in their shape or size and any puckering or dimpling of the skin.

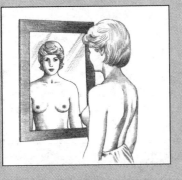

2. Have her raise her arms and press her hands together behind her head. She should observe her breasts as she did before.

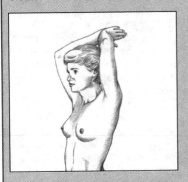

3. Next, have her press her palms firmly on her hips. She should observe her breasts again.

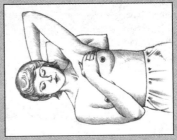

Lying down
1. Tell the patient that she should examine her breasts while lying flat on her back. Advise her to place a small pillow under her left shoulder, and to put her left hand behind her head.

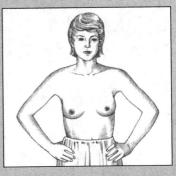

2. Instruct the patient to examine her left breast with her right hand, using a circular motion and progressing
(continued)

Teaching about breast self-examination *(continued)*

clockwise, until she's examined every portion. Explain that she'll notice a ridge of firm tissue in the lower curve of her breast.

Have her check the area under her arm with her elbow slightly bent. Point out that she shouldn't be alarmed if she feels a small lump under her armpit that moves freely; this area contains lymph glands, which may become swollen when she's ill. Advise her to check the size of the lump daily, and to call a doctor or nurse if it doesn't go away in a few days or if it gets larger.

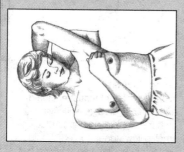

3. Next, instruct the patient to gently squeeze the nipple between her thumb and forefinger, and to note any discharge. Have her repeat this examination on her right breast, using her left hand.

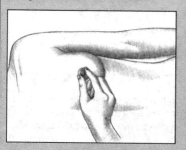

In the shower

Instruct the patient to examine her breasts while in the shower or bath, after first lubricating them with soap and water. Then, using the same circular, clockwise motion, she should gently inspect both breasts with her fingertips. After she's toweled dry, she should squeeze each nipple gently, noting any discharge.

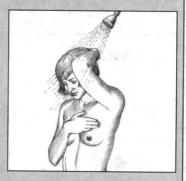

What to do about lumps

Tell your patient not to panic if she feels a lump while examining her breasts. Reassure her that most lumps aren't cancerous. Direct her to note whether she can easily lift the skin covering it and whether the lump moves when she does so.

Tell the patient to notify her doctor or nurse after she's examined the lump. Advise her to describe how the lump feels (hard or soft) and whether it moves easily under the skin.

Finally, remind your patient that although self-examination is important, it's not a substitute for examination by her doctor or nurse practitioner. Urge her to see her doctor or nurse annually — or semiannually, if she's considered at special risk.

Teaching about testicular self-examination

To help your patient detect testicular abnormalities early, urge him to examine his testicles once a month. Explain that eventually he will be able to recognize anything abnormal.

Checking appearance
Instruct the patient to remove his clothes and stand in front of a mirror. Tell him to lift his penis and check his scrotum for any change in shape or size and for red, distended veins. Tell him the scrotum's left side naturally hangs slightly lower than the right.

Palpating for lumps and masses
Tell the patient to palpate the testicles for lumps and masses. Have him begin by locating the epididymis and spermatic cord. Next, using his thumb and the first two fingers of his right hand, have him gently squeeze the spermatic cord above the right testicle. Then have him repeat the procedure with the spermatic cord above his left testicle. Have him check for lumps and masses by squeezing along the entire length of each cord.

Now tell the patient to examine his right testicle by placing his right thumb on the front of the testicle and

his index and middle fingers behind it, then gently pressing his thumb and fingers together; they should meet. Tell him to be sure he checks the entire testicle. Then have him use his left hand to examine his left testicle in the same manner. Advise him that his testicles should feel smooth, rubbery, and slightly tender and should move easily.

Finally, tell the patient to notify his doctor immediately if he feels any lumps, masses, or other changes.

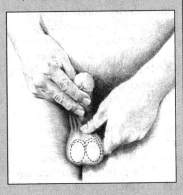

emphasize the importance of monthly self-examination, tell the patient that 88% of such cancers have already spread by the time they're diagnosed. Also teach him the warning signs of testicular cancer, such as a slight enlargement or a change in the consistency of the testes. (See *Teaching about testicular self-examination.*)

Prostate cancer ranks as the second most common cancer in adult males. Describe its warning signs and symptoms, such as weak or interrupted urine flow, an inability to urinate or control urine flow, urinary frequency (especially at night), blood-tinged urine, pain or burning on urination, and pain in the lower back, pelvis, or upper thighs. Instruct the patient to see his doctor if he experiences any of these.

Teach the patient to seek medical help immediately if he experiences an MI's cardinal symptom: persistent chest pain (commonly described as "heavy," "squeezing," or "crushing") that may radiate to the left side of the jaw or neck or to the left shoulder or arm. MI may also cause anxiety or a sense of impending doom, dizziness or fainting, sweating, nausea, and shortness of breath.

Describe the signs and symptoms of CVA to the patient: sudden, temporary weakness or numbness of the face, arm, or leg on one side of the body; temporary loss of speech or inability to understand speech; temporary loss of vision or blurred vision, usually in one eye; unexplained dizziness, unsteadiness, or sudden falls. Explain that many severe CVAs are preceded by transient ischemic attacks. These attacks produce signs and symptoms similar to a CVA and may occur days, weeks, or even months before a CVA. If the patient experiences any of these signs or symptoms, have him immediately seek medical attention.

GERIATRIC HEALTH PROMOTION

Reject the idea that being old means being unhealthy. Health problems in old age are *not* inevitable — many are preventable or can be effectively controlled. Life expectancy has increased tremendously in this century. Today, people who reach the age of 65 can expect to live well into their eighties. As the baby boom generation approaches retirement, our population of older adults will continue to grow dramatically. The fastest growing population segment in America is those individuals over 85 years of age.

This increased longevity makes attention to health promotion and disease prevention strategies for older adults highly important. Nurses can promote a state of health that combines maximal active life expectancy with a high level of function.

The U.S. Department of Health and Human Services and the Public Health Service have noted in *Healthy People 2000* that older Americans are a high priority population group to be targeted for health promotion. Maintenance of health and functional independence are essential to both healthy aging and enhanced quality of life. By educating, motivating, and supporting elders to actively promote their own health, nurses can reduce the incidence of disability and institutionalization in the 21st century.

Below you'll find advice on focusing your teaching on the following topics: immunization, tobacco use and alcohol consumption, polypharmacy, diet and exercise, and injury prevention including motor vehicle, burns and fire, asphyxiation, and heat emergencies. Also covered are dental health and advance directives.

Immunization

Immunization of geriatric patients is important to prevent the spread of infectious disease. Older adults are highly susceptible to lower respiratory tract infections. Influenza and pneumonia are the fifth leading cause of death in this population. Pneumococcal vaccine should be administered to all immunocompromised individuals ages 65 and over. The prevalence of immunity to tetanus declines with age, thus, a tetanus-diphtheria booster continues to be recommended every 10 years.

Tobacco and alcohol

The U.S. Preventive Services Task Force recommends that all older adults who use tobacco products should receive regular cessation counseling. Older adults will benefit from smoking cessation as well as from the reduction of environmental tobacco smoke. Not only does life expectancy increase significantly, but those already experiencing signs and symptoms of chronic lung disease, coronary artery disease, osteoporosis, or a reduction in exercise tolerance, will notice improvement.

To prevent the physical injury and medical problems associated with problem drinking, counsel any elder who you believe may be drinking excessively. All elders should be encouraged to limit their alcohol consumption. It's also important to stress the danger of operating a vehicle, boating, or swimming while under the influence of alcohol, and the need to avoid the use of alcohol while performing any such dangerous activity.

Polypharmacy

Today, 80% of the elderly population suffer from at least one chronic health problem and many from a number of health problems. With each health problem, a variety of medications may be prescribed leading to the possibility of polypharmacy — the administration of multiple medications to a patient. Complications of polypharmacy can be prevented by reviewing your patient's medication regime, including both old and new prescriptions. Educated about the proper use of their medication, and aware of potential adverse effects or drug interactions, patients are less likely to have adverse reactions.

Diet and exercise

Eating a healthy diet and engaging in regular exercise can help prevent or delay the onset of physical and psychological deficits. Both are effective therapies for stress, sleep disorders, depression, decreased self-esteem, anxiety, hypertension, obesity, diabetes mellitus, coronary artery disease, hyperlipidemia, osteoporosis, cancer, and constipation, just to name a few.

Injury prevention

Falls are the leading cause of nonfatal injuries and unintentional injury deaths in the United States. Counseling elderly patients on measures to reduce the chance of falling is vital.

To prevent asphyxiation, counsel older patients on how to help prevent aspiration of food. Advise them to correct denture fit and to change the size and consistency of their food as necessary. Also teach the Heimlich maneuver.

Fires and burns are also principle causes of death in elderly patients. *Healthy People 2000* suggests that every household have a working smoke detector on each floor. Teach patients about avoiding smoking in bed or around upholstered furniture. Also advise them to keep their hot water heater temperature set at 120° to 130° F (49° to 54° C).

Dental health

Today, over half the adults over age 65 in the United States are edentulous (without teeth). Tooth loss causes a financial burden and a decreased sense of well-being. Thus, counsel your older adults to visit a dental care provider annually, floss daily, and brush their teeth daily with a fluoride-containing toothpaste.

Advance directives

As a primary nurse, include an early and ongoing discussion of advance directives with your older patient to ensure that your patient receives desired terminal care. Advance directives include the living will, health care durable power of attorney, and health care proxy.

REFERENCES AND READINGS

Lifshitz, F. *Childhood Nutrition.* Boca Raton, Fla.: CRC Press, 1995.

Pender, N. *Health Promotion in Nursing Practice,* 3rd ed. Stamford, Conn.: Appleton & Lange, 1995

U.S. Department of Health and Human Services. *Healthy People 2000: Midcourse Review and 1995 Revisions.* Boston: Jones & Bartlett Publishers, 1996.

U.S. Preventative Services Taskforce. *Guide to Clinical Preventative Services,* 2nd ed. Baltimore: Williams & Wilkins, 1996.

Wong, D. *Clinical Manual of Pediatric Nursing,* 4th ed. St. Louis: Mosby-Year Book, 1996.

4

RESPIRATORY CARE

The respiratory system functions primarily to maintain the exchange of oxygen and carbon dioxide in the lungs and tissues and to regulate acid-base balance. Any change in this system affects every other body system. What's more, changes in other body systems may also reduce the lungs' ability to provide oxygen.

ASSESSMENT

Because the body depends on the respiratory system to survive, respiratory assessment is a critical nursing responsibility. By performing it thoroughly, you can evaluate subtle and obvious respiratory changes. This section reviews the techniques for performing a complete physical examination.

Physical examination

Before assessing your patient's respiratory system, inspect his skin. A dusky or bluish skin tint (cyanosis) may indicate decreased oxygen content in the arterial blood. (See *Effects of chronic ineffective gas exchange*, pages 46 and 47.)

Distinguishing central from peripheral cyanosis is important. Central cyanosis results from hypoxemia and affects all body organs. It may appear in patients with right-to-left cardiac shunting or a pulmonary disease that causes hypoxemia such as chronic bronchitis. The cyanosis appears on the skin; on the mucous membranes of the mouth, lips, and conjunctivae; or in other highly vascular areas, such as the earlobes or nail beds.

On the other hand, peripheral cyanosis results from vasoconstriction, vascular occlusion, or reduced cardiac output. Commonly seen in patients exposed to cold, peripheral cyanosis appears in the nail beds, nose, ears, and fingers and doesn't affect the mucous membranes.

In dark-skinned patients, inspect the oral mucous membranes and lips. If a dark-skinned patient has central cyanosis, these areas will

Effects of chronic ineffective gas exchange

Prolonged hypoxemia and hypercapnia, as seen in patients with chronic respiratory disorders, eventually take their toll on other vital systems.

Neurologic effects

Severe hypercapnia dulls the medullary respiratory center, forcing peripheral chemoreceptors in the aortic and carotid bodies to direct respiration. Because these receptors respond to low Pao_2, oxygen therapy must be strictly controlled in accordance with blood gas analysis.

Cardiovascular effects

Respiratory neuromuscular disorders or lung or pulmonary vascular disease can produce cor pulmonale, acute or chronic enlargement of the right ventricle. Usually, cor pulmonale is chronic, secondary to chronic obstructive disease. In acute form, cor pulmonale may develop from massive pulmonary embolism, or from acute pulmonary infection or another condition that worsens hypoxemia.

Cor pulmonale may result from widespread destruction of lung tissue or pulmonary capillaries, from increased pulmonary vascular resistance, from shunting of unoxygenated blood, or from pulmonary vasoconstriction and pulmonary artery hypertension. Pulmonary hypertension leads to right ventricular dilation and hypertrophy, followed by right-sided heart failure, reduced cardiac output, and shock.

Musculoskeletal effects

When Pao_2 is low, an increase in pulmonary vasculature in response to chronic hypoxemia may cause pulmonary osteoarthropathy, also called secondary hypertrophic osteoarthropathy. This condition shows up as bone and tissue changes in the extremities: arthralgia, clubbing, and proliferation of subperiosteal tissues in long bones.

Renal effects

Sustained hypercapnia causes renal retention of bicarbonate ions, sodium, and water, leading to fluid overload. Sustained hypoxemia stimulates the kidneys to release erythropoietic factor into the blood. This factor causes a plasma transport protein to yield erythropoietin, the compound that spurs red blood cell production and raises hematocrit.

Hematopoietic effects

Chronic hypoxemia commonly causes an increase in the number of red blood cells, which makes embolism and thrombosis more likely, and increases the heart's workload.

appear ashen, rather than bluish. Facial skin may appear pale gray, or ashen, in a cyanotic black-skinned patient and yellowish brown in a cyanotic brown-skinned patient.

Next, assess the patient's nail beds and toes for abnormal enlargement. This condition, called clubbing, results from chronic tissue

Prolonged hypoxemia and hypercapnia

Cardiovascular effects
Pulmonary capillary vaso-constriction
Increased pulmonary vascular resistance
Pulmonary hypertension
Shunting of unoxygenated blood
Cor pulmonale

Neurologic effects
Dulling of medullary respiratory center
Respiration stimulated by aortic and carotid bodies

Renal effects
Release of erythropoietin
Increased retention of bicarbonate ion, sodium, and water
Fluid overload

Musculoskeletal effects
Pulmonary osteoarthropathy (arthralgia, digital clubbing, subperiosteal proliferation of tissue of long bones)
Increased myoglobin in muscles

Hematopoietic effects
Polycythemia
Increased risk of embolism and thrombosis

hypoxia. Nail thinning accompanied by an abnormal alteration of the angle of the finger and toe bases distinguishes clubbing.

Preparing for respiratory assessment

After obtaining an overall picture of the patient's oxygenation, assess his respiratory system. You'll need a stethoscope with a diaphragm, a felt-tipped marking pen, a ruler, and a tape measure.

Have the patient sit in a position that allows access to the anterior and posterior thorax. Make sure the patient isn't cold because shivering may alter breathing patterns.

If the patient can't sit up, use the supine semi-Fowler position to assess the anterior chest wall and the side-lying position to assess the posterior thorax. Keep in mind that these positions may cause some distortion of findings.

When performing the assessment, you may find it easier to inspect, palpate, percuss, and auscultate the anterior chest before the posterior.

Inspection

Basic assessment of respiratory function requires determination of the rate, rhythm, and quality of the patient's respirations as well as inspection of chest configuration, chest symmetry, skin condition, and accessory muscle use. It should also include assessment for nasal flaring. Accomplish these steps by inspecting the patient's breathing and the anterior and posterior thorax, and noting any abnormal findings. (See *Recognizing common chest deformities.*)

Respiration. Count the number of respirations, each composed of an inspiration and an expiration, for 1 full minute. For a patient with periodic or irregular breathing, monitor the respirations for more than 1 minute to determine the rate accurately. Assess the duration of any periods lacking spontaneous respi-

ration (apnea) and note any abnormal respiratory patterns, such as tachypnea and bradypnea. (For more information, see *Assessing abnormal breath sounds,* page 51.)

Assess the quality of respiration by observing the type and depth of breathing. Also, assess the method of ventilation by having the patient lie supine to expose the chest and abdominal walls. Patients with chronic obstructive pulmonary disease (COPD) may exhibit pursed-lip breathing, which prevents small airway collapse during exhalation. Forced inspiration or expiration may alter assessment findings; therefore, ask the patient to breathe normally.

Note the depth of breathing, assessing for shallow chest wall expansion (hypopnea) or unusually deep chest wall expansion (hyperpnea). Use your judgment to assess the depth of breathing, but be sure to use the terms *hypopnea* or *hyperpnea,* not *hypoventilation* or *hyperventilation.* Detecting hypoventilation or hyperventilation requires a measurement of partial pressure of carbon dioxide in arterial blood ($PaCO_2$).

Anterior thorax. Inspect the thorax for structural deformities, such as a concave or convex curvature of the anterior chest wall over the sternum. Inspect between and around the ribs for visible sinking of soft tissues (retractions). Assess the patient's respiratory pattern for symmetry. Look for any abnormalities in skin color or alterations in muscle tone.

Initially, inspect the chest wall to identify the shape of the thoracic

Recognizing common chest deformities

Inspecting the patient's anterior chest for deviations in size or shape is important. Normally, the anteroposterior diameter is one-half the lateral diameter. The illustrations below demonstrate three common deformities and show signs, associated conditions, and characteristics typical of each. For each deformity, a cross-sectional view compares the anteroposterior and lateral diameters of the normal chest with that of the deformed chest (as indicated by the dotted line).

Funnel chest (pectus excavatum)

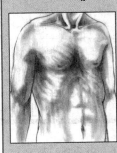

Signs and associated conditions
- Postural disorders such as forward displacement of neck and shoulders
- Upper thoracic kyphosis
- Protuberant abdomen
- Functional heart murmur

Characteristics
- Sinking or funnel-shaped depression of lower sternum
- Diminished anteroposterior chest diameter
- Slightly increased lateral diameter

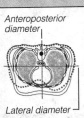

Pigeon chest (pectus carinatum)

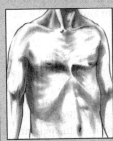

Signs and associated conditions
- Functional cardiovascular or respiratory disorders

Characteristics
- Projection of sternum beyond frontal plane of abdomen; evident in two variations: projection greatest at xiphoid process or projection greatest at or near center of sternum
- Increased anteroposterior diameter
- Greatly decreased lateral diameter at front of chest

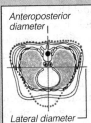

(continued)

Recognizing common chest deformities (continued)

Barrel chest

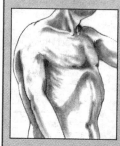

Signs and associated conditions
- Chronic respiratory disorders
- Increasing dyspnea
- Chronic cough
- Wheezing

Characteristics
- Enlarged anteroposterior and lateral chest dimensions; chest appears barrel-shaped
- Prominent accessory muscles
- Prominent sternal angle
- Thoracic kyphosis

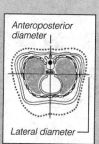

Anteroposterior diameter

Lateral diameter

---

cage. In an adult, the thorax should have a greater diameter laterally (from side to side) than anteroposteriorly (from front to back).

Note the angle between the ribs and the sternum at the point immediately above the xiphoid process. This angle, called the costal angle, should be less than 90 degrees in an adult; it widens if the chest wall is chronically expanded, as in increased anteroposterior diameter (barrel chest).

To inspect the anterior chest for symmetry of movement, have the patient lie supine. Stand at the foot of the bed and carefully observe the patient's deep breathing for equal expansion of the chest wall. Watch for the abnormal collapse of part of the chest wall during inspiration along with an abnormal expansion of the same area during expiration (paradoxical movement). Paradoxi-

cal movement indicates a loss of normal chest wall function.

Next, check for use of the accessory muscles of respiration by observing the sternocleidomastoid, scalene, and trapezius muscles in the shoulders and neck. During normal inspiration and expiration, the diaphragm and external intercostal muscles alone should easily maintain the breathing process. Hypertrophy of any of the accessory muscles may indicate frequent use, especially if found in an elderly patient, but may be normal in a well-conditioned athlete. Also observe the position the patient assumes to breathe. A patient who depends on accessory muscles may assume a "tripod position," which involves resting the arms on the knees or on the sides of a chair.

Observe the patient's skin on the anterior chest for any unusual color,

Assessing abnormal breath sounds

Type	Description	Location	Cause
Crackles	Light crackling, popping, nonmusical sound, like hairs being rubbed together; further classified by pitch: high, medium, or low	Anywhere; heard in lung bases initially, usually during inspiration; also in dependent lung portions of bedridden patients. If clear with coughing, they're not abnormal.	Air passing through moisture, especially in the small airways and alveoli, with pulmonary edema; also, alveoli "popping open" in atelectasis
Wheezes	Whistling sound; described as sonorous, moaning, musical, sibilant and rumbling, or groaning	Anywhere; heard during inspiration or expiration; if clear with coughing, they may originate in the larger upper airways	Fluid or secretions in the large airways or in airways narrowed by mucus, bronchospasm, or tumor
Rhonchi	Gurgling sound	Central airways; heard during inspiration and expiration	Air passing through fluid-filled airways, as in upper respiratory tract infection
Pleural friction rub	Superficial squeaking or grating sound, like pieces of sandpaper or leather being rubbed together	Lateral lung field; heard during inspiration and expiration (with patient in upright position)	Inflamed parietal and visceral pleural linings rubbing together
Grunting	Grunting noise	Central airways; heard during expiration in children	Physiologic retention of air in lungs to prevent alveolar collapse
Stridor	Crowing noise	Larynx or trachea; heard during inspiration	Forced movement of air through edematous upper airway; in adults, laryngoedema as in allergic reaction or smoke inhalation and laryngospasm, as in tetany

lumps, or lesions, and note the location of any abnormality.

Posterior thorax. To inspect the posterior chest, observe the patient's breathing again. If he can't sit in a backless chair or lean forward against a supporting structure, he can lie in a lateral position. However, this may distort findings.

Assess the posterior chest wall for the same characteristics as the anterior: chest structure, respiratory pattern, symmetry of expansion, skin color and muscle tone, and accessory muscle use.

Palpation

By carefully palpating the trachea and the anterior and posterior thorax, you can detect structural and skin abnormalities, areas of pain, and chest asymmetry.

Trachea and anterior thorax. First, palpate the trachea for position. Observe the patient to determine whether he uses accessory neck muscles to breathe.

Next, palpate the suprasternal notch. In most patients, the arch of the aorta lies close to the surface just behind the suprasternal notch. Use your fingertips to gently evaluate the strength and regularity of the patient's aortic pulsations there.

Then palpate the thorax to assess the skin and underlying structures.

Gentle palpation shouldn't be painful, so assess any complaints of pain for localization, radiation, and severity. Be especially careful to palpate any areas that looked abnormal during inspection. If necessary, support the patient during the procedure with one hand while using your other hand to palpate one side at a time, continuing to compare sides. Note any unusual findings, such as masses, crepitus, skin irregularities, or painful areas.

If the patient complains of chest pain, attempt to determine the cause by palpating the anterior chest. Palpation doesn't worsen pain caused by cardiac or pulmonary disorders, such as angina or pleurisy.

Next, palpate the costal angle. The area around the xiphoid process contains many nerve endings, so be gentle to avoid causing pain. If a patient frequently uses the internal intercostal muscles to breathe, these muscles will eventually pull the chest cavity upward and outward. If this has occurred, the costal angle will be greater than the normal 90 degrees.

Posterior thorax. Palpate the posterior thorax in a similar manner, using the palmar surface of the fingertips of one or both hands. Identify bony structures, such as the vertebrae and the scapulae.

To determine the location of any abnormalities, identify the first thoracic vertebra (with the patient's head tipped forward) and count the number of spinous processes from this landmark to the abnormal finding. Use this reference point for documentation. Also identify the inferior scapular tips and medial borders of both bones to define the margins of the upper and lower lung lobes posteriorly. Locate and describe all abnormalities in relation to these landmarks.

Palpating for tactile fremitus

Follow this procedure to assess for tactile fremitus:

1. Place your open palm flat against the patient's chest without touching the chest with your fingers.

2. Ask the patient to repeat a resonant phrase like "99" as you systematically move your hands over his chest from the central airways to the lung periphery and back. Always proceed in a systematic manner from the top of the suprascapular, interscapular, infrascapular, and hypochondriac areas (areas found from the fifth to tenth intercostal spaces to the right and left of midline).

3. Repeat this procedure on the posterior thorax. You should feel vibrations of equal intensity on either side of the chest. Fremitus usually occurs in the upper chest, close to the bronchi, and feels strongest at the

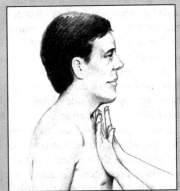

second intercostal space on either side of the sternum. Little or no fremitus should occur in the lower chest. The intensity of the vibrations varies according to the thickness and structure of the patient's chest wall as well as the patient's voice intensity and pitch.

Tactile fremitus. Because sound travels more easily through solid structures than through air, assessing for tactile fremitus (the palpation of vocalizations) informs you about the contents of the lungs. (See *Palpating for tactile fremitus.*)

The patient's vocalization should produce vibrations of equal intensity on both sides of the chest. Normally, vibrations should occur in the upper chest, close to the bronchi, and then decrease and finally disappear toward the periphery of the lungs.

Conditions that restrict air movement, such as pneumonia, pleural effusion, or COPD with overinflated lungs, decrease tactile fremitus. Conditions that consolidate tissue or fluid in a portion of the pleural area, such as a lung tumor, or pulmonary fibrosis, increase tactile fremitus. A grating feeling may signify a pleural friction rub.

Percussion

This assessment technique helps you determine the boundaries of the lungs and how much gas, liquid, or solid exists in them. Percussion can effectively assess structures as deep as $1^3/4''$ to $3''$ (4.5 to 7.5 cm). Perform percussion in a quiet environment, and proceed systematically, percussing the anterior, lateral, and posterior chest over the intercostal spaces. (For an illustrated procedure, see *Percussing the thorax.*) Avoid percussing over bones, which yields no useful information. Percussion over a healthy lung elicits a resonant sound (hollow and loud, with a low pitch and long duration).

To percuss the anterior chest, have the patient sit facing forward, hands resting at the side of the body. Following the anterior percussion sequence, percuss and compare sound variations from one side to the other. Anterior chest percussion should produce resonance from below the clavicle to the fifth intercostal space on the right (where dullness occurs close to the liver) and to the third intercostal space on the left (where dullness occurs near the heart).

Next, percuss the lateral chest to obtain information about the left upper and lower lobes and about the right upper, middle, and lower lobes. The patient's left arm should be positioned on his head. Repeat the same sequence on the right side. Lateral chest percussion should produce resonance to the sixth or eighth intercostal space.

Finally, percuss the posterior thorax according to the percussion sequence. Posterior percussion should sound resonant to the level of T10.

Auscultation

Auscultate the anterior, lateral, and posterior thorax to detect normal and abnormal breath sounds. To auscultate the thorax of an adult, first warm the stethoscope between your hands and then place the diaphragm of the stethoscope directly on the patient's skin.

If the patient has significant hair growth over the areas to be auscultated, wet the hair to decrease sound blurring. Instruct the patient to take deep breaths through the mouth and caution him against breathing too deeply or too rapidly to prevent light-headedness or dizziness.

During auscultation, first identify normal breath sounds and then assess and identify abnormal sounds. Specific breath sounds occur normally only in certain locations; therefore, the same sound heard anywhere else in the lung field constitutes an important abnormality requiring appropriate documentation.

Anterior and lateral thorax. Systematically auscultate the anterior and lateral thorax for normal as well as abnormal breath sounds, following the same sequence used for percussion. Begin at the upper lobes, and move from side to side and down.

Auscultate a point on one side of the chest, and then auscultate the same point on the other side of the chest, comparing findings. Always assess one full breath at each point.

To assess the right middle lung lobe, auscultate for breath sounds laterally at the level of the fourth to the sixth intercostal spaces, following the lateral auscultation sequence, which is the same as the lateral percussion sequence. The right middle lobe is a common site of aspiration pneumonia, so it requires special attention.

Normal breath sounds include tracheal, bronchial, bronchovesicular, and vesicular sounds. Tracheal

Percussing the thorax

When percussing a patient's thorax, you should always use mediate percussion and follow the same sequence, comparing sound variations from one side with the other. This helps ensure consistency and prevents you from overlooking any important findings. Auscultation follows the same sequence as percussion.

To percuss the anterior thorax, place your fingers over the lung apices in the supraclavicular area.

Then proceed downward, moving from side to side at 1½" to 2" (4- to 5-cm) intervals.

To percuss the lateral thorax, start at the axilla and move down the side of the rib cage, percussing between the ribs, as shown.

To percuss the posterior thorax, progress in a zigzag fashion from the suprascapular to the interscapular to the infrascapular areas, avoiding the spinal column and the scapulae, as shown.

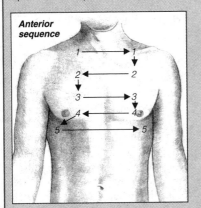

Anterior sequence

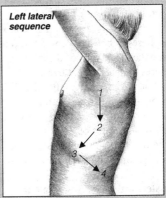

Left lateral sequence

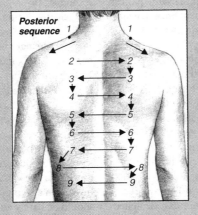

Posterior sequence

sounds, which are harsh and discontinuous, are heard equally during inspiration and expiration. Bronchial sounds, high-pitched and discontinuous, are prolonged during expiration. Bronchovesicular sounds, medium-pitched and continuous, are equally audible during inspiration and expiration. Vesicular sounds, low-pitched and continuous, are prolonged during inspiration. (See *Normal breath sounds.*)

Classify normal and abnormal breath sounds according to location, intensity (amplitude), characteristic sound, pitch (tone), and duration during the inspiratory and expiratory phases. When assessing duration, time the inspiratory and expiratory phases to determine the ratio.

For the last step in auscultation, identify the inspiratory and expiratory phase of normal and abnormal breath sounds. Also determine whether the sound occurs during inspiration, expiration, or both.

Posterior thorax. Auscultate the posterior thorax in the same pattern as the percussion sequence. During auscultation, remain aware of the patient's breathing pattern.

In a normal adult, bronchovesicular breath sounds (the sound of air moving through the bronchial airways) should occur over the interscapular area; vesicular breath sounds (the sound of air moving through the alveoli) should occur in the suprascapular and infrascapular areas. Note any absent, decreased, or adventitious breath sounds. For example, bronchovesicular sounds auscultated in the periphery of the lungs are adventitious. Crackles and rhonchi (gurgles) are also adventitious; if you hear them, instruct the patient to cough, and then listen again.

Diaphragmatic excursion. This technique allows you to evaluate your patient's diaphragm movement. (For an illustrated procedure, see *Measuring diaphragmatic excursion,* page 58.)

Normal diaphragmatic excursion is $1^{1}/4''$ to $2^{1}/4''$ (3 to 6 cm). Failure of the diaphragm to contract downward may indicate paralysis or muscle flattening, a condition that results from COPD.

Voice resonance. To assess voice resonance, instruct the patient to say "99." As he speaks, auscultate in the usual sequence. The voice normally sounds muffled and indistinct during auscultation. The sound appears loudest medially and softest in the lung periphery. However, conditions producing lung tissue consolidation cause bronchophony — the greater resonance that allows you to hear "99" clearly during auscultation.

To test increased resonance further, ask the patient to repeat the letter *e*, which should sound muffled and indistinct on auscultation. If the letter sounds like *a* and the voice sounds nasal or bleating, you've heard egophony, another indication of consolidation.

To perform another test for increased resonance, ask the patient to whisper the words "one-two-three." On auscultation, these words should be barely audible. If the words sound distinct and under-

Normal breath sounds

These illustrations show the location of the various breath sounds.

Tracheal sounds result from air passing through the glottis. They are heard best over the trachea as harsh, discontinuous sounds. Their ratio of inspiration to expiration is 1:1.

Bronchial sounds result from high rates of turbulent air flowing through the large bronchi. They are loud, high-pitched, hollow, harsh, or coarse sounds that are heard over the manubrium. Their inspiration-expiration ratio is 2:3.

Bronchovesicular sounds result from transitional airflow moving through the branches and convergences of the smaller bronchi and bronchioles. These soft, breezy sounds are pitched about two notes lower than bronchial sounds. Anteriorly, they are heard near the mainstem bronchi in the first and second intercostal spaces; posteriorly, between the scapulae. Their inspiration-expiration ratio is 1:1.

Vesicular sounds result from laminar airflow moving through the alveolar ducts and alveoli at low rates. They are heard best in the periphery of the lungs but are inaudible over the scapulae. These soft, swishy, breezy sounds are about two notes lower than bronchovesicular sounds. Their inspiration-expiration ratio is 3:1.

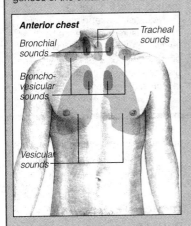

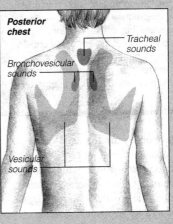

standable, you have heard whispered pectoriloquy, which suggests lung tissue consolidation from such conditions as a lung tumor, pneumonia, or pulmonary fibrosis.

DIAGNOSTIC TESTS

If the history and physical examination reveal evidence of respiratory dysfunction, diagnostic tests will be needed to help identify and evaluate such dysfunction. These tests include blood and sputum studies,

Measuring diaphragmatic excursion

Follow this procedure to measure the extent of diaphragmatic excursion — the distance that the diaphragm travels between inhalation and exhalation.

First instruct the patient to take a deep breath and hold it while you percuss down the right side of the posterior thorax. Begin at the lower border of the scapula and continue until the percussion note changes from resonance to dullness, which identifies the location of the diaphragm. Using a washable, felt-tipped pen, mark this point with a small line.

Now instruct the patient to take a few normal breaths. Then ask him to exhale completely and hold it while you percuss again to locate the point where the resonant sounds become dull. Mark this point with a small line.

Repeat this entire procedure on the left side of the posterior thorax. Keep in mind that the diaphragm

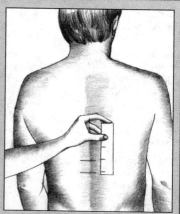

usually sits slightly higher on the right side than on the left because of the position of the liver.

Next, using a tape measure or ruler, measure the distance between the two marks on each side of the posterior thorax, as shown here. The distance between these two marks reflects diaphragmatic excursion.

---

pulmonary function studies, endoscopic and imaging tests, fluid aspiration, tissue monitoring, and pulse oximetry. (For more information about diagnostic tests, see *Diagnostic tests for respiratory disorders.*)

NURSING DIAGNOSES

After completing your assessment, you're ready to integrate the findings and select nursing diagnoses. Below you'll find nursing diagnoses commonly used in patients with respiratory problems. For each diagnosis, you'll also find expected outcomes

and nursing interventions along with rationales (which appear in italic type).

Ineffective breathing pattern

Related to decreased energy or fatigue, this nursing diagnosis can be associated with such conditions as COPD and pulmonary embolus.

Expected outcomes
• Patient's respiratory rate stays within ±5 breaths/minute of baseline.

(Text continues on page 64.)

Diagnostic tests for respiratory disorders

Test	Purpose	Nursing considerations
Blood tests		
Arterial blood gases (ABGs)	To evaluate gas exchange in the lungs	• Use an arterial line, if possible. • If a percutaneous puncture is done, perform Allen's test first. • After obtaining a specimen, apply pressure to the puncture site for 5 minutes and tape a gauze pad firmly in place. • Place a blood specimen on ice and send it immediately to a laboratory. • Document on a laboratory slip whether the patient is breathing room air or oxygen. • Regularly monitor the puncture site for bleeding.
Red blood cell (RBC) count and hemoglobin (Hg)	To assess perfusion and oxygen transport	• After obtaining a venipuncture specimen, apply pressure to the site to control bleeding. • Monitor the site periodically for bleeding.
Pulmonary function tests (PFT)		
The five PFTs are tidal volume and expiratory reserve volume (which use direct spirography), and minute volume, inspiratory reserve volume, and residual volume (which must be calculated from the results of other PFT). The pulmonary capacity tests are vital capacity and inspirato-	To evaluate ventilatory function through spirometric measurements, determine the cause of dyspnea, assess the effectiveness of such therapies as bronchodilators and steroids, and to determine if a respiratory abnormality	• Explain the procedure to the patient. • Explain that he'll be asked to breathe a certain way. • He may need to wear noseclips and sit upright. • Explain that he may experience dyspnea or fatigue but may have rest periods. • Tell him he should inform the technician if he experiences dizziness, chest pain, *(continued)*

Diagnostic tests for respiratory disorders *(continued)*

Test	Purpose	Nursing considerations
Pulmonary function tests (PFT) *(continued)*		
ry capacity, functional residual capacity, total lung capacity, maximal midexpiratory flow, forced vital capacity, forced expiratory volume, and maximal voluntary volume.	stems from an obstructive or restrictive disease process	palpitations, nausea, severe dyspnea, or wheezing.
Endoscopy		
Bronchoscopy	To provide direct inspection of the trachea and bronchi through a flexible fiberoptic or rigid bronchoscope; to allow the doctor to determine the location and extent of pathologic processes, assess resectability of a tumor, diagnose bleeding sites, collect tissue or sputum specimens, and remove foreign bodies, mucus plugs, or excessive secretions	• Explain that the patient will be placed supine on a bed or table. • Advise him that he'll receive medication to relax, and that the tube will be introduced through the nose or the mouth. • Explain that his vital signs will be monitored frequently. • After the test he should lie on his side or sit with head elevated until his gag reflex returns. • Food, fluid, and oral drugs will be withheld for about 2 hours. • Watch for subcutaneous crepitus around the face and neck which may indicate tracheal or bronchial perforation. • Monitor for breathing problems from laryngeal edema or laryngospasm. • Observe for signs of hypoxia, pneumothorax, bronchospasm, or bleeding.
Radiography		
Pulmonary angiography	To allow radiographic examination of the pulmonary circulation to	• The patient should receive nothing by mouth for 6 hours before the test, or as ordered.

Diagnostic tests for respiratory disorders *(continued)*

Test	Purpose	Nursing considerations
Radiography *(continued)*		
Pulmonary angiography *(continued)*	detect blood flow abnormalities, such as pulmonary emboli or infarction	• Explain the procedure: he will lie supine on a table; ECG electrodes will be attached; I.V. line will be started; and a blood pressure cuff applied. • He will be given a sedative and contrast dye. The dye may cause him to feel a warm flush when it's injected. • The doctor will insert a catheter in a selected vein. • After the test, monitor the catheter insertion site for bleeding, and arterial occlusion. • Monitor the patient for hypersensitivity to the contrast medium or the local anesthetic. Monitor vital signs.
Chest X-ray	To show the location and size of lesions and identify structural abnormalities that influence ventilation and diffusion	• Explain the procedure to the patient. • Tell him he'll be asked to take a deep breath and hold it for a few seconds. • Reassure him that the amount of radiation exposure is minimal.
Scanning tests		
Ventilation-perfusion scan	To evaluate ventilation-perfusion mismatch, to detect pulmonary emboli, and to evaluate pulmonary function, particularly in preoperative patients with marginal reserves	• Explain procedure to patient. • Explain he will lie supine on a table and that a radioactive contrast dye will be injected into a vein. • Instruct him that he will lie prone, supine, and sitting while the camera takes pictures.
Thoracic computed tomography	To provide cross-sectional views of the chest by passing an X-ray beam	• Explain the procedure and that it takes $1\frac{1}{2}$ hours to perform. *(continued)*

Diagnostic tests for respiratory disorders *(continued)*

Test	Purpose	Nursing considerations
Scanning tests *(continued)*		
Thoracic computed tomography *(continued)*	from a computerized scanner through the body at different angles; to allow assessment of abnormalities, masses, lesions, and abnormal lung shadows	• If a contrast dye will be used, instruct the patient to fast for 4 hours before the test. • When the dye is injected into his vein, he may experience nausea, flushing, or warmth. • Tell him not to move during the test, but to relax and breathe normally. Movement may invalidate the results and require repeat testing.
Magnetic resonance imaging (MRI)	To help diagnose respiratory disorders by using a powerful magnet, radiowaves, and a computer to provide high-resolution, cross-sectional images of lung structures and to trace blood flow	• Instruct the patient to remove all jewelry. Emphasize that there must be no metal in the test room. • Tell the patient that he'll be asked to lie on a table that slides into an 8′ (2.5-m) tunnel. • Instruct him that he should breathe normally but not talk or move during the test. • Tell him that the machinery will be noisy. • Encourage him to relax.
Specimen analysis		
Sputum analysis	To diagnose respiratory disease, identify the cause of pulmonary infection, identify abnormal lung cells and help manage lung disease	• Obtain a sputum specimen through voluntary coughing, sputum induction, nasotracheal suctioning, or bronchoscopy. • Collect specimen early in the morning. • Instruct the patient not to eat, brush his teeth, or use mouthwash before expectorating to prevent specimen contamination. He may rinse his mouth with water. • Before sending the specimen to the laboratory, make sure it's sputum, not saliva.

Diagnostic tests for respiratory disorders *(continued)*

Test	Purpose	Nursing considerations
Specimen analysis *(continued)*		
Thoracentesis	To obtain a specimen of pleural fluid for analysis; to relieve lung compression; to obtain a lung tissue biopsy specimen	• Explain the procedure. • Tell the patient he'll be positioned either sitting with his arms on pillows or an overbed table, or lying partially on his side in bed. • The doctor will clean the insertion site and then inject a local anesthetic. • Warn him that he will feel pressure during the needle insertion and withdrawal. • Instruct him to remain still during the test and not to cough or breathe deeply. • Notify the doctor if the patient experiences dyspnea, palpitations, wheezing, dizziness, weakness, or diaphoresis. • Monitor vital signs after the test. • Monitor the needle insertion site for fluid or blood leakage. • Be sure a chest X-ray is obtained following the test.
Monitoring		
Mixed venous oxygen saturation ($S\bar{v}O_2$ monitoring)	To help to evaluate the body's ability to deliver oxygen to tissues, a patient's response to drug administration, endotracheal tube suctioning, ventilator setting changes, and positive end-expiratory pressure by using a fiber-optic, flow-directed	• Explain the procedure, including risks and outcomes. • Monitor vital signs and cardiac rhythm during catheter insertion. • After catheter placement, the patient's activity will be restricted. • Monitor for problems that can interfere with accurate testing, such as malfunctioning equipment, loose connections, clot formations at catheter tip, or balloon rupture.

(continued)

Diagnostic tests for respiratory disorders (continued)

Test	Purpose	Nursing considerations
Monitoring (continued)		
Mixed venous oxygen saturation (continued)	thermodilution pulmonary artery catheter	• Change sterile dressing and I.V. tubing according to facility policy. • Maintain an airtight system. • Closely monitor the patient's hemodynamic status. • Record initial $S\bar{v}o_2$ reading and calibrate the oximeter to ensure accurate values. • Document hourly $S\bar{v}o_2$ readings and attach selected strips to the chart, as ordered.
Pulse and ear oximetry	To track arterial oxygen saturation (Sao_2) levels noninvasively and continuously monitor pulse rate and amplitude, by using light to measure Sao_2	• The selected site requires no specific preparation. • Attach the ear transducer to the fleshy part of the ear lobe. • Attach a finger transducer to the index finger and keep finger at heart level. • Don't attach a transducer to an extremity that has a blood pressure cuff or arterial catheter in place. • Protect the transducer from strong light. • Examine the skin periodically for abrasion and circulatory impairment. • Rotate the transducer at least every 4 hours to avoid skin irritation.

• Arterial blood gas (ABG) levels remain normal.
• Patient achieves comfort without depressing respirations.
• Auscultation reveals no adventitious breath sounds.

• Patient states understanding of importance of taking deep breaths periodically.
• Patient states understanding of taking rest periods frequently.

Nursing interventions and rationales

- Auscultate for breath sounds at least every 4 hours *to detect decreased or adventitious breath sounds.*
- Assess adequacy of ventilation *to detect early signs of respiratory compromise.*
- Teach breathing techniques *to help the patient improve ventilation.*
- Administer bronchodilators *to help relieve bronchospasm.*
- Administer oxygen, as ordered, *to help relieve respiratory distress.*

Ineffective airway clearance

Related to the presence of tracheo-bronchial secretions or obstruction, this nursing diagnosis can be associated with such conditions as asthma, COPD, interstitial lung disease, cystic fibrosis, pneumonia, and other problems.

Expected outcomes

- Patient coughs effectively.
- Patient expectorates sputum.
- Patient drinks 3 to 4 qt (3 to 4 L) of fluid daily.
- Physical examination and laboratory studies indicate adequate ventilation.
- Patient maintains patent airway.

Nursing interventions and rationales

- Teach coughing techniques *to promote chest expansion and ventilation, enhance clearance of secretions from airways, and involve patient in his own health care.*
- Perform postural drainage, percussion, and vibration *to facilitate secretion movement.*
- Encourage fluids *to ensure adequate hydration and liquefy secretions.*
- Give expectorants and mucolytics, as ordered, *to enhance airway clearance.*
- Provide an artificial airway, as needed, *to maintain airway patency and provide an airway seal if mechanical ventilation is required.*

Impaired gas exchange

Related to altered oxygen supply or oxygen-carrying capacity of the blood, this nursing diagnosis can be associated with acute respiratory failure, COPD, pneumonia, pulmonary embolism, and other respiratory problems.

Expected outcomes

- Patient states understanding of how to perform deep breathing.
- Patient demonstrates correct use of incentive spirometer.
- Patient maintains adequate ventilation.

Nursing interventions and rationales

- Give antibiotics, as ordered and indicated, *to treat infection and improve alveolar expansion.*
- Teach deep breathing and incentive spirometry *to enhance lung expansion and ventilation.*
- Monitor arterial blood gas (ABG) levels and notify the doctor immediately if partial pressure of oxygen in arterial blood (PaO_2) drops or $PaCO_2$ rises. If needed, start mechan-

ical ventilation *to improve ventilation.*

• Provide continuous positive airway pressure (CPAP) or positive-end-expiratory pressure (PEEP), as needed, *to improve the driving pressure of oxygen across the alveolocapillary membrane and enhance arterial blood oxygenation.*

Risk for infection

Related to external factors, this nursing diagnosis can be applied to almost any hospitalized patient. However, elderly, debilitated, and postoperative patients are at greatest risk.

Expected outcomes

• Respiratory secretions are clear and odorless.
• Patient demonstrates an understanding of bronchial hygiene techniques.
• Patient takes the prescribed amount of fluid and protein daily.
• Temperature, white blood cell (WBC) count, and differential stay within normal range.

Nursing interventions and rationales

• Provide hydration to help liquefy mucus secretions.
• Teach bronchial hygiene techniques *to prevent infection.*
• Teach equipment cleaning techniques *to prevent spread of infection.*
• Monitor WBC count, as ordered, *to detect infection.*
• At first sign of infection, give antibiotics, as ordered, *to treat and control infection.*

• Teach the patient how to avoid infection and symptoms to report immediately *to control infection.*

Decreased cardiac output

Related to reduced stroke volume, this nursing diagnosis can be associated with acute respiratory failure, pulmonary edema, and pulmonary embolism.

Expected outcomes

• Patient demonstrates no signs of edema.
• Patient maintains adequate intake and output.
• Patient demonstrates an understanding of signs and symptoms to report to doctor as well as an understanding of medication regimen.
• Patient tolerates exercise and activities at his usual level.
• Patient does not experience any tachycardia, restlessness, dyspnea, fainting, fatigue, or weakness.

Nursing interventions and rationales

• Monitor and record level of consciousness, heart rate and rhythm, and blood pressure at least every 4 hours, or more often if necessary, *to detect indications of hypoperfusion.*
• Auscultate heart and breath sounds at least every 4 hours. Report abnormal sounds as soon as they develop. *S_3 heart sounds may indicate early cardiac failure; adventitious breath sounds may indicate pulmonary congestion.*
• Measure fluid intake and output accurately, and record. *Decreasing urine output without decreasing fluid intake may indicate decreased renal*

perfusion, possibly from decreased cardiac output.
• Weigh the patient daily before breakfast *to detect fluid retention.*
• Inspect for pedal or sacral edema *to detect venous stasis and indication of right-sided heart failure.*
• Plan the patient's activities allowing frequent rest periods *to avoid increased myocardial workload.*
• Teach the patient about chest pain and other reportable symptoms, prescribed diet, medications, prescribed activity level, and stress-reduction techniques. *These measures involve patient and family in care.*

Activity intolerance

Related to an imbalance between oxygen supply and demand, this nursing diagnosis can be associated with COPD, interstitial lung disease, pulmonary edema, pulmonary embolism, respiratory infections, respiratory failure, and neoplasms.

Expected outcomes
• Patient participates in exercise and activities to the extent possible.
• Patient modifies exercise to adjust to decreased activity tolerance.
• Patient's pulse, respirations, and blood pressure remain within established parameters during periods of rest.

Nursing interventions and rationales
• Teach energy conservation techniques *to reduce the body's oxygen demand and prevent fatigue.*
• Teach exercises for physical reconditioning *to gradually increase activity level.*

• Teach coordination of breathing and activity *to improve efficiency and reduce oxygen demand.*

Sleep pattern disturbance

Related to internal factors (such as illness or stress), this nursing diagnosis can be associated with COPD and other problems.

Expected outcomes
• Patient reports getting adequate rest.
• Patient establishes a bedtime routine including relaxation techniques.
• Patient identifies factors that interfere with achieving undisturbed sleep.

Nursing interventions and rationales
• Allow patient to discuss any concerns that may be preventing sleep. *Active listening helps in determining causes of difficulty with sleep.*
• Plan nursing care routines to allow uninterrupted sleep. *This allows consistent nursing care and gives the patient uninterrupted sleep time.*
• Provide patient with sleep aids, such as pillows, bath before sleep, food or drink, and reading materials. *Milk and some high-protein snacks, such as cheese and nuts, contain tryptophan, a sleep promoter. Personal hygiene routine precedes sleep in many patients.*
• Create a quiet environment conducive to sleep; for example, close the curtains, adjust the lighting, and close the door. *These measures promote rest and sleep.*

• Administer medications that promote normal sleep patterns, as ordered. Monitor and record effectiveness and adverse reactions. *A hypnotic agent induces sleep; a tranquilizer reduces anxiety.*

• Promote involvement in diversional activities or an exercise program during the day. Discourage excessive napping. *Activity and exercise promote sleep by increasing fatigue and relaxation.*

• Ask the patient to describe in specific terms each morning the quality of sleep during the previous night. *This helps detect sleep-related behavioral problems.*

DISORDERS

Respiratory disorders include acute and chronic conditions.

Acute disorders

Acute respiratory disorders range from acute respiratory failure and adult respiratory distress syndrome (ARDS) to infectious disorders, such as pneumonia and lung abscess.

Acute respiratory failure

Acute respiratory failure occurs when the lungs no longer meet the body's metabolic needs. This disorder isn't easily defined because it has many causes and variable clinical presentation. ABG levels usually provide clues. For most patients, a PaO_2 of 50 mm Hg or less or a $PaCO_2$ of 50 mm Hg or above indicates acute respiratory failure. However, patients with COPD have a chronically low PaO_2 and high $PaCO_2$. Therefore, a PaO_2 that doesn't increase despite an increased fraction of inspired oxygen (FIO_2) or an increased $PaCO_2$ that results in a pH of less than 7.30 suggests acute respiratory failure. A pH of less than 7.25 is also significant because medications and enzymes don't function well in acidemia.

Causes. Acute respiratory failure may develop in patients from any condition that increases the work of breathing and decreases the respiratory drive. Such conditions include respiratory tract infection (such as bronchitis or pneumonia) — the most common precipitating factor — bronchospasm, or accumulating secretions secondary to cough suppression. Other causes of acute respiratory failure include head trauma or misuse of sedatives, narcotics, tranquilizers, or oxygen; myocardial infarction (MI), heart failure, or pulmonary emboli; airway irritants such as smoke or fumes; myxedema or metabolic alkalosis; and chest trauma, pneumothorax, or thoracic or abdominal surgery.

Assessment findings. In patients with acute respiratory failure, the resulting hypoxemia and acidemia affect all body organs, especially the central nervous, respiratory, and cardiovascular systems. Perform a thorough assessment because specific symptoms vary with the underlying cause. However, you should always assess for:

• altered respirations. Rate may be increased, decreased, or normal; respirations may be shallow, deep, or alternate between the two. Cyanosis may or may not be present. Auscultation of the chest may reveal crackles, rhonchi, wheezes, or diminished breath sounds.

• altered mentation. The patient shows evidence of restlessness, confusion, loss of concentration, irritability, tremulousness, diminished tendon reflexes, and papilledema.

• cardiac arrhythmias. Tachycardia, with increased cardiac output and mildly elevated blood pressure secondary to adrenal release of catecholamine, occurs early in response to low PaO_2. With myocardial hypoxia, arrhythmias may develop. Pulmonary hypertension also occurs.

Diagnostic tests. Progressive deterioration in ABG levels and pH, when compared with the patient's baseline values, strongly suggests acute respiratory failure. (In patients with essentially normal lung tissue, a pH below 7.35 usually indicates acute respiratory failure, but COPD patients display an even greater deviation from this normal value, as they do with $PaCO_2$ and PaO_2.) Other supporting findings include:

• Bicarbonate (HCO_3^-) level — increased level indicates metabolic alkalosis or reflects metabolic compensation for chronic respiratory acidosis.

• Serum electrolyte levels — hypokalemia may result from compensatory hyperventilation — an attempt to correct acidosis; hypochloremia commonly occurs in metabolic alkalosis.

• WBC count — count is elevated if acute respiratory failure results from bacterial infection; Gram stain and sputum culture can identify pathogens.

• Chest X-ray — findings identify pulmonary abnormalities, such as emphysema, atelectasis, lesions, pneumothorax, infiltrates, or effusions.

• Electrocardiogram (ECG) — arrhythmias commonly suggest cor pulmonale and myocardial hypoxia.

Treatment. In COPD patients, acute respiratory failure is an emergency that requires cautious oxygen therapy (using nasal prongs or Venturi mask) to raise the patient's arterial oxygen saturation (SaO_2) to approximately 90%. (See *COPD*, pages 70 to 73.) If significant respiratory acidosis persists, mechanical ventilation through an endotracheal or a tracheostomy tube may be necessary. Treatment routinely includes antibiotics for infection, bronchodilators, and bronchial hygiene measures.

Nursing interventions. To reverse hypoxemia, administer oxygen at appropriate concentrations to maintain SaO_2 at approximately 90%. Patients with COPD usually require only small amounts of supplemental oxygen. Watch for a positive response, such as improvement in the patient's breathing, color, and ABG results.

• Maintain a patent airway. If the patient is intubated and lethargic, turn him every 1 to 2 hours. Use postural drainage and chest physiotherapy to help clear secretions.

• In an intubated patient, suction

(Text continues on page 72.)

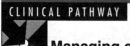

Managing chronic obstructive pulmonary disease

Diagnosis: COPD
Initiation:
Date:

DRG # 519.80
Average length of stay (LOS): 5 days
Actual LOS:

	DAY 1 Emergency care service (ECS)	DAY 1 Admission (Nursing Unit)

Medical interventions	• Brief history and physical (H & P)
	• Standing medications:
	  Bronchodilators
	  Antibiotics
	  Corticosteroids
	  Diuretics
	• Airway maintenance
	• Oxygen supplement (O_2 supp.)
	• Smoking restriction
		• H & P
		• Standing medications:
		  Bronchodilators
		  Antibiotics
		  Corticosteroids
		  Diuretics

Nursing interventions	• Brief data base • Auscultate lungs every 1 to 2 hr • Administer ordered O_2 • Vital signs (VS) every 15 min × 2, every 30 min × 2, every 1 to 2 hr, and as needed (p.r.n.) • Suction p.r.n. • Assess & help maintain airway	• Admission data base • VS and respiratory assessment every 8 hr • Intake and output (I&O) every 8 hr • Daily weight • Head of bed (HOB) up 45 degrees
Social work	• Consults	• Assessment of baseline home/community support system
Nutrition	• Nothing by mouth (NPO) • I.V. fluids	• Fluid restriction if needed • Diet advanced as tolerated
Tests	• Arterial blood gas (ABG) studies • Complete blood count (CBC), sequential multiple analyzer chemistry test (SMAC), coagulation studies • Chest X-ray (CXR), electrocardiogram (ECG) • Sputum analysis	• CXR, electrolytes, and ECG as needed • Pulmonary function tests (PFTs) if needed

Consults	• Respiratory
	  Nebulizer, treatments
	  Chest physiotherapy (PT)
		• Respiratory treatments
		• Chest PT

Activity	• Bedrest	• Out of bed (OOB) to chair
Patient education	• Explain purpose/importance of smoking cessation and smoke-free facility. • Explain emergency care service	• Continue previous teaching. • Review disease process and home care management with patient.

DAY 2-3	DAY 4	DAY 5
• Daily assessment • Review of standing meds • Regulation of O_2 supp.	• Daily assessment • Review of standing meds • Review of need for O_2 supp.	• Continued • Discharge instructions: Medications to pt Follow-up appts. given Activity & diet orders
• Respiratory assessment (according to pt's acuity) • I & O every 8 hr • Daily weight • Maintain elevated HOB • Provide bedside commode (BSC)	• Respiratory assessment every 24 hr and as needed according to acuity • VS and I & O every 8 hrs • Weight as ordered	• Continued • Discharge note: VS, patient status at discharge, teaching given, mode of transportation and destination, and follow-up with appts. given
• Continued	• Continued conference with patient and significant other	• Continued
• Diet continued	• Diet maintained as tolerated.	• Diet maintained as tolerated.
• Electrolytes, CBC, and ABGs as ordered	• CXR, electrolytes, and ECG as ordered and needed	
• Respiratory treatments	• Continued	
• OOB to chair	• Activity as tolerated	• Activity as tolerated • Rest encouraged as needed
• Discuss home health support system, health maintenance, medication routine, and follow-up appointment.	• Review prior teaching. • Explain importance of activity and rest, including planned rests, rest before	• Continued. *(continued)*

Managing chronic obstructive pulmonary disease *(continued)*

	DAY 1 (ECS)	DAY 1 Admission (Nursing Unit)
Patient education *(continued)*	(ECS) care and intervention. • Explain admission procedure. • Identify pertinent signs and symptoms.	• Explain importance of maintaining optimal respiratory function by taking medications, not smoking, and staying in smoke-free environment.
Discharge planning	• Initiate home health support system, home maintenance, medication routine, and follow-up appointment with primary care and smoking cessation clinics.	• Continue previous teaching. • Review disease process and home care management. • Explain importance of maintaining optimal respiratory function by taking meds, not smoking, and staying in smoke-free environment.
Key patient outcomes	• Demonstrates improved breath sounds and decreased respiratory effort and rate	

Adapted with permission from Veterans Affairs Maryland Health Care System, Baltimore.

the trachea, as required, after hyperoxygenation and hyperinflation. Observe for changes in quantity, consistency, and color of sputum. Provide humidification.
• Observe the patient closely for respiratory arrest. Auscultate for breath sounds. Monitor ABG levels, and report any changes immediately.
• Monitor and record serum electrolyte levels carefully, and correct imbalances. Record fluid intake and output or daily weights.

• Check the cardiac monitor for arrhythmias.

If the patient requires mechanical ventilation, take the following steps:
• Check ventilator settings, cuff pressures, and ABG values often because the FIO_2 setting depends on ABG values. Draw specimens for ABG analysis 20 to 30 minutes after every FIO_2 change.
• Prevent infection by using sterile technique while suctioning and by changing ventilator circuits every 48 to 72 hours or according to policy.

DAY 2-3	DAY 4	DAY 5
• Assess need for home nursing care and home O_2; arrange for consult if needed.	and after meals, limited activity on days with high air pollution, and slow deep breaths with activity.	
• Continued.	• Initiate ambulatory care teaching appointment.	• Discharge to home with significant other
• Patient verbalizes understanding of disease process and home care management by verbalizing signs and symptoms, need for regular follow-up, lifestyle changes, and need for home O_2 or nursing if needed.	• Patient demonstrates increased activity as evidenced by increased ability to perform activities of daily living (ADLs).	• Patient can identify activity, medication, diet, and follow-up care upon discharge. • Patient can demonstrate understanding of disease process and home management. • Lung sounds are clearer, returned to baseline. • Patient can demonstrate increasing ADLs. • Follow-up appointment with primary clinic arranged and patient and family can repeat appointment time.

• Check gastric secretions for evidence of bleeding if the patient has a nasogastric (NG) tube or complains of epigastric tenderness, nausea, or vomiting. Monitor hemoglobin levels and hematocrit, and check all stools for occult blood. Administer antacids or histamine$_2$-receptor antagonists, as ordered.

• Prevent tracheal erosion that can result from artificial airway cuff overinflation. Use minimal leak technique and a cuffed tube with high residual volume (low-pressure cuff), a foam cuff, or a pressure-regulating valve on the cuff.

• Keep the nasotracheal tube midline within the nostril, and provide good oral and nasal hygiene. Change the tape periodically to prevent skin breakdown. Avoid excessive movement of any tubes, and make sure the ventilator tubing is adequately supported.

Patient education. If the patient is not on mechanical ventilation and is retaining carbon dioxide, encourage him to breathe deeply with pursed lips. If the patient is alert, teach him how to use an incentive spirometer. Encourage the patient to cough if rhonchi are audible during auscultation.

Evaluation. The patient's ABG values are normal, with a PaO_2 greater than 50 mm Hg. The patient can make a normal respiratory effort.

Adult respiratory distress syndrome

A form of pulmonary edema that causes acute respiratory failure, ARDS results from increased permeability of the alveolocapillary membrane. Fluid accumulates in the lung interstitium, alveolar spaces, and small airways, causing the lung to stiffen. Effective ventilation is thus impaired.

Causes. ARDS may result from aspiration of gastric contents, sepsis (primarily gram-negative), trauma, oxygen toxicity, pneumonia, microemboli, drug overdose, blood transfusion, smoke or chemical inhalation, hydrocarbon or paraquat ingestion, pancreatitis, uremia, miliary tuberculosis (rare), or near drowning.

Assessment findings. Assess your patient for rapid, shallow breathing. Also look for dyspnea, tachycardia, hypoxemia, intercostal and suprasternal retractions, crackles and rhonchi, restlessness, apprehension, mental sluggishness, and motor dysfunction.

Diagnostic tests. Initially, ABG values on room air show decreased PaO_2 (less than 60 mm Hg) and $PaCO_2$ (less than 35 mm Hg). As ARDS becomes more severe, ABG values show respiratory acidosis (increasing $PaCO_2$ [more than 45 mm Hg]) and metabolic acidosis (decreasing HCO_3^- [less than 22 mEq/L]) and a decreasing PaO_2 despite oxygen therapy.

Pulmonary artery (PA) catheterization helps identify the cause of pulmonary edema by evaluating pulmonary artery wedge pressure (PAWP); allows collection of PA blood, which shows decreased mixed venous oxygen saturation, reflecting tissue hypoxia; measures PA pressure; and measures cardiac output by thermodilution techniques.

Serial chest X-rays initially show bilateral infiltrates; in later stages, ground-glass appearance and, eventually, "whiteouts" of both lung fields.

Treatment. When possible, treatment aims to correct the underlying cause of ARDS. Supportive medical care includes administering humidified oxygen by a tight-fitting mask, which allows for use of CPAP. Hypoxemia that responds poorly to these measures requires ventilatory support with intubation, mechanical ventilation, and PEEP. Other supportive measures include fluid restriction, diuretics, and correction of electrolyte and acid-base abnormalities.

When ARDS requires mechanical ventilation, sedatives, narcotics, neuromuscular blocking agents — such as tubocurarine or pancuronium — may be ordered to minimize restlessness and to facilitate ventilation. When ARDS results from fat emboli or chemical injuries to the lungs, a short course of high-dose steroids may help if given early. Use of fluids and vasopressors may be required to maintain blood pressure. Nonviral infections require antimicrobial drugs.

Nursing interventions. ARDS requires careful monitoring and supportive care.

• Frequently assess the patient's respiratory status. Be alert for retractions on inspiration. Note rate, rhythm, and depth of respirations, and watch for dyspnea and the use of accessory muscles of respiration. On auscultation, listen for adventitious or diminished breath sounds. Clear, frothy sputum may indicate pulmonary edema.

• Observe and document the hypoxemic patient's neurologic status.

• Maintain a patent airway with artificial airways and by suctioning, using sterile, nontraumatic technique — only as often as required.

• Closely monitor heart rate and rhythm, and blood pressure. With PA catheterization, know the desired PAWP level, and check readings often.

• Monitor serum electrolyte levels, and correct imbalances. Measure fluid intake and output and weigh the patient daily.

• Check ventilator settings frequently, and empty condensation from tubing promptly. Monitor ABG studies. Give sedatives, as needed, to reduce restlessness. If PEEP is used, check for hypotension, tachycardia, and decreased urine output. Use closed tracheal suction system so that PEEP is maintained. Reposition the patient often and record any increase in secretions, temperature, or hypotension that may indicate a deteriorating condition.

Patient education. Provide emotional support. Warn the patient who is recovering from ARDS that recovery will take some time and that he will feel weak for a while.

Evaluation. The patient has normal ABG values and a normal respiratory rate, depth, and pattern. Breath sounds are clear.

Atelectasis

In atelectasis, incomplete expansion of lobules (clusters of alveoli) or lung segments may result in partial or complete loss of lung expansion. The collapsed lobules, unable to perform gas exchange, allow unoxygenated blood to pass through the lung unchanged, thereby producing hypoxemia. Atelectasis may be chronic or acute. It occurs to some degree in many patients undergoing abdominal or thoracic surgery.

Causes. Atelectasis may result from bronchial occlusion by mucus plugs (a common problem in persons with COPD), bronchiectasis, cystic fibrosis, heavy smoking, occlusion by foreign bodies, bronchogenic carcinoma, inflammatory lung disease, or idiopathic respiratory distress syndrome of the newborn (hyaline membrane disease). Other causes include oxygen toxicity, pulmonary edema, any condition that inhibits full lung expansion or makes deep breathing painful, prolonged immobility, mechanical ventilation using constant small tidal volumes without intermittent deep breaths, and CNS depression, which eliminates periodic sighing.

Assessment findings. Your assessment findings will vary with the cause and degree of hypoxia and may include dyspnea (mild, subsiding without treatment if atelectasis involves only a small area of the lung; severe if massive collapse occurs), anxiety, cyanosis, diaphoresis, decreased breath sounds, dull sound on percussion if a large portion of the lung is collapsed, hypoxemia, and tachycardia. You may also find substernal or intercostal retraction, compensatory hyperinflation of unaffected areas of the lung, mediastinal shift to the affected side, and elevation of the ipsilateral hemidiaphragm.

Diagnostic tests. Chest X-ray shows characteristic horizontal lines in the lower lung zones and, with segmental or lobar collapse, characteristic dense shadows commonly associated with hyperinflation of neighboring lung zones in widespread atelectasis. However, extensive areas of "microatelectasis" may exist without abnormalities on chest X-ray.

Bronchoscopy may be included in diagnostic procedures to rule out an obstructing neoplasm or a foreign body if the cause is unknown.

Treatment. This disorder is treated with incentive spirometry and deep-breathing exercises. Encourage the patient to cough if rhonchi are audi-

ble. Postural drainage and percussion may be necessary. If these measures fail, bronchoscopy may help remove secretions. Humidity and bronchodilators (sometimes with a nebulizer) can improve mucociliary clearance and dilate airways.

Atelectasis secondary to an obstructing neoplasm may require surgery or radiation therapy.

Nursing interventions. Your goal is to keep the patient's airways clear and relieve hypoxia.
• To prevent atelectasis, encourage a high-risk patient to deep-breathe every 1 to 2 hours. Encourage coughing if rhonchi are audible. Have the patient splint his incision when coughing. *Gently* reposition a postoperative patient often, and help him walk as soon as possible. Give analgesics to control pain.
• During mechanical ventilation, tidal volume is usually maintained at 10 to 15 ml/kg of the patient's body weight. Use the sigh mechanism on the ventilator, if smaller tidal volume is used to intermittently increase tidal volume at the rate of three to four sighs per hour.
• Use an incentive spirometer to encourage deep inspiration through positive reinforcement.
• Humidify inspired air and encourage adequate fluid intake to mobilize secretions. Also, use postural drainage and chest percussion.
• If the patient is intubated or uncooperative, provide suctioning, as indicated. Use sedatives with discretion, but remember that the patient won't cooperate with treatment if he's in pain.

• Assess breath sounds and ventilatory status frequently and report any changes immediately.

Patient education. Provide reassurance because the patient will undoubtedly be frightened by his limited breathing capacity.

Teach the patient how to use the spirometer, and encourage him to use it every 1 to 2 hours. Explain how to deep-breathe and cough.

Encourage the patient to stop smoking, to lose weight, or both, as needed. Refer him to appropriate support groups for help.

Evaluation. The patient's secretions are clear, and he shows no symptoms of hypoxia.

Lung abscess

Lung abscess is accompanied by pus accumulation and tissue destruction. It often has a well-defined border. Lung abscess is a manifestation of necrotizing pneumonia, which commonly results from aspiration of oropharyngeal contents. Poor oral hygiene with dental or gingival (gum) disease is strongly associated with putrid lung abscess.

Causes. Anaerobic or aerobic bacteria can cause lung abscess.

Assessment findings. Assess your patient for cough (may produce bloody, purulent, or foul-smelling sputum), pleuritic chest pain, dyspnea, excessive sweating, chills, fever, headache, malaise, diaphoresis, weight loss, crackles, and diminished breath sounds.

Diagnostic tests. Chest X-ray shows a localized infiltrate. Percutaneous aspiration of an abscess may be attempted or bronchoscopy may be used to obtain cultures to identify the causative organism. Bronchoscopy is used only if abscess resolution occurs and the patient's condition permits it.

Blood cultures, Gram stain, and culture of sputum are also used to detect the causative organism. Leukocytosis (WBC count greater than 10,000/mm³) is commonly present.

Treatment. Prolonged antibiotic therapy, often lasting for months, is required. Oxygen therapy may relieve hypoxemia. Poor therapeutic response requires surgical treatment. All patients need rigorous follow-up and serial chest X-rays.

Nursing interventions. Care emphasizes performing chest physiotherapy, increasing fluid intake to loosen secretions, and providing a quiet, restful atmosphere.

Provide good mouth care and encourage the patient to practice good oral hygiene. Monitor the patient for complications such as rupture into the pleural space.

Evaluation. Secretions are thin, and breath sounds are clear bilaterally.

Pleural effusion

Transudative or exudative pleural effusion results from an excess of fluid in the pleural space.

Causes. *Transudative pleural effusion* can stem from heart failure, hepatic disease with ascites, peritoneal dialysis, hypoalbuminemia, and disorders resulting in overexpanded intravascular volume.

Exudative pleural effusion can stem from tuberculosis, subphrenic abscess, esophageal rupture, pancreatitis, and bacterial or fungal pneumonitis or empyema. Other causes include cancer, pulmonary embolism with or without infarction, collagen disorders (lupus erythematosus and rheumatoid arthritis), myxedema, and chest trauma.

Assessment findings. Assess your patient for dyspnea, pleural friction rub, possible pleuritic pain that worsens with coughing or deep breathing, dry cough, flatness on percussion, tachycardia, tachypnea, and decreased chest motion and breath sounds.

Diagnostic tests. Thoracentesis shows the following:
• In transudative effusions, specific gravity is usually less than 1.015 and protein less than 3 g/dl.
• In exudative effusions, the ratio of protein in pleural fluid to serum is equal to or greater than 0.5, pleural fluid lactate dehydrogenase (LD) is equal to or greater than 200 IU, and the ratio of LD in pleural fluid to LD in serum is equal to or greater than 0.6.
• If a pleural effusion results from esophageal rupture or pancreatitis, amylase levels in aspirated fluid are usually higher than serum levels.
• In empyema, cell analysis shows leukocytosis.
• Aspirated fluid also may be tested for lupus erythematosus cells, antinuclear antibodies, and neoplastic cells. It may be analyzed for color and consistency; acid-fast bacillus, fungal, and bacterial cultures; and triglycerides (in chylothorax).

Chest X-ray shows radiopaque fluid in dependent regions. Pleural biopsy may be useful for confirming tuberculosis or cancer.

Treatment. Symptomatic effusion may require either thoracentesis to remove fluid or careful monitoring of the patient's own reabsorption of the fluid. Hemothorax requires drainage to prevent fibrothorax formation. Hypoxemia requires oxygen administration.

Nursing interventions. Administer oxygen, as ordered. Provide meticulous chest tube care, and use aseptic technique for changing dressings around the tube insertion site in empyema. Record the amount, color, and consistency of any tube drainage.

If the patient has open drainage through a rib resection or an intercostal tube, use standard precautions.

If pleural effusion was a complication of pneumonia or influenza, advise prompt medical attention for chest colds.

Patient education. Explain thoracentesis to the patient. Reassure him during the procedure, and observe for complications during and after the procedure. (See *Calming the dyspneic patient.*)

Encourage the patient to do deep-breathing exercises to promote lung expansion. Teach him to use an incentive spirometer.

Evaluation. The patient has minimal chest discomfort, is afebrile, and has a normal respiratory pattern.

Pleurisy

An inflammation of the visceral and parietal pleurae that line the inside of the thoracic cage and envelop the lungs, pleurisy usually begins suddenly.

Causes. Pleurisy develops as a complication of pneumonia, tuberculosis, viruses, systemic lupus erythematosus, rheumatoid arthritis, uremia, Dressler's syndrome, cancer, pulmonary infarction, or chest trauma.

Assessment findings. Assess your patient for sharp, stabbing pain that increases with respiration and dyspnea. Auscultation reveals a characteristic pleural friction rub — a coarse, creaky sound heard directly over the area of pleural inflammation. Palpation over the affected area may reveal coarse vibration.

Other symptoms vary according to the underlying disease process.

Treatment. Treatment of pleurisy includes anti-inflammatory agents, analgesics, and bed rest. Severe pain may require intercostal nerve block. Pleurisy with pleural effusion calls for thoracentesis.

Nursing interventions. Stress the importance of bed rest. Plan your care to allow uninterrupted rest.

Administer antitussives and pain medication, as ordered, but don't overmedicate. Warn the patient about to be discharged that overuse

FOCUS ON CARING

Calming the dyspneic patient

When a patient is dyspneic, he may hypoventilate as he takes rapid but shallow breaths. You can help calm him by using slow, clearly enunciated speech.

Try breathing with him and then gradually slowing your breaths, to help slow him down with you.

Using imagery may also help. Ask him to close his eyes and envision a pleasant place where he was relaxed — perhaps at the mountains, the ocean, or a lake. (Images of water commonly have a relaxing effect.) Verbally describe the imaginary scene to help him relax.

of narcotic analgesics depresses coughing and respiration.

Encourage the patient to cough if rhonchi are audible. Apply firm pressure at the site of the pain during coughing exercises.

Evaluation. The patient has minimal chest discomfort, and his secretions are thin and white.

Pneumonia

Pneumonia is an acute infection of the lung parenchyma that often impairs gas exchange.

Causes. Primary pneumonia results from the inhalation or aspiration of a viral, bacterial, fungal, protozoal, mycobacterial, mycoplasmatic, or rickettsial pathogen. Pneumonias caused by cytomegaloviruses and the protozoan *Pneumocystis carinii* are more common in patients with acquired immunodeficiency syndrome.

Secondary pneumonia may follow initial lung damage from a noxious chemical or other insult (superinfection) or may result from hematogenous spread of bacteria from a distant focus. (See *Understanding types of pneumonia,* pages 82 to 85.)

Assessment findings. Assess your patient for the five cardinal signs or symptoms of early bacterial pneumonia: coughing, sputum production, pleuritic chest pain, shaking chills, and fever.

Physical signs vary widely, ranging from diffuse, fine crackles to signs of localized or extensive consolidation and pleural effusion.

Diagnostic tests. Chest X-rays showing infiltrates and a sputum smear demonstrating acute inflammatory cells support the diagnosis.

Positive blood cultures in patients with pulmonary infiltrates strongly suggest pneumonia produced by the organisms isolated from the blood cultures. Occasionally, a transtracheal aspirate of tracheobronchial secretions or bronchoscopy with brushings may be done to obtain material for smear and culture.

Early *P. carinii* pneumonia can be detected only by ventilation-perfusion scans.

Treatment. Antimicrobial therapy varies with the infecting agent. Therapy should be reevaluated early in the course of treatment. Support-

ive measures include humidified oxygen therapy for hypoxemia, mechanical ventilation for respiratory failure, a high-calorie diet and adequate fluid intake, bed rest, and an analgesic. Patients with severe pneumonia who are mechanically ventilated may require PEEP.

Nursing interventions. Maintain a patent airway and adequate oxygenation. Measure ABG levels, especially in hypoxic patients. Administer supplemental oxygen as ordered. (Usually, oxygen is administered if SaO_2 is less than 90%.) Patients with underlying chronic lung disease should be given oxygen cautiously to maintain SaO_2 of approximately 90%.

• In severe pneumonia that requires endotracheal intubation or tracheostomy with or without mechanical ventilation, maintain bronchial hygiene. Suction as needed to remove secretions using sterile technique.

• Give antibiotics, as ordered, and pain medication, as needed. Fever and dehydration may require I.V. fluids and electrolyte replacement.

• Maintain adequate nutrition. Ask the dietary department to provide a high-calorie, high-protein diet consisting of soft, easy-to-eat foods. As necessary, supplement oral feedings with enteral nutrition. Monitor fluid intake and output.

• Provide a quiet environment for the patient, with frequent rest periods.

• Dispose of secretions properly. Tell the patient to sneeze and cough into a disposable tissue; tape a waxed bag to the side of the bed for tissues.

• To prevent aspiration during NG tube feedings, elevate the patient's head, check the position of the tube, and administer feedings slowly. Avoid giving large volumes at one time to prevent vomiting. If the patient has a tracheostomy or an endotracheal tube, inflate the tube cuff. Keep his head elevated for at least 30 minutes after feeding.

Patient education. Explain all procedures (especially intubation and suctioning) to the patient and his family.

Teach the patient how to cough and perform deep-breathing exercises, and encourage him to do so often. Position patients properly to promote full aeration and drainage of secretions.

Evaluation. Chest X-rays are normal, and the patient's ABG levels show SaO_2 greater than 90%.

Pneumothorax

In pneumothorax, air or gas accumulates between the parietal and visceral pleurae. The amount of air or gas trapped in this intrapleural space determines the degree of lung collapse. In tension pneumothorax, air in the pleural space is under higher pressure than air in adjacent lung and vascular structures. Without prompt treatment, tension or large-volume pneumothorax results in fatal pulmonary and circulatory impairment.

Causes. *Spontaneous pneumothorax* can result from ruptured congenital blebs, ruptured emphysematous bullae, tubercular or malignant lesions that erode into the pleural space, and interstitial lung disease.

Traumatic pneumothorax can result from insertion of a central venous pressure line, thoracic surgery, bronchoscopy, penetrating chest injury, transbronchial biopsy, and thoracentesis or closed pleural biopsy.

Tension pneumothorax can result from positive pleural pressure, which develops from traumatic pneumothorax.

Assessment findings. Spontaneous pneumothorax may be asymptomatic or cause profound respiratory distress. Weak and rapid pulse, pallor, neck vein distention, and anxiety indicate tension pneumothorax. Look for sudden, sharp, pleuritic pain; asymmetrical chest wall movement; shortness of breath; cyanosis; decreased or absent breath sounds over the collapsed lung; hyperresonance on the affected side; and crackling beneath the skin on palpation (subcutaneous emphysema).

Diagnostic tests. Chest X-rays showing air in the pleural space and possibly mediastinal shift confirm the diagnosis. ABG findings include pH less than 7.35, PaO_2 less than 80 mm Hg, and $PaCO_2$ above 45 mm Hg, if the pneumothorax is significant.

Treatment. Treatment is conservative for spontaneous pneumothorax in which no signs of increased pleural pressure (indicating tension pneumothorax) appear, and the patient shows no signs of dyspnea or other indications of physiologic compromise. Such treatment consists of bed *(Text continues on page 86.)*

Understanding types of pneumonia

Type	Signs and symptoms
Viral	
Influenza (prognosis poor even with treatment; 50% mortality)	• Cough (initially nonproductive; later, producing purulent sputum), marked cyanosis, dyspnea, high fever, chills, substernal pain and discomfort, moist crackles, frontal headache, myalgia • Death from cardiopulmonary shock
Adenovirus (insidious onset; usually affects young adults)	• Sore throat, fever, cough, chills, malaise, small amounts of mucoid sputum, retrosternal chest pain, anorexia, rhinitis, adenopathy, scattered crackles, rhonchi
Respiratory syncytial virus (most prevalent in infants and children)	• Listlessness; irritability; tachypnea with retraction of intercostal muscles; slight sputum production; fine, moist crackles; fever; severe malaise; and, possibly, cough or croup
Measles (rubeola)	• Fever, dyspnea, cough, small amounts of sputum, coryza, rash, and cervical adenopathy
Chickenpox (varicella) (uncommon in children, but pneumonia is present in 30% of adults with varicella)	• Cough, dyspnea, cyanosis, tachypnea, pleuritic chest pain, hemoptysis and rhonchi 1 to 6 days after onset of rash
Cytomegalovirus (common complication of acquired immunodeficiency syndrome)	• Difficult to distinguish from other nonbacterial pneumonias • Fever, cough, shaking chills, dyspnea, cyanosis, weakness, and diffuse crackles • Occurs in neonates as devastating multisystemic infection; resembles mononucleosis in normal adults; varies in immunocompromised hosts from clinically inapparent to devastating infection

Diagnosis	Treatment
• *Chest X-ray:* diffuse bilateral bronchopneumonia radiating from hilus • *White blood cell (WBC) count:* normal to slightly elevated • *Sputum smears:* no specific organisms	• *Supportive:* for respiratory failure, endotracheal intubation and ventilator assistance; for fever, hypothermia blanket or antipyretics; for influenza A, amantadine
• *Chest X-ray:* patchy distribution of pneumonia, more severe than indicated by physical examination • *WBC count:* normal to slightly elevated	• Treatment aimed at symptoms only. • Mortality low; usually clears with no residual effects
• *Chest X-ray:* patchy bilateral consolidation • *WBC count:* normal to slightly elevated	• *Supportive:* humidified air, oxygen, antimicrobials commonly given until viral etiology confirmed
• *Chest X-ray:* reticular infiltrates, sometimes with hilar lymph node enlargement • *Lung tissue specimen:* characteristic giant cells	• *Supportive:* bed rest, adequate hydration, antimicrobials, assisted ventilation if necessary
• *Chest X-ray:* more extensive pneumonia than indicated by physical examination and bilateral, patchy, diffuse, nodular infiltrates • *Sputum analysis:* predominant mononuclear cells and characteristic intranuclear inclusion bodies, with characteristic rash	• *Supportive:* adequate hydration, oxygen therapy in critically ill patients
• *Chest X-ray:* in early stages, variable patchy infiltrates; later, bilateral, nodular, and more predominant in lower lobes • *Percutaneous aspiration of lung tissue, transbronchial biopsy or open lung biopsy:* microscopic examination shows typical intranuclear and cytoplasmic inclusions; virus can be cultured from lung tissue • Usually benign and self-limiting in mononucleosis-like form	• *Supportive:* adequate hydration and nutrition, oxygen therapy, bed rest • More severe and possibly fatal in immunosuppressed patients *(continued)*

Understanding types of pneumonia *(continued)*

Type	Signs and symptoms
Bacterial	
Streptococcus *(Diplococcus pneumoniae)*	• Sudden onset of a single, shaking chill and sustained temperature of 102° to 104° (38.9° to 40° C); often preceded by upper respiratory tract infection
Klebsiella	• Fever and recurrent chills; cough producing rusty, bloody, viscous sputum (currant jelly); cyanosis of lips and nail beds due to hypoxemia; shallow, grunting respirations • Likely in patients with chronic alcoholism, pulmonary disease, and diabetes
Staphylococcus	• Temperature of 102° to 104° F (38.9° to 40° C), recurrent shaking chills, bloody sputum, dyspnea, tachypnea, and hypoxemia • Should be suspected with viral illness, such as influenza or measles, and in patients with cystic fibrosis
Protozoan	
Pneumocystis carinii (PCP)	• History of immunocompromising conditions, such as human immunodeficiency virus infection, leukemia, or lymphoma • Begins insidiously, increasing shortness of breath, nonproductive cough, anorexia, generalized fatigue and weight loss, low-grade intermittent fever • Tachypnea, dyspnea, crackles, decreased breath sounds, cyanosis
Aspiration	
Results from vomiting and aspiration of gastric or oropharyngeal contents into trachea and lungs	• Noncardiogenic pulmonary edema may follow damage to respiratory epithelium from contact with stomach acid. • Crackles, dyspnea, cyanosis, hypotension, and tachycardia • May be subacute pneumonia with cavity formation, or lung abscess may occur if foreign body is present

Diagnosis	Treatment
• *Chest X-ray:* areas of consolidation, often lobar • *WBC count:* elevated • *Sputum culture:* may show gram-positive *Streptococcus pneumoniae;* this organism not always recovered	• *Antimicrobial therapy:* penicillin G (or erythromycin, if patient is allergic to penicillin) for 7 to 10 days to begin after obtaining culture specimen but without waiting for results
• *Chest X-ray:* typically, but not always, consolidation in the upper lobe that causes bulging of fissures • *WBC count:* elevated • *Sputum culture and Gram stain:* may show gram-negative cocci, *Klebsiella*	• *Antimicrobial therapy:* aminoglycoside and, in serious infections, a cephalosporin
• *Chest X-ray:* multiple abscesses and infiltrates; high incidence of empyema • *WBC count:* elevated • *Sputum culture and Gram stain:* may show gram-positive staphylococci	• *Antimicrobial therapy:* nafcillin or oxacillin for 14 days if staphylococci produce penicillinase • Chest tube drainage of empyema
• *Histologic studies:* confirm the diagnosis • *Bronchoscopy:* confirms PCP • *Chest X-ray:* slowly progressing fluffy infiltrates, nodular lesions, or spontaneous pneumothorax • *Gallium scan:* increased uptake over the lungs	• *Supportive:* oxygen therapy, mechanical ventilation, adequate hydration and nutrition • *Antimicrobial therapy:* co-trimoxazole or pentamidine isethionate
• *Chest X-ray:* locates areas of infiltrates, which suggest diagnosis	• *Supportive:* oxygen therapy, suctioning, coughing, deep breathing, adequate hydration, and I.V. corticosteroids • *Antimicrobial therapy:* penicillin G or clindamycin

rest or activity as tolerated; careful monitoring of blood pressure, pulse rate, and respirations; oxygen administration; and, possibly, needle aspiration of air with a large-bore needle attached to a syringe.

If more than 30% of the lung is collapsed, treatment to reexpand it includes placing a thoracostomy tube, connected to an underwater seal with suction at low pressures, in the second or third intercostal space at the midclavicular line.

Recurring spontaneous pneumothorax requires thoracotomy and pleurectomy. Traumatic or tension pneumothorax requires chest tube drainage. Traumatic pneumothorax may also require surgical repair.

Nursing interventions. Watch for pallor, gasping respirations, and sudden chest pain. Carefully monitor vital signs at least every hour for indications of shock, increasing respiratory distress, or mediastinal shift. Listen for breath sounds over both lungs. Falling blood pressure and rising pulse and respiratory rates may indicate tension pneumothorax, which could be fatal without prompt treatment.

Make the patient as comfortable as possible, usually sitting upright.

Urge the patient to control coughing and gasping during thoracostomy. However, after the chest tube is in place, encourage him to breathe deeply (at least once an hour) to facilitate lung expansion.

In the patient undergoing chest tube drainage, watch for continuing air leakage (bubbling) in the water-seal bottle or chamber, indicating

the lung defect has failed to close; this may require surgery. Also watch for increasing subcutaneous emphysema by checking around the neck or at the tube insertion site for crackling beneath the skin. If he's on a ventilator, watch for pressure changes on ventilator gauges.

Change dressings around the chest tube insertion site, as necessary. Be careful not to reposition or dislodge the tube. If the tube dislodges, place a petrolatum gauze dressing over the opening immediately to prevent rapid lung collapse.

Monitor vital signs frequently after thoracostomy. Also, for the first 24 hours, assess respiratory status by checking breath sounds hourly. Observe the chest tube site for leakage, and note the amount and color of drainage. Walk the patient, as ordered (usually on the first postoperative day).

Patient education. Reassure the patient. Explain pneumothorax, its causes, and all tests and procedures.

Evaluation. The patient's X-rays, respiratory rate and depth, and vital signs are normal.

Pulmonary embolism and infarction

Pulmonary embolism is an obstruction of the pulmonary arterial bed by a dislodged thrombus or foreign substance. Pulmonary infarction may be asymptomatic, but massive embolism and infarction can be rapidly fatal.

Causes. Pulmonary embolism usually results from dislodged thrombi originating in the leg veins. Less common sources of thrombi are the pelvic veins, renal veins, hepatic vein, right side of the heart, and arms.

Pulmonary infarction may evolve from pulmonary embolism, especially in patients with chronic cardiac or pulmonary disease.

Assessment findings. Total occlusion of the main pulmonary artery is rapidly fatal; smaller or fragmented emboli produce various symptoms.

Usually, the first symptom of pulmonary embolism is dyspnea. Other clinical features include anginal or pleuritic chest pain, tachycardia, productive cough (sputum may be blood-tinged), and low-grade fever.

Less common signs include massive hemoptysis, splinting of the chest, and leg edema.

With a large embolus, you'll find cyanosis, syncope, distended neck veins, signs of shock (weak, rapid pulse; hypotension), and signs of hypoxia (restlessness).

Auscultation may reveal a right ventricular S_3 and S_4 audible at the lower sternum and increased intensity of a pulmonary component of S_2. Crackles and a pleural friction rub also may be heard at the infarction site.

Diagnostic tests. The following test results can help confirm pulmonary embolism or infarction.
• Chest X-ray helps to rule out other pulmonary diseases; it shows areas of atelectasis, an elevated diaphragm, pleural effusion, a prominent pulmonary artery and, occasionally, the characteristic wedge-shaped infiltrate suggestive of pulmonary embolism.
• Lung scan shows perfusion defects in areas beyond occluded vessels; a normal lung scan rules out pulmonary embolism.
• Pulmonary angiography is the most definitive test. As it poses some risk to the patient, its use depends on the uncertainty of the diagnosis and the need to avoid unnecessary anticoagulant therapy in high-risk patients.
• ECG is inconclusive but helps distinguish pulmonary embolism from MI. In extensive embolism, the ECG may show right axis deviation; right bundle-branch block; tall, peaked P wave on lead II; depressed ST segments and T-wave inversions (indicating right heart strain) in V_1 and V_2, and supraventricular tachyarrhythmias.
• ABG measurements showing decreased PaO_2 and $PaCO_2$ are characteristic with respiratory alkalosis.

Treatment. Treatment aims to maintain adequate cardiovascular and pulmonary function during resolution of the obstruction and to prevent recurrence of emboli. Because most emboli resolve within 10 days, treatment consists of oxygen therapy, as needed, and anticoagulation with heparin.

Patients with massive pulmonary embolism and shock may require thrombolytic therapy with tissue plasminogen activator or streptokinase to enhance fibrinolysis.

ALTERNATIVE THERAPY

Music therapy

Music therapy has been used to achieve relaxation and reduce anxiety. Relaxation leads to a decrease in heart and respiratory rates. Also, relaxed muscles use less oxygen than tense muscles.

Involve the patient in the choice of music. What is relaxing to you may not be relaxing to the patient. Recordings of the ocean, rain, or a rambling brook may also help the patient feel more relaxed.

While you're adding pleasant sounds, try to eliminate unpleasant and stressful sounds. For example, turn off an unwatched television, encourage the nursing staff not to talk or laugh loudly in the patient's room or hallways, or have the wheels of a squeaky cart oiled.

Treatment for septic emboli requires antibiotic therapy, not anticoagulants, and evaluation of the source of infection, particularly endocarditis.

Surgery to interrupt the inferior vena cava is reserved for patients who cannot take anticoagulants or who have recurrent emboli during anticoagulant therapy. It should not be performed without angiographic demonstration of pulmonary embolism.

To prevent postoperative venous thromboembolism, low-dose heparin may be administered.

Nursing interventions. Give oxygen by nasal cannula or mask. Check ABG levels if dyspnea worsens. Be prepared to provide endotracheal intubation with assisted ventilation if the patient tires and $PaCO_2$ increases.

Administer heparin, as ordered, through I.V. push or continuous drip. Monitor coagulation studies daily and with any change in dose. Maintain adequate hydration to prevent hypercoagulability.

After the patient is stable, encourage him to move about often and assist with isometric and range-of-motion exercises. Check temperature and color of feet to detect venostasis. *Never* vigorously massage the patient's legs. Walk the patient as soon as possible after surgery to prevent venostasis. Report frequent pleuritic chest pain so that analgesics can be prescribed.

Patient education. Teach the patient incentive spirometry. Warn him not to cross his legs; this promotes thrombus formation.

Explain procedures and treatments and encourage the patient's family to participate in his care. (See *Music therapy*.) Most patients need treatment with an oral anticoagulant (warfarin) for 4 to 6 months after a pulmonary embolism.

Advise the patient to watch for signs of bleeding from anticoagulants (bloody stools, blood in urine, large ecchymoses), to take the prescribed medication exactly as ordered, and to avoid taking any additional medication (even for headaches or colds) or changing medication dosages without consulting his doctor. Stress the importance of follow-up laboratory tests to monitor anticoagulant therapy.

Evaluation. Vital signs are within normal limits, and the patient shows no signs of bleeding after anticoagulant therapy.

Pulmonary hypertension

In adults, pulmonary hypertension is indicated by a resting systolic pulmonary artery pressure above 30 mm Hg and a mean pulmonary artery pressure above 20 mm Hg. It may be primary (rare) or secondary (far more common). Primary, or idiopathic, pulmonary hypertension shows the highest mortality among pregnant women. Secondary pulmonary hypertension results from existing cardiac or pulmonary disease. Prognosis depends on the severity of the underlying disorder.

Causes. *Primary pulmonary hypertension* is thought to result from altered immune mechanisms because this form of pulmonary hypertension occurs in association with collagen diseases.

Secondary pulmonary hypertension can stem from:
• alveolar hypoventilation in COPD, sarcoidosis, diffuse interstitial pneumonia, malignant metastases, and scleroderma
• vascular obstruction from pulmonary embolism, vasculitis, and disorders that cause obstructions of small or large pulmonary veins, such as left atrial myxoma, idiopathic veno-occlusive disease,

fibrous mediastinitis, and mediastinal neoplasm
• primary cardiac disease, which may be congenital (such as patent ductus arteriosus and atrial or ventricular septal defect) or acquired (such as rheumatic valvular disease and mitral stenosis).

Assessment findings. Assess your patient for increasing dyspnea on exertion, weakness, syncope, fatigability, and possible signs of right-sided heart failure, including peripheral edema, ascites, neck vein distention, and hepatomegaly.

Diagnostic tests. ABG values show hypoxemia (decreased PaO_2). An ECG shows right axis deviation and tall, peaked P waves in lead II.

Cardiac catheterization shows increased pulmonary artery pressure — pulmonary systolic pressure is above 30 mm Hg; PAWP is increased if the underlying cause is left atrial myxoma, mitral stenosis, or left-sided heart failure.

Pulmonary angiography detects filling defects in pulmonary vasculature such as those that develop in patients with pulmonary emboli. Pulmonary function tests in underlying obstructive disease may show decreased flow rates and increased residual volume; in underlying restrictive disease, total lung capacity may decrease.

Treatment. Treatment usually includes oxygen therapy. For patients with right-sided heart failure, treatment also includes fluid restriction, digitalis glycosides to increase cardiac contractibility, and diuretics to decrease intravascular volume and extravascular fluid accumulation. Of course, an important goal of treatment is correction of the underlying cause.

Nursing interventions. Administer oxygen therapy, as ordered, and observe the response. Report any signs of increasing dyspnea. Monitor ABG levels for acidosis and hypoxemia. Report any change in level of consciousness immediately.

When caring for a patient with right-sided heart failure, especially one receiving diuretics, record weight daily, carefully measure fluid intake and output, and explain all medications and diet restrictions. Check for increasing neck vein distention.

Monitor vital signs, especially blood pressure and heart rate. Watch for hypotension and tachycardia. Check pulmonary artery pressure and PAWP, as ordered, and report any changes.

Patient education. Help the patient adjust to physical limitations. Suggest frequent rest periods. Refer the patient to the social services department if oxygen equipment is needed for home use. Make sure he understands the prescribed diet and medications.

Evaluation. The patient shows no signs of decreased cardiac output, and urine output is within normal limits.

Respiratory acidosis

An acid-base disturbance characterized by reduced alveolar ventilation and manifested by hypercapnia ($PaCO_2$ greater than 45 mm Hg), respiratory acidosis can be acute (from a sudden failure in ventilation) or chronic (as in long-term pulmonary disease).

Causes. Respiratory acidosis can result from such drugs as narcotics, anesthetics, hypnotics, and sedatives; CNS trauma; neuromuscular disease, such as myasthenia gravis, Guillain-Barré syndrome, and poliomyelitis; airway obstruction; and parenchymal lung disease that interferes with alveolar ventilation. Other causes include COPD, late ARDS, large pneumothorax, extensive pneumonia, and pulmonary edema.

Assessment findings. CNS effects include restlessness, confusion, apprehension, somnolence, asterixis, coma, possible headaches, dyspnea, and tachypnea with papilledema and depressed reflexes.

Cardiovascular effects include possible tachycardia, hypertension, and atrial and ventricular arrhythmias. In severe acidosis, findings may include hypotension with vasodilation (bounding pulse and warm periphery).

Diagnostic tests. ABG measurements confirm respiratory acidosis: $PaCO_2$ above 45mm Hg; pH usually below the normal range of 7.35 to 7.45; and HCO_3^- normal in the acute stage but elevated in the chronic stage.

Treatment. Effective treatment aims to correct the underlying source of alveolar hypoventilation — for example, brochodilators, oxygen, and antibiotics for COPD. Significantly reduced alveolar ventilation may require mechanical ventilation.

Nursing interventions. Be alert for critical changes in the patient's respiratory, CNS, and cardiovascular functions. Report any such changes immediately as well as any variations in ABG measurements and electrolyte status. Maintain adequate hydration.

Maintain a patent airway and provide adequate humidification. Perform tracheal suctioning, as indicated, and vigorous chest physiotherapy, if ordered. Continually monitor ventilator settings and respiratory status.

To detect respiratory acidosis, closely monitor patient with COPD and chronic carbon dioxide retention for signs of acidosis. Also, administer oxygen at flow rates to achieve SaO_2 of approximately 90% and closely monitor any patient who receives narcotics or sedatives.

Patient education. Instruct the patient who has received a general anesthetic to turn and perform deep-breathing exercises frequently.

Evaluation. The patient has normal serum electrolyte values, normal ABG levels, and normal mentation.

Respiratory alkalosis

This disorder is marked by a decrease in $PaCO_2$ to less than 35 mm Hg, which results from alveolar hyperventilation. Uncomplicated respiratory alkalosis causes elevated blood pH. Hypocapnia occurs when carbon dioxide elimination by the lungs exceeds carbon dioxide production at the cellular level.

Causes. Pulmonary causes include pneumonia, interstitial lung disease, pulmonary vascular disease, and acute asthma. Nonpulmonary causes include anxiety, fever, aspirin toxicity, metabolic acidosis, CNS inflammation or tumor, gram-negative septicemia, and hepatic failure.

Assessment findings. Clinical features include deep, rapid breathing, possibly above 40 breaths a minute and much like the Kussmaul's respiration of diabetic acidosis (the key symptom); light-headedness or dizziness; agitation; circumoral and peripheral paresthesias; carpopedal spasms; twitching (possibly progressing to tetany); muscle weakness; and cardiac arrhythmias in severe respiratory alkalosis.

Diagnostic tests. ABG measurements confirm respiratory alkalosis and rule out respiratory compensation for metabolic acidosis: $PaCO_2$ below 35 mm Hg; pH elevated in proportion to fall in $PaCO_2$ in the acute stage, but falling toward normal in the chronic stage; HCO_3^- normal in the acute stage, but below normal in the chronic stage.

Treatment. Treatment aims to eradicate the underlying condition — for example, removal of ingested toxins, treatment of fever or sepsis, and treatment of CNS disease. In severe respiratory alkalosis, the patient may be instructed to breathe into a paper bag, which helps relieve acute anxiety and increases carbon dioxide levels.

Prevention of hyperventilation in patients receiving mechanical ventilation requires monitoring ABG levels and adjusting minute ventilation volume.

Nursing interventions. Watch for and report any changes in neurologic, neuromuscular, or cardiovascular function.

Remember that twitching and cardiac arrhythmias may be associated with alkalemia and electrolyte imbalances. Monitor ABG and serum electrolyte levels closely, reporting any changes immediately.

Patient education. Explain all diagnostic tests and procedures.

Evaluation. The patient has normal ABG and serum electrolyte values.

Hemothorax

In hemothorax, blood from damaged vessels enters the pleural cavity. Depending on the amount of bleeding and the underlying cause, hemothorax may be associated with varying degrees of lung collapse and mediastinal shift. Pneumothorax usually accompanies hemothorax.

Causes. Hemothorax usually results from blunt or penetrating chest trauma. Less commonly, it results from thoracic surgery, pulmonary infarc-

tion, neoplasm, dissecting thoracic aneurysm, or anticoagulant therapy.

Assessment findings. Characteristic clinical signs and symptoms with a history of trauma strongly suggest hemothorax. Percussion reveals dullness, whereas auscultation reveals decreased to absent breath sounds over the affected side. Chest pain, tachypnea, and mild to severe dyspnea may be present.

If respiratory failure results, the patient may appear anxious, restless, possibly stuporous, and cyanotic; marked blood loss produces hypotension and shock. The affected side of the chest expands and stiffens, while the unaffected side rises and falls with the patient's gasping respirations.

Diagnostic tests. Thoracentesis yields blood or serosanguineous fluid. Chest X-ray shows pleural fluid with or without mediastinal shift.

ABG levels may document respiratory failure. Hemoglobin may be decreased, depending on blood loss.

Treatment. Treatment seeks to stabilize the patient's condition, stop the bleeding, evacuate blood from the pleural space, and reexpand the underlying lung. Mild hemothorax usually clears in 10 to 14 days, requiring only observation for further bleeding. In severe hemothorax, thoracentesis is a diagnostic tool and a method of removing fluid from the pleural cavity.

After diagnosis is confirmed, a chest tube is inserted quickly into the sixth intercostal space at the posterior axillary line. Suction may be used; a large-bore tube is used to prevent clot blockage. The patient may need thoracotomy to evacuate blood and clots and to control bleeding. Blood transfusions may be necessary; watch for indications of hypoperfusion and hypoxia.

Nursing interventions. Give oxygen by face mask or nasal cannula. Give I.V. fluids and blood transfusions (monitored by a central venous pressure line), as needed, to treat shock. Monitor ABG levels often.

Assist with thoracentesis. Observe chest tube drainage carefully and record volume drained (at least every hour). Milk the chest tube only as necessary to maintain patency if the water seal chamber fails to fluctuate. *Note:* If the tube is warm and full of blood and the bloody fluid level in the water-seal bottle is rising rapidly, report this immediately. The patient may need immediate surgery.

Watch the patient closely for pallor and gasping respirations. Monitor his vital signs diligently. Falling blood pressure, rising pulse rate, and rising respiration rate may indicate shock or massive bleeding.

Patient education. Explain all procedures to the patient. Warn him not to cough during procedures.

Evaluation. The patient's respiratory status is normal; he has no dyspnea and feels no chest pain.

Chronic disorders

Chronic pulmonary disorders include tuberculosis, COPD, bronchiectasis, and lung cancer.

Tuberculosis

Tuberculosis is an acute or chronic infection, characterized by pulmonary infiltrates, formation of granulomas with caseation, fibrosis, and cavitation. The disease spreads by inhalation of droplet nuclei when infected persons cough or sneeze. Sites of extrapulmonary tuberculosis include the pleura, meninges, joints, lymph nodes, peritoneum, genitourinary tract, and bowel.

Causes. *Mycobacterium tuberculosis* is the major cause; other strains of mycobacteria may be involved.

Risk factors for primary infection include poverty and crowded, poorly ventilated living conditions. Risk factors for reinfection include gastrectomy, uncontrolled diabetes mellitus, opportunistic infections, Hodgkin's disease, leukemia, corticosteroid therapy, immunosuppressant therapy, and silicosis.

Assessment findings. In primary infection, the disease is usually asymptomatic. It may produce nonspecific symptoms, such as fatigue, weakness, anorexia, weight loss, night sweats, or low-grade fever. In active tuberculosis, the patient may experience cough, productive mucopurulent sputum, and chest pain.

Diagnostic tests. Chest X-rays show nodular lesions, patchy infiltrates, cavity formation, scar tissue, and calcium deposits. However, they may not distinguish active from inactive tuberculosis. Tuberculin skin tests detect exposure to tuberculosis but don't distinguish the disease from uncomplicated infection.

Stains and cultures (of sputum, cerebrospinal fluid, urine, drainage from abscess, or pleural fluid) confirm the diagnosis.

Treatment. Antitubercular therapy with daily oral doses of isoniazid or rifampin (with ethambutol added in some cases) for at least 9 months usually cures tuberculosis. After 2 to 4 weeks, the disease is usually no longer infectious, and the patient can resume his normal lifestyle while continuing to take medication. Patients with atypical mycobacterial disease or drug-resistant tuberculosis may require second-line drugs, such as capreomycin, streptomycin, para-aminosalicylic acid, pyrazinamide, and cycloserine.

Nursing interventions. Isolate the infectious patient in a quiet, well-ventilated room until he's no longer contagious. Be alert for adverse effects of medications. Because isoniazid use sometimes leads to peripheral neuritis, give pyridoxine (vitamin B_6), as ordered. If the patient receives ethambutol, watch for optic neuritis; if it develops, discontinue the drug. If he receives rifampin, watch for hepatitis and purpura. Observe the patient for other complications.

Patient education. Teach the isolated patient to cough and sneeze into tissues and to dispose of all secretions properly. Place a covered trash can in his room, and tape a waxed bag to the side of the bed for used tissues. Instruct the patient to wear a mask before he leaves his room. Visitors and hospital personnel should also wear masks.

Remind the patient to get plenty of rest. If the patient is anorexic, urge him to eat small meals throughout the day. Record weight weekly.

Before discharge, teach the patient to watch for adverse effects of medication and warn him to report them immediately. Emphasize the importance of regular follow-up examinations, and instruct the patient and his family about the signs and symptoms of recurring tuberculosis. Stress the need to follow long-term treatment regimens.

Advise persons who have been exposed to infected patients to receive tuberculin tests and, if ordered, chest X-rays and prophylactic isoniazid.

Evaluation. The patient's sputum culture is negative. Secretions are thin and clear.

Chronic obstructive pulmonary disease

COPD includes emphysema, chronic bronchitis, asthma, or any combination of them. Usually, more than one of these underlying conditions coexist. In most cases, bronchitis and emphysema occur together.

Although COPD doesn't always produce symptoms and causes only minimal disability in many patients, it tends to worsen with time.

Causes. COPD may be brought on by cigarette smoking, recurrent or chronic respiratory infection, allergies, or deficiency of alpha$_1$-antitrypsin.

Assessment findings. A thorough patient history is important. The typical patient is asymptomatic until middle age, when his ability to exercise or do strenuous work gradually declines, and he begins to develop a productive cough. Eventually the patient develops dyspnea on minimal exertion.

Diagnostic tests. See *Comparing types of COPD,* pages 96 to 99, for specific diagnostic tests.

Treatment and nursing interventions. Treatment aims to relieve symptoms and prevent complications. Give antibiotics, as ordered, to treat respiratory infections. Also administer low concentrations of oxygen, as ordered. Check ABG levels regularly. (See *Oxygen by nasal cannula—how much?* page 100.)

Patient education. Because most COPD patients receive outpatient treatment, they need comprehensive teaching.
• If programs in pulmonary rehabilitation are available, encourage the patient to enroll.
• Urge the patient to stop smoking and to avoid respiratory irritants. Suggest that he install an air conditioner with an air filter in his home.
• Explain that bronchodilators alleviate bronchospasm and enhance mucociliary clearance of secretions.

Familiarize the patient with prescribed bronchodilators.
• Stress the need to complete antibiotic therapy.
• Teach the patient and his family how to recognize early signs and symptoms of infection. Warn the patient to avoid contact with persons with respiratory infections. Encourage good oral hygiene. Pneumococcal vaccination every 3 years and annual influenza vaccinations are also important.
• Teach the patient to take slow, deep breaths and to exhale through pursed lips.
• Teach the patient how to cough effectively. If the patient has difficulty mobilizing secretions, teach his family how to perform postural drainage and chest physiotherapy. If secretions are thick, urge the patient to drink 12 to 15 glasses of fluid a day. Suggest using a home humidifier, particularly in the winter.
• If the patient is to continue oxygen therapy at home, teach him how to use the equipment correctly. Patients with COPD rarely require more than 2 to 3 L/minute to maintain adequate oxygenation.
• Emphasize the importance of a balanced diet. Suggest frequent, small meals, and consider using oxygen, administered by nasal cannula, during meals. Diet should be high in protein and calories in the form of fat.
• Help the patient and his family adjust their lifestyles to accommodate the limitations imposed by this debilitating chronic disease. Instruct the patient to allow for daily rest
(Text continues on page 98.)

Comparing types of COPD

Description	Causes and physiology	Clinical features
Emphysema • Abnormal irreversible enlargement of air spaces distal to terminal bronchioles caused by destruction of alveolar walls, resulting in decreased elastic recoil properties of lungs • Most common cause of death from respiratory disease in the United States	• Cigarette smoking, deficiency of alpha₁-antitrypsin • Recurrent inflammation associated with release of proteolytic enzymes from lung cells causes bronchiolar and alveolar wall damage and, ultimately, destruction. Loss of lung supporting structure results in decreased elastic recoil and airway collapse on expiration. Destruction of alveolar walls decreases surface area for gas exchange.	• Insidious onset, with dyspnea the predominant symptom • *Other signs and symptoms* of long-term disease: chronic cough, anorexia, weight loss, malaise, barrel chest, use of accessory muscles of respiration, prolonged expiratory period with grunting, pursed-lip breathing and tachypnea, peripheral cyanosis, and digital clubbing • *Complications:* recurrent respiratory tract infections, cor pulmonale, and respiratory failure
Chronic bronchitis • Excessive mucus production with productive cough for at least 3 months a year for 2 successive years • Only a minority of patients with the clinical syndrome of chronic bronchitis develop significant airway obstruction.	• Severity of disease related to amount and duration of smoking; respiratory infection exacerbates symptoms. • Hypertrophy and hyperplasia of bronchial mucous glands, increased goblet cells, damage to cilia, squamous metaplasia of columnar epithelium, and chronic leukocytic and lymphocytic infiltration of bronchial walls; widespread inflammation, distortion, narrowing of airways, and mucus within the airways produce resistance in small airways and cause severe ventilation-perfusion imbalance.	• Insidious onset, with productive cough and exertional dyspnea the predominant symptoms • *Other signs and symptoms:* colds associated with increased sputum production and worsening dyspnea that take progressively longer to resolve, copious sputum (gray, white, or yellow), weight gain from edema, cyanosis, tachypnea, wheezing, prolonged expiratory time, use of accessory muscles of respiration

Diagnostic tests	Management
• *Physical examination:* hyperresonance on percussion, decreased breath sounds, prolonged expiratory period • *Chest X-ray:* in advanced disease, flattened diaphragm, reduced vascular markings at lung periphery, hyperinflation of lungs, vertical heart, enlarged anteroposterior chest diameter, large retrosternal air space • *Pulmonary function tests:* increased residual volume, total lung capacity, and compliance; decreased vital capacity, diffusing capacity, and forced expiratory volumes • *Arterial blood gas (ABG) levels:* reduced with normal partial pressure of arterial carbon dioxide ($Paco_2$) until late in disease • *Electrocardiogram (ECG):* tall, peaked P waves in leads II, III, and aV_F; right axis deviation; signs of right ventricular hypertrophy late in disease • *Red blood cell count:* increased hemoglobin late in disease when persistent severe hypoxia is present	• Antibiotics to treat respiratory infection, influenza vaccine to prevent influenza, and pneumococcal vaccine to prevent pneumococcal pneumonia • Adequate fluid intake and, in selected patients, chest physiotherapy to mobilize secretions • Oxygen at low-flow settings to treat hypoxemia • Avoidance of smoking and air pollutants
• *Physical examination:* rhonchi and wheezes on auscultation, prolonged expiratory period, neck vein distention, pedal edema • *Chest X-ray:* may show hyperinflation and increased bronchovesicular markings • *Pulmonary function tests:* increased residual volume, decreased vital capacity and forced expiratory volumes, normal static compliance and diffusing capacity • *ABG levels:* decreased partial pressure of arterial oxygen (Pao_2); normal or increased $Paco_2$ • *Sputum:* contains many organisms and neutrophils • *ECG:* may show atrial arrhythmias; tall, peaked P waves in leads II, III, and aV_F; and, eventually, right ventricular hypertrophy	• Antibiotics for infections • Avoidance of smoking and air pollutants • Bronchodilators to relieve bronchospasm and facilitate mucociliary clearance • Adequate fluid intake and chest physiotherapy to mobilize secretions • Ultrasonic or mechanical nebulizer treatments to loosen secretions and aid in mobilization • Diuretics for edema • Oxygen for hypoxemia

(continued)

Comparing types of COPD *(continued)*

Description	Causes and physiology	Clinical features
Asthma • Increased bronchial reactivity to various stimuli, which produces episodic bronchospasm and airway obstruction • Asthma with onset in adulthood: in most cases, without distinct allergies; asthma with onset in childhood: in most cases, associated with definite allergens. Status asthmaticus is an acute asthma attack with severe bronchospasm that fails to clear with bronchodilator therapy. • *Prognosis:* More than one-half of asthmatic children become asymptomatic as adults; more than one-half of asthmatics with onset after age 15 have persistent disease, with occasional severe attacks.	• Possible mechanisms include allergy (family tendency, seasonal occurrence); allergic reaction results in release of mast cell vasoactive and bronchospastic mediators. • Upper airway infection, exercise, anxiety, and, rarely, coughing or laughing can precipitate an asthma attack. • Paroxysmal airway obstruction associated with nasal polyps may be seen in response to aspirin or indomethacin ingestion. • Airway obstruction from spasm of bronchial smooth muscle narrows airways; inflammatory edema of the bronchial wall and inspissation of tenacious mucoid secretions are also important, particularly in status asthmaticus.	• History of intermittent attacks of dyspnea and wheezing • Mild wheezing progressing to severe dyspnea, audible wheezing, chest tightness (a feeling of not being able to breathe), and cough producing thick mucus • *Other signs:* prolonged expiration, intercostal and supraclavicular retraction on inspiration, use of accessory muscles of respiration, flaring nostrils, tachypnea, tachycardia, perspiration, and flushing; often symptoms of eczema and allergic rhinitis (hay fever) • Status asthmaticus, unless treated promptly, can progress to respiratory failure

periods and to exercise daily as his doctor directs.
• As COPD progresses, encourage the patient to discuss his fears.
• Assist in the early detection of COPD by urging persons to have periodic physical examinations, including spirometry and medical evaluation of a chronic cough, and to seek treatment for recurring respiratory infections promptly.

Evaluation. The patient's chest X-rays, respiratory rate and rhythm,

Diagnostic tests	Management
• *Physical examination:* usually normal between attacks; auscultation shows rhonchi and wheezing throughout lung fields on expiration and, at times, inspiration; absent or diminished breath sounds during severe obstruction; chest hyperinflated • *Chest X-ray:* hyperinflated lungs during attack; normal during remission • *Sputum:* presence of Curschmann's spirals (casts of airways), Charcot-Leyden crystals, and eosinophils • *Pulmonary function tests:* during attacks, decreased forced expiratory volume, which improves significantly after inhaled bronchodilator; increased residual volume and, occasionally, total lung capacity; may be normal between attacks • *ABG levels:* decreased PaO_2; decreased, normal, or increased $PaCO_2$ (in severe attack) • *ECG:* sinus tachycardia during an attack; severe attack may produce signs of cor pulmonale (right axis deviation, tall, peaked P wave in lead II), which resolve after the attack • *Skin tests:* identify allergens	• Inhaled, oral, or I.V. corticosteroids; aerosol containing beta-adrenergic agents such as metaproterenol or albuterol; inhaled anticholinergics (ipratropion bromide); oral beta-adrenergic agents (terbutaline); and oral methylxanthines (aminophylline) • *Emergency treatment:* oxygen therapy, I.V. corticosteroids, and bronchodilators, such as subcutaneous epinephrine, I.V. aminophylline, and inhaled agents such as metaproterenol • Monitor for deteriorating respiratory status, and note sputum characteristics; provide adequate fluid intake and oxygen, as ordered. • *Prevention:* Tell the patient to avoid possible allergens and to use antihistamines, decongestants, inhalation of cromolyn powder, and oral or aerosol bronchodilators, as ordered. Explain the influence of stress and anxiety on asthma and its frequent association with exercise (particularly running) and cold air.

ABG values, pH are normal; PaO_2 is approximately 50 to 60 mm Hg. Body weight and urine output are also normal.

Bronchiectasis

An irreversible condition marked by chronic abnormal dilation of bronchi and destruction of bronchial walls, bronchiectasis can occur throughout the tracheobronchial tree or can be confined to one segment or lobe.

CRITICAL THINKING

Oxygen by nasal cannula—how much?

John Rakes, 68 years old, has a long history of chronic bronchitis. He is cyanotic and restless. His pulse oximetry reads 86%. How would you determine how much oxygen he can safely receive by nasal cannula?

Suggested response

Because this patient chronically has a partial pressure of arterial carbon dioxide ($Paco_2$) above 50 mm Hg, his central chemoreceptors are no longer sensitive to elevated $Paco_2$ levels as the primary stimulus to breathe. His peripheral chemoreceptors, stimulated primarily by a low blood oxygen level, are now responsible for keeping him breathing. While you don't want to eliminate this drive, you do want to prevent hypoxia. Your goal is to maintain a partial pressure of oxygen of approximately 60 mm Hg or an oxygen saturation of 90%. Remember that those chemoreceptors have no idea what the flow meter is set at!

Use pulse oximetry as a guide to administer enough oxygen to ensure adequate blood oxygenation without eliminating the hypoxic drive.

Causes. This disease results from conditions associated with repeated damage to bronchial walls and abnormal mucociliary clearance, which cause a breakdown of supporting tissue adjacent to airways. Such conditions include:
- immunologic disorders (agammaglobulinemia, for example)
- recurrent, inadequately treated bacterial respiratory tract infections such as tuberculosis
- measles, pneumonia, pertussis, or influenza
- obstruction (by a foreign body, tumor, or stenosis) associated with recurrent infection
- inhalation of corrosive gas or repeated aspiration of gastric juices into the lungs.

Assessment findings. Initially, bronchiectasis may be asymptomatic. Assess your patient for a chronic cough that produces copious, foul-smelling, mucopurulent secretions, possibly totaling several cupfuls daily (classic symptom). Other characteristic findings include coarse rhonchi over involved lobes or segments, occasional wheezes, dyspnea, weight loss, malaise, clubbing, recurrent fever, chills, and other signs and symptoms of infection.

Diagnostic tests. Besides aiding diagnosis, these tests also help determine the severity of the disease and the effects of therapy, and help evaluate patients for surgery.
- Chest X-rays show peribronchial thickening, areas of atelectasis, and scattered cystic changes.

However, it is usually bilateral, involving the basilar segments of the lower lobes. Bronchiectasis has three forms: cylindrical (fusiform), varicose, and saccular (cystic). It affects people of both sexes and all ages.

• Bronchography (most reliable diagnostic test) reveals the location and extent of the disease.
• Bronchoscopy helps identify the source of secretions or the site of bleeding in hemoptysis.
• Sputum culture and Gram stain identify predominant organisms.
• Complete blood count and WBC differential check for possible anemia and leukocytosis.
• Pulmonary function studies detect decreased vital capacity and decreased forced expiratory volume.
• ABG studies show hypoxemia.

Treatment. Antibiotics are given by mouth or I.V. for 7 to 10 days or until sputum production decreases. Bronchodilators, with postural drainage and chest percussion, help remove secretions. Bronchoscopy may be used occasionally to aid mobilization of secretions. Hypoxemia requires oxygen therapy. Severe hemoptysis commonly requires lobectomy or segmental resection.

Nursing interventions. You'll need to provide supportive care and help the patient adjust to permanent lifestyle changes. Thorough patient education is vital.

Provide a warm, quiet environment, and urge the patient to rest. Give antibiotics, as ordered.

Perform chest physiotherapy, including postural drainage and chest percussion designed for involved lobes, several times a day. Early morning and just before bedtime are best. Have the patient maintain each position for 10 minutes; then perform percussion and tell him to cough.

Encourage balanced, high-protein meals. Provide frequent mouth care to remove foul-smelling sputum.

Patient education. Explain all diagnostic tests. Show family members how to perform postural drainage and percussion. Also, teach the patient coughing and deep-breathing techniques.

Advise the patient to stop smoking. Refer the patient to a local self-help group.

Teach the patient to dispose of all secretions properly. Tell the patient to avoid air pollutants and people with upper respiratory tract infections. Instruct him to take medications (especially antibiotics) as ordered.

Evaluation. The patient's secretions are thin and clear or white.

Lung cancer

The most common cause of cancer death, lung cancer usually develops within the wall or epithelium of the bronchial tree. Prognosis varies with cell type and the extent of spread at the time of diagnosis.

Causes. The cause of lung cancer is unknown. Risk factors include cigarette smoking, exposure to carcinogenic industrial and air pollutants, and genetic predisposition.

Assessment findings. Late-stage respiratory signs and symptoms with epidermoid and small-cell carcinomas include smoker's cough, hoarseness, wheezing, dyspnea, hemoptysis, and chest pain; with adenocarcinoma and large-cell carcinoma: fever, weakness, weight loss, anorexia, and shoulder pain.

Hormone-related changes include gynecomastia (large-cell carcinoma), bone and joint pain (large-cell carcinoma and adenocarcinoma), symptoms of Cushing's and carcinoid syndromes (small-cell carcinoma), and symptoms of hypercalcemia, such as muscle pain and weakness (epidermoid carcinoma).

Metastatic signs and symptoms with bronchial obstruction include hemoptysis, atelectasis, pneumonitis, and dyspnea; with recurrent nerve invasion, vocal cord paralysis; with chest wall invasion, piercing chest pain, increasing dyspnea, and severe shoulder pain radiating down the arm; with local lymphatic spread, cough, hemoptysis, stridor, and pleural effusion.

Other metastatic signs and symptoms include, with phrenic nerve involvement dyspnea, shoulder pain, unilateral paralyzed diaphragm, paradoxical motion; with esophageal compression, dysphagia; with vena caval obstruction, venous distention and edema of face, neck, chest, and back; with pericardial involvement, pericardial effusion, tamponade, arrhythmias; with cervical thoracic sympathetic nerve involvement, miosis, ptosis, exophthalmos, and reduced sweating.

Diagnostic tests. Chest X-ray usually shows an advanced lesion. It also indicates tumor size and location.

Sputum cytology, which is 75% reliable, requires a specimen coughed up from the lungs and tracheobronchial tree.

Bronchoscopy can locate the tumor site. Bronchoscopic washings provide material for cytologic and histologic examination. The flexible fiber-optic bronchoscope increases test effectiveness. Needle biopsy employs biplane fluoroscopic visual control to detect peripherally located tumors. Tissue biopsy of accessible metastatic sites includes supraclavicular and mediastinal node and pleural biopsy. Thoracentesis allows chemical and cytologic examination of pleural fluid.

Additional studies include chest tomography, bronchography, esophagography, and angiocardiography.

Tests to detect metastasis include bone scan, bone marrow biopsy, computed tomography scan of the brain, liver function studies, and gallium scan (noninvasive nuclear scan) of liver, spleen, and bone.

Staging determines the extent of the disease and helps in planning treatment and understanding the prognosis. (See *Staging lung cancer.*)

Treatment. Treatment consists of combinations of surgery, radiation, and chemotherapy and may prolong survival. However, because treatment usually begins at an advanced stage, it's largely palliative.

Surgery is the primary treatment for squamous cell carcinoma, adenocarcinoma, and large-cell carcinoma. Surgery may include partial or total removal of a lung.

Staging lung cancer

T$_0$
No evidence of primary tumor

T$_x$
Tumor proved by the presence of malignant cells in bronchopulmonary secretions but not visualized by X-rays or bronchoscopy, or any tumor that can't be assessed

T$_{is}$
Carcinoma in situ

T$_1$
A tumor that's 1¼″ (3 cm) or less in greatest diameter, surrounded by lung or visceral pleura, and without evidence of invasion proximal to a lobar bronchus at bronchoscopy

T$_2$
A tumor more than 1¼″ (3 cm) in greatest diameter, or a tumor of any size that invades the visceral pleura or has associated atelectasis or obstructive pneumonitis extending to the hilar region. At bronchoscopy, the proximal extent of demonstrable tumor that's within a lobar bronchus or at least ¾″ (2 cm) distal to the carina. Any associated atelectasis or obstructive pneumonitis must involve less than an entire lung, and there must be no pleural effusion.

T$_3$
A tumor of any size with direct extension into an adjacent structure, such as the parietal pleura, chest wall, diaphragm, or mediastinum; a tumor shown by bronchoscopy to involve a main bronchus less than 2 cm distal to the carina; or any tumor associated with atelectasis, obstructive pneumonitis of an entire lung, or pleural effusion

N$_0$
No demonstrable metastasis to regional lymph nodes

N$_1$
Metastasis to lymph nodes in the peribronchial or the ipsilateral hilar region, or both, including direct extension

N$_2$
Metastasis to lymph nodes in the mediastinum

M$_0$
No distant metastasis

M$_1$
Distant metastasis, such as in scalene, cervical, or contralateral hilar lymph nodes, brain, bones, liver, or contralateral lung

Radiation therapy is ordinarily recommended for stage I and stage II lesions if surgery is contraindicated and sometimnes for stage III lesions. Radiation is also used for palliation of metastatic lesions.

Chemotherapy may include a combination of fluorouracil, vincristine, and mitomycin for adenocarcinomas. Promising combinations for treating small-cell carcinomas include cyclophosphamide, doxorubicin, and vincristine; cyclophosphamide, doxorubicin, vincristine, and etoposide; and etoposide and cisplatin. Chemotherapy is the primary therapy for small-cell carcinomas.

Nursing interventions. Provide comprehensive supportive care to minimize complications and aid the patient's recovery from surgery, radiation, and chemotherapy.

Patient education. Before surgery, follow these patient education guidelines:
• Supplement and reinforce the doctor's explanation of the disease and the surgical procedure itself.
• Explain postoperative procedures, such as insertion of an indwelling catheter and chest tube, dressing changes, and I.V. therapy. Instruct the patient in coughing, deep breathing, and ROM exercises.
• Encourage patients with recurring or chronic respiratory infections and those with chronic lung disease who detect any change in the character of a cough to see their doctor promptly for evaluation.

Before discharge, teach patients about the use of home oxygen therapy and the signs and symptoms of pulmonary infection.

Evaluation. Uneventful recovery from surgery, radiation, or chemotherapy indicates successful treatment. The patient and his family understand risk factors and quit smoking. The patient follows the treatment regimen and understands the need for good pulmonary hygiene and follow-up. He also recognizes the signs and symptoms of

pulmonary infection and the need for immediate medical attention.

Pulmonary fibrotic disorders

Silicosis is a pulmonary fibrotic disorder.

Silicosis

Silicosis is a progressive disease that is characterized by nodular lesions and commonly progresses to fibrosis. It's the most common form of pneumoconiosis.

Silicosis can be classified according to the severity of pulmonary disease and the rapidity of onset and progression; it usually occurs as a simple asymptomatic illness. Acute silicosis develops after 1 to 3 years in workers (sandblasters, tunnel workers) exposed to high concentrations of respirable silica. Accelerated silicosis appears after an average of 10 years of exposure to lower concentrations of free silica. Chronic silicosis develops after 20 or more years of exposure to lower concentrations of free silica.

Prognosis is good, unless the disease progresses into the complicated fibrotic form, which causes respiratory insufficiency and cor pulmonale and is associated with pulmonary tuberculosis.

Causes. The disorder results from inhalation and pulmonary deposition of respirable crystalline silica dust, mostly from quartz.

Assessment findings. Silicosis may be asymptomatic in initial stages.

Assess your patient for dyspnea on exertion (worsening as the disease progresses), cough, tachypnea, weight loss, fatigue, weakness, and CNS changes such as confusion in the advanced stage.

In chronic silicosis, assess for possible decreased chest expansion, diminished intensity of breath sounds, and fine-to-medium crackles.

Diagnostic tests. Chest X-rays show small, discrete, nodular lesions distributed throughout both lung fields but typically concentrated in the upper lung zones; the hilar lung nodes may be enlarged and exhibit "eggshell" calcification in simple silicosis. In complicated silicosis, X-rays show one or more conglomerate masses of dense tissue.

Pulmonary function studies yield the following results:
• forced vital capacity (FVC): reduced in complicated silicosis
• FEV: reduced in obstructive disease (emphysematous areas of silicosis); also reduced in complicated silicosis, but with a ratio of FEV to FVC that's normal or high
• maximal voluntary ventilation: reduced in both restrictive and obstructive diseases
• Diffusing capacity for carbon monoxide: reduced when fibrosis destroys alveolar walls and obliterates pulmonary capillaries, or when fibrosis thickens the alveolocapillary membrane.

ABG studies show the following:
• PaO_2 normal in simple silicosis but may be significantly decreased in the late stages of chronic or compli-

cated disease, when the patient breathes room air
• $PaCO_2$: normal in early stages but may decrease because of hyperventilation; may increase as a restrictive pattern develops, particularly if the patient has severe impairment of alveolar ventilation.

Treatment. Treatment aims to relieve symptoms, to manage hypoxia and cor pulmonale, and to prevent respiratory tract irritation and infections. Treatment also includes careful observation for the development of tuberculosis.

Respiratory symptoms may be relieved by daily use of bronchodilating aerosols and increased fluid intake (at least 3 qt [3 L] daily).

Steam inhalation and chest physiotherapy techniques help clear secretions. In severe cases, it may be necessary to administer oxygen by cannula or mask for the patient with chronic hypoxemia or by mechanical ventilation if the patient is persistently hypercapnic and acidotic.

Respiratory infections require administration of antibiotics.

Nursing interventions. Encourage the patient to drink the recommended amount of fluids, and monitor intake and output daily. Keep the environment moist and provide oxygen, as ordered. Watch for complications such as pulmonary hypertension.

Patient education. Tell the patient to avoid crowds and other patients with respiratory infections.

Increase exercise tolerance by encouraging regular activity. Advise the patient to plan his daily activities to decrease the work of breathing. He should pace himself and rest often.

Evaluation. The patient is adequately hydrated, as evidenced by skin turgor and normal urine output. ABG values are normal.

TREATMENTS

Respiratory disorders interfere with airway clearance, breathing patterns, and gas exchange. If not corrected, they can adversely affect many other body systems and can be life-threatening. Treatments for respiratory disorders include drug therapy, physiotherapy, surgery, bronchoscopy, and mechanical ventilation.

Drugs are used for airway management in such disorders as bronchial asthma and chronic bronchitis. When secretions or mucus plugs obstruct the airways, chest physiotherapy or bronchoscopy may improve ventilation. Other treatments include endotracheal intubation, tracheostomy, mechanical ventilation, or oxygen therapy.

Drug therapy

Xanthines (such as aminophylline and theophylline) and adrenergics (such as albuterol sulfate and isoproterenol hydrochloride) dilate bronchial passages and reduce airway resistance. Corticosteroids (such as prednisone, flunisolide, and beclomethasone) reduce inflammation and make the airways more responsive to bronchodilators. Antihistamines (such as terfenadine and clemastine fumarate) and antitussives (such as acetylcysteine and benzonatate) help suppress coughing. Expectorants (such as guaifenesin and terpin) hydrate and mobilize secretions.

Surgery

If drugs or other therapeutic approaches fail to maintain airway patency and protect healthy tissues from disease, surgical intervention may be necessary. Respiratory surgeries include tracheotomy, chest tube insertion, and thoracotomy.

Tracheotomy

Tracheotomy is commonly done to provide an airway for an intubated patient who needs prolonged mechanical ventilation. It's also done to help remove lower tracheobronchial secretions in a patient who can't clear them. A tracheotomy is done when endotracheal intubation isn't possible, to prevent an unconscious or paralyzed patient from aspirating food or secretions, or to bypass upper airway obstruction caused by trauma, burns, epiglottitis, or a tumor.

After the doctor creates the surgical opening, he inserts a tracheostomy tube to permit access to the airway. He may select from several tube styles, depending on the patient's condition.

Patient preparation. For an emergency tracheotomy, briefly explain the procedure to the patient if time permits, and quickly obtain supplies or a tracheostomy tray.

For a scheduled tracheotomy, explain the procedure and the need for general anesthesia to the patient and the family. If possible, mention whether the tracheostomy will be temporary or permanent. Set up a communication system with the patient (Magic Slate, letter board, or flash cards), and have him practice using it so that he can communicate comfortably.

If the patient will be having a long-term or permanent tracheostomy, introduce him to someone who has undergone a similar procedure and has adjusted well to tube and stoma care.

Ensure that samples for ABG analysis and other diagnostic tests have been collected and that the patient or a responsible family member has signed a consent form.

Monitoring and aftercare. Auscultate for breath sounds every 2 hours after the procedure. Note crackles, rhonchi, or diminished breath sounds. Turn the patient every 2 hours to avoid pooling tracheal secretions. As ordered, provide chest physiotherapy and note the quantity, consistency, color, and odor of secretions. (See *Combating complications of tracheostomy,* pages 108 and 109, for how to prevent or recognize complications.)

Provide humidification to reduce the drying effects of oxygen on mucous membranes and to thin secretions. Give oxygen through a T-piece connected to a nebulizer or heated cascade humidifier. If your patient is an infant or a young child, be sure to warm the oxygen. Monitor ABG results and compare them with baseline values to check adequacy of oxygenation and carbon dioxide removal. Also monitor the patient's oximetry values, as ordered.

Suctioning. As ordered, suction the tracheostomy with sterile equipment and technique to remove excess secretions. Before and after suctioning, administer 100% oxygen for 2 minutes to reduce the risk of hypoxemia. Use a suction catheter no larger than one-half the diameter of the tracheostomy tube, and minimize oxygen deprivation and tracheal trauma by keeping the bypass port open while inserting the catheter. Use a gentle, twisting motion on withdrawal to help minimize tracheal and bronchial mucosal irritation. Apply suction for no longer than 10 seconds at a time, and discontinue suctioning if the patient develops respiratory distress. Monitor for arrhythmias, which can occur if suctioning decreases PaO_2 levels below 50 mm Hg. Administer 100% oxygen for 2 minutes between passes and after suctioning. Evaluate the effectiveness of suctioning by auscultating for breath sounds.

Cuffed tube cautions. A cuffed tube, usually kept inflated until the patient no longer needs controlled ventilation or no longer risks aspiration, may cause tracheal stenosis from excessive pressure or incorrect placement. Avoid traumatizing the interior tracheal wall by using pressures less than 25 cm H_2O (18 mm Hg) and minimal-leak technique when inflating the cuff. Reduce the risk of trau-

Combating complications of tracheostomy

Complication	Prevention	Detection	Treatment
Aspiration	• Evaluate patient's ability to swallow. • Elevate his head and inflate cuff during feeding and for 30 minutes afterward.	• Assess for dyspnea, tachypnea, rhonchi, crackles, excessive secretions, and fever.	• Suction excessive secretions. • Obtain chest X-ray, if ordered. • Give antibiotics or steroids if necessary.
Bleeding at tracheostomy site	• Don't pull on the tracheostomy tube or allow ventilator tubing to do so. • If dressing adheres to wound, wet it with hydrogen peroxide and remove gently.	• Check dressing regularly; slight bleeding is normal, especially if the patient has a bleeding disorder.	• Keep cuff inflated to prevent edema and blood aspiration. • Give humidified oxygen. • Document rate and amount of bleeding. Check for prolonged clotting time. • As ordered, assist with application of an absorbable gelatin sponge or ligation of a small bleeder.
Infection at tracheostomy site	• Always use strict aseptic technique. • Thoroughly clean all tubing. • Change nebulizer or humidifier jar and all tubing daily. • Collect sputum and wound drainage specimens for culture.	• Check for purulent, foul-smelling drainage from stoma. • Be alert for other signs and symptoms of infection: fever, malaise, increased white blood cell count, and local pain.	• As ordered, obtain culture specimens and give antibiotics. • Inflate tracheostomy cuff to prevent aspiration. • Suction the patient as indicated, maintaining sterile technique; avoid cross-contamination. • Change dressing whenever soiled.
Pneumothorax	• Assess for subcutaneous emphysema, which may indicate pneumothorax. Notify doctor if this occurs.	• Auscultate for decreased or absent breath sounds. • Check for tachypnea, pain, and subcutaneous emphysema.	• If ordered, prepare for chest tube insertion. • Obtain chest X-ray, as ordered.

Combating complications of tracheostomy (continued)

Complication	Prevention	Detection	Treatment
Subcutaneous emphysema	• Make sure cuffed tube is patent and properly inflated. • Avoid displacement by securing ties and using lightweight ventilator tubing and swivel valves.	• Expect to find in mechanically ventilated patients. • Palpate neck for crepitus, listen for escape of air around tube cuff, and check for excessive swelling at wound site.	• Inflate cuff correctly or use a larger tube. • Suction patient and clean tube to remove any blockage. • Document extent of crepitus.
Tracheal malacia	• Avoid excessive cuff pressures. • Avoid suctioning beyond end of tube.	• Be alert for dry, hacking cough and blood-streaked sputum when tube is being manipulated.	• Minimize trauma from tube movement. • Keep cuff pressure below 18 mm Hg.

ma to the stoma site and internal tracheal wall by using lightweight corrugated tubing for the ventilator or nebulizer and providing a swivel adapter for the ventilator circuit.

Make sure the tracheostomy ties are secure but not too tight. Avoid changing the ties unnecessarily until the stoma track is more stable to help prevent accidental tube dislodgment or expulsion. Report any tube pulsation to the doctor because this may mean it's near the innominate artery, risking hemorrhage.

Using aseptic technique, change the tracheostomy dressing when soiled or once per shift, and check the color, odor, amount, and type of any drainage. Check for swelling, erythema, and bleeding at the site, and report excessive bleeding or unusual drainage immediately.

Keep two sterile tracheostomy tubes with obturators (one that's one size smaller than the tube currently being used) at the patient's bedside. Be prepared to replace an expelled or contaminated tube. Because the trachea begins to close after tube expulsion, you may need to insert the smaller tube.

Patient education. Before discharge, tell the patient to notify his doctor if he develops any breathing problems or chest or stoma pain or notices any change in the amount or color of secretions.

Ensure that he can care for his stoma and tracheostomy tube effectively. Instruct him to wash the skin around his stoma with a moist cloth. Emphasize the importance of not getting water in the stoma. He should, of course, avoid swimming. When he showers, he should wear a stoma shield or direct the water below his stoma.

Tell the patient to place a foam filter over his stoma in winter to warm the inspired air and to wear a bib over the filter.

Teach the patient to bend at his waist during coughing to help expel secretions. Tell him to keep a tissue handy to catch expelled secretions.

Chest tube insertion

A chest tube may be required to help treat pneumothorax, hemothorax, empyema, pleural effusion, or chylothorax. Inserted into the pleural space, the tube allows blood, fluid, pus, or air to drain and allows the lung to reinflate. In pneumothorax, the tube restores negative pressure to the pleural space by means of an underwater-seal drainage system. The water in the system prevents air from being sucked back into the pleural space during inspiration. (If a leak occurs through the bronchi and cannot be sealed, suction applied to the underwater-seal system removes air from the pleural space faster than it can collect.)

Because a collapsed lung is life-threatening, chest tube insertion is often an emergency treatment. Complications include lung puncture, bleeding, or additional hemothorax at the insertion site. Tension pneumothorax, a life-threatening complication, may result from an obstructed chest tube or from a blocked air vent in the underwater-seal drainage system.

Patient preparation. If time permits, explain the procedure to the patient. Take his vital signs to serve as a baseline, and obtain a signed consent form. Then administer a sedative, as ordered.

Collect necessary equipment, including a thoracotomy tray and an underwater-seal drainage system. Prepare lidocaine for local anesthesia, as directed. Clean the insertion site with povidone-iodine solution. Set up the underwater-seal drainage system according to the manufacturer's instructions, and place it at bedside, below the patient's chest level. Stabilize the unit to avoid knocking it over. (See *Comparing closed chest drainage systems.*)

Monitoring and aftercare. Once the patient's chest tube is stabilized, have him take several deep breaths to inflate his lungs fully and help push pleural air out through the tube. Obtain vital signs immediately after tube insertion and then every 15 minutes or as ordered. Change the dressing daily to clean the site and remove any drainage.

Prepare the patient for a chest X-ray to verify tube placement and to assess the outcome of treatment. As ordered, arrange for daily X-rays to monitor his progress.

Routinely assess chest tube function. Describe and record the amount of drainage on the intake and output sheet. After most of the air has been removed, the drainage

Comparing closed chest drainage systems

A *one-bottle system,* which drains by gravity, combines drainage and water-seal chambers in one. It's the easiest system to use, but it doesn't allow suction control and can't handle copious drainage.

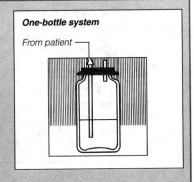

One-bottle system

From patient

A *two-bottle system* uses the first bottle for drainage and water-sealing and the second for suction. Don't use this system for excessive drainage.

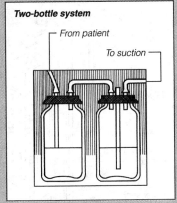

Two-bottle system

From patient

To suction

A *three-bottle system* uses the first bottle for drainage, the second for water-sealing, and the third for suction control. Use this system for copious drainage.

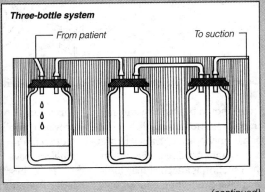

Three-bottle system

From patient

To suction

(continued)

Comparing closed chest drainage systems *(continued)*

A one-piece, disposable plastic device, the *Pleur-evac* (among others) has three chambers that mimic a three-bottle collection system. The drainage chamber, on the right, has three calibrated columns that display the amount of drainage collected. When the first column fills, it empties into the second and then into the third. The water-seal chamber is located in the center.

The suction control chamber, which you can fill with water to achieve various suction levels, is located on the left. You can change the water level or remove a drainage sample through rubber diaphragms at the rear. A positive-pressure relief valve at the top of the water-seal chamber vents excess pressure into the atmosphere, preventing pressure buildup.

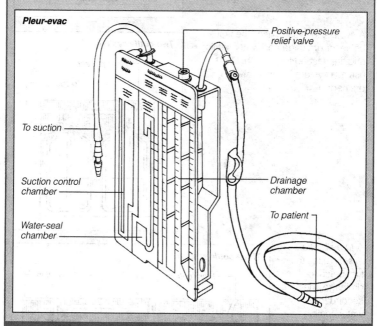

Pleur-evac

Positive-pressure relief valve

To suction

Suction control chamber

Water-seal chamber

Drainage chamber

To patient

system should bubble only during forced expiration unless the patient has a bronchopleural fistula. However, constant bubbling in the system when suction is attached may indicate that a connection is loose, or that the tube has advanced slightly out of the patient's chest. Promptly

correct any loose connections to prevent complications. (See *No fluctuation in the water-seal chamber—a problem?* page 114.)

If the chest tube becomes dislodged, cover the opening immediately with petrolatum gauze and apply pressure. Call the doctor and have an assistant collect equipment for tube reinsertion while you keep the opening closed. Reassure the patient and monitor him closely for signs of tension pneumothorax. (See *Combating tension pneumothorax,* page 115.)

The doctor will remove the patient's chest tube when the lung has reexpanded fully. As soon as the tube is removed, apply an airtight, sterile petroleum dressing.

Patient education. Typically, the patient will be discharged with a chest tube only if it's being used to drain a loculated empyema, which doesn't require an underwater-seal drainage system. Teach this patient how to care for his tube, dispose of drainage and soiled dressings properly, and perform wound care and dressing changes.

Teach the patient with a recently removed chest tube how to clean the wound site and change dressings. Tell him to report any signs of infection.

Thoracotomy

The surgical removal of all or part of a lung, thoracotomy aims to spare healthy lung tissue. Excision may involve pneumonectomy, lobectomy, segmental resection, or wedge resection.

Pneumonectomy is excision of an entire lung. Usually performed for bronchogenic carcinoma, it may also be used with tuberculosis, bronchiectasis, or lung abscess.

Lobectomy, the removal of one of the five lung lobes, treats bronchogenic carcinoma, tuberculosis, lung abscess, emphysematous blebs or bullae, benign tumors, or localized fungal infections.

Segmental resection, removal of one or more lung segments, is commonly used to treat bronchiectasis.

Wedge resection, removal of a small portion of the lung without regard to segments, can treat only a small, well-circumscribed lesion.

Complications include hemorrhage, infection, tension pneumothorax, bronchopleural fistula, empyema, and a persistent air space that the remaining lung tissue doesn't expand to fill. In the last instance, removal of up to three ribs may be necessary to reduce chest cavity size.

Patient preparation. Explain the anticipated lung excision to the patient, and inform him that he'll receive a general anesthetic. Prepare him psychologically. A patient with lung cancer faces the fear of dying and needs ongoing emotional support. In contrast, a patient with a chronic lung disorder may view the surgery as a cure.

Inform the patient that postoperatively he may have chest tubes in place and may be receiving oxygen. Teach him deep-breathing techniques. Also teach how to use an incentive spirometer; record the volumes achieved to provide a baseline.

As ordered, arrange for laboratory studies, such as pulmonary function tests, ECG, chest X-ray, ABG analysis, bronchoscopy, and possibly cardiac catheterization before pneumonectomy.

No fluctuation in the water-seal chamber— a problem?

Mr. Jason Green, 61 years old, had a lobectomy yesterday. In evaluating his chest tube and Pleur-evac, you note that there's no fluctuation in the water-seal chamber.

Is there a problem?
The reason for loss of fluctuation is reexpansion of the lung (because the tube is compressed between two layers of the pleura and intrapleural pressure changes are not transmitted) or an occlusion in the drainage system. Check the morning's chest X-ray for reexpansion, but this is unlikely (remember: surgery was just yesterday). Next, see if you can find any kinks or occlusions in the tube. If the water-seal is still not fluctuating, a blood clot has occluded the tube.

What should you do?
Begin with gentle maneuvers such as hand-over-hand milking. If there's still no fluctuation, strip short sections of the chest drainage tubing. Although milking and stripping do create excessive negative pressure on the pleural space and can potentially cause pleural trauma, a non-patent chest tube predisposes your patient to a potentially life-threatening tension pneumothorax.

How can you prevent this from recurring?
Remember "good lung down" in unilateral lung conditions (except pneumothorax). Positioning the patient with the "good lung down" (on his side with the unaffected lung closest to the mattress) increases ventilation to the affected lung. This encourages reexpansion and sends more blood to the lung that wasn't operated on to optimize ventilation-perfusion matching in the good lung.

Make sure that the patient or a responsible family member has signed a consent form.

Monitoring and aftercare. After a pneumonectomy, position the patient only on his operative side or on his back until he's stabilized. This prevents fluid from draining into the unaffected lung if the sutured bronchus opens. After a thoracotomy, position the patient on his nonoperative side or back. Make sure his chest tube is func-

tioning, and monitor him for signs of tension pneumothorax. Provide analgesics, as ordered.

Have the patient begin deep-breathing exercises as soon as he's stabilized. Auscultate his lungs, place him in semi-Fowler's position, and have him splint his incision to facilitate deep breathing. Have him cough every 4 hours if rhonchi are audible.

Perform passive ROM exercises the evening of surgery and two to three times daily thereafter. Progress to active ROM exercises.

Patient education. Tell the patient to continue deep-breathing exercises to prevent complications. Advise him to report any changes in sputum characteristics.

Instruct him to continue performing ROM exercises to maintain shoulder and chest wall mobility. Tell the patient to avoid contact with people who have upper respiratory tract infections and to refrain from smoking. Provide instructions for wound care and dressing changes, as necessary.

Inhalation therapy

Inhalation therapy employs carefully controlled ventilation techniques to help the patient maintain optimal ventilation after respiratory failure. Techniques include manual ventilation, mechanical ventilation, CPAP, oxygen therapy, humidification and aerosol treatments, and incentive spirometry.

Manual ventilation

A handheld resuscitation bag is an inflatable device that can be attached to a face mask or directly to an ET or tracheostomy tube to allow manual delivery of oxygen or room air to the lungs of a patient who can't breathe by himself. Usually used in an emergency, manual ventilation may be performed during transport or tubing changes or before suctioning to maintain ventilation.

Combating tension pneumothorax

Fatal if not treated promptly, tension pneumothorax refers to the entrapment of air within the pleural space.

What causes it?

Tension pneumothorax can result from dislodgment or obstruction of the chest tube. In both of these cases, increasing positive pressure within the patient's chest cavity compresses the affected lung and the mediastinum, shifting them toward the opposite lung. This leads to markedly impaired venous return and cardiac output and possible lung collapse.

Telltale signs

Suspect tension pneumothorax if your patient develops any of the following signs or symptoms: dyspnea, chest pain, an irritating cough, vertigo, syncope, or anxiety. Is his skin cold, pale, and clammy? Are his respiratory and pulse rates unusually rapid? Do the intercostal spaces bulge during respiration?

If the patient develops any of these signs or symptoms, palpate his neck, face, and chest wall for subcutaneous emphysema, and palpate his trachea for deviation from midline. Auscultate his lungs for decreased or absent breath sounds on the affected side. Then percuss them for hyperresonance.

If you suspect tension pneumothorax, notify the doctor at once and help him to identify the cause.

Patient preparation. Select a mask that fits snugly over the mouth and nose (unless the patient is intubated or has a tracheostomy) and attach it to the resuscitation bag.

If oxygen is available, connect the handheld resuscitation bag to it, turn it on, and adjust the flow rate according to the patient's condition. For example, if the patient has a low partial pressure of oxygen in arterial blood, he'll need a higher fraction of inspired oxygen (FIO_2). To increase the concentration of inspired oxygen, add an oxygen accumulator (or *reservoir*). Attached to an adapter on the bag, this device permits an FIO_2 of up to 100%. If time allows, set up suction equipment.

Procedure. Before using the handheld resuscitation bag, check the patient's upper airway for foreign objects. If present, remove them because this alone may restore spontaneous respirations. Suction the patient. If necessary, insert an oropharyngeal or nasopharyngeal airway to maintain airway patency. If a tracheostomy or ET tube is in place, suction it.

• If appropriate, remove the bed's headboard and stand at the head of the bed to help keep the patient's neck extended and to free space for activities such as cardiopulmonary resuscitation.

• Tilt the patient's head backward, if not contraindicated, and pull his jaw forward to move the tongue away from the pharynx and prevent airway obstruction.

• Keeping your nondominant hand on the patient's mask, exert downward pressure to seal the mask against his face. For the adult patient, use your dominant hand to compress the bag every 5 seconds to deliver about 500 ml of air. For a child, deliver 15 breaths/minute, or one compression of the bag every 4 seconds; for the infant, 20 breaths/minute, or one compression every 3 seconds. Infants and children should receive 250 to 500 cc of air with each bag compression.

• Deliver breaths with the patient's own inspiratory effort, if any. Don't attempt it during exhalation.

• Observe the patient's chest to ensure that it rises and falls with each compression. If ventilation fails to occur, check the fit of the mask and the patency of the airway; if necessary, reposition his head and ensure patency with an oral airway.

Monitoring and aftercare. Avoid neck hyperextension if the patient has a possible cervical injury; instead, use the jaw-thrust technique to open the airway. If you need both hands to keep the patient's mask in place and maintain hyperextension, use the lower part of your arm to compress the bag against your side.

Observe for vomiting through the mask. If it occurs, stop the procedure immediately, lift the mask, wipe and suction vomitus, and resume resuscitation.

Underventilation commonly occurs because the handheld resuscitation bag is difficult to keep positioned tightly on the patient's face while ensuring an open airway.

Have someone assist with the procedure, if possible.

In an emergency, record the date and time of the procedure, manual ventilation efforts, any complications and the nursing action taken, and the patient's response to treatment, according to your facility's protocol for respiratory arrest.

If it's not an emergency, record the date and time, reason for the procedure, duration of manual ventilation and disconnection from mechanical ventilator, any complications and the nursing action taken, and the patient's tolerance for the procedure. (See *How to document mechanical ventilation.*)

Mechanical ventilation

Mechanical ventilation controls or assists the patient's respirations. Typically requiring an ET or tracheostomy tube, this treatment delivers room air under positive pressure or oxygen-enriched air in concentrations of up to 100% and corrects profoundly impaired ventilation, as evidenced by hypercapnia and symptoms of breathing difficulty.

Major types of mechanical ventilation systems include positive-pressure and negative-pressure. Positive-pressure systems, the most commonly used, can be volume-cycled or pressure-cycled and may deliver PEEP or CPAP. Negative-pressure systems provide ventilation for patients unable to generate adequate inspiratory pressures. (See *Reviewing types of positive-pressure ventilation,* page 118.)

Mechanical ventilators can be used as controllers, assisters, or

---

CHARTING TIPS

How to document mechanical ventilation

Keep these areas in mind when documenting ET tube insertion and mechanical ventilation.

Endotracheal tube
• Size of the ET tube
• Centimeter mark of the ET tube at the teeth (or at the nare if nasotracheal tube)
• Assessment of the oral or nasal mucosa
• Cuff pressure
• Breath sounds

Spontaneous parameters
• Tidal volume
• Minute ventilation
• Vital capacity
• Negative inspiratory pressure

Mechanical ventilator
• Ventilatory mode (control, assist-control, synchronized intermittent mandatory ventilation, pressure support ventilation)
• Tidal volume
• Rate (ventilator and spontaneous)
• Fraction of inspired oxygen
• Positive end-expiratory pressure
• Peak inspiratory flow

---

assister-controllers. In the control mode, a ventilator can deliver a set tidal volume at a prescribed rate, using predetermined inspiratory and expiratory times.

In the assist mode, the patient initiates inspiration and receives a preset tidal volume from the machine, which augments his venti-

Reviewing types of positive-pressure ventilation

Below are several types of mechanical ventilation that use positive-pressure ventilation.

Type	Description	Nursing considerations
Continuous positive-airway pressure	Applies positive pressure during entire respiratory cycle	• Useful for patients who are breathing spontaneously but have hypoxemic respiratory failure; also useful during weaning from positive end-expiratory pressure
Positive end-expiratory pressure	Applies positive pressure during expiration	• Useful for treating hypoxemic respiratory failure • Adults usually receive 5 to 20 cm H_2O of pressure, although higher pressures may be used
Pressure-cycled	Flow continues until a preset pressure is achieved	• Useful when excessive inspiratory pressure may damage lungs, as with neonates • Tidal volume varies with airway resistance and lung compliance • Alveolar ventilation may not be adequate but decrease on shearing forces might damage alveoli
Volume-cycled	Delivers a preset volume to the patient	• Effectively treats respiratory failure in adults because it delivers consistent tidal volume despite changes in airway resistance or lung compliance • Shearing forces, especially if high tidal volumes are used, may injure alveoli

latory effort while letting him determine his own minute ventilation. In the assist-control mode, the patient initiates breathing but a backup control delivers a preset number of breaths at a set volume.

In synchronized intermittent mandatory ventilation (SIMV), the ventilator delivers a set number of specific-volume breaths. The patient may breathe spontaneously between the SIMV breaths at volumes that differ from those on the machine. Often used as a weaning tool, SIMV may be used for ventilation and helps to condition ventilatory muscles.

Nursing care aims to provide emotional support, prevent machine failure, and avert such complications as pneumothorax, atelectasis, decreased cardiac output, pulmonary barotrauma, stress ulcer, and infection.

Patient preparation. Usually, the patient is ventilated using a positive-pressure system. Explain the system to the patient. Set up a communication system with him (such as a Magic Slate or a letter board) and reassure him that a nurse will always be nearby. Keep in mind that an apprehensive patient may fight the machine, defeating its purpose.

Place him in semi-Fowler's position, if possible, to promote lung expansion. Obtain baseline blood pressure and ABG readings.

Monitoring and aftercare. If the patient doesn't have an ET or tracheostomy tube in place, he'll be intubated to establish an artificial airway. A bite block may be used with an oral ET tube to prevent the patient from biting the tube. Arrange for a chest X-ray after intubation to evaluate tube placement. If necessary, use soft restraints to prevent the patient from extubating himself. Be sure a communication device is within reach.

Check ABG levels periodically. Overventilation may cause respiratory alkalosis from decreased carbon dioxide levels. Inadequate alveolar ventilation or atelectasis from an inappropriate tidal volume may cause respiratory acidosis.

Perform the following steps every 1 to 2 hours:
• Check all connections between the ventilator and the patient. Make sure critical alarms are turned on. This includes the low-pressure alarm (not less than 3 cm H_2O), which indicates a disconnection in the system, and the high-pressure alarm (set 20 to 30 cm H_2O greater than the patient's peak airway pressure) to prevent excessive airway pressures. Volume alarms should also be used if available. Ensure that the patient can reach the call bell.
• Verify that ventilator settings are correct and that the ventilator is operating at those settings; compare the patient's respiratory rate with the setting and, for a volume-cycled machine, watch that the spirometer reaches the correct volume. For a pressure-cycled machine, use a respirometer to check exhaled tidal volume.
• Check the humidifier and refill it if necessary. Check the corrugated tubing for condensation; drain any into another container and discard. (*Don't* drain condensation into the humidifier because it may be contaminated with bacteria.)
• Check the temperature gauges, which should be set between 89.6° F (32° C) and 98.6° F (37° C). Also check that gas is being delivered at the correct temperature.
• If ordered, give the patient several deep breaths (usually two or three) each hour by setting the sigh mechanism on the ventilator or by using a handheld resuscitation bag.

Subsequently, check oxygen concentration every 8 hours and overall

ABG values whenever ventilator settings are changed. Assess respiratory status at least every 2 hours in the acutely ill patient and every 4 hours in the stable chronically ill patient. Suction the patient as necessary, noting the amount, color, odor, and consistency of secretions. Auscultate for decreased breath sounds on the left side — an indication of tube slippage into the right mainstem bronchus. Arrange for chest X-rays, as ordered.

Monitor the patient's fluid intake and output and his electrolyte balance. Weigh him as ordered. Using aseptic technique, change the humidifier, nebulizer, and ventilator tubing every 48 hours; ventilate the patient manually during this time. Change his position frequently, and perform chest physiotherapy as necessary. Provide emotional support. Give antacids and other medications, as ordered. Monitor for decreased bowel sounds and distention, which may indicate paralytic ileus. Check nasogastric aspiration and stools for blood, since stress ulcer is a common complication.

If the patient is receiving high-pressure ventilation, assess for pneumothorax, signaled by absent or diminished breath sounds on the affected side, acute chest pain, and possibly tracheal deviation or subcutaneous or mediastinal emphysema. With a high oxygen concentration, watch for signs and symptoms of toxicity: substernal chest pain, increased coughing, tachypnea, decreased lung compliance and vital capacity, and decreased PaO_2 without a change in oxygen concentration.

If the patient fights the ventilator and ineffective ventilation results, give a sedative or a neuromuscular blocking agent, as ordered, and observe him closely.

Wean the patient, as ordered, based on his respiratory status. (See *Weaning the patient from mechanical ventilation.*)

Patient education. If the patient will need to use a ventilator at home, teach him and a family member to check the device and its settings, the nebulizer, and the oxygen equipment at least once a day. Tell the patient to refill his humidifier as necessary. Explain that his ABG levels will need to be measured periodically.

Inform the patient that he should call the doctor if he experiences chest pain, fever, dyspnea, or swollen extremities. Teach him to count his pulse rate, and urge him to report any changes in rate or rhythm. Instruct him to report a weight gain of 5 lb or more within a week.

Tell the patient to clean his tracheostomy daily, using the technique he learned from the nurse or respiratory therapist. Teach him how to clean nondisposable items.

Instruct the patient to try to bring his ventilator with him if he needs treatment for an acute problem. He may be stabilized without hospital admission. Provide the patient with emergency telephone numbers, and tell him to call his doctor or respiratory therapist if he

Weaning the patient from mechanical ventilation

To ensure successful weaning, the patient should have:
• a partial pressure of arterial carbon dioxide ($PaCO_2$) level under 50 mm Hg or whatever is normal for the patient
• an oxygen concentration of 40% or below with a $PaCO_2$ of 60 mm Hg or more
• a vital capacity greater than 10 ml/kg of body weight
• a negative inspiratory force greater than 20 cm H_2O
• minute ventilation of less than 10 L/minute with a tidal volume equal to 5 ml/kg of body weight
• an ability to double his spontaneous resting minute ventilation
• a spontaneous respiratory effort
• successful cessation of neuromuscular blocking drugs and absence of infection, acid-base or electrolyte imbalance, hyperglycemia, fever, arrhythmias, renal failure, shock, anemia, and excessive fatigue.

Once these criteria are met, wean the patient using a conventional T-piece or tracheostomy collar connected to humidified oxygen. Or use continuous positive-airway pressure (CPAP), synchronized intermittent mandatory ventilation (SIMV), or pressure support ventilation.

Conventional weaning
• Obtain baseline arterial blood gas (ABG) levels, pulse rate, breath sounds, and spontaneous tidal volume, minute ventilation, and negative inspiratory force. Connect a T-piece or tracheostomy collar to a separate humidified oxygen system, and adjust the flow rate or concentration. Deflate the cuff for a T-piece trial unless it's needed to prevent aspiration of saliva or stomach contents.
• If possible, place the patient in semi-Fowler's position. Give a bronchodilator, as ordered, and suction 15 minutes before disconnecting the patient from the ventilator.
• Turn on the oxygen source, detach the patient from the ventilator, and connect his tube to the oxygen source for 5 to 10 minutes/hour at the start, gradually increasing by 5 to 15 minutes/hour.
• Watch closely for signs of hypoxia: restlessness, dyspnea, accessory muscle use, altered skin color and level of consciousness, tachycardia, electrocardiogram (ECG) changes, and altered ABG values.

Notify the doctor if the patient's respiratory rate exceeds 30 breaths/minute, his pulse rate rises more than 20 beats/minute, his systolic pressure rises or falls more than 15 mm Hg, or his ECG shows a depressed ST segment or more than six extrasystoles per minute. Draw an ABG sample and reconnect the patient to the ventilator.
• Obtain ABG samples, as ordered, while the patient is breathing spontaneously. Compare results with baseline levels and report changes. When the prescribed amount of time for the weaning session has elapsed, return the patient to the ventilator. Increase weaning times as tolerated. (Weaning at night is usually attempted last, to allow the patient rest.)

Weaning with CPAP
As ordered, use CPAP to help maintain functional residual capacity and

(continued)

Weaning the patient from mechanical ventilation (continued)

partial pressure of arterial oxygen when the patient is breathing spontaneously during weaning. Using a T-piece and a high-flow, air-oxygen blend, CPAP maintains positive airway pressure throughout the respiratory cycle. Before and during treatment, assess the respiratory rate and check for accessory muscle use. Increased rate, reduced volume, and accessory muscle use indicate fatigue.

Weaning with SIMV
In many cases, patients are placed on an SIMV mode for periods during the day and then returned to an assist-control mode for sleep or if they can't sustain spontaneous efforts. Expect to use SIMV if the

patient fails to progress satisfactorily with traditional weaning. This method delivers breaths at preset volumes and intervals but also allows the patient to breathe spontaneously in between.

As ordered, gradually decrease the number of machine-delivered breaths per minute until the patient can breathe on his own. Keep in mind that machine weaning doesn't eliminate the risk of hypoxia, so be sure to evaluate the patient's respiratory status and ABG levels. Know the patient's total minute ventilation necessary to maintain stable ABG levels. Monitor spontaneous minute ventilation carefully as SIMV is reduced. Acidosis and hypercapnia may stem from inadequate ventilation.

doctor or respiratory therapist if he has any questions or problems.

Continuous positive-airway pressure
As its name suggests, CPAP ventilation maintains positive pressure in the airways throughout the patient's entire respiratory cycle. CPAP may be used for either intubated or non-intubated patients. This treatment may be delivered through an artificial airway, a mask, or nasal prongs by means of a ventilator or a separate high-flow generating system.

CPAP is available as a demand system and as a continuous-flow system. In the demand system, a valve opens in response to the patient's inspiratory flow. In the continuous-flow system, an air-oxy-

gen blend flows through a humidifier and a reservoir bag into a T-piece.

CPAP can also be used to help wean a patient from mechanical ventilation. Nasal CPAP is useful or long-term treatment of obstructive sleep apnea. High-flow compressed air is directed into a mask that covers only the patient's nose.

CPAP may cause gastric distress if the patient swallows air during the treatment (most common when CPAP is delivered without intubation). The patient may feel claustrophobic. Mask CPAP shouldn't be used in patients who are unresponsive or at risk for vomiting and aspiration. Rarely, CPAP causes barotrauma or lowers cardiac output.

Patient preparation. If the patient is intubated, attach the CPAP device to his ET or tracheostomy tube. Assess his vital signs and lung sounds to provide a baseline.

If CPAP will be delivered through a mask, a respiratory therapist usually sets up the system. After setup, place the mask on the patient. (The mask should be transparent and lightweight and should have a soft, pliable seal.) Obtain ABG determinations and pulmonary function studies, as ordered, to serve as a baseline.

Procedure. For the intubated adult, set the ventilator to CPAP and adjust the desired setting; the flow required to maintain constant pressure usually is three to four times the patient's minute ventilation. Attach the T-piece on the CPAP device to the patient's ET or tracheostomy tube.

For mask CPAP, adjust the cm H_2O settings to exceed the patient's maximum inspiratory flow rate.

Monitoring and aftercare. If the patient is undergoing CPAP for an acute condition, monitor his heart rate, blood pressure, PAWP, and urine output hourly. Continue to monitor him until he's stable at a CPAP setting necessary to maintain a PaO_2 level greater than 60 mm Hg with an FIO_2 of 0.50 or less. Check for decreased cardiac output. Watch closely for changes in respiratory rate and pattern. Uncoordinated breathing patterns may indicate severe respiratory muscle fatigue

that can't be helped by CPAP. Report this to the doctor; the patient may need mechanical ventilation.

Check the CPAP system for pressure fluctuations. Keep in mind that high airway pressures increase the risk of pneumothorax, so monitor for chest pain and decreased breath sounds. Use oximetry, if possible, to monitor oxygen saturations, especially when you remove the CPAP mask to provide routine care. If the patient is stable, remove his mask briefly every 2 to 4 hours to provide mouth and skin care and fluids. Increase the length of time the mask is off, as the patient's ability to maintain oxygenation without CPAP improves.

Between treatments, apply benzoin to the skin under the edge of the mask to reduce the risk of breakdown and necrosis. Check closely for air leaks around the mask near the eyes; escaping air can dry the eyes, causing conjunctivitis or other problems. Check air intake ports (if present) to detect any obstructions.

If the patient is using a nasal CPAP device for sleep apnea, observe for decreased snoring and mouth breathing while he sleeps. If these symptoms don't subside, notify the doctor; either the system is leaking or the pressure is inadequate.

Patient education. CPAP for sleep apnea is the only treatment requiring instructions for home care.
• Ask the patient to demonstrate use of the system to make sure he can prevent excess leakage and maintain

the prescribed pressures. Teach him how to clean the mask and change the air filter.

• Explain to the patient that he must use nasal CPAP every night, even if he feels well after the initial treatments. Apneic episodes will recur if he doesn't use CPAP as directed. He should call his doctor if his symptoms recur despite consistent use.

• If the patient is obese, explain that he might have less frequent CPAP treatments if he loses weight.

Oxygen therapy

In oxygen therapy, oxygen is delivered by nasal prongs or catheter, mask, or transtracheal catheter to prevent or reverse hypoxemia and reduce the work of breathing. Possible causes of hypoxemia include emphysema, pneumonia, Guillain-Barré syndrome, heart failure, and MI.

The type of equipment used depends on the patient's condition and on the required FIO_2. High-flow systems, such as the Venturi mask and ventilators, deliver a precisely controlled air-oxygen mixture. Low-flow systems, such as nasal prongs or catheter, simple mask, partial rebreather mask, and nonrebreather mask, allow variation in the oxygen percentage delivered, depending on the patient's respiratory pattern.

Nasal prongs deliver low concentrations of oxygen. The prongs permit talking, eating, and suctioning without removal. However, they may cause nasal drying and can't deliver high oxygen concentrations.

In contrast, a nasal catheter can deliver low-flow oxygen at some-

what higher concentrations, but it isn't commonly used because it causes discomfort and dries the mucous membranes. Masks can deliver oxygen concentrations of up to 100%. Transtracheal catheters permit highly efficient oxygen delivery and increased mobility with portable oxygen systems. They also avoid the adverse effects of nasal delivery systems.

Oxygen therapy can cause severe complications. For example, high oxygen concentrations over 24 or more hours can lead to oxygen toxicity, causing possibly permanent cellular damage. High oxygen concentrations in the patient with chronic hypercapnia can eliminate the patient's stimulus to breathe, causing acute respiratory failure.

Patient preparation. Instruct the patient, his roommates, and any visitors not to smoke or use an improperly grounded radio, television, electric razor, or other equipment. Place an "oxygen precautions" sign on the outside of the patient's door.

Perform a cardiopulmonary assessment, and check that baseline ABG values or oximetry values have been obtained. Check the patency of the patient's nostrils (he may need a mask if they're blocked). Consult the doctor if a change in administration route is necessary.

Assemble the equipment, check all the connections, and turn on the oxygen source. Make sure that the humidifier is bubbling and that oxygen is flowing through the prongs, catheter, or mask. Set the flow rate, as ordered. If necessary, have the respiratory therapist check the flowmeter for accuracy.

Procedure. If you're inserting a *nasal cannula,* direct the curved prongs inward, following the nostrils' natural curvature. Hook the tubing behind the patient's ears and under his chin. Set the flow rate, as ordered.

If you're inserting a *nasal catheter,* determine the length to insert by stretching one end of the catheter from the tip of the patient's nose to his earlobe. Mark this spot. Then lubricate the catheter with sterile water or water-soluble lubricant, and gently insert the catheter through the nostril into the nasopharynx to the premeasured length. Use a flashlight and a tongue depressor to check that the catheter is positioned correctly: It should be directly behind the uvula but not beyond it (misdirected airflow may cause gastric distention). If the catheter causes the patient to gag or choke, withdraw it slightly. Secure the catheter by taping it at the nose and cheek, and set the flow rate, as ordered.

If you're using a *mask,* make sure the flow rate is at least 5 L/minute. Lower flow rates won't flush carbon dioxide from any mask. Now place the mask over the patient's nose, mouth, and chin, and press the flexible metal edge so that it fits the bridge of the patient's nose. Use gauze padding, as necessary, to ensure comfort and a proper fit.

The *partial rebreather mask* has an attached reservoir bag that conserves the first portion of the patient's exhalation and also fills with 100% oxygen before the next breath, delivering oxygen concentrations ranging from 40% at a flow rate of 8 L/minute to 60% at a flow rate of 15 L/minute. The *nonrebreather mask* also has a reservoir bag and can deliver oxygen concentrations ranging from 60% at a flow rate of 8 L/minute to 90% at a flow rate of 15 L/minute. Set flow rates for these masks, as ordered, but keep in mind that the reservoir bag should deflate only slightly during inspiration. If it deflates completely or markedly, increase the flow rate as necessary.

The *Venturi mask* delivers the most precise oxygen concentrations—to within 1% of the setting. If you use this mask, make sure its air entrainment ports don't become blocked. Otherwise, the patient's FIO_2 level could rise dangerously.

If a *transtracheal oxygen catheter* will be used to deliver oxygen, the doctor will give the patient a local anesthetic before inserting this device into the trachea.

Monitoring and aftercare. Periodically perform a cardiopulmonary assessment on the patient receiving any form of oxygen therapy. If the patient is on bed rest, change his position frequently. Provide good skin care to prevent irritation and breakdown caused by the tubing, prongs, or mask. Humidify any oxygen flow exceeding 3 L/minute to prevent drying of mucous membranes.

Assess for signs of hypoxia, including decreased level of consciousness, tachycardia, arrhythmias, diaphoresis, restlessness, altered blood pressure or respiratory rate, clammy skin, and cyanosis. If any of these occurs, notify the doctor and check the oxygen delivery equipment for malfunction. Be especially alert for changes in respiratory status when you change or discontinue oxygen therapy.

If your patient is using a nonrebreather mask, periodically check the valves to see if they're functioning properly. If the valves stick closed, the patient will not receive adequate oxygen. Replace the mask, if necessary.

If the patient is receiving high oxygen concentrations (exceeding 50%) for more than 24 hours, ask about symptoms of oxygen toxicity, such as burning, substernal chest pain, dyspnea, and dry cough. Atelectasis and pulmonary edema may also occur. (Encourage coughing and deep breathing.) Monitor ABG levels frequently, and reduce oxygen concentrations as soon as ABG results indicate that this is feasible.

If your patient has chronic pulmonary disease, use a flow rate that will provide an SaO_2 of about 90% by pulse oximetry. A greater O_2 saturation may eliminate the patient's hypoxic drive and cause respiratory depression and possibly apnea. However, *don't* use a simple face mask because low flow rates will not flush carbon dioxide from the mask. Watch for alterations in level of consciousness, heart rate, and respiratory rate.

Patient education. If the patient needs oxygen at home, the doctor will order the flow rate, the number of hours per day to be used, and the conditions of use if less than 24 hours. Several types of delivery systems are available, including a tank, a concentrator, and a liquid oxygen system. The choice of system will depend on the patient's needs and on the availability and cost of each system. Make sure the patient can use the prescribed system safely and effectively. Regular follow-up care is necessary to evaluate response.

Humidification and aerosol treatments

In humidification, water vapor is added to inspired gas to maintain airway moisture during inspiration of dry gases. Aerosols (fine particles of liquid suspended in a gas) can be used to deliver medications.

Humidity may be added directly to the air by a room humidifier or it may be given with oxygen, using an in-line device such as a cold bubble diffuser or a cascade humidifier. Some type of humidification device can be used with every oxygen delivery device, except for the Venturi mask. (If the patient with a Venturi mask needs humidification, entrained room air, rather than the oxygen, is humidified.)

A large-volume nebulizer supplies cool or heated moisture to the patient whose upper airway has been bypassed by ET intubation or a tracheostomy, or who has recently been extubated. The ultrasonic nebulizer provides intermittent therapy for the patient with thick secretions, helping to mobilize them and promote a productive cough. The small-volume nebulizer is typically used to deliver aerosolized medications, such as bronchodilators, mucolytics, and antibiotics.

Aerosols should be used cautiously in patients susceptible to fluid accumulation and atelectasis, especially those with heart failure, respiratory distress, or a depressed cough reflex. Because they can precipitate bronchospasm, aerosols should also be given cautiously to asthmatic patients.

Patient preparation. Explain the procedure to the patient. Allow him to used to the mask. Explain that it may obscure his vision.

Procedure. For a room humidifier, direct the nozzle away from the patient's face and look for visible mist at the nozzle's mouth. Close all doors and windows to maintain humidity in the room.

For a cold bubble diffuser, set the oxygen flowmeter at the prescribed rate and check the device for positive pressure release. If this doesn't occur, tighten the connections and check again. Then apply the oxygen delivery device to the patient. The water in the humidifier should bubble as oxygen passes through it.

For a cascade humidifier, adjust the temperature to 89.6° to 98.6° F (32° to 37° C), as ordered, and arrange the tubing so that condensation flows away from the patient.

For a large-volume nebulizer, attach the nebulizer to the flowmeter and set the flowmeter to at least 10 L.

For an ultrasonic nebulizer, turn on the machine and check for misting at the outflow port. Have the patient breathe slowly and deeply.

If needed, teach the patient to use a handheld nebulizer. Stress that he should inhale the medication slowly and deeply, then hold his breath for 3 to 5 seconds.

Monitoring and aftercare. After an aerosol treatment, encourage the patient to cough and deep-breathe to mobilize secretions. Suction him if necessary. Evaluate therapy by comparing current breath sounds with pretreatment findings. Document the amount, color, and consistency of his sputum. If no improvement occurs or the patient's condition worsens, notify the doctor.

Check the water level in the device frequently and refill or replace it, as needed. Change and clean the equipment regularly, according to policy. If the patient tires, stop the treatment and turn off the equipment briefly.

If you're using a cascade humidifier, monitor the temperature closely, and replace the water if it's too hot. Make sure the tubing is placed to prevent condensation from flowing toward the patient, where it may be aspirated. When water collects in the tubing, disconnect the tubing from the nebulizer and drain the water into a waste container.

If you're using a heated large-volume nebulizer, frequently monitor the temperature, using an in-line thermometer. Tell the patient to report any discomfort, and turn off the heater when the equipment is turned off. Check the patient for signs of overhydration, such as sudden weight gain, crackles, or electrolyte imbalance.

If the patient is receiving ultrasonic nebulizer treatment, watch him for bronchospasm and dyspnea. Stay with him for the duration of treatment (usually 15 to 20 minutes). Be ready to discontinue treatment promptly.

When administering medication by side-stream nebulizer or mininebulizer, take the patient's vital signs before treatment begins and monitor for drug reactions.

Patient education. Before discharge, tell the patient using a room humidifier at home that he can fill it with plain tap water or distilled water. Also tell him to run a solution of vinegar and water through the unit daily. Instruct him to do this in a well-ventilated room and to rinse the unit well afterward.

Tell the patient to report sudden weight gain, a change in his cough or sputum production, congestion, edema, or dyspnea.

Incentive spirometry

Primarily used postoperatively to prevent respiratory complications, incentive spirometry measures respiratory flow or volume. A *flow-incentive* spirometer measures the patient's inspiratory effort, or flow rate, in cubic centimeters per second. A *volume-incentive* spirometer does this and also calculates the volume of inspired air.

Both types aim to encourage the patient to produce the deep, sustained inspiratory efforts that normally occur as yawns or sighs. As he steadily strives to meet his target flow or volume, he prevents or reverses atelectasis.

Patient preparation. If you plan to use incentive spirometry postoperatively, explain the procedure and familiarize the patient with the device before surgery, when he can practice. Adjust the target respiratory flow or volume, as ordered. Before the patient practices deep breathing, auscultate his lungs to obtain a baseline.

Procedure. Tell the patient the target flow or volume, and instruct him to exhale slowly and completely after each breath. Have him place the mouthpiece between his teeth and close to his lips. Then have him take a slow, deep breath through his mouth until he reaches the preset goal. Tell him to remove the mouthpiece, hold his breath for 3 to 5 seconds, and exhale slowly. Encourage him to repeat this procedure 10 times each hour or as ordered.

Monitoring and aftercare. Your patient may understand the need to perform incentive spirometry, but when he's weak, sedated, or in pain, you'll need to encourage him. He should show progressive improvement in volume: a daily increase of 20% if he doesn't have underlying lung disease. Document the volume and repetitions he achieves and auscultate his lungs after each treatment. If he doesn't show the expected improvement, notify the doctor and check the patient's temperature, lung sounds, and sputum production. He may be developing a pulmonary infection.

When your patient has met his goal and maintained it for 2 to 3 days, expect to discontinue incentive spirometry. However, continue to encourage deep breathing, coughing, and ambulation.

Physiotherapy and bronchoscopy

Physiotherapy or bronchoscopy may be used to promote drainage of secretions or to remove a foreign body or a mucus plug.

Chest physiotherapy

Chest physiotherapy includes postural drainage, chest percussion and vibration, and coughing and deep-breathing exercises. *Postural drainage* uses gravity to promote drainage of secretions from the lungs and bronchi into the trachea. *Percussion*, which involves cupping the hands and fingers together and clapping them alternately over the patient's lung fields, loosens secretions, as does the gentler technique of *vibration*. *Coughing* helps clear the lungs, bronchi, and trachea of secretions and prevents aspiration. *Deep-breathing exercises* help loosen secretions and promote more effective coughing. Especially important for the bedridden patient, these treatments improve secretion clearance and ventilation and help prevent or treat atelectasis and pneumonia.

Indications for chest physiotherapy include the presence of secretions (from such conditions as bronchitis or pneumonia), COPD, diseases that have increased the risk of aspiration (such as muscular dystrophy and cerebral palsy), postoperative incisional pain that restricts breathing, and prolonged immobility. Chest physiotherapy is usually performed with other treatments, such as suctioning, incentive spirometry, and administration of medications such as expectorants.

Contraindications include active or recent pulmonary hemorrhage, untreated pneumothorax, lung contusion, recent MI, pulmonary tuberculosis, pulmonary tumor or abscess, osteoporosis, fractured ribs, or an unstable chest wall. Perform chest physiotherapy cautiously in patients with head injuries or with recent eye or cranial surgery.

Patient preparation. Explain the procedure. As ordered, give pain medication and teach the patient to splint his incision. Auscultate the lungs to determine baseline status, and check the doctor's order to determine which lung areas require treatment.

Obtain pillows and a tilt board if necessary. *Don't* schedule therapy immediately after a meal. Make sure the patient is adequately hydrated before you begin. If ordered, first administer bronchodilator and mist therapy.

Provide tissues, an emesis basin, and a cup for sputum. If the patient doesn't have an adequate cough to clear secretions, set up suction equipment. If he needs oxygen therapy or is borderline hypoxemic without it, use adequate flow rates of oxygen during therapy.

Procedure. For *postural drainage,* position the patient as ordered. (The doctor usually determines a position sequence after auscultation and chest X-ray review.) If the patient has a localized condition such as pneumonia in a specific lobe, expect to start with that area first. If the patient has a diffuse disorder such as bronchiectasis, expect to start with the lower lobes and work toward the upper ones. Move through the positions in a way that minimizes the patient's repositioning efforts. Tell him to remain in each position for 10 to 15 minutes. During this time, perform percussion and vibration, as ordered.

For *percussion,* place your cupped hands against the patient's chest wall and rapidly flex and extend your wrists, generating a rhythmic, popping sound (a hollow sound helps verify correct performance of the technique). Percuss each segment for a minimum of 3 minutes. The vibrations you generate pass through the chest wall and help loosen secretions from the airways. Perform percussion throughout both inspiration and expiration, and encourage the patient to take slow, deep breaths. *Don't* percuss over the spine, sternum, liver, kidneys, or the female patient's breasts because you may cause trauma, especially in elderly patients.

For *vibration,* hold your hand flat against the patient's chest wall and, during exhalation, vibrate your hands rapidly by tensing your arm and shoulder muscles. This rapid oscillation aids secretion movement by increasing the velocity and turbulence of exhaled air. Repeat vibration for five exhalations over each chest segment. When the patient says "ah" on exhalation, you should hear a quaver in his voice.

After you complete postural drainage, percussion, or vibration, instruct the patient in *coughing* to remove loosened secretions. Have him take slow, deep breaths, and place your hands on his chest wall to help him direct air to the lower and peripheral areas of his lungs. Tell him to push his abdomen out on inspiration, which will give his diaphragm more room to move downward. Tell him to inhale deeply through his mouth or nose and then exhale in three short huffs or coughs through a slightly open mouth. An effective cough sounds deep and almost hollow; an ineffective cough, shallow and high-pitched. Have him repeat the coughing sequence at least two or three times.

For *deep breathing,* place the patient in a sitting position with feet well supported. Have him inhale slowly and deeply, pushing his abdomen out against his hand to maximize air distribution. Tell him to exhale through pursed lips and to contract his abdomen. Initially, have him do this exercise for 1 minute and then rest for 2 minutes. Gradually increase this to 10 minutes four times each day.

After chest physiotherapy, auscultate the patient's lungs.

Monitoring and aftercare. Evaluate the patient's tolerance for therapy and make adjustments as needed.

Assess for any difficulty in expectorating secretions, and use suction if the patient has an ineffective cough or a diminished gag reflex. Provide oral hygiene after therapy because secretions may taste foul or have an unpleasant odor.

Patient education. The patient with chronic bronchitis, or bronchiectasis, may need chest physiotherapy at home. Teach him and his family the appropriate techniques and positions. Arrange for the patient to get a mechanical percussion and vibration device if necessary.

Bronchoscopy

A foreign body or mucus lodged in the tracheobronchial tree can be removed with a rigid metal or flexible fiber-optic bronchoscope. Although the rigid bronchoscope allows more room for foreign body removal, it's usually used only in the operating room. The flexible fiber-optic bronchoscope, a slender tube containing fine glass fibers that transmit light, effectively removes mucus plugs and secretions.

Usually done with a local anesthetic, bronchoscopic removal of a foreign body or mucus may also be performed on a patient on a ventilator who has an ET or tracheostomy tube in place.

Possible complications of bronchoscopy include hypoxemia, hemorrhage (most likely when a biopsy is done concurrently), respiratory distress, pneumothorax, bronchospasm, and infection.

Patient preparation. Describe the treatment to the patient and explain its purpose. Assess his condition and obtain baseline vital signs. If possible, have him fast for 6 to 12 hours before treatment.

The room where bronchoscopy will be performed will be darkened. Advise the patient that he may receive a sedative to help him relax. Inform him that a local anesthetic will be sprayed into his nose and mouth. The spray has an unpleasant taste and the patient may have a sensation of pharyngeal fullness during treatment. Reassure him that he'll be able to breathe but won't be able to speak.

Procedure. Place the patient in a sitting position on an examination table or a bed. If he wears dentures, have him remove them. Tell him to remain relaxed, to hyperextend his neck, to place his arms at his side, and to breathe through his nose. As ordered, give medications such as atropine and an I.V. barbiturate or narcotic.

Assemble equipment, including intubation equipment and a high-flow oxygen source in case of emergency. Typical equipment consists of a flexible fiber-optic bronchoscope, 2% to 4% lidocaine, sterile gloves, an emesis basin, a handheld resuscitation bag with face mask, oral and ET airways, a laryngoscope, suction equipment, and masks and eye protectors for the staff. If the patient requires controlled mechanical ventilation, obtain a bronchoscopy adapter.

Monitoring and aftercare. Check the patient's vital signs during the procedure and every 15 minutes afterward until they're stable. Place him in semi-Fowler's position. Keep resuscitation equipment and a tracheotomy tray at hand for 24 hours.

Watch for and immediately report symptoms of respiratory difficulty, such as stridor and dyspnea resulting from laryngeal edema or laryngospasm. Observe for bleeding and listen for wheezing, a sign of bronchospasm. Monitor for dyspnea and diminished breath sounds on one side, which may indicate pneumothorax. Report any abnormal findings to the doctor, and prepare for a chest X-ray, if ordered.

Provide an emesis basin and instruct the patient to spit out saliva rather than swallow it. Expect to find blood-tinged sputum for up to several hours. However, report prolonged bleeding or persistent hemoptysis to the doctor.

Restrict all oral intake until after the patient's gag reflex returns. If he experiences hoarseness and a sore throat, provide medicated lozenges when allowed and encourage him not to talk, to rest his vocal cords.

Patient education. If the procedure was performed on an outpatient basis or in the emergency room, tell the patient that he should report any shortness of breath, pain, or prolonged bleeding.

Advise the patient not to strain his voice, but reassure him that his sore throat and hoarseness are temporary. Tell him to report signs of infection, such as fever or thick, yellow sputum.

REFERENCES AND READINGS

Bolton, P. and Kline K. "Understanding Modes of Mechanical Ventilation," *AJN* 94(6):36, 1994.

Guyton, A.C. and Hall, J. *Textbook of Medical Physiology,* 9th ed. Philadelphia: W.B. Saunders Co., 1996.

Ignatavicius, D., et al. *Medical Surgical Nursing: A Nursing Process Approach,* 2nd ed. Philadelphia: W.B. Saunders Co., 1995.

Illustrated Guide to Diagnostic Tests, 2nd ed. Springhouse, Pa.: Springhouse Corp., 1997.

Jones, M., et al. "ARDS — New Ways to Fight An Old Enemy Revisited," *Nursing94* 24(12):34, 1994.

Taylor, C.M., et al. *Nursing Diagnosis Pocket Manual.* Springhouse, Pa.: Springhouse Corp., 1996.

Thelan, L., et al. *Textbook of Critical Care Nursing: Diagnosis and Management,* 2nd ed. St. Louis: Mosby, 1994.

5

CARDIOVASCULAR CARE

In North America, more than 70 million people suffer from some form of cardiovascular disorder, and many of them suffer from a combination of disorders. Year after year, the number of affected patients continues to rise.

This chapter will help you provide effective care for these patients, promote recovery, improve patient compliance, and ensure adequate home care.

ASSESSMENT

Performed correctly, assessment helps identify and evaluate changes in the patient's cardiac function—changes that may disrupt or threaten his life. Baseline information obtained during assessment will help guide your intervention and follow-up care. (See *Key questions for assessing cardiac function*, page 134.)

Note, however, that if your patient is in a cardiac crisis you'll have to rethink your assessment priorities. The patient's condition and the clinical situation will dictate what steps to take. See the section on cardiac emergencies at the end of this chapter.

Inspection

Inspect the patient's chest and thorax. Expose the anterior chest and observe its general appearance. Normally, the lateral diameter is twice the anteroposterior diameter. Note deviations from typical chest shape.

Checking for jugular vein distention. When the patient is supine, the neck veins normally protrude; when the patient stands, they normally lie flat. To check for jugular vein distention, place the patient in semi-Fowler's position with the head turned slightly away from the side being examined. Use tangential lighting (lighting from the side) to cast small shadows along the neck. This will allow you to see pulse wave movement better. If jugular veins appear distended, it indicates high

Key questions for assessing cardiac function

Ask the following questions to help the patient more accurately describe the symptoms of cardiovascular illness:

• Can you point to the site of your pain?
• Do you get a burning or squeezing sensation in your chest?
• What relieves the pain?
• Do you ever feel short of breath? Does a particular body position seem to bring this on? Which one? How long does any shortness of breath last? What relieves it?
• Has sudden breathing trouble ever woken you up?
• Do you ever wake up coughing? How often?
• Have you ever coughed up blood?
• Does your heart ever pound or skip a beat? If so, when does this happen?
• Do you ever get dizzy or faint? What brings this on?
• Do your feet or ankles swell? At what time of day? Does anything relieve the swelling?
• Do you urinate more frequently at night?
• Do any activities tire you? Which ones? Have you had to limit your activities or rest more often while doing them?

right atrial pressure and an increase in fluid volume caused by right heart dysfunction.

Characterize distention as mild, moderate, or severe. Determine the level of distention in fingerbreadths above the clavicle or in relation to the jaw or clavicle. Also, note the amount of distention in relation to head elevation.

You can use jugular vein distention to obtain a rough estimate of central venous pressure (CVP). In addition, observing pulsations of the right internal jugular vein will help to assess right heart dynamics. (See *Assessing jugular venous pulse.*)

Inspecting the precordium. Place the patient in a supine position with the head flat or elevated for respiratory comfort. Stand to the right of the patient. Then identify the necessary anatomic landmarks. (See *Inspecting and palpating the precordium,* page 136.)

Using tangential lighting to cast shadows across the chest, watch for chest wall movement, visible pulsations, and exaggerated lifts or heaves (strong outward thrusts palpated over the chest during systole) in all areas of the precordium.

Normally, you'll see pulsations at the point of maximal impulse (PMI) of the apical impulse. The apical impulse (pulsations at the apex of the heart) normally appears in the fifth intercostal space at or just medial to the midclavicular line. This impulse reflects the location and size of the heart, especially of the left ventricle.

Palpation

Palpate the peripheral pulses and precordium. Also, warm your hands and remember to use gentle to moderate pressure.

Assessing jugular venous pulse

Inspecting the right jugular venous pulse can provide information about the dynamics of the right side of the heart. The jugular venous pulse consists of five waves: three positive, or ascending, waves (a, c, and v) and two negative, or descending, waves (x and y).

The following pulsations of the positive waves occur 3/8" to 3/4" (1 to 2 cm) above the clavicle, just medial to the sternocleidomastoid muscle. Use the carotid pulse or heart sounds to time venous pulsations with the cardiac cycle:

• The a wave marks the initial pulsation of the jugular vein. Occurring just before the first heart sound, it results from right atrial contraction and transmission of pressure to the jugular veins.

• The c wave occurs shortly after the first heart sound. It results from tricuspid valve closing at the beginning of ventricular systole.

• The v wave peaks during ventricular contraction as the tricuspid valve bulges into the right atrium.

Although the negative waves aren't visible as pulsations, they help define the ascending pulses and are shown when the jugular venous pulse is recorded as a waveform. The negative waves occur as follows:

• The x descent follows the a and c waves. It results from right atrial relaxation, ventricular filling, and falling right atrial pressure.

• The y descent reflects the drop in right atrial pressure from the v wave peak that occurs with ventricular systole and the opening of the tricuspid valve.

Implications

Abnormal jugular vein pulsations may signal an arrhythmia. For example, an exaggerated a wave may indicate pulmonary or tricuspid stenosis—conditions that elevate right atrial pressure. A giant a wave, or cannon wave, may signal serious conduction defects. A giant v wave may indicate tricuspid valve insufficiency with regurgitant blood flow.

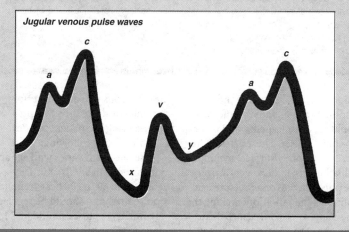

Jugular venous pulse waves

Inspecting and palpating the precordium

Use the following guidelines when inspecting and palpating the precordium:

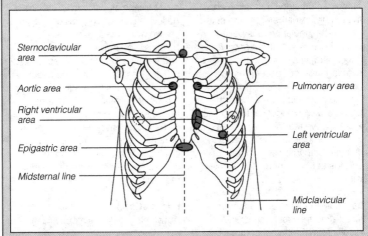

Sternoclavicular area

Aortic area

Right ventricular area

Epigastric area

Midsternal line

Pulmonary area

Left ventricular area

Midclavicular line

- Locate the six precordial areas by using the anatomic landmarks named for the *underlying structures.*
- Palpate (or inspect) the *sternoclavicular area,* which lies at the top of the sternum at the junction of the clavicles.
- Move to the *aortic area,* located in the second intercostal space on the right sternal border.
- Assess the *pulmonary area,* found in the second intercostal space on the left sternal border.

- Palpate the *right ventricular area*—the point where the fifth rib joins the left sternal border.
- Then assess the *left ventricular area (apical area),* which falls at the fifth intercostal space at the midclavicular line.
- Finally, palpate the *epigastric area* at the base of the sternum between the cartilage of the left and right seventh ribs.

Palpating pulses. Palpate the carotid, brachial, radial, femoral, popliteal, dorsalis pedis, and posterior tibial pulses. These arteries are close to the body surface, making palpation easier. Press gently over the pulse sites; excess pressure can obliterate the pulsation, making the pulse appear absent. Also, palpate only one carotid artery at a time;

simultaneous palpation can slow the pulse or decrease blood pressure, causing the patient to faint.

Look for the following:
- pulse rate—this varies with age and other factors; in adults, it usually ranges from 60 to 100 beats/minute
- pulse rhythm—should be regular
- symmetry—pulses should be equally strong bilaterally

• contour—the wavelike flow of the pulse, the upstroke and downstroke, should be smooth
• strength—pulses should be easily palpable; obliterating the pulse should require strong finger pressure.

Grade the pulse amplitude bilaterally at each site. Use a pulse rating scale, such as a 3+ scale in which 0 is absent; 1 is weak; 2 is normal; and 3 is bounding. Document any variations in rate, rhythm, contour, symmetry, and strength.

Palpating the precordium. Follow a systematic palpation sequence covering the sternoclavicular, aortic, pulmonary, right ventricular, left ventricular (apical), and epigastric areas. Use the pads of the fingers to effectively assess large pulse sites. Finger pads prove especially sensitive to vibrations.

Start at the sternoclavicular area and move methodically through the palpation sequence down to the epigastric area. At the sternoclavicular area, you may feel pulsation of the aortic arch, especially in a thin or average-build patient.

To locate the apical impulse, place your fingers in the fifth intercostal space at or just medial to the midclavicular line. Usually, you palpate the apical pulse best at the PMI; light palpation should reveal a tap with each heartbeat over a space roughly $3/4''$ (2 cm) in diameter.

Moderately strong, the apical impulse demonstrates a swift upstroke and downstroke early in systole, caused by left ventricular movement. It normally lasts for about one-third of the cardiac cycle, if the heart rate is under 100 beats/minute. It should correlate with the first heart sound and carotid pulsation.

You should not be able to palpate pulsations over the aortic, pulmonary, or right ventricular area.

Auscultation

The cardiovascular system requires more auscultation than any other body system.

Auscultating the precordium. Practice auscultating and identifying heart sounds in the precordium. First practice identifying normal heart sounds, rates, and rhythms. Then auscultate patients with known abnormal sounds, seeking help from experts to identify findings.

Expect some difficulty. Fat, muscle, and air tend to reduce sound transmission.

Make sure the room is quiet. Use the diaphragm of the stethoscope to detect the normal higher-pitched heart sounds (S_1 and S_2). Use the bell to identify low-pitched sounds, such as mitral murmurs and gallops.

Help the patient into a supine position. Use alternative positions, as needed, to improve heart sound auscultation.

Instruct the patient to breathe normally, inhaling through the nose and exhaling through the mouth. Warm the stethoscope chestpiece by rubbing it between your hands.

Identify cardiac auscultation sites. Most normal heart sounds result from vibrations created by the opening and closing of the heart valves. Auscultation sites don't lie directly over the valves, but over the pathways the blood takes as it flows through chambers and valves. (See *Auscultation sites.*)

Now auscultate, listening selectively for each cardiac cycle component. Move the stethoscope slowly and methodically over the four main auscultation sites.

You must concentrate to hear these relatively quiet sounds. Keep your hand steady, and ask the patient to remain as still as possible.

Begin by listening for a few cycles to become accustomed to the rate and rhythm of the sounds. Two sounds normally occur: the first heart sound (S_1) and the second heart sound (S_2). They sound relatively high pitched and are separated by a silent period.

You'll characterize heart sounds by their pitch (frequency), intensity (loudness), duration, quality (such as musical or harsh), location, and radiation. The timing of heart sounds in relation to the cardiac cycle is particularly important. Normal heart sounds last only a fraction of a second, followed by slightly longer periods of silence.

The first heart sound. The first heart sound—the *lub* of *lub-dub*—marks the beginning of systole. It occurs as the mitral and tricuspid valves close. The closing of these valves immediately precedes elevation of ventricular pressure, aortic and pulmonary valve opening, and ejection of blood into the circula-

tion. All this occurs within one-third of a second.

The mitral valve actually closes slightly before the tricuspid valve. An experienced examiner may be able to discriminate the corresponding sound (split S_1), which sounds somewhat like *li-lub*. However, an inexperienced examiner may confuse a split S_1 with an abnormal extra sound occurring just before S_1.

The first heart sound is louder in the mitral and tricuspid listening areas (*LUB-dub*) and softer in the aortic and pulmonary areas (*lub-DUB*). Comparing the loudness of the normal heart sounds at each site will help you differentiate systole from diastole. Learning to identify phases of the cardiac cycle will help you to time abnormal sounds.

The second heart sound. The *dub* of *lub-dub*—occurs at the beginning of diastole. The S_2 sound coincides with the closing of the aortic and pulmonic valves; it's louder in the aortic and pulmonary areas of the chest. At these sites, the sequence sounds like *lub-DUB*. The second heart sound coincides with the pulse downstroke. At normal rates, the diastolic pause between S_2 and the next S_1 exceeds the systolic pause between S_1 and S_2.

During auscultation, S_2 may have a split sound, like that of a broken syllable. This may occur normally when aortic and pulmonic valves don't close at exactly the same time. Split S_2 commonly occurs in healthy children and young adults.

Auscultation sites

When auscultating for heart sounds, place the stethoscope over four different sites. Follow the same auscultation sequence during every cardiovascular assessment:

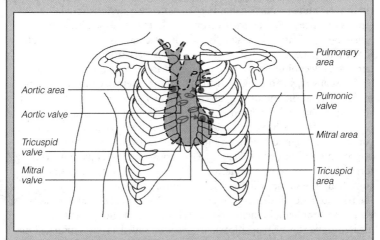

- Place the stethoscope in the second intercostal space along the right sternal border. In the aortic area, blood moves from the left ventricle during systole, crossing the aortic valve and flowing through the aortic arch.
- Move to the pulmonary area, located in the second intercostal space at the left sternal border. In the pulmonary area, blood ejected from the right ventricle during systole crosses the pulmonary valve and flows through the main pulmonary artery.
- Assess in the third auscultation site, the tricuspid area, which lies in the fifth intercostal space along the left sternal border. In the tricuspid area, sounds reflect blood movement from the right atrium across the tricuspid valve, filling the right ventricle during diastole.
- Finally, listen in the mitral area, located in the fifth intercostal space near the midclavicular line. (If the patient's heart is enlarged, the mitral area may be closer to the anterior axillary line.) In the mitral, or apical, area, sounds represent blood flow across the mitral valve and left ventricular filling during diastole.

At each auscultatory site, use the diaphragm to listen closely to S_1 and S_2 and compare them. Next, listen to the systolic period and the diastolic period. Then, auscultate again, using the bell of the stethoscope. If you hear any sounds during the systolic or diastolic period, or any variations in S_1 and S_2, document the characteristics of the sound. Note the auscultatory site and part of the cardiac cycle in which it occurred.

The third heart sound. Also known as S_3 or a ventricular gallop, its rhythm resembles a horse galloping, and its cadence resembles the word *Ken-tuc-ky* (*lub-dub-by*). Listen for S_3 with the patient supine or in the left-lateral decubitus position.

S_3 usually occurs during early to middiastole, at the end of the passive filling phase of either ventricle. It may signify that the ventricle isn't compliant enough to accept the filling volume without additional force. If the right ventricle is noncompliant, the sound will occur in the tricuspid area; if the left ventricle is noncompliant, in the mitral area. A heave may be palpable when the sound occurs.

An S_3 may occur normally in a child or young adult. In a patient over age 30, it usually indicates a disorder such as right-sided heart failure (HF), left-sided HF, pulmonary congestion, intracardiac shunting of blood, myocardial infarction (MI), anemia, or thyrotoxicosis.

The fourth heart sound. This heart sound is S_4 and occurs late in diastole, just before the pulse upstroke. It immediately precedes the S_1 of the next cycle and is associated with acceleration and deceleration of blood entering a chamber that resists additional filling. Known as the atrial or presystolic gallop, it occurs during atrial contraction.

The fourth heart sound shares the same cadence as the word *Ten-nes-see* (*le-lub-dub*). Heard best with the bell of the stethoscope and with the patient in a supine position, S_4 may occur in the tricuspid or mitral area, depending on which ventricle is dysfunctional.

In many cases, it indicates cardiovascular disease, such as acute MI, hypertension, coronary artery disease (CAD), cardiomyopathy, angina, anemia, elevated left ventricular pressure, or aortic stenosis. If the sound persists, it may indicate impaired ventricular compliance or volume overload. It commonly appears in elderly patients with age-related systolic hypertension and aortic stenosis.

Occasionally, a patient may have both a third and a fourth heart sound called a summation gallop. Auscultation may reveal two separate abnormal heart sounds and two normal sounds. Usually, the patient has tachycardia and diastole is shortened. S_3 and S_4 occur so close together that they appear to be one sound—a summation gallop.

Murmurs. Murmurs are longer than a heart sound and occur as a vibrating, blowing, or rumbling noise. Turbulent blood flow produces a murmur.

If you detect a murmur, identify where it is loudest, pinpoint the time it occurs during the cardiac cycle, and describe its pitch, pattern, quality, and intensity.

Abnormal heart sounds. During auscultation, three other abnormal sounds may occur: clicks, snaps, and rubs. These sounds may indicate a need for diagnostic examination.

Clicks. A click usually precedes a late systolic murmur caused by regurgitation of a little blood from the left ventricle into the left atrium.

To detect the high-pitched click of mitral valve prolapse, place the stethoscope diaphragm at the apex and listen during midsystole to late systole. To enhance the sound, change the patient's position to sitting or standing, and listen along the lower left sternal border.

Snaps. Upon placing the stethoscope diaphragm medial to the apex along the lower left sternal border, you may detect an opening snap immediately after S_2. The snap resembles the normal S_1 and S_2 in quality; its high pitch helps differentiate it from an S_3. The opening snap usually precedes a midsystole to late diastolic murmur—a classic sign of stenosis.

Rubs. To detect a pericardial friction rub, use the diaphragm of the stethoscope to auscultate in the third left intercostal space along the lower left sternal border. Listen for a harsh, scratchy, scraping, or squeaking sound that occurs throughout systole, diastole, or both. Have the patient sit upright and lean forward or exhale to enhance the sound. A rub usually indicates pericarditis.

Auscultating the arteries. Auscultate the carotid, femoral, and popliteal arteries as well as the abdominal aorta. Over the carotid, femoral, and popliteal arteries, auscultation should reveal no sounds; over the abdominal aorta, it may detect bowel sounds, but no vascular sounds.

During auscultation of the central and peripheral arteries, you may notice a bruit—a continuous sound caused by turbulent blood flow. A bruit over the carotid artery usually indicates atherosclerosis; over the femoral or popliteal arteries, narrowed vessels; over the abdominal aorta, an aneurysm or a dissection.

DIAGNOSTIC TESTS

Today, safe and effective nursing care means, in part, becoming fully familiar with commonly performed diagnostic tests and keeping up with rapid advances in testing. (See *Diagnostic tests for cardiovascular disorders,* pages 142 to 147.)

NURSING DIAGNOSES

When caring for patients with cardiovascular disorders, you'll find that several nursing diagnoses are commonly used. These diagnoses appear below, along with appropriate nursing interventions and rationales. (Rationales appear in italic type.)

Decreased cardiac output

Related to reduced stroke volume, decreased cardiac output may be associated with such conditions as angina, infective endocarditis, HF, MI, valvular heart disease, and other ailments.

(Text continues on page 147.)

Diagnostic tests for cardiovascular disorders

Tests	Purpose	Nursing considerations
Chest X-ray	To help detect cardiac enlargement, pulmonary congestion, pleural effusion and calcium deposits in or on the heart and show placement of a pacemaker, hemodynamic monitoring or tracheal tubes	• Explain the procedure to the patient. • No food or fluid restriction. • Explain that he'll have to hold his breath during the X-ray.
Serum electrolytes	To help detect cardiac arrhythmias and evaluate fluid balance and acid-base balance.	• Explain the procedure. • Note on the laboratory slip if patient is taking diuretics or other medications that may influence test results. • After the test, observe the venipuncture site for bleeding.
Total cholesterol	To assess patient's risk for coronary artery disease (CAD) and to evaluate fat metabolism	• Explain the procedure. • Have the patient fast overnight and abstain from alcohol for 24 hours before the test. • After the test, observe venipuncture site for bleeding.
Serum triglycerides	To determine patient's risk for CAD	• Explain the procedure. • Advise the patient not to eat for 12 hours and to abstain from alcohol for 24 hours before the test. • After the test, observe the venipuncture site for bleeding.
Lipoprotein-cholesterol fractionation	To assess the risk of CAD	• Advise the patient to abstain from alcohol for 24 hours and to fast and avoid exercise for 12 to 14 hours before the test. • After the test, observe the venipuncture site for bleeding.

Diagnostic tests for cardiovascular disorders *(continued)*

Tests	Purpose	Nursing considerations
Cardiac enzymes	To aid diagnosis of acute myocardial infarction	• Explain the procedure. • Draw the venipuncture specimen before or within 1 hour of giving I.M. injections.
Electrocardiography (ECG)	To help identify primary conduction abnormalities, arrhythmias, cardiac hypertrophy, pericarditis, electrolyte imbalance, myocardial infarction (MI) and the site and extent of MI	• Tell patient ECG will take about 10 minutes. • Explain he must lie still, relax, and breathe normally.
Exercise ECG	To help assess cardiovascular response to an increased workload	• Explain the procedure. • Instruct patient not to eat, smoke, or drink alcohol or caffeine for 3 hours before the test. • Emphasize that he should stop the test if he feels chest pain, leg discomfort, breathlessness, or severe fatigue. • Suggest that he wear loose, lightweight clothing and comfortable walking shoes. • Inform him that he may receive an injection of thallium during the test but that the radiation exposure is minimal. • After the test, monitor blood pressure and ECG for 10 to 15 minutes. • Explain that he should wait an hour before showering.
Continuous ambulatory ECG	To capture the effect of daily physical and psychological stresses on heart activity and possibly to detect intermittent arrhythmias	• Explain to the patient that the test lasts 24 hours. • Demonstrate how to check the recorder for proper functioning. • Emphasize the importance of keeping track of his activities. *(continued)*

Diagnostic tests for cardiovascular disorders (continued)

Tests	Purpose	Nursing considerations
Echocardiography	To evaluate size, shape, and motion of various cardiac structures	• Explain the procedure. • Inform the patient that he may be asked to inhale a gas with a slightly sweet odor (amyl nitrite). • Describe possible effects of amyl nitrite (dizziness, flushing, tachycardia) but assure the patient that they subside quickly. • Inform patient that he may be asked to lie on his left side, to inhale and exhale slowly or to hold his breath.
Magnetic resonance imaging (MRI)	To visualize valves, pericardial abnormalities, ventricular hypertrophy, cardiac neoplasm, infarcted tissue, anatomic malformations, and structural deformities	• Explain the procedure and that it may take up to 90 minutes. • Instruct the patient to remove all metal objects before the test. • Inform him that he will be lying on a narrow bed which slides into a large cylinder. • Explain to him that he will be able to communicate with the technician at all times and that the procedure will be stopped if he feels claustrophobic.
Technetium pyrophosphate scanning	To help diagnose acute MI injury by showing the location and size of newly damaged myocardial tissue	• Explain the procedure and that the isotope will be injected into an arm vein 1 to 3 hours before the start of the 45-minute test. • Instruct him to remain still during the test. • If stress imaging is done, tell patient to restrict alcohol and tobacco for 24 hours and fast for 3 hours before the test.
Multiple-gated acquisition scan (MUGA)	To help assess left ventricular function and the extent of muscle impairment of an MI, and help diagnose heart failure	• Explain the procedure. • Encourage the patient to reduce his stress and activity levels and to avoid heavy meals before the test. • If he is to exercise during the test, tell him to wear comfortable clothing and shoes.

Diagnostic tests for cardiovascular disorders *(continued)*

Tests	Purpose	Nursing considerations
Cardiac catheterization and coronary angiography	To determine a coronary lesion's size and location, evaluate ventricular function and measure heart pressures and oxygen saturation	• Explain the procedure and take baseline vital signs. • Document the presence of peripheral pulses. • Identify allergies, especially to iodine or shellfish. • Explain that the patient may feel warm, flushed, or nauseated following dye injection. • Restrict food and fluid for at least 6 hours before the test. • Tell him that he may receive a mild sedative but will remain conscious. • Inform him that he will have an I.V. inserted in his arm. • Advise him that the catheter will be inserted into an artery or vein in his arm or leg and that the site will be shaved and cleaned. • Assure him that if he experiences any chest discomfort he will be given medication. • After the test, monitor vital signs, color, temperature and pulse distal to the puncture site, as ordered. • Observe the insertion site for hematoma or bleeding and reinforce the dressing, as needed. • Enforce bed rest for 8 hours if the femoral route was used for catheter insertion; keep the leg extended for 6 to 8 hours. If the antecubital fossa was used, keep the patient's arm extended for at least 3 hours.
Digital subtraction angiography	To help evaluate coronary arterial flow, myocardial perfusion, and left ventricular function	• Explain the procedure. • Ask about allergies to shellfish or iodine. • Tell the patient that he may *(continued)*

Diagnostic tests for cardiovascular disorders *(continued)*

Tests	Purpose	Nursing considerations
Digital subtraction angiography *(continued)*		feel warm or flushed when the contrast medium is injected. • Caution him to lie still on the X-ray table. • After the test, observe the venipuncture site for signs of bleeding. If bleeding occurs, apply pressure to the puncture site.
Hemodynamic monitoring	To assess cardiac function and determine effectiveness of therapy by measuring cardiac output, mixed venous oxygen saturation, and intracardiac pressures	• Explain the catheterization and that it takes about 30 minutes and shouldn't cause discomfort. • After catheter insertion, inflate the balloon with a syringe with no more than 1.5 ml air to take the PAWP reading. Then remove the syringe to deflate the balloon. Never leave the balloon inflated. • After each PAWP reading, flush the line with the heparinized saline solution. • Recalibrate the monitoring system every 8 to 24 hours. • Make sure the stopcocks are properly positioned and connections are secure. • Be sure the lumen hubs are properly identified to serve the appropriate catheter ports.
Cardiac radiography	To reveal the size, shape, and appearance of the heart and lungs	• Instruct the patient to remove jewelry, other metal objects, and clothing above his waist and put on a hospital gown. • Explain that he may be asked to take a deep breath and hold it while the film is being taken.
Transesophageal echocardiography with color flow Doppler	To allow visual examination of the heart function and structures and the	• Restrict food and fluids for 6 hours before the test. • Remove any dentures or oral prostheses.

Diagnostic tests for cardiovascular disorders (continued)

Tests	Purpose	Nursing considerations
Transesophageal echocardiography with color flow Doppler (continued)	flow of blood through the heart valves and great vessels	• Connect patient to heart monitor, blood pressure machine, and pulse oximeter to allow monitoring during the procedure. • Explain that his throat will be sprayed with a topical anesthetic and that he may gag when the tube is inserted. • Inform him that an I.V. line will be inserted. • After the test, keep him supine until sedation wears off. • Withhold food and fluids until the patient's gag response has returned.

Expected outcomes

• Patient doesn't experience tachypnea, restlessness, anxiety, dyspnea, confusion, fainting, dizzy spells, light-headedness, nausea, fatigue, or weakness.

• Patient tolerates exercise and activities at usual level, taking into account any cardiac damage.

• Patient maintains respiratory status within established parameters.

• Patient or family members state signs and symptoms of possible cardiac problems.

• Patient's cardiac status stabilizes, with no evidence of arrhythmias.

Nursing interventions and rationales

• Monitor and record level of consciousness (LOC), heart rate and rhythm, and blood pressure at least every 4 hours, or more often if necessary, *to detect cerebral hypoxia.*

• Auscultate heart and breath sounds at least every 4 hours. Report abnormal sounds as soon as they develop. *Extra heart sounds may indicate early cardiac decompensation. Adventitious breath sounds suggest pulmonary congestion and diminished cardiac output.*

• Measure intake and output accurately and record. *Lowered urine output without reduced fluid intake may indicate reduced renal perfusion.*

• Promptly treat life-threatening arrhythmias.

• Weigh patient daily before breakfast *to detect fluid retention.*

• Inspect for pedal or sacral edema *to detect venous stasis.*

• Provide skin care every 4 hours *to enhance perfusion and venous flow.*

• Gradually increase patient's activities within limits of prescribed heart rate *to allow heart to adjust to increased oxygen demand.* Monitor pulse rate before and after activity *to compare rates and gauge tolerance.*
• Plan patient's activities *to avoid increased myocardial workload.*
• Maintain dietary restrictions, as ordered, *to avert cardiac disease.*
• Explain all procedures and tests.
• Teach patient about chest pain and other reportable symptoms, prescribed diet, medications, prescribed activity level, simple methods for lifting and bending, and stress-reduction techniques. *These measures involve patient in care.*
• Administer oxygen, as ordered, *to increase supply to myocardium.*

Activity intolerance

Related to an imbalance between oxygen supply and demand, this diagnosis may be associated with such conditions as acute MI, congenital cardiac and valvular disorders, HF, peripheral vascular disorders, and other ailments.

Expected outcomes

• Patient uses assistive devices to carry out activities.
• Patient expresses feelings about decreased energy levels.
• Patient develops a plan to incorporate meaningful activities into his daily routine.
• Patient's pulse, respirations, and blood pressure remain within established parameters during activity.
• Patient modifies activity to adjust to decreased activity tolerance.

• Patient takes incremental steps to gradually increase activity level.
• Patient discusses importance of good nutrition and adequate rest.

Nursing interventions and rationales

• Discuss with the patient the need for activity, *which improves physical and psychosocial well-being.*
• Encourage him to help plan activity progression. *Participation in planning helps ensure compliance.*
• Instruct and help patient to alternate periods of rest and activity *to reduce the body's oxygen demand.*
• Identify and minimize factors that diminish exercise tolerance *to help increase the activity level.*
• Monitor physiologic responses to increased activity (including respirations, heart rate and rhythm, and blood pressure), *to ensure return to normal a few minutes after activity.*
• Teach patient how to conserve energy while performing activities of daily living (ADLs)—for example, sitting in a chair while dressing. *These measures reduce cellular metabolism and oxygen demand.*
• Demonstrate exercises for increasing strength and endurance, *which will improve breathing.*
• Support and encourage activity to patient's level of tolerance. *This helps develop independence.*
• Before discharge, formulate a plan with patient and caregivers that will enable patient either to continue functioning at maximum activity tolerance or to gradually increase the tolerance. For example, teach patient and caregivers to monitor patient's pulse during activities; to

recognize need for oxygen, if prescribed; and to use oxygen equipment properly. *Participation in planning encourages compliance.*

Anxiety

Related to situational crisis, anxiety can apply to any hospitalized patient. It's used most commonly in patients with conditions requiring surgery or use of sophisticated technologic devices or techniques. The diagnosis also applies to patients with newly diagnosed chronic or terminal cardiovascular disorders.

Expected outcomes

- Patient states feelings of anxiety.
- Patient identifies factors that elicit anxious behavior.
- Patient maintains normal sleep and nutritional patterns.
- Patient discusses activities that tend to decrease anxious behavior.
- Patient is involved in decisions about care.
- Patient practices progressive relaxation techniques twice daily.
- Patient begins to gain self-control over anxiety.

Nursing interventions and rationales

- Spend a designated amount of time with patient twice a shift. Convey a willingness to listen. Offer verbal reassurance—for example, "I know you're frightened. I'll stay with you." *Specific amount of uninterrupted, non-care-related time spent with an anxious patient reduces tension. Active listening helps the patient express feelings.*

- Give patient clear, concise explanations of anything about to occur. *Anxiety may impair patient's cognitive abilities.*
- Listen attentively; allow patient to express feelings. *This may allow patient to identify anxious behaviors and discover the source of anxiety.*
- Make no demands on patient. *An anxious patient may respond to excessive demands with hostility .*
- Identify and reduce as many environmental stressors as possible. This may apply to people as well as other stimuli. *Anxiety commonly results from lack of trust.*
- Have patient state what kinds of activities promote feelings of comfort, and encourage patient to perform them (specify). *This gives patient a sense of control.*
- Remain with patient during periods of severe anxiety. *Anxiety may step from a fear of being left alone.*
- Include patient in decisions related to care when feasible. *Involvement in decision making may reduce anxious behaviors.*
- Allow extra visiting periods with family if this seems to allay patient's anxiety. *This allows anxious patient and family to support each other.*
- Teach patient relaxation techniques to be performed at least every 4 hours, such as guided imagery, progressive muscle relaxation, and meditation. *These measures can decrease the autonomic response to anxiety.*
- Refer patient to community or professional mental health resources, *to provide ongoing mental health assistance.*

DISORDERS

This section discusses common cardiovascular disorders—from inflammatory heart disease such as myocarditis to vascular disorders such as arterial occlusive disease. For each disorder, you'll find information on causes, assessment findings, diagnostic tests, treatments, nursing interventions, patient education, and evaluation criteria.

Inflammatory heart disease

Although inflammation is normally a protective mechanism, its effects on the heart are potentially devastating. For instance, in myocarditis, pericarditis, endocarditis, and rheumatic heart disease, scar formation and other healing processes cause debilitating structural damage, especially in the valves.

Myocarditis

Myocarditis, a focal or diffuse inflammation of the cardiac muscle (myocardium), may be acute or chronic and may strike at any age. In many cases, myocarditis fails to produce specific cardiovascular symptoms or electrocardiogram (ECG) abnormalities. Many patients experience spontaneous recovery, without residual defects. Occasionally, myocarditis is complicated by HF and, rarely, leads to cardiomyopathy.

Causes. Potential causes of this disorder include:

• viral infections (most common cause in the United States), such as coxsackievirus A and B strains and, possibly, poliomyelitis, influenza, rubeola, rubella, and adenoviruses and echoviruses
• bacterial infections, such as diphtheria, tuberculosis, typhoid fever, tetanus, and staphylococcal, pneumococcal, and gonococcal infections
• hypersensitivity reactions, such as acute rheumatic fever and postcardiotomy syndrome
• radiation therapy to the chest in treating lung or breast cancer
• chronic alcoholism
• parasitic infections, especially South American trypanosomiasis (Chagas' disease) in infants and immunosuppressed adults; also toxoplasmosis
• helminthic infections such as trichinosis.

Assessment findings. Look for fatigue, dyspnea, palpitations, fever and, occasionally, mild continuous pressure or soreness in the chest.

On auscultation, be alert for supraventricular and ventricular arrhythmias, S_3 and S_4 gallops, a faint S_1, possibly a murmur of mitral regurgitation (from papillary muscle dysfunction) and, if pericarditis is present, a pericardial friction rub.

Diagnostic tests. A definitive diagnosis requires endomyocardial biopsy. ECG changes provide the most reliable diagnostic aid. Typically, the ECG shows diffuse ST-segment and T-wave abnormalities as in pericarditis, conduction defects (prolonged PR interval), and other supraventricular ectopic arrhythmias.

Laboratory tests cannot unequivocally confirm myocarditis. Results may reveal elevated cardiac enzymes, an increased white blood cell (WBC) count and erythrocyte sedimentation rate (ESR), and elevated antibody titers (such as anti-streptolysin-O [ASO] titer in rheumatic fever).

Treatment. Treatment includes antibiotics for bacterial infection, modified bed rest to decrease heart workload, and careful management of complications.

Nursing interventions. Assess cardiovascular status frequently, watching for signs of HF, such as dyspnea, hypotension, and tachycardia. Check for changes in cardiac rhythm or conduction.

Assist the patient with bathing, as necessary. Provide a bedside commode because this stresses the heart less than using a bedpan.

Patient education. Reassure the patient that activity limitations are temporary. Offer quiet diversionary activities.

Stress the importance of bed rest. During recovery, recommend that the patient resume normal activities slowly and avoid competitive sports.

Evaluation. The patient's cardiac output should be adequate as evidenced by normal blood pressure, warm and dry skin, normal LOC, and absence of dizziness. He should be able to tolerate a normal level of activity. His temperature should be normal, and he shouldn't be dyspneic.

Endocarditis

An infection of the endocardium, heart valves, or cardiac prosthesis, endocarditis results from bacterial invasion. In I.V. drug abusers, it may also result from fungal invasion. This invasion produces vegetative growths on the heart valves, endocardial lining of a heart chamber, or the endothelium of a blood vessel that may embolize to the spleen, kidneys, central nervous system, and lungs.

Acute infective endocarditis usually follows open-heart surgery involving prosthetic valves, septic thrombophlebitis, or skin, bone, and pulmonary infections. This form of endocarditis also occurs in I.V. drug abusers.

Subacute infective endocarditis typically occurs in individuals with acquired valvular or congenital cardiac lesions. It can also follow dental, genitourinary, gynecologic, and GI procedures.

Rheumatic endocarditis commonly affects the mitral valve; less commonly, the aortic or tricuspid valve; and, rarely, the pulmonic valve. Preexisting rheumatic endocardial lesions are a common predisposing factor.

Untreated endocarditis usually proves fatal, but with proper treatment, 70% of patients recover.

Causes. In acute infective endocarditis, causative organisms include group A nonhemolytic streptococcus (rheumatic endocarditis), pneumococcus, staphylococcus, and rarely gonococcus.

Causes of acute endocarditis in I.V. drug abusers include *Staphylococcus aureus, Pseudomonas, Candida,* or usually harmless skin saprophytes. In subacute infective endocarditis, infecting organisms include *Streptococcus viridans,* which normally inhabits the upper respiratory tract, and *Streptococcus faecalis* (enterococcus), usually found in GI and perineal flora.

Assessment findings. Early clinical features are usually nonspecific and include weakness, fatigue, weight loss, anorexia, arthralgia, night sweats, intermittent fever (may recur for weeks), and a loud, regurgitant murmur. This murmur is typical of the underlying rheumatic or congenital heart disease. A suddenly changing murmur or the discovery of a new murmur along with fever is a classic sign of endocarditis.

Other signs include petechiae on the skin (especially on the upper anterior trunk); the buccal, pharyngeal, or conjunctival mucosa; and the nails (splinter hemorrhages).

In subacute endocarditis, embolization may produce the following clinical features:
• splenic infarction (pain in the left upper quadrant, radiating to the left shoulder; abdominal rigidity)
• renal infarction (hematuria, pyuria, flank pain, decreased urine output)
• cerebral infarction (hemiparesis, aphasia, or other neurologic deficits)
• pulmonary infarction (most common in right-sided endocarditis, which commonly occurs among I.V. drug abusers and after cardiac surgery; cough, pleuritic pain, pleural friction rub, dyspnea, and hemoptysis)
• peripheral vascular occlusion (numbness and tingling in an arm, leg, finger, or toe, or signs of impending peripheral gangrene).

Diagnostic tests. Three or more blood cultures during a 24- to 48-hour period identify the causative organism in up to 90% of patients. The remaining 10% may have negative blood cultures, possibly suggesting fungal infection. Echocardiography may identify valvular damage. ECG readings may show atrial fibrillation and other arrhythmias that accompany valvular disease. Other indications of the disorder include elevated WBC count; abnormal histocytes (macrophages); elevated ESR; normocytic, normochromic anemia (in subacute bacterial endocarditis); and rheumatoid factor (occurs in about one-half of all patients).

Treatment. Antibiotic therapy, the primary treatment, should start promptly and continue over several weeks. I.V. antibiotic therapy usually lasts about 4 weeks. Supportive treatment includes bed rest, aspirin for fever and aches, and sufficient fluid intake. Severe valvular damage, especially aortic insufficiency, or infection of a cardiac prosthesis may require corrective surgery if refractory HF develops.

Nursing interventions. Before giving antibiotics, obtain a patient history of allergies. Administer antibiotics on time to maintain consistent blood levels. Check dilutions for compatibility with other patient medications, and use a compatible solution (for example, add methicillin to a buffered solution). To reduce the risk of I.V. site complications, rotate venous access sites. In addition, follow these guidelines:
• Watch for signs of embolization (hematuria, pleuritic chest pain, left upper quadrant pain, or paresis), a common occurrence during the first 3 months of treatment. Embolization may indicate impending peripheral vascular occlusion or splenic, renal, cerebral, or pulmonary infarction.
• Monitor the patient's renal status (including blood urea nitrogen [BUN] and serum creatinine levels, and urine output) to check for signs of renal emboli or drug toxicity.
• Observe for signs of HF.

Patient education. Teach the patient to watch for and report signs of embolization and to watch closely for fever, anorexia, and other signs and symptoms of relapse about 2 weeks after treatment stops. During the recovery period, recommend quiet diversionary activities.

Tell susceptible patients they need prophylactic antibiotics before, during, and after dental work, childbirth, and genitourinary, GI, or gynecologic procedures.

Evaluation. Evidence of recovery includes normal temperature, lungs clear to auscultation, and adequate cardiac output shown by normal blood pressure and no increase in valve dysfunction. The patient should have adequate tissue perfusion and be able to tolerate activity for a reasonable period and to maintain normal weight.

Pericarditis

Pericarditis is an acute or chronic inflammation affecting the pericardium, the fibroserous sac that envelops, supports, and protects the heart. *Acute pericarditis* can be fibrinous or effusive, with purulent serous or hemorrhagic exudate. *Chronic constrictive pericarditis* leads to dense fibrous pericardial thickening. Diagnosis of acute pericarditis depends on identifying typical clinical features and ruling out other possible causes. Most patients recover from acute pericarditis, unless constriction occurs.

Causes. Pericarditis may result from:
• bacterial, fungal, or viral infection (infectious pericarditis)
• neoplasms (primary or metastatic)
• high-dose radiation to the chest
• uremia
• hypersensitivity or autoimmune diseases such as rheumatic fever (the most common cause of pericarditis in children), systemic lupus erythematosus, and rheumatoid arthritis

• postcardiac injury, such as MI (which later causes an autoimmune reaction [Dressler's syndrome] in the pericardium), trauma, or surgery that leaves the pericardium intact but causes blood to leak into the pericardial cavity
• drugs, such as hydralazine or procainamide
• idiopathic factors (most common in acute pericarditis)
• less commonly, aortic aneurysm with pericardial leakage, and myxedema with cholesterol deposits in the pericardium.

Assessment findings. Many patients experience sharp and sudden pain that usually starts over the sternum and radiates to the neck, shoulders, back, and arms. Unlike the pain of MI, pericardial pain is often pleuritic, increasing with deep inspiration and decreasing when the patient sits up and leans forward.

You may hear a pericardial friction rub. A classic sign, this grating sound occurs as the heart moves. You'll usually hear the friction rub best during forced expiration while the patient leans forward or is on his hands and knees in bed. It may have up to three components, corresponding to the timing of atrial systole, ventricular systole, and the rapid-filling phase of ventricular diastole. Occasionally, friction rub is heard only briefly or not at all.

When assessing for *chronic constrictive pericarditis,* look for a gradual increase in systemic venous pressure and signs and symptoms similar to those of chronic right-sided HF, including fluid retention, ascites, and hepatomegaly.

Diagnostic tests. Look for these ECG changes in acute pericarditis:
• elevation of ST segments in the standard limb leads and most precordial leads without significant changes in QRS morphology that occur with MI
• atrial ectopic rhythms such as atrial fibrillation
• in pericardial effusion, diminished QRS voltage.

In pericardial effusion, echocardiography may establish diagnosis.

Laboratory results don't establish diagnosis. They reflect inflammation and may identify its cause. They may include normal or elevated WBC count, especially in infectious pericarditis; an elevated ESR; and with associated myocarditis, slightly elevated cardiac enzymes.

Other pertinent laboratory data include checking BUN level for uremia, ASO titers to detect rheumatic fever, and a purified protein derivative skin test to check for tuberculosis. A culture of pericardial fluid may be obtained by open surgical drainage or cardiocentesis.

Treatment. Treatment seeks to relieve symptoms and manage underlying systemic disease. In acute idiopathic pericarditis, post-MI pericarditis, and postthoracotomy pericarditis, treatment consists of bed rest as long as fever and pain persist, and nonsteroidal drugs, such as aspirin and indomethacin, to relieve pain and reduce inflammation. If these drugs fail to relieve symptoms, expect to administer corticosteroids.

Infectious pericarditis resulting from disease of the left pleural space, mediastinal abscesses, or septicemia requires antibiotics, surgical drainage, or both. If cardiac tamponade develops, the doctor may perform emergency pericardiocentesis.

Recurrent pericarditis may necessitate partial pericardiectomy, which creates a "window" that allows fluid to drain into the pleural space. In constrictive pericarditis, total pericardiectomy to permit adequate filling and contraction of the heart may be necessary. Treatment must also include management of rheumatic fever, uremia, tuberculosis, and other underlying disorders.

Nursing interventions. A patient with pericarditis usually needs complete bed rest. Assess pain in relation to respiration and body position to distinguish pericardial pain from myocardial ischemic pain.

Place the patient in an upright position to relieve dyspnea and chest pain, provide analgesics and oxygen, and reassure the patient with acute pericarditis that this condition is temporary.

Monitor for signs of cardiac compression or cardiac tamponade, which are possible complications of pericardial effusion. Signs and symptoms include decreased blood pressure, increased CVP, pulsus paradoxus, neck vein distention, and dyspnea. Because cardiac tamponade requires immediate treatment, keep a pericardiocentesis set

at bedside whenever pericardial effusion is suspected.

Patient education. Explain tests and treatments to the patient.

Evaluation. Evidence of successful treatment includes normal temperature, absence of pain and shortness of breath, adequate blood pressure, warm and dry skin.

Rheumatic fever and heart disease

Rheumatic fever is a systemic inflammatory disease of childhood that follows a group A beta-hemolytic streptococcal infection. Rheumatic heart disease refers to the cardiac manifestations of rheumatic fever. It includes pancarditis (myocarditis, pericarditis, and endocarditis) during the early acute phase and chronic valvular disease in the later phases. Long-term antibiotic therapy can minimize recurrence of rheumatic fever, reducing the risk of permanent cardiac damage and eventual valvular deformity. However, severe pancarditis occasionally produces fatal HF during the acute phase.

Causes. Apparently, a hypersensitivity reaction to a group A beta-hemolytic streptococcal infection causes rheumatic fever. Rheumatic heart disease results from episodes of rheumatic fever.

Assessment findings. Signs and symptoms may include fever; migratory joint pain; skin lesions; firm, movable, nontender subcutaneous nodules near tendons or bony prominences of joints; chorea (later symptom); or pleural friction rub and pain.

The patient may also have a heart murmur. This may be a systolic murmur of mitral insufficiency (high-pitched, blowing, holosystolic, loudest at apex, possibly radiating to the anterior axillary line). Alternatively, the patient may have a midsystolic murmur or, occasionally, a diastolic murmur of aortic insufficiency (low-pitched, rumbling, almost inaudible).

Diagnostic tests. The following results indicate rheumatic fever and rheumatic heart disease:
• elevated WBC count and ESR (especially during the acute phase)
• blood studies showing slight anemia because of suppressed erythropoiesis during inflammation
• positive C-reactive protein (especially during acute phase)
• increased cardiac enzyme levels (in severe carditis)
• elevated ASO titer
• a prolonged PR interval (occurs in 20% of patients).

In addition, chest X-rays show normal heart size, except with myocarditis, HF, or pericardial effusion. Echocardiography helps evaluate valvular damage, chamber size, and ventricular function, and cardiac catheterization helps to evaluate valvular damage and left ventricular function.

Treatment. Effective management reduces the chance of permanent cardiac damage. During the acute phase, treatment includes penicillin or erythromycin for patients with penicillin hypersensitivity. Salicylates such as aspirin relieve fever and minimize joint swelling and pain; if the patient has carditis or salicylates fail to relieve pain and inflammation, expect to administer corticosteroids. Supportive treatment requires strict bed rest for about 5 weeks during the acute phase with active carditis, followed by a progressive increase in physical activity, as appropriate.

After the acute phase subsides, the patient may receive oral sulfadiazine or penicillin G to prevent recurrence. Such preventive treatment usually continues for at least 5 years or until age 25. HF requires continued bed rest and diuretics.

Severe mitral or aortic valvular dysfunction causing persistent HF requires corrective valvular surgery, including commissurotomy (separation of the adherent, thickened leaflets of the mitral valve), valvuloplasty (repair of valve), or valve replacement (with prosthetic valve).

Nursing interventions. Before giving penicillin, ask the patient or his parents if he has ever had a hypersensitivity reaction to it. Tell them to stop the drug and call the doctor immediately if the patient develops a rash, fever, or chills.

After the acute phase, encourage the family and friends to spend as much time as possible with the patient to minimize boredom. The patient is usually discharged after stabilization. Then a home health nurse provides I.V. antibiotic therapy and continued assessment.

Patient education. Instruct the patient and his family to watch for and report early signs of HF, such as dyspnea and a hacking, nonproductive cough.

• Stress the need for bed rest during the acute phase and suggest appropriate diversions.

• Advise parents to secure tutorial services to help the child keep up with schoolwork.

• Help parents overcome any guilt feelings.

• Encourage the parents and the child to vent their frustrations during the long convalescence. If the child has severe carditis, help parents prepare for permanent changes in his lifestyle.

• Warn parents to watch for and immediately report signs and symptoms of recurrent streptococcal infection—sudden sore throat, diffuse throat redness and oropharyngeal exudate, swollen and tender cervical lymph glands, pain on swallowing, temperature of 101° to 104° F (38.3° to 40° C), headache, and nausea. Urge them to keep the child away from persons with respiratory tract infections.

• Promote good dental hygiene to prevent gingival infection. Make sure the patient and his family understand the need to comply with prolonged antibiotic therapy and follow-up care and the need for additional antibiotics during dental surgery.

Evaluation. The patient should experience no joint pain and no decrease in activity tolerance. Signs of infection should be absent.

Valvular heart disease

Preventing efficient blood flow through the heart, valvular disease includes *stenosis* and *insufficiency.* Valvular heart disease may affect any of the four valves of the heart: mitral, aortic, pulmonary, or tricuspid. Severe valvular heart disease can eventually lead to HF.

Mitral insufficiency

In mitral insufficiency, blood from the left ventricle flows back into the left atrium during systole, causing the atrium to enlarge to accommodate the backflow. As a result, the left ventricle also dilates to accommodate the increased volume of blood from the atrium and to compensate for diminishing cardiac output. Ventricular hypertrophy and increased end-diastolic pressure result in increased pulmonary artery (PA) pressure, eventually leading to left- and right-sided HF.

Causes. Mitral insufficiency may result from rheumatic fever, hypertrophic cardiomyopathy, mitral valve prolapse, MI, severe left-sided HF, or ruptured chordae tendineae. It's also associated with congenital anomalies such as transposition of the great vessels.

Assessment findings. The patient experiences orthopnea, dyspnea, fatigue, angina, and palpitations. Other findings include:

• peripheral edema, jugular vein distention, hepatomegaly (right-sided HF)
• possible tachycardia, crackles, and pulmonary edema
• auscultation of a holosystolic murmur at apex, possible split S_2, and an S_3.

Diagnostic tests. Cardiac catheterization may reveal mitral insufficiency, with increased left ventricular end-diastolic volume and pressure; elevated atrial and pulmonary artery wedge pressures (PAWP); reduced cardiac output.

X-ray may indicate left atrial and ventricular enlargement, pulmonary vein congestion. Echocardiography may reveal abnormal valve leaflet motion, left atrial enlargement. ECG may show left atrial and ventricular hypertrophy, sinus tachycardia, and atrial fibrillation.

Mitral stenosis

Mitral stenosis, a narrowing of the valve by valvular abnormalities, fibrosis, or calcification, obstructs blood flow from the left atrium to the left ventricle. Consequently, left atrial volume and pressure rise and the chamber dilates. Greater resistance to blood flow causes pulmonary hypertension, right ventricular hypertrophy, and eventually right-sided HF. Also, inadequate filling of the left ventricle produces low cardiac output.

Causes. Most commonly, rheumatic fever leads to mitral stenosis. It may be associated with congenital anomalies.

Assessment findings. The patient experiences dyspnea on exertion, paroxysmal nocturnal dyspnea, orthopnea, weakness, fatigue, and palpitations. Your assessment findings include:
• peripheral edema, jugular vein distention, ascites, hepatomegaly (right-sided HF in severe pulmonary hypertension)
• crackles, cardiac arrhythmias (atrial fibrillation), and systemic emboli
• auscultation of a loud S_1 or opening snap and a diastolic murmur at the apex.

Diagnostic tests. Cardiac catheterization reveals diastolic pressure gradient across valve, elevated left atrial pressure and PAWP (greater than 15) with severe pulmonary hypertension and pulmonary arterial pressures, elevated right heart pressure, diminished cardiac output, and abnormal contraction of the left ventricle.

X-ray shows left atrial and ventricular enlargement, enlarged pulmonary arteries, and mitral valve calcification. Echocardiography reveals thickened mitral valve leaflets and left atrial enlargement. ECG shows left atrial hypertrophy, atrial fibrillation, right ventricular hypertrophy, and right axis deviation.

Aortic insufficiency

In aortic insufficiency, blood flows back into the left ventricle during diastole, causing a fluid overload in the ventricle, which, in turn, dilates and, ultimately, hypertrophies. The excess volume causes a fluid overload in the left atrium and finally in the pulmonary system. Left-sided HF and pulmonary edema eventually result.

Causes. Rheumatic fever, syphilis, hypertension, and endocarditis may all lead to aortic insufficiency. The condition may also be idiopathic. It's associated with Marfan syndrome and ventricular septal defect, even after surgical closure.

Assessment findings. The patient experiences dyspnea, cough, fatigue, palpitations, angina, and syncope. Other findings include:
• pulmonary vein congestion, HF, pulmonary edema, "pulsating" nail beds (Quincke's pulse)
• rapidly rising and collapsing pulses (pulsus biferiens), cardiac arrhythmias, and wide pulse pressure in severe regurgitation
• auscultation of an S_3 and a diastolic blowing murmur at left sternal border
• palpation and visualization of apical impulse in chronic disease.

Diagnostic tests. Cardiac catheterization reveals reduction in arterial diastolic pressures, aortic insufficiency, other valvular abnormalities, and increased left ventricular end-diastolic pressure.

X-ray shows left ventricular enlargement, and pulmonary vein congestion. Echocardiography reveals left ventricular enlargement, alterations in mitral valve movement (indirect indication of aortic valve disease), and mitral thickening. ECG shows sinus tachycardia, left ventricular hypertrophy, and left atrial hypertrophy in severe disease.

Aortic stenosis

In aortic stenosis, elevated left ventricular pressure attempts to overcome the resistance of the narrowed valvular opening. The added workload causes a greater demand for oxygen, while diminished cardiac output causes poor coronary artery perfusion, ischemia of the left ventricle, and eventually left-sided HF.

Causes. Possible causes include congenital aortic bicuspid valve (associated with coarctation of the aorta), congenital stenosis of valve cusps, rheumatic fever, or atherosclerosis.

Assessment findings. The patient experiences dyspnea on exertion, paroxysmal nocturnal dyspnea, fatigue, syncope, angina, and palpitations. Other findings include:
• pulmonary vein congestion, HF, pulmonary edema
• diminished carotid pulses, decreased cardiac output, cardiac arrhythmias or, possibly, pulsus alternans
• auscultation of systolic murmur at base or in carotids and possibly an S_4.

Diagnostic tests. Cardiac catheterization reveals pressure gradient across valve (indicating obstruction) and increased left ventricular end-diastolic pressures.

X-ray shows valvular calcification, left ventricular enlargement and pulmonary vein congestion.

Echocardiography reveals thickened aortic valve and left ventricular wall, possibly coexistent with mitral valve stenosis. ECG shows left ventricular hypertrophy.

Pulmonary insufficiency

In pulmonary insufficiency, blood ejected into the PA during systole flows back into the right ventricle during diastole, causing a fluid overload in the ventricle, ventricular hypertrophy, and finally right-sided HF.

Causes. In many cases congenital, pulmonary insufficiency may also result from pulmonary hypertension.

Assessment findings. The patient experiences dyspnea, weakness, fatigue, and chest pain. Other findings include:
• peripheral edema, jugular vein distention, and hepatomegaly (right-sided HF)
• auscultation of diastolic murmur in pulmonary area.

Diagnostic tests. Cardiac catheterization reveals pulmonary insufficiency, increased right ventricular pressure, and associated cardiac defects.

X-ray shows right ventricular and pulmonary arterial enlargement. ECG reveals right ventricular or right atrial enlargement.

Pulmonary stenosis

In pulmonary stenosis, obstructed right ventricular outflow causes right ventricular hypertrophy in an attempt to overcome resistance to the narrow valvular opening. Right-sided HF ultimately results.

Causes. The disorder may result from congenital stenosis of valve cusps or, less commonly, rheumatic heart disease. It's associated with congenital heart defects such as tetralogy of Fallot.

Assessment findings. The patient is asymptomatic or symptomatic with dyspnea on exertion, fatigue, chest pain, and syncope. Other findings include:
• possible peripheral edema, jugular vein distention, and hepatomegaly (right-sided HF)
• auscultation of a systolic murmur at the left sternal border and a split S_2 with a delayed or absent pulmonary component.

Diagnostic tests. Cardiac catheterization shows elevated right ventricular pressure, reduced PA pressure, and abnormal valve orifice.

ECG may show right ventricular hypertrophy, right axis deviation, right atrial hypertrophy, and atrial fibrillation.

Tricuspid insufficiency

In tricuspid insufficiency, blood flows back into the right atrium during systole, reducing blood flow to the lungs and left side of the heart. Cardiac output also lessens. Fluid overload in the right side of the heart can eventually lead to right-side HF.

Causes. Right-sided HF or rheumatic fever may lead to tricuspid insufficiency. So may permanent placement of a transvenous pacing catheter. This disorder is associated with congenital disorders.

Assessment findings. The patient experiences dyspnea and fatigue. Other findings include:
• possible peripheral edema, jugular vein distention, hepatomegaly, and ascites (right-sided HF)
• auscultation of a possible S_3 and a systolic murmur at the lower left sternal border that increases with inspiration.

Diagnostic tests. Catheterization on the right side of the heart reveals high atrial pressure, tricuspid insufficiency, and decreased or normal cardiac output.

X-ray shows right atrial dilation and right ventricular enlargement. Echocardiography reveals systolic prolapse of tricuspid valve and right atrial enlargement. ECG shows right atrial or right ventricular hypertrophy and atrial fibrillation.

Tricuspid stenosis

In tricuspid stenosis, obstructed blood flow from the right atrium to the right ventricle causes the right atrium to dilate and hypertrophy. Eventually, this leads to right-sided HF and increases pressure in the superior vena cava.

Causes. Tricuspid stenosis may result from rheumatic fever or congenital causes. It's associated with mitral or aortic valve disease.

Assessment findings. The patient may be symptomatic with dyspnea, fatigue, and syncope. Other findings include:
• possible peripheral edema, jugular vein distention, hepatomegaly, and ascites (right-sided HF).
• auscultation of a diastolic murmur at the lower left sternal border that increases with inspiration.

Diagnostic tests. Cardiac catheterization reveals heightened pressure gradient across valve, elevated right atrial pressure, and reduced cardiac output.

X-ray reveals right atrial enlargement. Echocardiography shows leaflet abnormality and right atrial enlargement. ECG shows right atrial hypertrophy, right or left ventricular hypertrophy, and atrial fibrillation.

Treatment. Treatment of valvular heart disease depends on the nature and severity of associated symptoms. For example, HF requires digoxin, diuretics, a sodium-restricted diet, and, in acute cases, oxygen. Other appropriate measures include anticoagulant therapy to prevent thrombus formation and prophylactic antibiotics before and after surgery or dental care.

If the patient has severe disease, he may undergo open-heart surgery using cardiopulmonary bypass for valve replacement. Elderly patients and others who pose a high surgical risk may undergo valvuloplasty.

Nursing interventions. Watch closely for signs of HF or pulmonary edema and adverse effects of drug therapy.

Patient education. Teach the patient about diet restrictions, medications, and the importance of reporting symptoms and consistent follow-up care. Monitor activity level to assess worsening of the valve disorder.

Evaluation. The patient should maintain normal blood pressure and clear lungs (as revealed by auscultation). Peripheral edema should be absent and the patient should be able to tolerate activity.

Degenerative disorders

The most common cardiovascular ailments, degenerative disorders include hypertension, CAD, MI, and HF.

Hypertension

Hypertension refers to an intermittent or sustained elevation in diastolic or systolic blood pressure. *Essential,* or idiopathic, hypertension occurs most commonly. *Secondary* hypertension results from a number of disorders. Malignant hypertension is a severe fulminant form of hypertension common to both types.

Hypertension represents a major cause of cerebrovascular accident (CVA), cardiac disease, and renal failure. Early detection and treatment greatly improve the patient's prognosis. Severely elevated blood pressure may become fatal.

Causes. Essential hypertension probably results from an interaction of multiple homeostatic forces, including changes in renal regulation of sodium and extracellular fluids, in aldosterone secretion and metabolism, and in norepinephrine secretion and metabolism.

Secondary hypertension may be caused by renal vascular disease, pheochromocytoma, primary hyperaldosteronism, Cushing's syndrome, or dysfunction of the thyroid, pituitary, or parathyroid glands. It may also result from coarctation of the aorta, pregnancy, and neurologic disorders.

Certain risk factors appear to increase the likelihood of hypertension. These include family history of hypertension, race (more common in African Americans), stress, obesity, and diabetes. Other risk factors include high dietary intake of saturated fats or sodium, tobacco use, oral contraceptive use, sedentary lifestyle, and aging.

Assessment findings. Serial resting blood pressure measurements of more than 140/90 mm Hg confirm hypertension. Other clinical effects don't appear until complications develop from vascular changes.

Diagnostic tests. Along with patient history, the following additional tests may show predisposing factors and help identify an underlying cause:

• Urinalysis: Protein, red blood cells, and WBCs may indicate glomerulonephritis.

• Intravenous pyelography: Renal atrophy indicates chronic renal disease; one kidney more than $5/8''$ (1.5 cm) shorter than the other suggests unilateral renal disease.

• Serum potassium level: Levels less than 3.5 mEq/L may indicate adrenal dysfunction (primary hyperaldosteronism).

• BUN and creatinine levels: BUN level normal or elevated to more than 20 mg/dl and creatinine level normal or elevated to more than 1.5 mg/dl suggest renal disease.

Other tests help detect cardiovascular damage and other complications. ECG may show left ventricular hypertrophy or ischemia. Chest X-ray may show cardiomegaly.

Treatment. Although essential hypertension has no cure, modifications in diet and lifestyle as well as drug therapy can control it. Drug therapy usually begins with a diuretic, beta-adrenergic blockers, other sympathetic blockers, vasodilators or angiotensin-converting enzyme (ACE) and calcium channel blockers. If the patient doesn't receive desired results from one drug, a second (from another classification) is usually added.

Lifestyle and dietary changes may include weight loss, relaxation techniques, exercise, and restriction of sodium and saturated fat intake.

Treatment of secondary hypertension includes correcting the underlying cause and controlling hypertensive effects.

Nursing interventions. If a patient is admitted with hypertension, find out if he was taking prescribed medication. If not, ask why. If the patient can't afford the medication, refer him to an appropriate social service agency. If he suffered severe adverse reactions, he may need different medication. Routinely screen all patients for hypertension, especially those at high risk.

Patient education. Warn the patient that uncontrolled hypertension may cause CVA and MI, retinal damage and renal failure. To encourage compliance with antihypertensive therapy, suggest that the patient establish a daily routine for taking medication. Tell him to report drug adverse effects. Instruct him and his family to keep a record of drugs used, noting their effectiveness. Also, advise him to avoid high-sodium antacids and over-the-counter cold and sinus medications, which contain harmful vasoconstrictors.

Help the patient examine and modify his lifestyle—for example, by exercising regularly. Teach stress management methods. (See *Biofeedback and imagery,* page 164.) Encourage any necessary changes in dietary habits. Help the obese patient plan a reducing diet; tell him to avoid high-sodium foods and table salt.

Evaluation. The patient should demonstrate blood pressure under 140/90 mm Hg at rest and the absence of enlargement of the left ventricle (as revealed by ECG or

Biofeedback and imagery

Two alternative therapies with a long record of success, biofeedback and imagery have been successfully used to reduce hypertension. Biofeedback and imagery have been proven to decrease the stress response and moderate the sympathetic nervous system response, thus reducing the blood pressure.

Biofeedback utilizes electronic monitors to measure psychophysiologic functions for the express purpose of feeding these functions back to the patient so that he can learn to control his body responses.

Imagery engages the patient's imagination in the process of self-healing. It may involve visualization or any of the other senses. Guided imagery helps the patient imagine a restful place such as a beach by a lake. The patient is then encouraged to use the technique whenever needed to reduce stress.

chest X-ray). He should be able to tolerate activity.

Coronary artery disease

CAD refers to any narrowing or obstruction of arterial lumina that interferes with cardiac perfusion. Deprived of sufficient blood, the myocardium can develop various ischemic diseases, including angina pectoris, MI, HF, sudden death, and cardiac arrhythmias.

Causes. Most commonly, atherosclerosis leads to CAD. Other possible causes include arteritis, coronary artery spasm, certain infectious diseases, and congenital defects in the coronary vascular system.

Patients with certain risk factors appear to face a greater likelihood of developing CAD. These factors include family history of heart disease, smoking, hypertension, hyperlipoproteinemia, sedentary lifestyle, high-fat diet, diabetes, and obesity.

Assessment findings. Angina, the classic symptom of CAD, occurs as a burning, squeezing, or crushing tightness in the substernal or precordial chest. It may radiate to the left arm, neck, jaw, or shoulder blade. Angina most commonly follows physical exertion but may also follow emotional excitement, exposure to cold, or a large meal. Less severe and shorter than the pain associated with acute MI, angina is commonly relieved by nitroglycerin.

Other possible signs and symptoms include nausea, vomiting, weakness, diaphoresis, and cool extremities.

Diagnostic tests. An ECG taken during an anginal episode shows ischemia and possibly arrhythmias such as premature ventricular contraction. A pain-free patient may have a normal ECG. Arrhythmias may occur without infarction, secondary to ischemia. An exercise ECG may provoke chest pain and signs of myocardial ischemia in response to physical exertion.

Coronary angiography reveals coronary artery stenosis or obstruction and collateral circulation, and shows the condition of the arteries beyond the narrowing. Myocardial perfusion imaging with thallium-201 during treadmill exercise detects ischemic areas of the myocardium.

The patient may also undergo serum lipid studies to detect and classify hyperlipemia.

Treatment. For patients with angina, treatment seeks either to reduce myocardial oxygen demand or increase oxygen supply. Therapy consists primarily of nitrates, such as nitroglycerin (given sublingually, orally, transdermally, or topically in ointment form), isosorbide dinitrate (sublingually or orally), beta-adrenergic blockers (orally), or calcium channel blockers (orally).

Percutaneous transluminal coronary angioplasty (PTCA) and laser angioplasty are alternatives to surgical treatments. Obstructive lesions may necessitate coronary artery bypass grafting (CABG).

Nursing interventions. During anginal episodes, monitor blood pressure and heart rate. Take an ECG before giving nitroglycerin or other nitrates. Record duration of pain, amount of medication required to relieve it, and accompanying symptoms. Keep nitroglycerin on hand.

After cardiac catheterization, monitor the catheter site for bleeding. Also, check for distal pulses. To counter the diuretic effect of the dye, make sure the patient drinks plenty of fluids. Assess potassium levels.

If the patient must undergo surgery, give the patient and his family a tour of the intensive care unit (ICU).

Patient education. Instruct the hospitalized patient to call immediately whenever he feels chest, arm, or neck pain.

Before cardiac catheterization, explain the procedure. Make sure the patient understands the risks and realizes that it may indicate a need for surgery. After catheterization, review the course of treatment with the patient and family.

Before discharge, stress the need to follow the prescribed drug regimen (antihypertensives, nitrates, antilipemics, for example), exercise program, and diet. Encourage regular, moderate exercise. Refer the patient to a smoking cessation program if necessary.

Teach the patient to stop and rest when angina occurs and to take his nitroglycerin, as prescribed: one every three minutes until the pain subsides or the patient has taken three to five nitroglycerin pills. The patient should call 911 and then the doctor if the pain continues or if the pattern of chest pain changes, occurs with less effort, or increases.

Evaluation. Note if the patient experiences pain or shortness of breath at rest or with usual activity. Assess whether he can tolerate activity. ECG and blood pressure should be normal.

Myocardial infarction

A myocardial infarction is an occlusion of a coronary artery that leads to oxygen deprivation, myocardial ischemia, and eventual necrosis. The extent of functional impairment depends on the size and location of the infarct, the condition of the uninvolved myocardium, the potential for collateral circulation, and the effectiveness of compensatory mechanisms. In the United States, MI is the leading cause of death.

Causes. An MI can arise whenever myocardial oxygen supply can't keep pace with demand and myocardial cells die. CAD, coronary artery emboli, thrombus, coronary artery spasm, and severe hematologic and coagulation disorders may all lead to MI. Other causes include myocardial contusion and congenital coronary artery anomalies.

Certain risk factors increase a patient's vulnerability to MI. These include family history of MI; hypertension; smoking; elevated serum triglyceride, cholesterol, and low-density lipoprotein levels; diabetes mellitus; obesity or excessive intake of saturated fats, carbohydrates, or salt. Other risk factors include sedentary lifestyle, aging, stress or Type A personality, and oral contraceptive use.

Assessment findings. The patient often experiences severe, persistent chest pain that's unrelieved by rest or nitroglycerin. He may describe pain as crushing or squeezing. Usually substernal, pain may radiate to left arm, jaw, neck, or shoulder blades. Other signs and symptoms include a feeling of impending doom, fatigue, nausea and vomiting, shortness of breath, cool extremities, perspiration, anxiety, hypotension or hypertension, palpable precordial pulse and, possibly, muffled heart sounds. (See *Detecting and treating MI complications.*)

Diagnostic tests. A serial 12-lead ECG may show no abnormalities or may prove inconclusive during the first few hours after MI. When present, characteristic abnormalities show serial ST-T changes in subendocardial MI, and Q waves representing transmural MI.

Noninvasive, but highly sensitive, ST-segment monitoring tracks the heart's response to MI. Continuous monitoring can immediately detect ischemic episodes. ST-segment monitoring can identify patients at high risk for reocclusion after PTCA or MI—and permits prompt intervention.

Serial serum enzyme measurements show elevated creatine kinase (CK), especially the CK-MB isoenzyme (the cardiac muscle fraction of CK).

With a transmural MI, echocardiography shows ventricular wall dyskinesia. To evaluate MI effects, the patient may undergo thallium scans, technetium Tc 99m pyrophosphate scans, or radionuclide ventriculography.

Treatment. The following treatment seeks to relieve pain, stabilize heart rhythm, and reduce cardiac workload:

Detecting and treating MI complications

Complication	Diagnosis	Treatment
Cardiogenic shock	Cardiac catheterization shows decreased cardiac output and increased pulmonary artery (PA) pressure and pulmonary artery wedge pressure (PAWP). Signs include hypotension, tachycardia, decreased level of consciousness, reduced urine output, neck vein distention, and cool, pale skin.	• I.V. fluids • Vasodilators • Cardiotonics • Digitalis glycosides • Intra-aortic balloon pump (IABP) • Beta-adrenergic stimulants
Heart failure (HF)	In left-sided HF, chest X-rays show venous congestion and cardiomegaly. Cardiac catheterization shows increased PA pressure, PAWP, and central venous pressure.	• Angiotensin converting enzyme inhibitor • Diuretics • Vasodilators • Inotropics • Digitalis glycosides
Arrhythmias	Electrocardiogram (ECG) shows premature ventricular contractions, ventricular tachycardia, or ventricular fibrillation; in inferior wall, myocardial infarction (MI), bradycardia, and junctional rhythms or atrioventricular block; in anterior wall, MI, tachycardia, or heart block.	• Antiarrhythmics • Atropine • Cardioversion • Pacemaker
Mitral regurgitation	Auscultation reveals crackles and apical holosystolic murmur. Dyspnea is prominent. Cardiac catheterization shows increased PA pressure and PAWP. Echocardiogram shows valve dysfunction.	• Nitroglycerin • Nitroprusside • IABP • Surgical replacement of the mitral valve and concomitant myocardial revascularization
Pericarditis or Dressler's syndrome	Auscultation reveals a friction rub. Chest pain is relieved by sitting up.	• Anti-inflammatory agents, such as aspirin, corticosteroids, or nonsteroidal anti-inflammatory drugs
Thromboembolism	Severe dyspnea and chest pain or neurologic changes occur. Magnetic resonance imaging	• Oxygen • Heparin *(continued)*

Detecting and treating MI complications *(continued)*

Complication	Diagnosis	Treatment
Thromboembolism *(continued)*	scan shows ventilation-perfusion mismatch. Angiography shows arterial blockage.	• Endarterectomy
Ventricular aneurysm	Chest X-ray may show cardiomegaly. ECG may show arrhythmias and persistent ST-segment elevation. Left ventriculography shows altered or paradoxical left ventricular motion.	• Cardioversion • Antiarrhythmics • Vasodilators • Anticoagulants • Digitalis glycosides • Diuretics • Surgical resection, if necessary
Ventricular septal rupture	In left-to-right shunt, examination reveals a harsh holosystolic murmur and thrill. Cardiac catheterization shows increased PA pressure and PAWP. Increased oxygen saturation of right ventricle and PA occurs.	• Surgical correction (may be postponed several weeks) • IABP • Nitroglycerin • Nitroprusside

• morphine or meperidine I.V. for pain and sedation
• bed rest with a bedside commode
• oxygen administration (by face mask or nasal cannula) at a modest flow rate for 24 to 48 hours
• thrombolytic therapy up to 6 hours after infarction, using intracoronary or systemic (I.V.) streptokinase, urokinase, alteplase, or anistreplase
• PTCA to dilate the artery narrowed from plaque
• nitroglycerin (sublingual, topical, transdermal, or I.V.); isosorbide dinitrate or calcium channel blockers, such as nifedipine, verapamil, and diltiazem (sublingual, by mouth, or I.V.), to relieve pain and reduce myocardial workload

• lidocaine for ventricular arrhythmias, or drugs such as procainamide, quinidine, bretylium, or disopyramide
• PA catheterization to detect left- and right-sided HF to monitor response to treatment
• atropine I.V. or a temporary pacemaker to treat heart block or bradycardia
• beta-adrenergic blockers, such as propranolol and timolol, after acute MI to help prevent reinfarction
• an inotropic drug, dobutamine, to treat reduced myocardial contractility.

Nursing interventions. Most patients with MI receive treatment in the ICU, under constant observation for complications. Expect to perform the following nursing care measures:

• Monitor and record ECG, blood pressure, temperature, and heart and breath sounds.

• Assess pain, and administer analgesics, as ordered. Always record the severity and duration of pain. Avoid giving I.M. injections. Muscle damage increases CK and lactate dehydrogenase (LD) levels, making diagnosis of MI more difficult.

• Check the patient's blood pressure after giving nitroglycerin, especially the first dose.

• Frequently monitor ECG to detect rate changes or arrhythmias. Place rhythm strips in the patient's chart periodically for evaluation.

• During episodes of chest pain, obtain ECG, blood pressure, and PA catheter measurements to determine changes.

• Watch for signs and symptoms of fluid retention (crackles, cough, tachypnea, edema), which may indicate impending HF. Carefully monitor daily weight, intake and output, respirations, serum enzyme levels, and blood pressure. Auscultate for adventitious breath sounds periodically (many patients on bed rest have atelectatic crackles), and for S_3 or S_4 gallops.

• Organize patient care and activities to maximize rest.

• Ask the dietary department to provide a clear liquid diet until nausea subsides. A low-cholesterol, low-sodium diet, without caffeine-containing beverages, may be ordered.

• Provide a stool softener to prevent straining at stool, which may slow

heart rate. Allow the patient to use a bedside commode, and provide as much privacy as possible.

• Assist with range-of-motion (ROM) exercises. If the patient is completely immobilized by a severe MI, turn him often. Antiembolism stockings help prevent venostasis and thrombophlebitis.

• Provide emotional support; administer tranquilizers, as needed. Involve the family as much as possible in his care. (See *Indigestion or angina?*, page 170.)

Patient education. Explain procedures and answer questions. Explain the ICU environment and routine to lessen the patient's anxiety.

Carefully prepare the MI patient for discharge. Thoroughly explain dosages and therapy. Warn about drug adverse effects, and advise the patient to watch for and report signs of toxicity. If the patient has a Holter monitor in place, explain its purpose and use.

Counsel the patient about lifestyle changes. Provide a referral to a cardiac rehabilitation program. Review dietary restrictions. If the patient must follow a low-sodium or low-fat and low-cholesterol diet, provide a list of undesirable foods. Ask the dietitian to speak to the patient and his family. Advise the patient to resume sexual activity progressively. Stress the need to stop smoking. If necessary, refer him to a smoking cessation group.

Instruct the patient to report chest pain. Postinfarction syndrome may develop, producing chest pain that

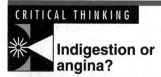

Indigestion or angina?

Three days after a routine chole-cystectomy, David Morton, age 52, was scheduled for discharge the next morning.

A problem or not?
You find him sitting up in his bed, anxious and slightly diaphoretic. His skin is pale and cool. "I have indigestion," he says.

Questioning him further, you learn that his discomfort is located in the lower half of the sternum and left chest. The patient describes pain that is local and doesn't radiate. His vital signs are stable and his breath sounds are normal.

Suggested response
You call for a stat, 12-lead electrocardiogram, start oxygen by nasal cannula, insert an intermittent infusion device and notify the doctor.

must be differentiated from recurrent MI, pulmonary infarct, or HF.

Evaluation. Look for absence of arrhythmias, chest pain, shortness of breath, fatigue, and edema; clear lung sounds; normal heart sounds and blood pressure; and evidence of ability to tolerate exercise. In addition, cardiac output should be adequate, as shown by a normal LOC; warm, dry skin; and an absence of dizziness.

Heart failure

HF is the major cause of hospitalization of adults. As more people survive MI and valvular disease, they eventually develop HF from the primary heart disease. In this disorder, abnormal circulatory congestion and impaired pump performance result from myocardial dysfunction. Congestion of systemic venous circulation may cause peripheral edema or hepatomegaly. Congestion of pulmonary circulation may cause pulmonary edema, an acute life-threatening emergency. (See *Managing pulmonary edema,* page 172.)

Pump failure usually occurs in a damaged left ventricle (left-sided HF) but may happen in the right ventricle, either as primary failure or secondary to left-sided HF. Sometimes, left- and right-sided HF develop simultaneously. HF may be classified as systolic or diastolic. Systolic failure is the ineffective pumping of blood during contraction while diastolic failure results from ineffective ventricular filling.

Acute HF may result from MI, CAD, cardiomyopathy, or other disorders. The chronic form of the disorder is associated with renal retention of sodium and water.

Causes. Cardiovascular disorders that lead to HF include atherosclerotic heart disease, MI, hypertension, rheumatic heart disease, congenital heart disease, ischemic heart disease, cardiomyopathy, valvular diseases, and arrhythmias.

Noncardiovascular causes of HF include postpartum cardiomyopathy, thyrotoxicosis, pulmonary embolism, and chronic obstructive pulmonary disease.

Assessment findings. Fatigue is the hallmark assessment finding. Other clinical signs of left-sided HF include dyspnea, initially upon exertion. The patient also develops paroxysmal nocturnal dyspnea, Cheyne-Stokes respirations, and orthopnea. Check also for tachycardia, fatigue, muscle weakness, edema and weight gain, irritability, restlessness, and a shortened attention span. Auscultate for a ventricular gallop (heard over the apex) and bibasilar crackles.

The patient with right-sided HF may develop edema. Initially dependent, edema may progress. His neck veins may become distended and rigid. Hepatomegaly may eventually lead to anorexia, nausea, and vague abdominal pain. Observe also for ascites or a ventricular heave.

Diagnostic tests. ECG reflects heart strain or ventricular enlargement, or ischemia. It may also reveal atrial enlargement, tachycardia, and extrasystoles, suggesting HF.

Chest X-ray shows increased pulmonary vascular markings, interstitial edema, or pleural effusion and cardiomegaly.

PA monitoring demonstrates elevated PA pressure and PAWP, which reflect left ventricular end-diastolic pressure, in left-sided HF, and elevated right atrial pressure or CVP in right-sided HF.

A multiple-gated acquisition scan (cardiac blood pool imaging) shows a decreased ejection fraction in left-sided HF.

Cardiac catheterization may show ventricular dilation, coronary artery occlusion, and valvular disorders (such as aortic stenosis) in both left- and right-sided HF.

Echocardiography may show ventricular hypertrophy, decreased contractility, and valvular disorders in both left- and right-sided HF. Serial echocardiograms may help assess the patient's response.

Treatment. ACE inhibitors are the first line of pharmacologic intervention. Other measures include diuretics, vasodilators, and digitalis glycosides. Acute failure may call for a positive inotropic agent, such as I.V. dopamine or dobutamine.

The patient must also get plenty of bed rest and follow a sodium-restricted diet with smaller, more frequent meals. He may have to wear antiembolism stockings to prevent venostasis and possible thromboembolism formation. The doctor may order oxygen therapy.

After recovery, the patient usually remains under medical supervision. If the patient with valve dysfunction has recurrent acute HF, he may undergo surgical valve replacement. When these treatments fail, carefully selected patients may undergo a heart transplant.

Nursing interventions. During the acute phase of HF, place the patient in Fowler's position and give him supplemental oxygen to help him breathe more easily. Weigh him daily, and check for peripheral

Managing pulmonary edema

Because of left-sided heart failure, fluid may accumulate in the extravascular spaces of the lungs. To intervene appropriately, you must accurately assess the severity of the patient's edema. Provide emotional support to the patient and family through all stages of illness.

Initial stage

At first, the patient may develop persistent cough, slight dyspnea or orthopnea, exercise intolerance, restlessness, and anxiety. Assessment may reveal crackles at lung bases and a diastolic gallop.

Take the following steps:
• Check color and amount of expectoration.
• Position patient for comfort and elevate head of bed.
• Auscultate chest for crackles and S_3.
• Administer prescribed medications.
• Monitor apical and radial pulses.
• Assist patient to conserve strength.

Acute stage

As edema progresses, the patient may develop acute shortness of breath. Respirations may become rapid and noisy, with audible wheezes and crackles. His cough intensifies and produces a frothy, blood-tinged sputum. Skin may become cyanotic, cold, and clammy. Other clinical signs include tachycardia, arrhythmias, and hypotension.

During the acute stage, expect to take these steps:
• Administer supplemental oxygen, as necessary (preferably in high concentrations by Venturi mask or intermittent positive-pressure breathing).
• Insert I.V. line, if not already done.
• Aspirate nasopharynx, as needed.
• Give inotropic agents, such as digoxin, dopamine, or dobutamine, as ordered.
• Give nitrates, morphine, and potent diuretics such as furosemide, as ordered.
• Insert an indwelling urinary catheter.
• Calculate intake and output accurately.
• Draw blood to measure arterial blood gas levels.
• Attach cardiac monitor leads, and observe electrocardiogram.
• Reassure the patient.
• Keep resuscitation equipment available at all times.

Advanced stage

If edema goes unchecked, the patient may suffer decreased level of consciousness, ventricular arrhythmias, and shock. Your assessment may also reveal diminished breath sounds.

Be prepared for cardioversion. Assist with intubation and mechanical ventilation, and resuscitate the patient, if necessary.

edema. Monitor I.V. intake and urine output, vital signs (for increased respiratory rate, heart rate, and narrowing pulse pressure), and mental status. Auscultate the heart for abnormal sounds (S_3 gallop) and the lungs for crackles and rhonchi. Report changes immediately.

Frequently monitor BUN, serum creatinine, potassium, sodium, chloride, and magnesium levels.

To prevent deep vein thrombosis from vascular congestion, assist the patient with ROM exercises. Enforce bed rest during exacerbations, and apply antiembolism stockings. Watch for calf pain and tenderness. (See *Managing heart failure*, pages 174 to 179.)

Patient education. Teach the patient about lifestyle changes. Advise him to avoid foods high in sodium. Explain that the potassium he loses through diuretic therapy must be replaced by taking a prescribed potassium supplement and eating high-potassium foods. Stress the need for regular checkups. Emphasize continuing low levels of activity as tolerated. Encourage cardiac rehabilitation as applicable.

Stress the importance of taking digitalis glycosides exactly as prescribed. Tell the patient to watch for and immediately report signs and symptoms of toxicity, such as anorexia, vomiting, and yellow vision.

Tell the patient to notify the doctor if his pulse is unusually irregular or less than 60 beats/minute; if he experiences dizziness, shortness of breath, blurred vision, a persistent dry cough, palpitations, increased fatigue, paroxysmal nocturnal dyspnea, swollen ankles, or decreased urine output; or if he gains 3 to 5 lb (1.35 to 2.25 kg) in a week.

Evaluation. Assessment of the patient should reveal clear lungs, normal heart sounds, adequate blood pressure, and absence of dyspnea or edema. The patient should be able to perform ADLs and maintain his normal weight.

Cardiac complications

Cardiac complications include cardiac arrhythmias, hypovolemic and cardiogenic shock, and cardiac tamponade.

Cardiac arrhythmias

Cardiac arrhythmias occur when abnormal electrical conduction or automaticity changes heart rate or rhythm or both. Arrhythmias vary in severity from mild, asymptomatic disturbances to catastrophic ventricular fibrillation, which necessitates immediate resuscitation. Arrhythmias are usually classified according to their origin (ventricular or supraventricular). Their clinical significance depends on their effect on cardiac output and blood pressure.

Causes. Arrhythmias may be congenital or may result from myocardial anoxia, MI, hypertrophy of heart muscle fiber because of hypertension or valvular heart disease, or degeneration of conductive tissue necessary to maintain normal heart rhythm (sick sinus syndrome). Toxic doses of cardioactive drugs, such as digoxin and other digitalis glycosides, may also lead to arrhythmias. (See *Reviewing cardiac arrhythmias*, pages 180 to 186.)

(Text continues on page 178.)

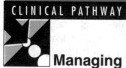

CLINICAL PATHWAY

Managing heart failure

(Excluding intra-aortic balloon pump)
* Note all allergies and check to ensure patient receives no medication that he is allergic to.
Call service to obtain alternative medications.

Care element	Admission Day 1 Date:	Day 2 Date:
Care unit	Cardiac catheter laboratory Medical intensive care unit (MICU)/coronary care unit (CCU) Intermediate care (IMC)	MICU IMC
Consults	• Nutrition • Social services	→→→→ • Social services • Physical therapist (PT) to evaluate patient for cardiac rehabilitation
Tests/lab work Notify house officer (HO) for: _____ Partial thromboplastin time (PTT) < 40 or > 100	• Renal disease battery (RDB), complete blood count (CBC), liver function tests (LFT), prothrombin time (PT)/international normalized ratio (INR) if on warfarin • Partial thromboplastin time (PTT) every 6 hr, if anticoagulated until PTT > 60 • Chest X-ray: anterior, posterior, and lateral views on admission per order • 12-lead electrocardiogram on admission per order	• RDB in a.m. • PTT if heparinized
Assessments Notify doctor if: • Systolic blood pressure (SBP) < 80 or > 140 • Heart rate (HR) < 60 or > 120 • Respiratory rate (RR) < 30 • Oxygen saturation (O_2 sat) > 90% • Ventricular tachycardia (VT), > 10 premature ventricular contractions (PVCs) per min- ute, frequent multifocal PVCs • Pulmonary artery wedge pressure (PAWP) < 15 or > 25 mm Hg • Cardiac index (CI) < 2.5 • Systemic vascular resis- tance (SVR) < 800 or > 1,200 dynes/sec/cm-⁵	• Vital signs (VS) every 15 min when titrating medications; then every hr • PAWP & pulmonary artery dias- tolic (PAD) pressure initially; if wedge within 1-2 of PAD, don't wedge; do readings every 4 hr • Assessment of inotropic drug effects every 4 hr • Systems assessment every shift • Intake and output (I & O) record- ing every shift • Weight on admission • Rhythm monitoring	→→→→ • Swan-Ganz catheter readings every 4 hr • Assessment of inotrop- ic drug effects every 4 hr • Systems assessment every shift • I & O recording every shift • Weight check daily • Rhythm monitoring

Day 3 Date:	Day 4 Date:	Day 5 Date:
MICU IMC	IMC	IMC
• RDB • PTT if heparinized • PT/INR if on warfarin	• RDB • PTT if heparinized	• RDB • PTT if heparinized
• VS every 15 min when titrating meds; then every hr • Assessment of inotropic drug effects every 4 hr • Systems assessment every shift • I & O recording every shift • Daily weight check • Rhythm monitoring	• VS every 2 to 4 hr after weaned from inotropic support • Systems assessment every shift • I & O recording every shift • Daily weight check	• VS every 4 hr • Systems assessment every shift • I & O recording every shift • Daily weight check

Managing heart failure *(continued)*

Care element	Admission Day 1 Date:	Day 2 Date:
Treatments	• I.V. midline (ML) or peripherally inserted central catheter (PICC)—flush every shift with normal saline solution (NSS) • If applicable, Swan-Ganz catheter (MICU) • Cardiac monitor • O₂ at _____ liters per minute (LPM) • O₂ sat monitor • O₂ titrated to keep sat > 92% • Evaluation for discontinuing O₂ and sat monitor once stable; may be discontinued if O₂ sat > 92% on room air	• I.V. ML or PICC—flush every shift with NSS • If hemodynamic goal achieved, discontinue Swan-Ganz catheter (MICU) • Cardiac monitor • O₂ at _____ LPM • O₂ sat monitor • O₂ titrated to keep sat > 92% • Evaluation for discontinuing O₂ and sat monitor once stable; may be discontinued if O₂ sat > 92% on room air

Medication	• Electrolyte replacements per protocol
	• Inotropic drugs titrated to keep SBP 85-110, PAWP 18-20, Woods units mean pulse pressure minus pulse cap wedge pressure (PCWP) divided by cardiac output < 3.0, urine output (UO) > 30 ml/hr
	• Medications per doctor order:
	  • ACE inhibitors
	  • Vasodilators
	  • Diuretics
	  • Digoxin
	  • Anticoagulant
		• Electrolyte replacements per MICU protocol
		• Inotropic drugs titrated to keep SBP 85-110, PAWP 18-20, Woods units < 3.0, UO > 30 ml/hr
		• Medications per doctor order:
		  • ACE inhibitors
		  • Vasodilators
		  • Diuretics
		  • Digoxin
		  • Anticoagulant

Pain/symptom control	• Tylenol 650 mg P.O. every 6 hr as needed for pain or headache • Maalox TC 15 ml P.O. every 6 hr for indigestion • Milk of Magnesia (MOM) 30 ml P.O. every 8 hr for constipation • Benadryl 25 to 50 mg P.O. every evening at bedtime (qHS) for sleep • Xanax 0.125 mg P.O. every 8 hr for anxiety	• Tylenol 650 mg P.O. every 6 hr as needed for pain or headache • Maalox TC 15 ml P.O. every 6 hr for indigestion • MOM 30 ml P.O. every 8 hr for constipation • Benadryl 25-50 mg P.O. qHS sleep • Xanax 0.125 mg P.O. every 8 hr for anxiety
Activity	• Bed rest while Swan-Ganz catheter in place or titrating inotropic drugs • Bedside commode (BSC) if stable • Assistance with activities of daily living (ADLs)	• Out of bed (OOB) to chair with assist and BSC if stable • Progress with ADLs

Day 3 Date:	Day 4 Date:	Day 5 Date:
• I.V. ML or PICC—flush every shift with NSS • If hemodynamic goal achieved, Swan-Ganz catheter (MICU) discontinued • Cardiac monitor • O_2 at _____ LPM; may discontinue O_2 and monitor if O_2 sat > 92% on room air	• I.V. ML or PICC—flush every shift with NSS • Swan-Ganz catheter discontinued per doctor order • Cardiac monitor • O_2 at _____ LPM; may discontinue O_2 and monitor if O_2 sat > 92% on room air • Indwelling urinary catheter discontinued, if applicable	• ML discontinued before discharge • Telemetry if ordered • O_2 discontinued per doctor's order

• Electrolytes as needed
• Inotropic support titrated/weaned
• Medications per doctor's order:
  • ACE inhibitors
  • Vasodilators
  • Diuretics
  • Digoxin
  • Anticoagulant
	• P.O. meds
	• Inotropic support weaned over 2 to 6 hrs
	• Medications per doctor's orders:
	  • ACE inhibitors
	  • Vasodilators
	  • Diuretics
	  • Digoxin
	  • Anticoagulant
		• Aspirin 1 P.O. daily
		• P.O. meds
		• Medications per doctor's orders:
		  • ACE inhibitors
		  • Vasodilators
		  • Diuretics
		  • Digoxin
		  • Anticoagulant

• Tylenol 650 mg P.O. every 6 hr as needed for pain or headache • Maalox TC 15 ml P.O. every 6 hr for indigestion • MOM 30 ml P.O. every 8 hr for constipation • Benadryl 25-50 mg P.O. qHS for sleep • Xanax 0.125 mg P.O. every 8 hr for anxiety	• Tylenol 650 mg P.O. every 6 hr as needed for pain or headache • Maalox TC 15 ml P.O. every 6 hr for indigestion • MOM 30 ml P.O. every 8 hr for constipation • Benadryl 25-50 mg P.O. qHS for sleep • Xanax 0.125 mg P.O. every 8 hr for anxiety	• Tylenol 650 mg P.O. every 6 hr as needed for pain or headache • Maalox TC 15 ml P.O. every 6 hr for indigestion • MOM 30 ml P.O. every 8 hr for constipation • Benadryl 25-50 mg P.O. qHS for sleep • Xanax 0.125 mg P.O. every 8 hr for anxiety
• OOB to chair three times daily with meals and a.m. care • Ambulation with assistance in room • Progress with ADLs	• OOB to chair with meals and a.m. care • Ambulation in hallway as tolerated • Progress with ADLs	• Patient to resume usual activity level • Ambulation in hallway as tolerated • Progress with ADLs

(continued)

Managing heart failure (continued)

Care element	Admission Day 1 Date:	Day 2 Date:
Nutrition	• CCU 2 g Na, low fat, no caffeine or stimulants (NCS) • Fluid restriction (FR) 1,500 ml	• CCU 2 gm Na, low fat, NCS • FR 1,500 ml
Discharge planning/teaching	• Assess patient's knowledge deficit about congestive heart failure. • Explain monitors, tubes, lines. • Explain purpose of meds and ionotropic support. • Explain to patient and significant other purpose of sodium and fluid restriction and need for daily weight checks. • Assist Heart Transplant Coordinator with preoperative teaching (if indicated).	• Explain low-sodium, low-fat diet, and caffeine and stimulant restrictions. • Explain meds as they are converted from I.V. to P.O. • Reinforce purpose of daily weight checks, I & O recording, and fluid restriction. • Teach about knowledge deficits and cardiac treatment, if applicable.

Adapted with permission from SHANDS at the University of Florida, Gainesville.

Assessment findings and nursing interventions. If you suspect arrhythmia in an unmonitored patient, assess for rhythm disturbances. If the patient's pulse is abnormally rapid, slow, or irregular, watch for signs of hypoperfusion, such as hypotension and diminished urine output. Look for indications of predisposing factors—such as fluid and electrolyte imbalance—and signs of drug toxicity, especially with digoxin. Report suspected drug toxicity to the doctor immediately and withhold the next dose.

Document any arrhythmias in a monitored patient and assess for possible causes and effects.

Evaluate the patient experiencing an arrhythmia for altered cardiac output. Consider whether the arrhythmia is potentially progressive or ominous. If the arrhythmia appears to be life-threatening, follow the life-support procedures outlined later in this chapter.

Hypovolemic shock

In hypovolemic shock, reduced intravascular blood volume causes circulatory dysfunction and inadequate tissue perfusion. Without suf-

Day 3 Date:	Day 4 Date:	Day 5 Date:
• CCU 2 g Na, low-fat, NCS • FR 1,500 ml	• CCU 2 g Na, low-fat, NCS • FR 1,500 ml	• CCU 2 g Na, low-fat, NCS • FR 1,500 ml
• Reinforce diet instruction in low-sodium, low-fat diet. • Instruct patient to identify meds as they're given. • Ask patient to explain purpose of I & O and weight checks and fluid restriction. • Have patient monitor own fluid restriction. • Teach signs and symptoms of worsening CHF: shortness of breath, dyspnea on exertion, activity intolerance, increased heart rate, increased edema, decreased urine output, weight gain. • Evaluate for home care follow-up.	• Have patient list foods high in sodium. • Have patient identify and explain purpose of each medication. • Teach patient major side effects of each drug. • Have patient state signs and symptoms of worsening CHF. • Contact home care if needed.	• Ask patient to explain fluid and dietary restrictions. • Have patient state purpose and major side effects of each discharge medication. • Have patient list at least 5 signs and symptoms of worsening CHF. • Have patient or significant other verbalize plan for follow-up care.

ficient blood or fluid replacement, hypovolemic shock syndrome may lead to irreversible cerebral and renal damage, cardiac arrest and, ultimately, death.

Causes. Most commonly, patients develop hypovolemic shock after acute blood loss. Other causes include severe burns, intestinal obstruction, peritonitis, acute pancreatitis, ascites, dehydration from excessive perspiration, severe diarrhea or protracted vomiting, or excessive fluid loss through gastric suction, diabetes insipidus, diuresis, and inadequate fluid intake.

Assessment findings. The patient develops hypotension with narrowing pulse pressure; decreased sensorium; tachycardia; and rapid, shallow respirations. Assess also for reduced urine output (less than 25 ml/hour) and cold, pale, clammy skin. Metabolic acidosis with an accumulation of lactic acid develops as a result of tissue anoxia, as cellular metabolism shifts from aerobic to anaerobic pathways. Disseminated intravascular coagulation (DIC) is a possible complication of hypovolemic shock.

(*Text continues on page 187.*)

Reviewing cardiac arrhythmias

Normal sinus rhythm in adults

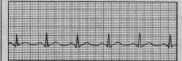

- Ventricular and atrial rates of 60 to 100 beats/minute (BPM)
- QRS complexes and P waves regular and uniform
- PR interval 0.12 to 0.2 second
- QRS duration < 0.12 second
- Identical atrial and ventricular rates, with constant PR interval

Sinus arrhythmia

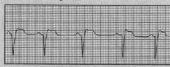

Causes
Sinus arrhythmia usually occurs as a normal variation of normal sinus rhythm (NSR). It's associated with sinus bradycardia.
Description
- Slight irregularity of heartbeat
- Rate increases with inspiration; decreases with expiration
Treatment
- Treated only if signs or symptoms develop

Sinus tachycardia

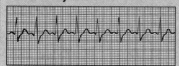

Causes
Sinus tachycardia occurs as a normal physiologic response to fever, exercise, anxiety, pain, dehydration; may also accompany shock, left-sided heart failure (HF), cardiac tamponade, anemia, hyperthyroidism, hypovolemia, and pulmonary embolus. It may also result from treatment with vagolytic and sympathetic stimulating drugs.
Description
- Rate >100 BPM; rarely, >160 BPM
- Every QRS wave follows a P wave
Treatment
Correct underlying cause

Sinus bradycardia

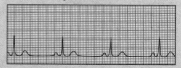

Causes
Sinus bradycardia may result from increased intracranial pressure; increased vagal tone from bowel straining, vomiting, intubation, or mechanical ventilation; sick sinus syndrome; or hypothyroidism. It may also follow treatment with beta blockers and sympatholytic drugs. Sinus bradycardia may be normal in athletes.
Description
- Rate < 60 BPM
- A QRS complex follows each P wave
Treatment
- For low cardiac output, dizziness, weakness, altered level of consciousness, or low blood pressure, 0.5 mg atropine every 5 minutes to total of 2 mg
- Temporary pacemaker or isoproterenol, if atropine fails

Reviewing cardiac arrhythmias *(continued)*

Sinoatrial arrest or block (sinus arrest)

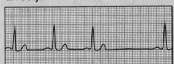

Causes
This arrhythmia may result from vagal stimulation or digitalis or quinidine toxicity. In many cases, it's a sign of sick sinus syndrome.

Description
• NSR interrupted by unexpectedly prolonged P-P interval, commonly terminated by an escape beat or return to NSR
• QRS complexes uniform but irregular

Treatment
• A pacemaker for repeated episodes

Wandering atrial pacemaker

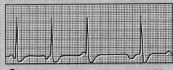

Causes
Wandering atrial pacemaker results from inflammation involving the sinoatrial node, digitalis toxicity, and sick sinus syndrome.

Description
• Rate varies
• QRS complexes uniform in shape but irregular in rhythm
• P waves irregular with changing configuration
• PR interval varies from short to normal

Treatment
• Treated if bradycardia develops

Premature atrial contraction

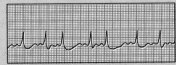

Causes
Premature atrial contraction may result from HF, ischemic heart disease, acute respiratory failure, or chronic obstructive pulmonary disease (COPD). It may also result from treatment with a digitalis glycoside, aminophylline, or adrenergic drugs or from anxiety or caffeine ingestion. Occasional premature atrial contraction (PAC) may occur normally.

Description
• Premature, abnormal-looking P waves; QRS complexes follow, except in early or blocked PACs
• P wave commonly buried in the preceding T wave or can be identified in the preceding T wave

Treatment
• If more than six times per minute or frequency is increasing, give a digitalis glycoside, quinidine, or propranolol; after revascularization surgery, propranolol
• Eliminate known causes, such as caffeine or drugs

Paroxysmal atrial tachycardia or paroxysmal supraventricular tachycardia

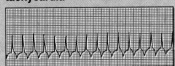

Causes
This arrhythmia may occur as an

(continued)

Reviewing cardiac arrhythmias *(continued)*

intrinsic abnormality of atrioventricular (AV) conduction system or as a congenital accessory atrial conduction pathway. It may also result from physical or psychological stress, hypoxia, hypokalemia, caffeine, marijuana, stimulants, or digitalis toxicity.

Description
• Heart rate >140 BPM; rarely exceeds 250 BPM
• P waves regular but aberrant; difficult to differentiate from preceding T wave
• Onset and termination of arrhythmia occur suddenly
• May cause palpitations and lightheadedness

Treatment
• Vagal maneuvers, sympathetic blockers (propranolol, quinidine), or calcium blocker (verapamil) to alter AV node conduction
• Elective cardioversion, if patient is symptomatic and unresponsive to drugs

Atrial flutter

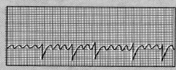

Causes
Atrial flutter may result from HF, valvular heart disease, pulmonary embolism, digitalis toxicity, or postoperative revascularization.

Description
• Ventricular rate depends on degree of AV block (usually 60 to 100 BPM)
• Atrial rate 250 to 400 BPM and regular

• QRS complexes uniform in shape, but many are irregular in rate
• P waves may have sawtooth configuration (F waves)

Treatment
• A digitalis glycoside (unless arrhythmia is caused by digitalis toxicity), propranolol, or quinidine
• May require synchronized cardioversion or atrial pacemaker

Atrial fibrillation

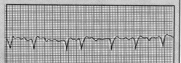

Causes
Atrial fibrillation may result from HF, COPD, hyperthyroidism, sepsis, pulmonary embolus, mitral stenosis, digitalis toxicity (rarely), atrial irritation, postcoronary bypass or valve replacement surgery.

Description
• Atrial rate >400 BPM
• Ventricular rate varies
• QRS complexes uniform in shape but at irregular intervals
• PR interval indiscernible
• No P waves, or P waves appear as erratic, irregular baseline f waves
• Irregular QRS rate

Treatment
• A digitalis glycoside, verapamil, or propranolol to increase atrial refractoriness
• Quinidine to slow or procainamide to prolong atrial refractoriness
• May require elective cardioversion for rapid rate

Reviewing cardiac arrhythmias *(continued)*

AV junctional rhythm (nodal rhythm)

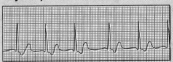

Causes
This arrhythmia may result from digitalis toxicity, inferior wall myocardial infarction (MI) or ischemia, hypoxia, vagal stimulation, acute rheumatic fever, or valve surgery.

Description
• Ventricular rate usually 40 to 60 BPM (60 to 100 BPM is accelerated junctional rhythm)
• P waves may precede, be hidden within (absent), or follow QRS; if visible, they're altered
• QRS duration is normal, except in aberrant conduction
• Patient may be asymptomatic unless ventricular rate is slow

Treatment
• Symptomatic
• Atropine or pacemaker for slow rate
• If patient is taking a digitalis glycoside, it's discontinued

Premature junctional contractions (premature nodal contractions)

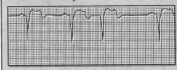

Causes
Premature junctional contractions (premature nodal contractions) may result from myocardial ischemia or MI, digitalis toxicity, or caffeine or amphetamine ingestion.

Description
• QRS complexes of uniform shape, but premature
• P waves irregular, with premature beat; may precede, be hidden within, or follow QRS

Treatment
• Correct underlying cause
• Quinidine or disopyramide, as ordered
• If patient is taking a digitalis glycoside, it may be discontinued

First-degree AV block

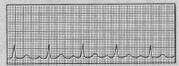

Causes
First-degree AV block may result from inferior myocardial ischemia or MI, hypothyroidism, digitalis toxicity, or potassium imbalance.

Description
• PR interval prolonged >0.20 second
• QRS complex normal

Treatment
• Patient should use digitalis glycosides cautiously
• Correct underlying cause. Otherwise, be alert for increasing block

Second-degree AV block Mobitz Type I (Wenckebach)

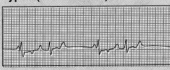

(continued)

Reviewing cardiac arrhythmias *(continued)*

Causes

This arrhythmia may result from inferior wall MI, digitalis toxicity, or vagal stimulation.

Description

- PR interval becomes longer with each cycle until QRS disappears (dropped beat); after a dropped beat, PR interval the shortest
- Atrial rhythm is regular
- Ventricular interval shortens as the PR interval lengthens, until the dropped beat is seen

Treatment

- Atropine, if patient is symptomatic
- May discontinue the digitalis glycoside

Second-degree AV block Mobitz Type II

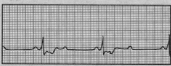

Causes

Second-degree AV block Mobitz Type II may result from degenerative disease of the conduction system, ischemia of the AV node in anterior MI, digitalis toxicity, or anteroseptal infarction.

Description

- PR interval is constant, with QRS complexes dropped
- Ventricular rhythm may be irregular, with varying degree of block
- Atrial rate regular

Treatment

- Temporary pacemaker, sometimes followed by permanent pacemaker
- Atropine for slow rate
- Isoproterenol if patient is hypotensive

- If patient is taking a digitalis glycoside, it's discontinued

Third-degree AV block (complete heart block)

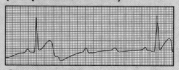

Causes

Third-degree AV block may result from ischemic heart disease or MI, postsurgical complications of mitral valve replacement, or digitalis toxicity. It may also result from hypoxia, which may lead to syncope from decreased cerebral blood flow (as in Stokes-Adams syndrome).

Description

- Atrial rate regular; ventricular rate, slow and regular
- No relationship between P waves and QRS complexes
- No constant PR interval
- QRS interval normal (nodal pacemaker); wide and bizarre (ventricular pacemaker)

Treatment

- Usually requires temporary pacemaker, followed by permanent pacemaker
- Atropine or isoproterenol

Junctional tachycardia (nodal tachycardia)

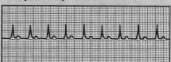

Causes

Junctional tachycardia (nodal tachycardia) may result from digitalis toxi-

Reviewing cardiac arrhythmias *(continued)*

city, myocarditis, cardiomyopathy, myocardial ischemia, or MI.

Description
• In many cases, onset of rhythm sudden, occurring in bursts
• Ventricular rate >100 BPM
• Other characteristics same as junctional rhythm

Treatment
• Vagal stimulation
• Propranolol, quinidine, a digitalis glycoside (if cause isn't digitalis toxicity), verapamil, or edrophonium
• Elective cardioversion

Premature ventricular contraction

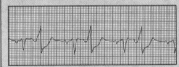

Causes
Premature ventricular contraction (PVC) may result from HF; old or acute MI or contusion with trauma; myocardial irritation by ventricular catheter such as a pacemaker; hypoxia, as in anemia and acute respiratory failure; drug toxicity (a digitalis glycoside, aminophylline, tricyclic antidepressants, beta adrenergics [isoproterenol or dopamine]); electrolyte imbalances (especially hypokalemia); or stress.

Description
• Beat occurs prematurely, usually followed by a complete compensatory pause after PVC; irregular pulse
• QRS complex wide and distorted
• Can occur singly, in pairs, or in threes; can alternate with normal beats; focus can be from one or more sites

• PVCs are ominous when clustered, multifocal, with R wave on T pattern

Treatment
• Lidocaine I.V. bolus and drip infusion; procainamide I.V. If induced by digitalis toxicity, stop this drug; if induced by hypokalemia, give potassium chloride I.V. Other drugs used depend on the cause of arrhythmia

Ventricular tachycardia

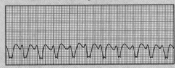

Causes
Ventricular tachycardia may result from myocardial ischemia or MI, aneurysm, ventricular catheters, digitalis or quinidine toxicity, hypokalemia, hypercalcemia, or anxiety.

Description
• Ventricular rate 140 to 220 BPM; may be regular
• Three or more PVCs in a row
• QRS complexes are wide, bizarre, and independent of P waves
• Usually no visible P waves
• Can produce chest pain, anxiety, palpitations, dyspnea, shock, coma, and death

Treatment
• If pulses are absent, cardiopulmonary resuscitation (CPR) followed by lidocaine I.V. (bolus and drip infusion) and countershock; if pulse is present, use synchronized cardioversion
• Bretylium tosylate and procainamide

(continued)

Reviewing cardiac arrhythmias *(continued)*

• Patients who survive should be evaluated for an implanted cardioverter/defibrillator

Ventricular fibrillation

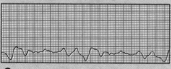

Causes

Ventricular fibrillation may result from myocardial ischemia or MI, untreated ventricular tachycardia, electrolyte imbalances (hypokalemia and alkalosis, hyperkalemia and hypercalcemia), digitalis or quinidine toxicity, electric shock, or hypothermia.

Description

• Ventricular rhythm rapid and chaotic
• QRS complexes wide and irregular; no visible P waves
• Loss of consciousness, with no peripheral pulses, blood pressure, or respirations; possible seizures; sudden death

Treatment

• CPR
• Asynchronized countershock (200 to 300 watts/second) twice; if rhythm does not return, reshock (300 to 400 watts/second)
• Epinephrine, lidocaine, or bretylium tosylate
• Patients who survive should be evaluated for an implanted cardioverter/defibrillator

Electromechanical dissociation

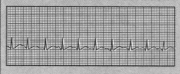

Causes

Electromechanical dissociation may indicate a failure in the calcium transport system. It may be associated with profound hypovolemia, cardiac tamponade, myocardial rupture, massive MI, or tension pneumothorax.

Description

• Organized electrical activity without pulse or other evidence of effective myocardial contraction

Treatment

• CPR
• Epinephrine

Ventricular standstill (asystole)

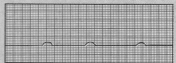

Causes

Ventricular standstill may result from acute respiratory failure, myocardial ischemia or MI, ruptured ventricular aneurysm, aortic valve disease, or hyperkalemia.

Description

• Primary ventricular standstill—regular P waves, no QRS complexes
• Secondary ventricular standstill—QRS complexes wide and slurred, occurring at irregular intervals; agonal heart rhythm
• Loss of consciousness, with no peripheral pulses, blood pressure, or respirations

Treatment

• CPR
• Endotracheal intubation; pacemaker should be available
• Epinephrine, isoproterenol, and atropine

Diagnostic tests. No single symptom or diagnostic test establishes the diagnosis or severity of hypovolemic shock. Laboratory findings include elevated serum potassium, serum lactate, and BUN levels; decreased blood pH level and partial pressure of arterial oxygen; and an increased partial pressure of arterial carbon dioxide. The patient will also exhibit an increase in urine specific gravity (more than 1.020) and urine osmolality.

In addition, the doctor may order gastroscopy, aspiration of gastric contents through a nasogastric (NG) tube, and X-rays to identify internal bleeding sites. Coagulation studies may detect coagulopathy from DIC. The doctor may also insert a PA catheter to obtain right atrial pressure and monitor PAWP.

Treatment. Emergency measures consist of prompt, adequate blood and fluid replacement to restore intravascular volume and raise blood pressure. Saline solutions, then possibly plasma proteins (albumin), other plasma expanders, or lactated Ringer's solution may produce volume expansion until whole blood can be matched.

Treatment may also include oxygen administration, identification of any bleeding sites, control of bleeding by direct measures, and possibly surgery. For some patients, autotransfusion of salvaged blood may be possible.

Nursing interventions. Follow these priorities:

• Check for a patent airway and adequate circulation. Administer oxygen, as ordered. If blood pressure and heart rate are absent, start cardiopulmonary resuscitation (CPR).
• Place the patient flat in bed to increase blood flow by promoting venous return to the heart.
• Record blood pressure, pulse rate, peripheral pulses, respirations, and other vital signs every 15 minutes. Monitor continuous ECG recording. When systolic blood pressure drops below 80 mm Hg, increase the oxygen flow rate, and notify the doctor immediately. A progressive drop in blood pressure, accompanied by a thready pulse, generally signals inadequate cardiac output from reduced intravascular volume. Notify the doctor, and increase the infusion rate.
• Start an I.V. infusion with normal saline or lactated Ringer's solution, using a large-bore catheter (14G), which allows easier administration of later blood transfusions. (**Caution:** Don't start an I.V. infusion in the legs of a patient in shock who has suffered abdominal trauma.)
• You may insert an indwelling urinary catheter to measure hourly urine output. If output is less than 30 ml/hour in adults, increase the fluid infusion rate, but watch for signs of fluid overload. Notify the doctor if urine output does not improve. He may order an osmotic diuretic to increase renal blood flow and urine output. Determine how much fluid to give by checking blood pressure, urine output, CVP, or PAWP.

• Draw an arterial blood sample to measure arterial blood gas (ABG) levels. Give oxygen by face mask or airway to ensure adequate oxygenation. Adjust the oxygen flow rate to a higher or lower level, as ABG measurements indicate.

• Watch for signs of impending coagulopathy (petechiae, bruising, and bleeding or oozing from gums or venipuncture sites).

Patient education. Explain all procedures and their purposes.

Evaluation. Look for adequate blood pressure, pulse, respirations, and urine output. Also note adequate tissue perfusion (normal LOC; warm, dry skin; and absence of cyanosis).

Cardiogenic shock

Also called pump failure, cardiogenic shock refers to a condition of diminished cardiac output that severely impairs tissue perfusion. It reflects severe left-sided HF and occurs as a serious complication in nearly 15% of all patients hospitalized with acute MI. Severe end-stage HF eventually can lead to cardiogenic shock. Most patients with cardiogenic shock die within 24 hours of onset.

Causes. Most commonly the result of MI, cardiogenic shock may follow any condition that causes significant left ventricular dysfunction with reduced cardiac output. Other conditions that lead to cardiogenic shock include myocardial ischemia,

papillary muscle dysfunction, cardiomyopathy and end-stage HF.

Assessment findings. Cardiogenic shock produces cold, pale, clammy skin; a drop in systolic blood pressure to 30 mm Hg below baseline; or a sustained reading below 80 mm Hg not attributable to medication. It also causes tachycardia; rapid, shallow respirations; oliguria (less than 20 ml urine/hour); restlessness; mental confusion; narrowing pulse pressure; narrowing left ventricular end-diastolic pressure; and cyanosis.

Auscultation may reveal gallop rhythm and faint heart sounds. If shock is from ventricular septum or papillary muscle rupture, you may detect a holosystolic murmur.

Diagnostic tests. PA pressure monitoring shows increased PA pressure and PAWP, reflecting a rise in left ventricular end-diastolic pressure (preload) and enhanced resistance to left ventricular emptying (afterload) caused by ineffective pumping and heightened peripheral vascular resistance. Thermodilution technique measures decreased cardiac index (less than 2.2 L/minute).

Elevated enzyme levels (CK, LD, aspartate aminotransferase, and alanine aminotransferase) point to MI or ischemia and suggest HF or shock. CK and LD isoenzyme assays may confirm acute MI.

Other tests include invasive arterial pressure monitoring, which may reveal hypotension from impaired ventricular ejection, and ABG measurements, which may show metabolic acidosis and hypoxia.

Treatment. Treatment aims to enhance cardiovascular status by increasing cardiac output, improving myocardial perfusion, and decreasing cardiac workload with various cardiovascular drugs and mechanical-assist techniques.

Drug therapy may include dopamine or dobutamine I.V.; vasopressors that increase cardiac output, blood pressure, and renal blood flow; and norepinephrine, a more potent vasoconstrictor. Along with a vasopressor, the doctor may order nitroprusside I.V., a vasodilator, to further improve cardiac output by decreasing peripheral vascular resistance (afterload) and reducing left ventricular end-diastolic pressure (preload). However, nitroprusside therapy requires that the patient have adequate blood pressure and be closely monitored.

A mechanical-assist device, the intra-aortic balloon pump (IABP) may improve coronary artery perfusion and reduce cardiac work load.

When drug therapy and IABP insertion fail, treatment may require a ventricular assist pump, cardiopulmonary support system, or the artificial heart or cardiac transplant.

Nursing interventions. At the first sign of cardiogenic shock, take the following steps:
• Check the patient's blood pressure and heart rate.
• If the patient is hypotensive or has difficulty breathing, make sure he has a patent I.V. line and a patent airway, and provide oxygen to promote tissue oxygenation.
• Notify the doctor immediately.
• Monitor ABG levels to measure oxygenation and detect acidosis from poor tissue perfusion. Increase oxygen flow as indicated by ABG measurements.
• Check complete blood count (CBC) and electrolytes.

After diagnosis, take these measures:
• Monitor cardiac rhythm continuously. Assess skin color, temperature, and other vital signs often. Watch for a drop in systolic blood pressure to less than 80 mm Hg. Report hypertension immediately.
• To measure urine output, insert an indwelling urinary catheter. Notify the doctor if urine output drops below 30 ml/hour.
• Using a PA catheter, closely monitor PA pressure, PAWP and, if equipment is available, cardiac output. A high PAWP indicates HF and should be reported immediately.
• Plan your care to allow frequent rest periods. Provide for privacy.

Evaluation. The patient should have adequate tissue perfusion, evidenced by a normal LOC; warm, dry skin; and absence of cyanosis. Blood pressure and urine output should be adequate, and heart sounds normal.

Cardiac tamponade

In cardiac tamponade, a rapid, unchecked rise in intrapericardial pressure impairs diastolic filling of the heart. The rise in pressure usually results from blood or fluid accumulation in the pericardial sac. If fluid accumulates rapidly, the patient requires emergency lifesaving measures.

Causes. Cardiac tamponade may be idiopathic (Dressler's syndrome) or may result from effusion (in cancer, bacterial infection, tuberculosis and, rarely, acute rheumatic fever), hemorrhage, acute MI, or uremia.

Assessment findings. Classic signs include neck vein distention, reduced arterial blood pressure, muffled heart sounds on auscultation, and pulsus paradoxus (an abnormal inspiratory drop in systemic blood pressure greater than 15 mm Hg).

You may also detect dyspnea, tachycardia, narrow pulse pressure, restlessness, or hepatomegaly.

Diagnostic tests. Chest X-ray shows slightly widened mediastinum and cardiomegaly. PA catheterization detects increased right atrial pressure, right ventricular diastolic pressure, and CVP. Echocardiography records pericardial effusion with signs of right ventricular and atrial compression.

ECG proves useful in ruling out other cardiac disorders. It may reveal changes produced by acute pericarditis.

Treatment. These patients require measures to remove accumulated blood or fluid, thereby relieving intrapericardial pressure and cardiac compression. Pericardiocente-

sis (needle aspiration of the pericardial fluid) or surgical creation of an opening improves systemic arterial pressure and cardiac output with aspiration of as little as 25 ml of fluid. Such treatment necessitates continuous hemodynamic and ECG monitoring in the ICU.

To maintain cardiac output, the hypotensive patient requires trial volume loading with temporary I.V. normal saline solution with albumin, and perhaps an inotropic drug, such as isoproterenol or dopamine. Although these drugs normally improve myocardial function, they may further compromise an ischemic myocardium after MI.

In traumatic injury, the patient may need a blood transfusion or a thoracotomy to drain accumulated fluid or to repair bleeding sites. Heparin-induced tamponade may call for the heparin antagonist protamine sulfate while warfarin-induced tamponade may call for vitamin K.

Nursing interventions. If the patient needs pericardiocentesis, follow these guidelines:
• Keep a pericardial aspiration needle or catheter attached to a 50-ml syringe by a three-way stopcock, an ECG machine, and an emergency cart with a defibrillator at the bedside. Make sure equipment is turned on and ready for use.
• Position the patient at a 45- to 60-degree angle. Connect the precordial ECG lead to the hub of the aspiration needle with an alligator clamp and connecting wire. Assist with fluid aspiration. When the nee-

dle touches the myocardium, you'll see an ST-segment elevation or premature ventricular contractions.
• Monitor blood pressure and CVP during and after pericardiocentesis. Infuse I.V. solutions, as ordered, to maintain blood pressure. A decrease in CVP and a concomitant rise in blood pressure indicate relief of cardiac compression.
• Watch for complications of pericardiocentesis, such as ventricular fibrillation, vagovagal arrest, or coronary artery or cardiac chamber puncture. Closely monitor ECG changes, blood pressure, pulse rate, LOC, and urine output.

If the patient needs thoracotomy, follow these guidelines:
• Give antibiotics, protamine sulfate, or vitamin K, as ordered.
• Postoperatively, monitor critical factors such as vital signs and ABG measurements, and assess heart and breath sounds.
• Give pain medication, as ordered.
• Maintain the chest drainage system. Watch for complications such as hemorrhage and arrhythmias.

Patient education. As appropriate, explain pericardiocentesis or thoracotomy to the patient. Tell the patient what to expect after thoracotomy (chest tubes, drainage bottles, administration of oxygen). Teach him how to turn, deep-breathe, and cough.

Evaluation. Look for adequate tissue perfusion as evidenced by normal LOC, absence of cyanosis, and warm, dry skin. The patient should have adequate blood pressure and shouldn't show signs of pulsus paradoxus.

Vascular disorders

Besides abdominal aortic aneurysm, vascular disorders include thrombophlebitis, arterial occlusive disease, and Raynaud's disease.

Abdominal aortic aneurysm

Abdominal aneurysm, an abnormal dilation in the arterial wall, most commonly occurs in the aorta between the renal arteries and iliac branches.

Causes. Typically, the aneurysm results from atherosclerosis. Other causes include cystic medial necrosis, trauma, syphilis, and infection.

Assessment findings. When aneurysmal rupture isn't imminent, you may be able to see an asymptomatic pulsating mass in the periumbilical area. Auscultation may reveal a systolic bruit over the aorta, and tenderness may be present on deep palpation.

When aneurysmal rupture is imminent, pressure on lumbar nerves may lead to lumbar pain that radiates to the flank and groin.

If the aneurysm ruptures into the peritoneal cavity, it causes severe, persistent abdominal and back pain, mimicking renal or ureteral colic. The patient may hemorrhage; however, retroperitoneal bleeding may make such signs and symptoms as weakness, sweating, tachycardia, and hypotension appear rather subtle.

Diagnostic tests. Several tests can confirm suspected abdominal aneurysm. Serial ultrasonography, for instance, allows determination of aneurysm size, shape, and location. Anteroposterior and lateral X-rays of the abdomen can detect aortic calcification, which outlines the mass, in at least 75% of patients. Aortography shows the condition of vessels proximal and distal to the aneurysm and the extent of the aneurysm but may underestimate aneurysm diameter.

Treatment. Usually, abdominal aneurysm requires resection of the aneurysm and replacement of the damaged aortic section with a Dacron graft. Some aneurysms necessitate immediate repair. Patients with poor distal runoff may undergo external grafting.

If the aneurysm appears small and asymptomatic, the doctor may delay surgery. Note, however, that small aneurysms may rupture. The patient must undergo regular physical examination and ultrasound checks to detect enlargement, which may forewarn rupture.

Nursing interventions. Abdominal aneurysm requires meticulous preoperative and postoperative care, psychological support, and comprehensive patient education. For more information, see "Vascular repair," page 206.

Be alert for signs of rupture, which may cause immediate death. Watch closely for any signs or symptoms of acute blood loss, such as hypotension, increasing pulse and respiratory rate, cool and clammy skin, restlessness, and decreased sensorium.

If rupture occurs, get the patient to surgery immediately. Consider using medical antishock trousers during transport. Surgery allows direct compression of the aorta to control hemorrhage. During the resuscitative period, the patient may require large transfusions. Postoperative renal failure from ischemia may require hemodialysis.

Patient education. Provide appropriate education to help the patient and his family cope with their fears.

Evaluation. Note whether the patient has experienced pain relief. Verify that tissue perfusion is adequate.

Thrombophlebitis

An acute condition characterized by inflammation and thrombus formation, thrombophlebitis may occur in deep (intermuscular or intramuscular) or superficial veins.

Deep vein thrombophlebitis affects small veins such as the lesser saphenous or large veins such as the venae cavae, and the femoral, iliac, and subclavian veins. Usually progressive, this disorder may lead to pulmonary embolism.

Superficial thrombophlebitis is usually self-limiting and rarely leads to pulmonary embolism.

Causes. While deep vein thrombophlebitis may be idiopathic, it usually results from endothelial damage, accelerated blood clotting, or reduced blood flow.

Superficial thrombophlebitis may follow trauma, infection, or I.V. drug abuse. It may also stem from chemical irritation caused by extensive I.V. use.

Risk factors include prolonged bed rest, trauma, childbirth, and use of oral contraceptives.

Assessment findings. Clinical features vary with the site and length of the affected vein. Deep vein thrombophlebitis may produce severe pain, fever, chills, malaise, and swelling and cyanosis of the affected arm or leg. Complications of this disorder include chronic venous insufficiency and varicose veins.

Superficial thrombophlebitis leads to heat, pain, swelling, rubor, tenderness, and induration along the length of the affected vein. Extensive vein involvement may cause lymphadenitis.

Diagnostic tests. Doppler ultrasonography identifies reduced blood flow to a specific area and any obstruction to venous flow, particularly in iliofemoral deep vein thrombophlebitis. Plethysmography shows decreased circulation distal to the affected area. Phlebography, which usually confirms diagnosis, shows filling defects and diverted blood flow.

Treatment. Treatment aims to control thrombus development, prevent complications, relieve pain, and prevent recurrence. Symptomatic measures include bed rest, with elevation of the affected arm or leg; warm, moist soaks to the affected area; and analgesics, as ordered. After an acute episode of deep vein thrombophlebitis subsides, the patient may begin to walk while wearing antiembolism stockings.

Treatment for thrombophlebitis may also include anticoagulants (initially, heparin; later, warfarin) to prolong clotting time. Before any surgical procedure, discontinue the full anticoagulant dose, as ordered, to lessen the risk of hemorrhage. After some types of surgery, especially major abdominal or pelvic operations, prophylactic doses of anticoagulants may reduce the risk of deep vein thrombophlebitis and pulmonary embolism.

For lysis of acute, extensive deep vein thrombosis, treatment should include streptokinase.

Therapy for severe superficial thrombophlebitis may include an anti-inflammatory drug such as indomethacin, along with antiembolism stockings, warm soaks, and elevation of the patient's leg.

Nursing interventions. Remain alert for signs and symptoms of pulmonary emboli, such as crackles, dyspnea, hemoptysis, sudden changes in mental status, restlessness, and hypotension.

Closely monitor anticoagulant therapy to prevent such serious complications as internal hemorrhage. Measure partial thromboplastin time (PTT) regularly for the patient on heparin therapy; prothrombin time (PT) for the patient on warfarin. (Therapeutic blood levels for both drugs are $1^{1}/_{2}$ to 2 times control values.) Watch for signs and symptoms of bleeding, such as dark, tarry stools; coffee-ground vomitus; and ecchymoses. Encourage the patient to use an electric razor and to avoid medications that contain aspirin.

To prevent venostasis in patients with thrombophlebitis, take the following steps:
• Enforce bed rest, as ordered, and elevate the patient's affected arm or leg. If you use pillows to elevate the leg, place them under the entire length of the affected extremity.
• Apply warm soaks to improve circulation to the affected area. Give analgesics to relieve pain, as ordered.
• Measure and record the circumference of the affected arm or leg daily, and compare this with the circumference of the other arm or leg. To ensure accuracy and consistency of serial measurements, mark the skin over the area and measure at the same spot daily.
• Administer heparin I.V., as ordered, with an infusion monitor or pump to control the flow rate, if necessary.

Patient education. Before discharge, emphasize the importance of follow-up blood studies to monitor anticoagulant therapy. If the doctor has ordered postdischarge heparin therapy, teach the patient or a family member how to give subcutaneous injections. If he requires further assistance, arrange for a home health nurse.

Tell the patient to avoid prolonged sitting or standing to help prevent recurrence. Teach him how to apply and use antiembolism stockings properly. He should also know to report any complications such as cold, blue toes.

Evaluation. The patient shouldn't feel pain in the affected area or have a fever. Skin temperature and pulses in the affected arm or leg should be normal.

Arterial occlusive disease
In this disorder, obstruction or narrowing of the lumen of the aorta and its major branches interrupts blood flow, usually to the legs and feet. A frequent complication of atherosclerosis, arterial occlusive disease may affect the carotid, vertebral, innominate, subclavian, mesenteric, and celiac arteries.

Causes. Emboli formation, thrombosis, and trauma or fracture may lead to arterial occlusive disease. Risk factors include smoking, aging, hypertension, hyperlipemia, diabetes mellitus, and a family history of vascular disorders, MI, or CVA.

Assessment findings. Signs and symptoms depend on the severity and site of the arterial occlusion. A multiple-segment occlusion commonly causes severe ischemia, leading to intermittent claudication, severe burning pain in the toes, ulcers, and gangrene.

Other signs include dependent rubor, pallor on elevation, delayed capillary filling or hair loss, and trophic nail changes. Progressive arterial disease can cause diminished or absent pedal pulses.

Progressive narrowing of the arterial lumen stimulates the development of collateral circulation in surrounding blood vessels. With insufficient collateral development, thrombosis or total occlusion may occur, jeopardizing the limb.

Diagnostic tests. Supportive diagnostic tests include the following:
• Arteriography demonstrates the type (thrombus or embolus), location, and degree of obstruction and the collateral circulation. This test proves particularly useful for diagnosing chronic forms of the disease and for evaluating candidates for reconstructive surgery.
• Doppler ultrasonography and plethysmography show reduced blood flow distal to the occlusion in acute disease.
• Ophthalmodynamometry helps determine degree of obstruction in the internal carotid artery by comparing ophthalmic artery pressure with brachial artery pressure on the affected side. A difference greater than 20% suggests insufficiency.

Treatment. Typically, treatment depends on the cause, location, and size of the obstruction. For patients with mild chronic disease, it usually consists of supportive measures, such as elimination of smoking, hypertension control, and walking exercise. For patients with carotid artery occlusion, antiplatelet therapy may begin with dipyridamole and aspirin. For those with inter-

mittent claudication caused by chronic arterial occlusive disease, pentoxifylline may improve capillary perfusion.

Acute arterial occlusive disease usually necessitates surgery to restore circulation to the affected area. Appropriate surgical procedures may include embolectomy, thromboendarterectomy, patch grafting, bypass grafting, and lumbar sympathectomy. Amputation becomes necessary with failure of arterial reconstructive surgery or if complications develop.

Other therapy includes heparin to prevent emboli (for embolic occlusion) and bowel resection after restoration of blood flow (for mesenteric artery occlusion).

Nursing interventions. For information on nursing care measures, see "Vascular repair," page 206.

Patient education. Teach proper foot care or other appropriate measures, depending on the affected area. Advise the patient to stop smoking and to follow his prescribed medical regimen closely.

Evaluation. The patient should be able to increase exercise tolerance without developing pain. Peripheral pulses should be normal. He should maintain good skin color and temperature in his extremities.

Raynaud's disease
One of several primary arteriospastic diseases characterized by episodic vasospasm in the small peripheral arteries and arterioles, Raynaud's

disease occurs bilaterally and usually affects the hands or, less commonly, the feet. Upon exposure to cold or stress, the patient experiences skin color changes. He may develop minimal cutaneous gangrene or no gangrene at all. Arterial pulses are normal. This benign condition requires no treatment.

Raynaud's phenomenon, however, a condition often associated with several connective tissue disorders, has a progressive course, leading to ischemia, gangrene, and amputation. Distinction between the two disorders is difficult; some patients who experience mild symptoms of Raynaud's disease for several years may later develop overt connective tissue disease.

Causes. Although the cause of Raynaud's disease remains unknown, several theories account for reduced digital blood flow. Probably, it results from an antigen-antibody immune response because most patients with Raynaud's phenomenon have abnormal immunologic test results. Other explanations for reduced digital blood flow include intrinsic vascular wall hyperactivity caused by cold and increased vasomotor tone from sympathetic stimulation.

Assessment findings. After exposure to cold or stress, the skin on the patient's fingers typically blanches, then becomes cyanotic before changing to red and before changing from cold to normal temperature. Numbness and tingling may

also occur. Note whether warmth brings about symptom relief.

In long-standing disease, assess for trophic changes, such as sclerodactyly, ulcerations, or chronic paronychia.

Diagnostic tests. Diagnosis requires that clinical symptoms last at least 2 years. The patient may undergo tests to rule out secondary disease processes, such as chronic arterial occlusive or connective tissue disease.

Treatment. Initially, the patient must avoid cold, safeguard against mechanical or chemical injury, and quit smoking.

Expect the doctor to reserve drug therapy for patients with unusually severe symptoms; adverse reactions, especially from vasodilators, may prove more bothersome than the disease itself. When ordered, therapy may include phenoxybenzamine or reserpine. If conservative measures fail to prevent ischemic ulcers, the patient may undergo sympathectomy.

Nursing interventions. For a patient with a less advanced form of illness, provide reassurance that symptoms are benign. As the disorder progresses, try to allay fears regarding disfigurement.

Patient education. Warn against exposure to the cold. Tell the patient to wear mittens or gloves in cold weather or when handling cold items or defrosting the freezer.

Advise him to avoid stressful situations and to stop smoking.

Instruct the patient to inspect his skin frequently and to seek immediate care for signs of skin breakdown or infection. Finally, teach him about prescribed drugs and their adverse effects.

Evaluation. The patient should have warm hands and feet. The skin of his hands and feet should retain its normal color.

TREATMENTS

Advances in cardiovascular treatment have been dramatic. This section details the advanced treatments that allow cardiovascular patients to live longer than ever before.

Drug therapy

Many types of drugs are used to treat or prevent cardiac abnormalities. Digitalis glycosides (such as amrinone lactate and digoxin) assist in the management of HF and certain arrhythmias. Adrenergics (such as norepinephrine) may help treat serious hypotension. Antiarrhythmics (such as amiodarone and procainamide) can prevent an arrhythmia from developing into a more serious condition. Antianginals (such as nitroglycerin and nifedipine) are effective in treating pain from myocardial oxygen imbalance; antihypertensives (such as captopril, doxazosin, and enalapril maleate) act to reduce cardiac output or decrease peripheral vascular resistance, thereby lowering blood pressure. Diuretics (such as chloro-thiazide, bumetanide, and amiloride) treat edema and hypertension by reducing circulatory plasma volume. Drug therapy may also include antilipemics (such as colestipol and simvastatin) to prevent the development of complications from hyperlipidemia and thrombolytics (such as alteplase and streptokinase).

Surgery

This section covers organ transplants, advanced ventricular assist devices, coronary artery bypass surgery, and vascular repair. (See *Bypassing coronary occlusions*, page 198.)

Coronary artery bypass grafting

CABG circumvents an occluded coronary artery with an autogenous graft (usually a segment of the saphenous vein or internal mammarian artery), thereby restoring blood flow to the myocardium. CABG techniques vary according to the patient's condition and the number of arteries being bypassed.

CABG is one of the most common cardiac surgeries. Prime candidates include patients with severe angina from atherosclerosis and others with CAD with a high MI risk. Successful CABG can relieve anginal pain, improve cardiac function, and possibly enhance the patient's quality of life. But although the surgery relieves pain in about 90% of patients, its long-term effectiveness remains uncertain. Its benefits may prove temporary; problems such as graft closure and development of atherosclerosis in other coronary arteries may require

Bypassing coronary occlusions

In this example of coronary artery bypass grafting, the surgeon has used saphenous vein segments to bypass occlusions in three sections of coronary artery.

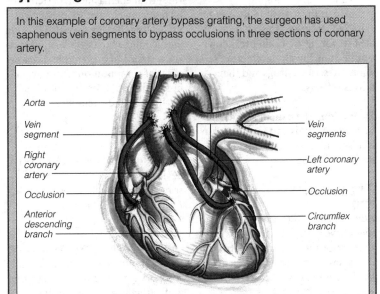

Aorta

Vein segment

Right coronary artery

Occlusion

Anterior descending branch

Vein segments

Left coronary artery

Occlusion

Circumflex branch

more surgery. No clear evidence exists that CABG reduces the risk of MI, although angina is reduced. A new minimally invasive form of CABG is being performed in some centers. Using fiber-optic and video technology, this procedure permits grafts with several small incisions, leaving the sternum intact.

Patient preparation. Begin by reinforcing the doctor's explanation of the surgery. Next, explain the complex equipment and procedures used in the ICU or recovery room. If possible, arrange a tour of the unit for the patient and his family.

Tell the patient that he'll awaken from surgery with an endotracheal (ET) tube in place and be connected

to a mechanical ventilator. He'll also be connected to a cardiac monitor and have in place an NG tube, a chest tube, an indwelling catheter, arterial lines, epicardial pacing wires, and possibly a PA catheter. Reassure him that this equipment should cause little discomfort and will be removed as soon as possible.

The evening before surgery, have the patient shower with antiseptic soap and shave him from his chin to his toes. Restrict food and fluids after midnight and provide a sedative, if ordered. On the morning of surgery, also provide a sedative, as ordered, to help him relax.

Before surgery, assist with PA catheterization and insertion of arterial lines. Then begin cardiac monitoring.

Monitoring and aftercare. After CABG, assess the patient for signs of hemodynamic compromise, such as severe hypotension, decreased cardiac output, and shock. Check and record vital signs every 15 minutes until the patient's condition stabilizes. Monitor the ECG for disturbances in heart rate and rhythm. If you detect abnormalities, notify the doctor and prepare to assist with epicardial pacing or, if necessary, cardioversion or defibrillation.

To ensure adequate myocardial perfusion, maintain arterial pressure within the guidelines set by the doctor. Usually, mean arterial pressure below 60 to 70 mm Hg results in inadequate tissue perfusion; pressure above 100 to 110 mm Hg can cause hemorrhage and increase the risk of graft rupture. Also monitor PA, central venous, and left atrial pressure, as ordered.

Frequently evaluate the patient's peripheral pulses, capillary refill time, and skin temperature and color, and auscultate for heart sounds. Notify the doctor of any abnormalities. Also evaluate tissue oxygenation by assessing breath sounds, chest excursion, and symmetry of chest expansion. Check ABG and pulse oximetry routinely. Adjust ventilator settings as needed to maintain ABG and arterial oxygen saturation values within prescribed limits. Monitor the patient's intake and output and assess him for electrolyte imbalance, especially

hypokalemia. If a saphenous vein was used, check the graft site.

Maintain chest tube drainage at the prescribed negative pressure (usually –10 to –40 cm H_2O). Monitor chest tubes every hour for patency, and assess regularly for hemorrhage, excessive drainage (greater than 200 ml/hour), and sudden decrease or cessation of drainage. Autotransfuse drainage according to protocol.

As the pain from the incision worsens, give an analgesic or use patient-controlled analgesia, as ordered.

Throughout the recovery period, assess for signs and symptoms of CVA (altered LOC, pupillary changes, weakness and loss of movement in extremities, ataxia, aphasia, dysphagia, sensory disturbances), pulmonary embolism (chest pain, dyspnea, hemoptysis, pleural friction rub, cyanosis, hypoxemia), and impaired renal perfusion (decreased urine output, elevated BUN and serum creatinine levels). Assess for wound infection.

After weaning the patient from the ventilator and removing the ET tube, promote chest physiotherapy. Start him on incentive spirometry, and encourage him to cough, turn frequently, and deep-breathe. Assist him with ROM exercises, as ordered.

Patient education. Instruct the patient to watch for and immediately notify the doctor of any signs or symptoms of infection (fever, sore throat, or redness, swelling, or drainage from the leg or chest incisions) or possible arterial reocclusion (angina, dizziness, dyspnea, rapid or irregular pulse, or prolonged recovery time from exercise).

Remind him to follow his prescribed diet, especially with regard to any sodium and cholesterol restrictions. Explain that this diet can help reduce the risk of recurrent arterial occlusion.

Stress the need to maintain a balance between activity and rest. Tell him to try to sleep at least 8 hours a night, to schedule a short rest period for each afternoon, and to rest frequently when engaging in tiring physical activity. Tell him he can climb stairs, engage in sexual activity, take baths and showers, and do light chores. Tell him to avoid lifting heavy objects (greater than 20 lb [9 kg]), driving a car, or doing heavy work that may place stress on the sternum (such as mowing the lawn or vacuuming) until his doctor grants permission. If the doctor has prescribed an exercise program, encourage the patient to follow it.

Have the patient contact a local chapter of the Mended Hearts Club and the American Heart Association (AHA) for information and support. Most patients should be referred to an outpatient cardiac rehabilitation program.

Explain to the patient that post-pericardiotomy syndrome often develops after open-heart surgery. Tell him to call his doctor if such signs and symptoms as fever, muscle and joint pain, weakness, or chest discomfort occur. You'll also have to prepare the patient for the possibility of postoperative depression, which may not develop until weeks after discharge. Reassure him that this depression is normal and should pass quickly. Finally, make sure the patient understands the dose, frequency of administration, and possible adverse effects of all prescribed medications.

Heart transplantation

Heart transplantation is a complex and controversial procedure that involves the replacement of a diseased heart with a healthy one from a brain-dead donor. Replacement with an artificial heart offers an even more controversial alternative. Limited to patients with end-stage cardiac disease, heart transplantation offers a last hope for survival after more conservative medical or surgical therapies have failed. Most candidates for this surgery have severe CAD or widespread left ventricular dysfunction caused by MI and associated fibrosis. Others suffer from hypertrophic cardiomyopathy, myotonic muscular dystrophy, or cardiomyopathy caused by viral infection.

Transplantation doesn't guarantee a cure. Postoperatively, most patients experience infection and tissue rejection. Rejection, caused by the patient's immune response to foreign antigens from the donor heart, usually occurs within the first 6 weeks after surgery. It's treated with monoclonal antibodies and potent immunosuppressive drugs, such as azathioprine, corticosteroids, and cyclosporine—sometimes in massive doses. The resulting immunosuppression leaves the patient vulnerable.

Patient preparation. The patient and his family need emotional support. Begin to address their fears by discussing the procedure, possible complications, and the impact of transplantation and a prolonged recovery period on his life. This surgery affects the entire family; encourage all family members to express their concerns and to ask questions. If necessary, refer them for psychological counseling.

Discuss the prospects of a successful transplantation and of postoperative complications. Make sure the patient and family understand that transplantation requires lifelong follow-up care.

Counsel the patient and family on what to expect before surgery, including food and fluid restrictions and the need for intubation and mechanical ventilation. Prepare them for the sights and sounds of the recovery room and ICU. If possible, arrange for them to tour these facilities and meet the staff. Describe postoperative isolation measures and the tests used to detect tissue rejection and other complications. Explain the expected immunosuppressive drug regimen.

Monitoring and aftercare. After surgery, maintain reverse isolation, according to hospital protocol. Administer immunosuppressive drugs, as ordered. Remember that these drugs typically mask obvious signs of infection. Watch for more subtle signs such as fever above

100° F (37.8° C). Expect to give prophylactic antibiotics and maintain strict asepsis when caring for incision and drainage sites.

Assess the patient for signs of hemodynamic compromise, such as severe hypotension, decreased cardiac output, and shock. Check and record vital signs every 15 minutes until his condition stabilizes.

Monitor the ECG for disturbances in heart rate and rhythm, such as bradycardia, ventricular tachycardia, and heart block. Such disturbances may result from myocardial irritability or ischemia, fluid and electrolyte imbalance, hypoxemia, or hypothermia. If you detect abnormalities, notify the doctor and assist with epicardial pacing.

To ensure adequate myocardial perfusion, maintain arterial pressure within the guidelines set by the doctor. Usually, mean arterial pressure below 70 mm Hg results in inadequate tissue perfusion. Also monitor PA, central venous, and left atrial pressures, as ordered.

Frequently evaluate peripheral pulses, capillary refill time, and skin temperature and color, and auscultate heart sounds. Notify the doctor of any abnormalities. Evaluate tissue oxygenation by assessing breath sounds, chest excursion, and symmetry of chest expansion. Check ABG and pulse oximetry levels routinely and adjust ventilator settings as needed to maintain them within prescribed limits.

Maintain chest tube drainage at the prescribed negative pressure (usually −10 to −40 cm H_2O). Milk chest tubes every hour to maintain patency, and regularly assess for hemorrhage, excessive drainage (greater than 200 ml/hour), or sudden decrease or cessation of drainage.

Continually assess the patient for signs of tissue rejection. Be alert for decreased electrical activity on ECG, right axis shift, atrial arrhythmias, conduction defects, ventricular gallop, HF, jugular vein distention, malaise, lethargy, weight gain, and increased T cell count. Report any of these signs immediately.

As ordered, administer antiarrhythmic, inotropic, pressor, and analgesic medications as well as I.V. fluids and blood products. Monitor intake and output, and assess for hypokalemia or other electrolyte imbalances.

Evaluate for the effects of denervation. Look for an elevated resting heart rate or a sinus rhythm that's unaffected by respirations. A lack of heart rate variation in response to changes in position, Valsalva's maneuver, or a carotid massage indicates complete denervation. Remember that atropine, anticholinergics, and edrophonium may have no effect on a denervated heart and that the effects of quinidine, digoxin, and verapamil may vary.

Throughout the patient's recovery period, assess carefully for complications. Watch especially for signs and symptoms of CVA (altered LOC, pupillary changes, weakness and loss of movement in the extremities, ataxia, aphasia, dysphagia, sensory disturbances), pulmonary embolism (dyspnea, cough, hemoptysis, chest pain, pleural friction rub, cyanosis, hypoxemia), and impaired renal perfusion (decreased urine output, elevated BUN and serum creatinine levels).

After weaning the patient from the ventilator and removing the ET tube, promote chest physiotherapy. Start him on incentive spirometry and encourage him to cough, turn frequently, and deep-breathe. Also assist him with ROM exercises, as ordered.

Patient education. Explain that the doctor will schedule frequent (weekly to monthly) myocardial biopsies to check for signs of tissue rejection. Stress the importance of keeping these appointments.

Instruct the patient to immediately report any signs and symptoms of rejection (fever, weight gain, dyspnea, lethargy, weakness) or infection (chest pain, fever, sore throat, or redness, swelling, or drainage from the incision site).

Explain that postpericardiotomy syndrome often develops after open-heart surgery. Tell him to call his doctor if he experiences its characteristic signs and symptoms: fever, muscle and joint pain, weakness, and chest discomfort.

During the initial recovery, instruct the patient to maintain a balance between activity and rest. Tell him to try to sleep at least 8 hours a night, to rest briefly each afternoon, and to take breaks when he's engaging in tiring physical activity. Tell him he can climb stairs, engage in sexual activity, take baths and showers, and do light housework and other chores. Tell him to avoid lifting heavy objects (greater than 20 lb [9 kg]), driving, or doing heavy work (such as mowing the lawn or vacuuming) until his doctor grants permission. He should also follow a home exercise program.

If the patient shows signs of denervation, advise him to rise slowly from a sitting or lying position to minimize orthostatic hypotension. Make sure he knows the dose, schedule, and adverse effects of prescribed drugs. Encourage him to follow his prescribed diet, especially noting sodium and fat restrictions.

Ventricular assist device

A temporary life-sustaining treatment for a failing heart, the ventricular assist device (VAD) diverts systemic blood flow from a diseased ventricle into a centrifugal pump. The VAD *assists* the heart rather than replaces it, and, the pumping chambers of the VAD usually aren't implanted.

A permanent VAD (unlike other VADs) is implanted in the chest cavity and receives power through the skin by a belt of electrical transformer coils surrounding the patient's waist. Despite its name, like other VADs, the permanent VAD provides only temporary support. It can run off an implanted rechargeable battery for up to an hour at a time.

Candidates for a VAD include patients with massive MI, irreversible cardiomyopathy, acute myocarditis, inability to wean from cardiopulmonary bypass, valvular disease, bacterial endocarditis, or rejection of a heart transplant. The device also benefits patients awaiting a heart transplant.

The VAD carries a high risk of complications. Despite the use of anticoagulants and special Dacron linings, the VAD commonly causes formation of thrombi, leading to pulmonary embolism, CVA, and other ominous complications. If ventricular function hasn't improved in 96 hours, the doctor may consider a heart transplant.

Patient preparation. Reinforce the doctor's explanation of the procedure and answer any questions.

Explain to the patient that you must restrict his food and fluid intake before surgery and that you'll continuously monitor his cardiac function, using an ECG, a PA catheter, and an arterial line. If time allows, you may have to shave the patient's chest and scrub it with an antiseptic solution.

Monitoring and aftercare. Before the patient returns to the ICU following the operation, place an air mattress or sheepskin on his bed; it will help prevent skin breakdown.

Expect the patient to be sedated when he arrives. As the anesthetic wears off, administer analgesics, as ordered.

Keep the patient immobilized to prevent accidental extubation, contamination, or disconnection of the device. Use soft restraints on both hands.

If you've been trained to adjust the device's pump, maintain cardiac output at 5 to 8 L/minute, PAWP at 10 to 20 mm Hg, CVP at 8 to 16 mm Hg, mean blood pressure above 60 mm Hg, and left atrial pressure at 4 to 12 mm Hg. Also monitor the patient for signs and symptoms of poor perfusion and ineffective pumping. These include arrhythmias, hypotension, cool skin, slow capillary refill, oliguria or anuria, confusion, restlessness, and anxiety.

Administer heparin, as ordered, to prevent clotting in the pump head and thrombus formation. Be sure to check for bleeding, especially at the operative sites. Monitor PT, PTT, hemoglobin level, and hematocrit every 4 hours. Notify the doctor of abnormal findings.

Assess incisions and the cannula insertion site for signs of infection, and culture any suspicious exudate. Monitor the patient's WBC count and differential daily, and take rectal or core temperatures every 4 hours. Using aseptic technique, change the dressing over the cannula insertion sites daily.

Provide supportive care such as lubricating the skin every 4 hours. Perform passive ROM exercises every 2 hours.

Valve replacement

In many cases, severe valvular stenosis or insufficiency requires excision of the affected valve and replacement with a mechanical or biological prosthesis. Because of the high pressure generated by the left ventricle during contraction, stenosis and insufficiency most commonly affect the mitral and aortic valves.

If a patient with a valvular defect has severe symptoms that can't be managed with drugs and dietary restrictions, he will require valve replacement (or commissurotomy) to prevent life-threatening HF. Other indications for valve replacement depend on the patient's symptoms and on the affected valve.

Although valve replacement surgery has a low mortality, it can cause serious complications. Hemorrhage, for instance, may result from unligated vessels, anticoagulant therapy, or coagulopathy due to cardiopulmonary bypass during surgery. CVA may result from thrombus formation caused by turbulent blood flow through the prosthetic valve or from poor cerebral perfusion during cardiopulmonary bypass. Bacterial endocarditis can develop within days of implantation or months later. Valve dysfunction or failure may occur as the prosthetic device wears out.

Patient preparation. Reinforce and supplement the doctor's explanation of the procedure. Listen to the patient's concerns and encourage him to ask questions. Tell him that he'll awaken from surgery in an ICU or recovery room. Mention that he'll be connected to a cardiac monitor and have I.V. lines, an arterial line, and possibly a PA or left atrial catheter in place. Explain that he'll breathe through an ET tube that's connected to a mechanical ventilator and that he'll have a chest tube in place.

Before surgery, expect to assist with insertion of an arterial line and possibly a PA catheter. As ordered, initiate cardiac monitoring.

Monitoring and aftercare. After surgery, closely monitor the patient's hemodynamic status for signs of compromise. Watch especially for severe hypotension, decreased cardiac output, and shock. Check and record vital signs every 15 minutes until his condition stabilizes. Frequently assess heart sounds; report distant heart sounds or new murmurs, which may indicate prosthetic valve failure.

Monitor the ECG for disturbances in heart rate and rhythm, such as bradycardia, ventricular tachycardia, and heart block. Such disturbances may point to injury of the conduction system, which may occur during valve replacement because of the proximity of the atrial and mitral valves to the atrioventricular node. Arrhythmias also may result from myocardial irritability or ischemia, fluid and electrolyte imbalance, hypoxemia, or hypothermia. If you detect abnormalities, notify the doctor and be prepared to assist with temporary epicardial pacing.

To ensure adequate myocardial perfusion, maintain mean arterial pressure within the guidelines set by the doctor. For adults, this range is usually between 70 and 100 mm Hg. Also monitor PA and left atrial pressures, as ordered.

Frequently assess the patient's peripheral pulses, capillary refill time, and skin temperature and color, and auscultate for heart sounds. Evaluate tissue oxygenation by assessing breath sounds, chest excursion, and symmetry of chest expansion. Report any abnormalities. Check ABG levels frequently, and adjust ventilator settings as needed.

Maintain chest tube drainage at the prescribed negative pressure (usually −10 to −40 cm H_2O for adults). Milk chest tubes every hour to maintain patency, and assess regularly for hemorrhage, excessive drainage (more than 200 ml/hour), and sudden decrease or cessation of drainage. Prepare and monitor autotransfusion, as ordered.

As ordered, administer analgesic, anticoagulant, antibiotic, antiarrhythmic, inotropic, and pressor medications as well as I.V. fluids and blood products. Monitor intake and output and assess for electrolyte imbalances, especially hypokalemia. Once anticoagulant therapy begins, evaluate its effectiveness by monitoring PT daily.

Throughout the patient's recovery period, observe him carefully for complications. Watch especially for signs and symptoms of CVA (altered LOC, pupillary changes, weakness and loss of movement in the extremities, ataxia, aphasia, dysphagia, sensory disturbances), pulmonary embolism (dyspnea, cough, hemoptysis, chest pain, pleural friction rub, cyanosis, hypoxemia), and impaired renal perfusion (decreased urine output and elevated BUN and serum creatinine levels). Other possible complications include cachexia and impaired hearing.

After weaning the patient from the ventilator and removing the ET tube, promote chest physiotherapy. Start him on incentive spirometry, and encourage him to cough, turn frequently, and deep-breathe. Gradually increase his activities.

Patient education. Tell the patient to immediately report chest pain, fever, or redness, swelling, or drainage at the incision site. Have him notify the doctor if signs or symptoms of postpericardiotomy syndrome (fever, muscle and joint pain, weakness, and chest discomfort) develop after surgery.

Make sure he understands the dose, schedule, and adverse effects of all prescribed drugs. Tell him to wear a medical identification bracelet and carry a card with information and instructions on anticoagulant and antibiotic therapy.

Remind him to follow the prescribed diet, especially with regard to sodium and fat restrictions. Tell him to inform his dentist or any other doctors that he has a prosthetic valve before undergoing any surgery or dental work. He'll probably need to take prophylactic antibiotics.

Also tell him to maintain a balance between activity and rest. Tell him to try to sleep at least 8 hours a night, to schedule a short rest period for each afternoon, and to rest frequently when engaging in tiring physical activity. Tell him he can climb stairs, engage in sexual activity, take baths and showers, and do light housework and other chores. Tell him to avoid lifting heavy objects (greater than 20 lb [9 kg]), driving a car, or doing heavy work (such as mowing the lawn or vacuuming) until the doctor grants permission. If an exercise program has been prescribed, encourage the patient to follow it carefully.

Vascular repair

Surgical repair may treat vessels damaged by arteriosclerotic or thromboembolic disorders (such as aortic aneurysm or arterial occlusive disease), trauma, infections, or congenital defects; vascular obstructions that severely compromise circulation; vascular disease that does not respond to drug therapy or nonsurgical treatments such as balloon catheterization; life-threatening dissecting or ruptured aortic aneurysms; and limb-threatening acute arterial occlusion.

Vascular repair includes aneurysm resection, grafting, embolectomy, interruption of venae caval blood flow, and vein stripping. The specific surgery used depends on the type, location, and extent of vascular occlusion or damage.

In all vascular surgeries, the potential for vessel trauma, emboli, hemorrhage, infection, and other complications exists. Grafting carries added risks: The graft may occlude, narrow, dilate, or rupture.

Patient preparation. If the patient requires emergency surgery, briefly explain the procedure to him, if possible. If he doesn't require immediate surgery, make sure that he and his family understand the doctor's explanation of the surgery and its possible complications.

If the patient is undergoing vein stripping, tell him that he'll receive a local anesthetic before the procedure. If he's undergoing other vascular surgery, inform him that he'll receive a general anesthetic. Mention that he'll awaken from the anesthetic in the ICU or recovery room. Explain that he'll have an I.V. line in place to provide access for fluids and drugs, ECG electrodes for continuous cardiac monitoring, and an arterial line or a PA catheter to provide continuous pressure monitoring. He may have a urinary catheter in place to allow accurate output measurement. If appropriate, explain that he'll be intubated and placed on mechanical ventilation.

On the day before scheduled surgery, perform a complete vascular assessment. Take vital signs to provide a baseline. Evaluate the strength and sound of the blood flow and the symmetry of the pulses, and note any bruits. Record the temperature of the extremities, their sensitivity to motor and sensory stimuli, and any pallor, cyanosis, or redness. Rate peripheral pulse volume and strength on a scale of 0 (pulse absent) to 4 (bounding, strong), and check capillary refill time by blanching the fingernail or toenail (normal refill time is under 3 seconds).

As ordered, instruct the patient to restrict food and fluids for at least 12 hours before surgery. Tell him that he probably will receive a sedative the night before surgery.

If the patient is awaiting surgery for aortic aneurysm repair, be on guard for signs and symptoms of acute dissection or rupture. Note especially sudden severe pain in the chest, abdomen, or lower back; severe weakness; diaphoresis; tachy-cardia; or a precipitous drop in blood pressure. If any of these life-threatening signs or symptoms occur, call the doctor immediately.

Monitoring and aftercare. After surgery, check and record the patient's vital signs every 15 minutes until his condition stabilizes and every 30 minutes to 1 hour thereafter. Monitor the ECG for abnormalities in heart rate or rhythm. Also monitor other pressure readings and carefully record intake and output. Check the patient's dressing regularly for excessive bleeding. Position the patient as ordered, and instruct him on recommended levels of activity during early stages of recovery. Provide analgesics, as ordered.

Frequently assess peripheral pulses, using Doppler ultrasonography if palpation proves difficult. Check all extremities for muscle strength and movement, color, temperature, and capillary refill time.

Throughout the patient's recovery period, assess him often for signs and symptoms of complications. Report any of the following signs and symptoms immediately:
• fever, cough, congestion, or dyspnea
• low urine output and elevated BUN and serum creatinine levels (possible signs of renal dysfunction)
• severe pain and cyanosis (possible indications of occlusion)
• hypotension, tachycardia, restlessness and confusion, shallow respirations, abdominal pain, and increased abdominal girth (possible indications of hemorrhage).

In addition, frequently check the incision site for drainage and signs of infection.

As the patient's condition improves, help wean him from the ventilator, if appropriate. To promote good pulmonary hygiene, encourage him to cough, turn, and deep-breathe frequently. Assist him with ROM exercises, as ordered, to help prevent thrombus formation.

Patient education. If appropriate, instruct the patient or a family member to check his pulse in the affected extremity before rising from bed each morning. Tell the patient to notify the doctor if he can't palpate his pulse or if he develops coldness, pallor, or pain in the extremity.

Stress the need for strict compliance with any prescribed medication regimen. Make sure the patient understands the schedule and the expected drug adverse effects. Also stress the importance of regular checkups to monitor his condition.

Balloon catheter treatments

Balloon catheter treatments range from life-support measures such as intra-aortic balloon counterpulsation (IABC) to nonsurgical alternatives to coronary artery bypass surgery such as PTCA.

Intra-aortic balloon counterpulsation

IABC temporarily reduces left ventricular workload and improves coronary perfusion. It may benefit patients with cardiogenic shock resulting from acute MI, septic shock, intractable angina pectoris before surgery, intractable ventricular arrhythmias, or ventricular septal or papillary muscle ruptures. It's also used for patients who suffer pump failure before or after cardiac surgery.

The doctor may perform balloon catheter insertion at the bedside as an emergency procedure or in the operating room—for example, when the patient can't be weaned from a cardiopulmonary bypass machine. The intra-aortic balloon pump consists of a single-chambered or multichambered polyurethane balloon attached to an external pump console by means of a large-lumen catheter.

Patient preparation. If time permits, explain to the patient that the doctor will place a special catheter in the aorta to help his heart pump more easily. Explain the insertion procedure. Discuss how the catheter will be connected to a large console next to his bed. Mention that the console has an alarm system. The console normally makes a pumping sound; make sure the patient understands that this doesn't mean his heart has stopped beating. Communicate to him that, because of the catheter, he won't be able to sit up, bend his knee, or flex his hip more than 30 degrees.

Next, attach the patient to an ECG for continuous monitoring, and make sure that he has an arterial line, a PA catheter, and a peripheral I.V. line in place. If the procedure is performed at the bedside, gather the appropriate equipment, including a surgical tray for percutaneous catheter insertion, heparin, normal saline solution, the IABC catheter, and the pump console. Connect the ECG monitor to the pump console. Then shave, disinfect, and drape the femoral site.

Monitoring and aftercare. If you're responsible for monitoring the pump's console, you can select any of three signals to regulate inflation and deflation of the balloon: the ECG, the arterial waveform, or the intrinsic pump rate. With the ECG, the pump inflates the balloon in the middle of the T wave (diastole) and deflates it just before the QRS complex (systole). With the arterial waveform, the upstroke of the arterial wave triggers balloon inflation. (See *Timing the balloon pump*, page 210.) You can also set the pump to inflate and deflate at a predetermined intrinsic rate. Expect to use this method when the patient has no intrinsic heartbeat such as during cardiopulmonary bypass.

Many complications may occur with IABC. The most common one, arterial embolism, stems from clot formation on the balloon's surface. Other complications include extension or rupture of an aortic aneurysm, perforation of the femoral or iliac artery, femoral artery occlusion, and sepsis. Bleeding at the insertion site may become aggravated by pump-induced thrombocytopenia.

To help prevent complications, use strict aseptic technique, maintain the catheterized leg in good alignment and prevent hip flexion, and frequently assess the insertion site. Don't elevate the head of the bed more than 30 degrees, to prevent upward migration of the catheter and occlusion of the left subclavian artery. If the balloon does occlude the artery, you may see a diminished left radial pulse, and the patient may report dizziness. Incorrect balloon placement may also cause flank pain or a sudden drop in urine output.

Also assess distal pulses and note the color, temperature, and capillary refill time of the patient's extremities. Assess the affected leg's warmth, color, and pulses, and the patient's ability to move his toes, at 15- to 30-minute intervals for the first 4 hours after insertion, then every 30 to 60 minutes for the duration of IABC. In many cases, arterial flow to the involved extremity diminishes during insertion, but the pulse should strengthen once pumping begins.

If the patient is receiving heparin or low-molecular-weight dextran to inhibit thrombosis, keep in mind that he's still at risk for thrombus formation. Watch for such indications as a sudden weakening of pedal pulses, pain, and motor or sensory loss. If indicated, apply antiembolism stockings for 8 hours, remove them, and then reapply them. Encourage active ROM exercises every 2 hours for the arms, the unaffected leg, and the affected ankle. Also be sure to maintain adequate hydration to help prevent thrombus formation. If bleeding occurs at the catheter insertion site,

Timing the balloon pump

Although intra-aortic balloon counterpulsation (IABC) can be synchronized with the electrocardiogram (ECG), you will usually use the arterial waveform to precisely adjust balloon-pump timing. The reason: The arterial waveform directly reflects diastole and systole. In contrast, the ECG shows *electrical* activity, which may not always correlate with the cardiac cycle—especially with a diseased heart.

Ideally, balloon inflation should begin when the aortic valve closes—at the dicrotic notch on the arterial waveform. Deflation should occur just before systole. Proper timing is crucial: Early inflation may damage the aortic valve by forcing it closed, whereas late inflation permits most of the blood emerging from the ventricle to flow past the balloon, reducing pump effectiveness. What's worse, late deflation increases the resistance against which the left ventricle must pump, possibly causing cardiac arrest.

The illustration at the top of the next column shows how IABC boosts peak diastolic pressure and lowers peak systolic and end-diastolic pressures.

Arterial waveforms

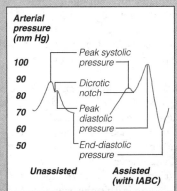

Arterial pressure (mm Hg)

Peak systolic pressure
Dicrotic notch
Peak diastolic pressure
End-diastolic pressure

Unassisted   **Assisted (with IABC)**

How timing affects waveforms

The arterial waveforms below show correctly and incorrectly timed balloon inflation and deflation.

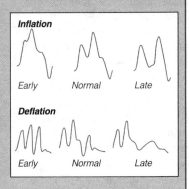

Inflation

Early   Normal   Late

Deflation

Early   Normal   Late

apply direct pressure over it and notify the doctor.

Once the signs and symptoms of left-sided HF have diminished and the patient requires only minimal drug support, the doctor will begin weaning him from IABC. To discontinue IABC, the doctor will deflate the balloon, clip the sutures, and remove the catheter. Then he'll allow the site to bleed for 5 seconds to expel clots, after which you'll apply direct pressure for 30 minutes. Afterward, apply a pressure dressing and evaluate the site for bleeding and hematoma formation hourly for the next 4 hours.

An alarm on the console may detect gas leaks from a damaged catheter or ruptured balloon. If the alarm sounds or if you note blood in the catheter, shut down the pump console and immediately place the patient in Trendelenburg's position to prevent an embolus from reaching the brain. Then notify the doctor.

Percutaneous transluminal coronary angioplasty

PTCA offers a nonsurgical alternative to coronary artery bypass surgery. The doctor uses this sophisticated radiologic technique to dilate a coronary artery narrowed by atherosclerotic plaque.

Performed in the cardiac catheterization laboratory under local anesthesia, PTCA doesn't involve a thoracotomy. Hospitalization lasts 2 to 4 days, rather than the 1- to 2-week stay for coronary artery bypass, and PCTA can be done for one-fifth of the cost. Patients can usually walk the next day and go to work in 2 weeks.

Only a small percentage of candidates for coronary artery bypass can benefit from PTCA. Usually, this treatment is indicated for patients who have myocardial ischemia and a lesion in the proximal portion of a single coronary artery. Because of higher risk of mortality and of coronary artery spasm, patients with lesions in the left main coronary artery rarely undergo PTCA.

Complications of PTCA are acute vessel closure and late restenosis. To prevent this, doctors insert a stent—a stainless steel tube used to support the artery and help prevent restenosis. Stenting is used in patients at risk for abrupt clotting after PTCA.

Although PTCA avoids many of the risks of surgery, it can cause arterial dissection during dilation, leading to coronary artery rupture, cardiac tamponade, myocardial ischemia or MI, or death. Other complications include coronary artery spasm, decreased coronary artery blood flow, allergic reactions to the contrast medium, and arrhythmias during catheter manipulation. Infrequently, thrombi may embolize and cause a CVA.

Patient preparation. Reinforce the doctor's explanation of the procedure, including its risks and alternatives. Tell the patient that a catheter will be inserted into an artery or vein in the groin area and that he may feel pressure as the catheter moves along the vessel. Also explain that he'll be awake during the procedure and may have to take deep breaths to allow visualization of the radiopaque balloon catheter. He may also have to answer questions about how he's feeling during the procedure and will have to notify the cardiologist if he experiences any angina. Advise him that the entire procedure lasts from 1 to 4 hours and that he'll have to lie flat on a hard table during that time.

Tell the patient that before the procedure you'll insert an I.V. line and shave the groin area of both legs and clean it with an antiseptic.

Explain that he'll experience a brief stinging sensation during injection of a local anesthetic.

Discuss how the doctor will order injection of a contrast medium to outline the lesion's location. Warn him that during the injection he may feel a hot, flushing sensation or transient nausea. Check his history for allergies; if he's had allergic reactions to shellfish, iodine, or contrast medium, notify the doctor.

Restrict the patient's food and fluid intake for at least 6 hours before the procedure or as ordered. Ensure that coagulation studies, CBC, serum electrolyte studies, and blood typing and crossmatching have been performed. Also palpate the bilateral distal pulses (usually the dorsalis pedis or posterior tibial pulses) and mark them with indelible marker to help you locate them later. Take vital signs and assess the color, temperature, and sensation in the patient's extremities to serve as a baseline for posttreatment assessment. Before the patient is taken to the catheterization laboratory, sedate him as ordered. Put a 5-lb (2.5 kg) sandbag on the bed, which you'll use later to apply direct pressure to the arterial puncture site.

Monitoring and aftercare. When the patient returns from the cardiac catheterization laboratory, he may be receiving I.V. heparin or nitroglycerin. In addition, he'll need to keep the leg immobilized to minimize bleeding until the femoral catheter sheaths are removed. He'll require continuous arterial and ECG monitoring.

To prevent excessive hip flexion and migration of the catheter, keep the patient's leg straight and elevate the head of the bed no more than 15 degrees; at mealtimes, elevate the head of the bed 15 to 30 degrees. For the first hour, monitor vital signs every 15 minutes, then every 30 minutes for 2 hours, and then hourly for the next 5 hours. If vital signs are unstable, notify the doctor and continue to check them every 5 minutes.

When you take vital signs, assess the peripheral pulses distal to the catheter insertion site and the color, temperature, and capillary refill time of the extremity. If pulses are difficult to palpate because of the size of the arterial catheter, use a Doppler stethoscope to hear them. Notify the doctor if pulses are absent.

Assess the catheter insertion site for hematoma formation, ecchymosis, or hemorrhage. If an expanding ecchymotic area appears, mark the area to see how fast it expands. If bleeding occurs, apply direct pressure and notify the doctor.

Monitor cardiac rate and rhythm continuously and notify the doctor of any changes or if the patient reports chest pain; it may signal vasospasm or coronary occlusion.

Give I.V. fluids at a rate of at least 100 ml/hour to promote excretion of the contrast medium, but be sure to assess the patient for signs of fluid overload (distended neck veins, atrial and ventricular gallops, dyspnea, pulmonary congestion, tachycardia, hypertension, and hypoxemia).

The doctor will remove the arterial catheter 2 to 6 hours after the procedure. Afterward, apply direct pressure over the insertion site for at least 30 minutes. A mechanical device that maintains pressure over the femoral puncture sites can be used. Then apply a pressure dressing and assess the patient's vital signs according to the same schedule you used when he first returned to the unit.

Patient education. Counsel the patient to call the doctor if he experiences any bleeding or bruising at the arterial puncture site. Emphasize the need to take all prescribed medications, and make sure he understands their intended effects.

Tell the patient that he can resume normal activity but advise him to avoid excessive bending at the hip for 1 to 4 days. If PTCA is successful, he may experience an increased exercise tolerance. Finally, remind him to return for a thallium stress test and follow-up angiography, as recommended by his doctor.

Balloon valvuloplasty

Balloon valvuloplasty seeks to enlarge the orifice of a heart valve that's stenotic because of a congenital defect, calcification, rheumatic fever, or aging, thereby improving valvular function.

While not the treatment of choice, valvuloplasty offers an alternative for individuals considered poor candidates for surgery.

The procedure can worsen valvular insufficiency by misshaping the valve so that it doesn't close completely. Pieces of the calcified valve may break off and travel to the brain or lungs, thereby leading to embolism. Valvuloplasty can cause severe damage to the delicate valve leaflets, requiring immediate surgery to replace the valve. Other complications include bleeding and hematoma at the arterial puncture site, arrhythmias, myocardial ischemia, MI, and circulatory defects distal to the catheter entry site. Many elderly patients with aortic disease experience restenosis 1 to 2 years after undergoing valvuloplasty. The most serious complications of valvuloplasty (valvular destruction, MI, and calcium emboli) are not common.

Patient preparation. Reinforce the doctor's explanation of the procedure, including its risks and alternatives, to the patient or his parents. Restrict food and fluid intake for at least 6 hours before valvuloplasty, or as ordered.

Explain that the patient will have an I.V. line inserted to provide access for any medications. Mention that you'll shave the patient's groin area and clean it with an antiseptic. He'll feel a brief stinging sensation upon injection of a local anesthetic.

Because it's done under a local anesthetic, the procedure can be frightening to a pediatric patient. Explain that the doctor will insert a catheter into an artery or vein in the groin area and that the patient may feel pressure as the catheter moves along the vessel. Also explain to the patient that he needs to be awake because the doctor may need him to take deep breaths (to allow visualization of the catheter) and to answer questions about how he's feeling. Warn him that the procedure lasts up to 4 hours and that he may feel discomfort from lying flat on a hard table during that time.

Make sure that you have the results of routine laboratory studies and blood typing and crossmatching. Just before the procedure, palpate the bilateral distal pulses and mark them with indelible ink. Take vital signs and assess color, temperature, and sensation in the patient's extremities to serve as a baseline for posttreatment assessment. Administer a sedative, as ordered.

Once you've prepared the patient, place a 5-lb (2.5 kg) sandbag on his bed. You'll use this later for applying pressure over the puncture site.

Monitoring and aftercare. When the patient returns to the ICU or recovery area, he may be receiving I.V. heparin or nitroglycerin. He'll also have the sandbag placed over the cannulation site to minimize bleeding until the arterial catheter is removed and will require continuous arterial and ECG monitoring.

To prevent excessive hip flexion and migration of the catheter, keep the affected leg straight and elevate the head of the bed no more than 15 degrees (at mealtimes, 15 to 30 degrees). For the first hour, monitor vital signs every 15 minutes, then every 30 minutes for 2 hours, and then hourly for the next 5 hours. If vital signs are unstable, notify the doctor and continue to check them every 5 minutes.

When you take vital signs, assess peripheral pulses distal to the insertion site and the color, temperature,

and capillary refill time of the extremity. If pulses are difficult to palpate because of the size of the arterial catheter, use a Doppler stethoscope. Notify the doctor if pulses are absent.

Observe the catheter insertion site for hematoma formation, ecchymosis, or hemorrhage. If an expanding ecchymotic area appears, mark the area to help determine the pace of expansion. If bleeding occurs, apply direct pressure and notify the doctor.

Following the doctor's orders or your hospital's protocol, auscultate regularly for murmurs, which may indicate worsening valvular insufficiency. Notify the doctor if you detect a new or worsening murmur.

Provide I.V. fluids at a rate of at least 100 ml/hour to help the kidneys excrete the contrast medium. Assess for signs of fluid overload: distended neck veins, atrial and ventricular gallops, dyspnea, pulmonary congestion, tachycardia, hypertension, and hypoxemia.

The doctor will remove the catheter 6 to 12 hours after valvuloplasty. Afterward, apply direct pressure over the puncture site for at least 30 minutes. Then apply a pressure dressing and assess vital signs according to the schedule used when the patient first returned to the unit.

Patient education. Tell the patient that he can resume normal activity. Most patients with successful valvuloplasties experience increased exercise tolerance. Instruct him to call his doctor if he experiences any bleeding or increased bruising at the puncture site or any recurrence of symptoms of valvular insufficiency, such as breathlessness or decreased exercise tolerance. Finally, stress the need for regular follow-up visits.

Basic life support

Basic life support (BLS) is the first of two types of emergency life-support procedures designated by the AHA. In BLS, emergency first aid focuses on recognizing respiratory or cardiac arrest and providing CPR to maintain life until the victim recovers or until advanced cardiac life support is available. You can perform BLS procedures quickly, in almost any situation, without assistance or equipment.

The critical factor is *time*—the quicker you start BLS, the better your patient's chances of survival.

Indications. Expect to use BLS during cardiac or respiratory arrest. In primary respiratory arrest, the heart will continue to pump blood for several minutes, while existing stores of oxygen in the lungs and blood continue to circulate to the brain and other vital organs. By intervening quickly once respirations have stopped or the airway has become obstructed, you can prevent cardiac arrest.

Respiratory arrest may result from drowning, stroke, foreign-body airway obstruction, smoke inhalation, drug overdose, electrocution, suffocation, injuries, MI, injury by lightning, and coma leading to airway obstruction.

In primary cardiac arrest, oxygen doesn't circulate, and oxygen stored in the vital organs becomes depleted in a few seconds. Cardiac arrest may be accompanied by ventricular fibrillation, ventricular tachycardia, asystole, or electromechanical dissociation.

Before performing CPR, you'll assess the patient to see if he's gone into respiratory or cardiac arrest. Use the ABC sequence: Open his *a*irway. Check to see if he's *b*reathing. Assess his *c*irculation.

Cardiopulmonary resuscitation

Cardiopulmonary resuscitation is an emergency procedure that seeks to restore and maintain a patient's respiration and circulation after his heartbeat and breathing have stopped. The goal is to provide oxygen and blood flow to the heart, brain, and other vital organs until help arrives. You must initiate CPR as soon as possible after cardiac and respiratory arrest begin. If the victim's heartbeat and respirations have stopped for less than 4 minutes before you intervene, he'll have a much better chance for complete recovery, as long as the resuscitation is effective. If his circulation has been stopped for 4 to 6 minutes, brain damage may have occurred. After 6 minutes without circulation, brain damage will almost certainly occur. However, there are exceptions—a drowning victim who's been in cold water or someone who's suffered hypothermia, for instance. If you have any doubt about how long the patient's pulse and respirations have been absent, you should still go ahead and perform CPR.

The easiest way to remember the basic CPR procedure is to follow the ABC scheme: **a**irway open, **b**reathing restored, then **c**irculation restored. After airway has been opened and breathing and circulation have been restored, drug therapy, diagnosis by ECG, or defibrillation may follow. CPR is contraindicated in no-code patients.

The following illustrated instructions will guide you through the CPR steps currently recommended by the AHA. Consider also becoming certified in CPR through a course sponsored by the AHA or the American Red Cross. Use this guide to review the correct steps. Also be sure to keep your CPR certification current and practice regularly. For some of your patients, it could mean the difference between life and death.

One-person rescue

If you're the sole rescuer, expect to open the patient's airway, check for breathing, and assess for circulation before beginning compressions.

Open the airway. Follow these steps:
1. Assess the victim to determine if he's unconscious. Gently shake his shoulders and shout, "Are you okay?" This simple action helps ensure that you don't start CPR on a person who's conscious. Check whether he's suffered an injury, particularly to the head or neck. If you suspect a head or neck injury, move him as little as possible to reduce the risk of paralysis.

2. Call out for help. Send someone to contact the emergency medical service (EMS), or if necessary contact the EMS yourself before beginning CPR.

3. Place him in a supine position on a hard, flat surface. When moving him, roll his head and torso as a unit. Avoid twisting or pulling his neck, shoulders, or hips.

4. Kneel near his shoulders. This position will give you easy access to his head and chest.

5. In many cases, the muscles controlling the victim's tongue will be relaxed, causing the tongue to obstruct the airway. If he doesn't appear to have a neck injury, use the *head-tilt, chin-lift maneuver* to open his airway. Place your hand that's closer to his head on his forehead. Then apply firm pressure to tilt his head back. Place the fingertips of your other hand under the bony part of his lower jaw near the chin. Lift the chin while keeping the mouth partially open. Avoid placing your fingertips on the soft tissue under the chin; this may inadvertently obstruct the airway you're trying to open.

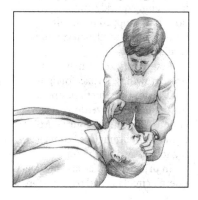

6. If you suspect a neck injury, use the *jaw-thrust maneuver* instead of the *head-tilt, chin-lift maneuver*. Kneel at his head with your elbows on the ground. Rest your thumbs on his lower jaw near the corners of the mouth, pointing your thumbs toward his feet. Then place your fingertips around the lower jaw. To open the airway, lift the lower jaw with your fingertips.

Check for breathing. Follow these steps:
1. While maintaining the open airway, place your ear over the victim's mouth and nose. Now, listen for the sound of air moving and note whether his chest rises and falls. You may also feel air flow on your cheek. If he starts to breathe, keep the airway open, place the victim in the recovery position on his side to protect the airway, and continue checking his breathing until help arrives.

2. If he doesn't start breathing after you open his airway, begin rescue breathing. Pinch his nostrils shut with the thumb and index finger of the hand you've had on his forehead.

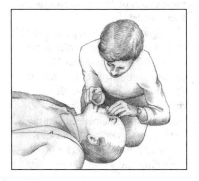

Because of the risk of acquired immunodeficiency syndrome (AIDS), the AHA now advocates teaching health care professionals how to use disposable airway equipment and recommends its use if available. However, given the fragile nature of the AIDS virus, transmission by saliva is highly unlikely.

3. Take a deep breath and place your mouth over his mouth, creating a tight seal. Give two full ventilations, taking a deep breath after each to allow enough time for his chest to expand and relax and to prevent gastric distention. Each ventilation should last $1^1/2$ to 2 seconds.

If the first ventilation isn't successful, reposition his head and try again. If you're still not successful, he may have a foreign-body airway obstruction. Check for loose dentures. If dentures or any other object is blocking the airway, follow the procedure for clearing an airway obstruction (see page 220).

Assess circulation. Follow these steps:
1. Keep one hand on the victim's forehead so his airway remains open. With your other hand, palpate the carotid artery that's closer to you. To do so, place your index and middle fingers in the groove between the trachea and the sternocleidomastoid muscle. Palpate for 5 to 10 seconds.

If you detect a pulse, don't begin chest compressions. Instead, perform rescue breathing by giving the victim 12 ventilations/minute (or one every 5 seconds). After every 12 ventilations, recheck his pulse.

2. If there's no pulse, start giving chest compressions. Make sure your knees are apart for a wide base of support. Using the hand closer to his feet, locate the lower margin of the rib cage. Then move your fingertips along the margin to the notch where the ribs meet the sternum.

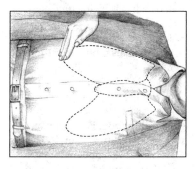

3. Place your middle finger on the notch and your index finger next to your middle finger. Your index finger will now be on the bottom of the sternum.

4. Put the heel of your other hand on the sternum, next to the index finger. The long axis of the heel of your hand will be aligned with the long axis of the sternum.

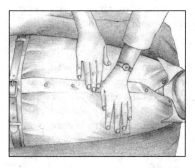

5. Take the first hand off the notch and put it on top of the hand on the sternum. Make sure you have one hand directly on top of the other and your fingers aren't on his chest. This position will keep the force of the compression on the sternum and reduce the risk of a rib fracture, lung puncture, or liver laceration.

6. With your elbows locked, arms straight, and your shoulders directly over your hands, you're ready to give chest compressions. Using the weight of your upper body, compress the victim's sternum $1^{1}/2''$ to $2''$ (4 to 5 cm), delivering the pressure through the heels of your hands. After each compression, release the pressure and allow the chest to return to its normal position so the heart can fill with blood. Don't change your hand position during compressions—you might injure the victim.

Give 15 chest compressions at a rate of 80 to 100/minute. Count, "One and two and three and. . ." up to 15. Open the airway and give two ventilations. Then find the proper hand position again and deliver 15 more compressions. Do four complete cycles of 15 compressions and two ventilations.

Palpate the carotid pulse again. If there's still no pulse, continue performing CPR in cycles of 15 compressions and two ventilations. If you're alone, perform CPR for 1 minute, check the victim's pulse, then try to get help. Return quickly to the victim and continue CPR. Every few minutes, check for breathing and a pulse. If you detect a pulse but he isn't breathing, give 12 ventilations/minute and monitor his pulse. If he has a pulse and is breathing, monitor his respirations and pulse closely. You should stop performing CPR only when his respirations and pulse return; he's turned over to the EMS; or you're exhausted.

Two-person rescue

If another rescuer arrives while you're giving CPR, follow these steps:
1. If he's not a health care professional, ask him to stand by. Then, if you become fatigued, he can take over one-person CPR. Have him begin by checking the pulse for 5 seconds after you've given two ventilations. If he doesn't feel a pulse, he should give two ventilations and begin chest compressions.

If the rescuer is another health care professional, the two of you can perform two-person CPR. He should start assisting after you've finished a cycle of 15 compressions, two ventilations, and a pulse check.

Sometimes when a health care professional arrives as a second rescuer, he'll instinctively take the victim's pulse without waiting to the end of a cycle. This is *not* part of the AHA recommendations and may confuse some rescuers. The aim of the AHA recommendations is to have all rescuers act in the same manner so precious time isn't wasted and all efforts help restore the victim's pulse and respirations.

2. The second rescuer should get into place opposite you. While you're checking for a pulse, he should be

finding the proper hand placement for delivering chest compressions.

3. If you don't detect a pulse, say, "No pulse, continue CPR" and give one ventilation. Then the second rescuer should begin delivering compressions at a rate of 80 to 100/minute. Compressions and ventilations should be administered at a 5:1 ratio. The compressor (at this point, the second rescuer) should count out loud so the ventilator can anticipate when to give ventilations. To ensure that ventilations are effective, the compressor should stop long enough for the chest to rise.

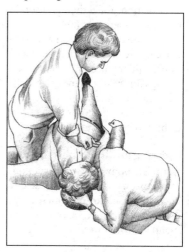

4. As the ventilator, you must check for breathing and a pulse. Signal the compressor to stop giving compressions for 5 seconds so you can make these assessments.

5. After a minimum of 10 cycles, the compressor (second rescuer) may call for a switch. This should be done clearly to allow for a smooth transition. The compressor can substitute the word *switch* for the word *one* as he counts compressions. In other words, he'd say, "Switch and two and three and four and five." You'd then give a ventilation and become the compressor by moving down to the victim's chest and placing your hands in the proper position.

6. The second rescuer would become the ventilator and move to the victim's head. He'd check the pulse for 5 seconds. If he found no pulse, he'd say, "No pulse," and give a ventilation. You'd then give compressions at a rate of 80 to 100/minute, using the same ratio of five compressions to each ventilation. Both of you should continue giving CPR in this manner until the victim's respirations and pulse return, he's turned over to the EMS, or both of you are exhausted.

Clearing an airway obstruction

A foreign-body airway obstruction may cause cardiopulmonary arrest. To give first aid for this emergency, use the following AHA-recommended procedures.

For a conscious victim. Follow these steps:

1. Ask the victim, "Are you choking?" If there's a complete airway obstruction, airflow to the vocal cords will be blocked, and she won't be able to speak. If she makes crowing sounds, her airway is partially obstructed. In this case, encourage her to cough, but don't attempt any other measures.

She'll either clear her airway herself or the obstruction will become complete. If the airway becomes completely obstructed, follow these steps:

2. Tell her that you know CPR and can help her. Wrap your arms around her waist and make a fist with one hand. Place the top of your fist against her abdomen, slightly above the umbilicus. To avoid injuring her, keep your hand well below the xiphoid process. Then grasp your fist with the other hand.

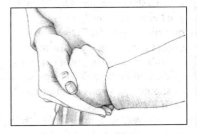

3. Squeeze her abdomen 6 to 10 times with quick inward and upward thrusts (called subdiaphragmatic abdominal thrusts, abdominal thrusts, or the Heimlich maneuver). Each thrust should be forceful enough to dislodge the obstruction. The thrusts will create an artificial cough, using air in the lungs. Giving 6 to 10 thrusts in rapid succession should create enough force to propel the obstruction out of the airway.

Be sure you have a firm grasp on the victim because she may lose consciousness and need to be lowered to the floor. You should also be aware of any objects in the area that could harm her if she's lowered to the floor.

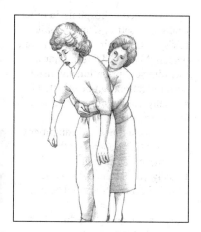

4. If she does lose consciousness during the rescue, lower her to the floor carefully.

5. Support her head and neck to prevent injury. Then continue your efforts by following steps 2 through 5 for the unconscious victim.

For an unconscious victim. Follow these steps:

1. If you come upon an unconscious victim, ask bystanders what happened. Begin CPR, using the procedure for one-person rescue (see page 216). If you're unable to ventilate, reposition the victim's head and try again. If you're still unable to ventilate the airway, follow steps 2 through 5.

2. Kneel astride her thighs. Then place the heel of one hand on top of the other and put your hands between her umbilicus and the tip of her xiphoid process at the midline. Push inward and upward 6 to 10 times. Each thrust should be

forceful enough to dislodge the obstruction.

3. After administering 6 to 10 abdominal thrusts, open her airway by grasping the tongue and lower jaw between your thumb and fingers and lifting the jaw.

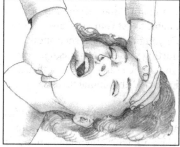

4. Insert the index finger of your other hand deep into her throat at the base of the tongue. With a hooking motion, remove the obstruction. Now, try to ventilate. If you can't remove the obstruction and can't ventilate, give another 6 to 10 abdominal thrusts. Then try to remove the obstruction and ventilate again.

Controversy: Some health care professionals contend that you shouldn't try sweeping the mouth with your finger unless you can see the obstruction and you're sure you can remove it. Sometimes, they point out, opening the airway will be enough to dislodge the obstruction. Then, by putting your finger in the victim's mouth, you create another obstruction.

5. After removing the foreign body, assess whether the victim is breathing and whether she has a pulse. Proceed as you would for a one-person rescue. Once your rescue has been successful, ensure that the victim is taken for follow-up medical care.

For an obese or pregnant victim. Sometimes, you won't be able to use abdominal thrusts. With an obese victim, for instance, you may be unable to get your arms around him. Or you may be concerned about hurting the fetus of a pregnant victim. In such cases, use chest thrusts instead of abdominal thrusts.

1. Place the top of your clenched fist against the middle of the sternum. Then put your other hand on top of your clenched fist. Perform chest thrusts until the obstruction is expelled or she loses consciousness.

2. If the victim is unconscious, give chest compressions as you would for a victim without a pulse.

Advanced cardiac life support

Advanced cardiac life support (ACLS) treats the physical changes and complications that can occur after cardiac arrest. These measures include the use of special techniques and equipment to help establish and maintain ventilation and circulation, the use of cardiac monitors to detect abnormal heart rate and rhythm, the insertion of peripheral and central I.V. lines, drug therapy, cardiac defibrillation, and the insertion of an artificial pacemaker. When the patient's condition stabilizes, the medical team can treat the cause of cardiac arrest.

Performed in hospitals, in other health care settings, or in mobile ICUs, ACLS requires more than one person. Many ACLS techniques, including defibrillation and drug administration, can be initiated by a specially trained nurse under standing orders.

The techniques and equipment used in ACLS depend on the patient's needs and on the setting. Usually, you'll follow the sequence of ACLS procedures listed below.

Preparation and procedure. First, alert code-team members and obtain a crash cart, which usually contains all equipment necessary for ACLS. Then take the following steps:
• Because CPR requires a firm surface to be effective, place a cardiac arrest board or other flat, rigid support under the patient's back. Start CPR immediately to ensure oxygenation and perfusion of vital organs. Continue CPR while other ACLS equipment is being set up. During later ACLS procedures, avoid interrupting CPR for longer than 15 seconds.
• Set up the ECG monitor to review cardiovascular status continuously and to help determine proper therapy. Because the ECG doesn't indicate the effectiveness of cardiac compression, take central (carotid or femoral) pulses frequently.
• Attempt to obtain a medical history from the patient's family or companion to learn the probable cause of the arrest and to determine contraindications for resuscitation.

• Insert a peripheral I.V. line for fluid and emergency drug administration. Use a large blood vessel such as the brachial vein because smaller peripheral vessels tend to collapse quickly during arrest. Use a large-gauge needle to prevent dislodgment or injury to the vein, with extravasation and vessel collapse. Use normal saline solution or other nonglucose fluids to start the infusion to preserve cerebral tissue.

• Perform defibrillation and administer appropriate drugs. (See *Common emergency cardiac drugs*, pages 224 to 226.) Although cardiac monitoring should be started before defibrillation, the automatic defibrillators available today have "quick-look" options built into them.

• If the patient fails to respond quickly to CPR, a single countershock, and basic drug therapy, insert a ventilatory device, such as an ET tube or oxygen cannula. After the device is in place, discontinue mouth-to-mouth breathing, but maintain respiratory assistance with a resuscitation bag. You'll use oxygen jointly with most of these devices.

• Remove oral secretions with portable or wall suction, and insert an NG tube to relieve or prevent gastric distention.

• If the patient responds to the preceding treatments and has severe bradycardia with reduced cardiac output (as in acute heart block), vasopressors may be given. If these aren't sufficient, the doctor may use a temporary transcutaneous or transvenous cardiac pacemaker.

Monitoring and aftercare. In most cases, when the patient begins to stabilize or when preliminary ACLS steps have been taken, he may be transported to a special-care area. (See *Charting codes effectively*, page 227.)

Begin direct therapy as ordered to treat the underlying cause of the patient's arrest. For example, use acute dialysis to clear endogenous or exogenous toxins that may have caused the arrest.

Defibrillation

In defibrillation, paddles applied to the patent's chest deliver a strong burst of electric current to the heart. This brief electric shock completely depolarizes the myocardium, allowing the heart's natural pacemaker to regain control of cardiac rhythm.

The treatment of choice for ventricular fibrillation and pulseless ventricular tachycardia, defibrillation may also benefit patients with monitored asystole when ventricular fibrillation is suspected. It proves successful about 40% of the time. You must perform defibrillation as soon as possible—even before intubation or drug administration. If ventricular fibrillation lasts for more than a few minutes, it causes irreparable brain damage. Note that for patients with certain arrhythmias such as unstable ventricular tachycardia, you may employ a technique similar to defibrillation, called synchronized cardioversion. (See *Performing synchronized cardioversion*, pages 228 and 229.)

(Text continues on page 226.)

Common emergency cardiac drugs

The following drugs and dosages are recommended for adult advanced cardiac life support by the American Heart Association.

Drug, route, and dosage	Nursing considerations
adenosine ***To treat paroxysmal supraventricular tachycardia (PSVT)*** *I.V. push:* 6 mg I.V. initially by rapid bolus over 1 to 3 seconds. If no response in 1 to 2 min, give 12 mg I.V	• Contraindicated in patients receiving dipyridamole and carbamazepine. • Patients receiving theophylline may require larger doses. • Follow each dose with a 20-ml saline flush.
atropine ***To treat symptomatic bradycardia*** *I.V. push:* 0.5 to 1 mg I.V. q 5 min, up to 3 mg total. ***To treat asystole*** *I.V. push:* 1 mg I.V.; repeat in 3 to 5 min if asystole persists. *I.V. infusion:* Not recommended. *Endotracheal:* May be used 2 to 2½ times the I.V. dose diluted in 10 ml of normal saline solution or sterile water.	• Lower doses (< 0.5 mg) may cause bradycardia. • Higher doses (>3 mg) may cause full vagal blockage. • Use cautiously in presence of acute myocardial infarction or ischemia.
bretylium ***To treat ventricular fibrillation (VF) and unstable ventricular tachycardia (VT) unresponsive to other therapy including electrical countershock*** *I.V. push:* Rapidly administer 5 mg/kg; can be increased to 10 mg/kg and repeated q 5 min. Maximum dose is 35 mg/kg. ***To treat persistent, recurrent VT*** *I.V. infusion:* 5 to 10 mg/kg diluted to 50 ml in dextrose 5% in water (D_5W) injected over 8 to 10 min. If VT persists, administer a second dose in 10 to 30 min and, if necessary, q 6 to 8 hours thereafter.	• Not typically used to treat VF or VT unless other drugs or countershock fail. • May lower blood pressure. • Follow each I.V. push dose with 20-ml I.V. fluid flush if peripheral site.
dobutamine hydrochloride ***To treat heart failure and low cardiac output*** *I.V. infusion:* Reconstitute with D_5W or normal saline solution; then prepare	• Don't use with beta blockers such as propranolol. • Drug is incompatible with alkaline solutions. • Patients with atrial fibrillation should

Common emergency cardiac drugs *(continued)*

Drug, route, and dosage	Nursing considerations
dobutamine hydrochloride *(continued)* standard dilution, and administer 2 to 20 mcg/kg/min.	receive digoxin first, or they may develop rapid ventricular response. • Infiltration may cause severe tissue damage.
dopamine hydrochloride ***To treat shock and correct hemodynamic imbalances; to improve perfusion to vital organs; to correct hypotension*** *I.V. infusion:* Standard dilution. May use with D_5W, dextrose 5% in normal saline solution, or combination of D_5W and normal saline solution; administer 1 to 5 mcg/kg/min; then titrate to desired effect with a final dosage of 5 to 20 mcg/kg/min. To improve perfusion to vital organs, infuse at a rate of 1 to 2 mcg/kg/min.	• May precipitate vasoconstriction in high doses. • May induce tachycardia. • Drug is incompatible with alkaline solutions. Do not mix with sodium bicarbonate in I.V. line. • Infiltration may cause severe tissue damage. • Norepinephrine should be added if dopamine dosage exceeds 20 mcg/kg/min.
epinephrine ***To restore cardiac rhythm in cardiac arrest*** *I.V. push:* Administer 10 ml of 1:10,000 solution (1 mg) q 3 to 5 min; then flush with 20 ml of I.V. fluid to ensure delivery. *Intracardiac:* Use only during open cardiac massage or when other routes are unavailable. *Endotracheal:* 2 to 2½ times the I.V. dose.	• Increases intraocular pressure. • May exacerbate heart failure (HF), arrhythmias, angina pectoris, hyperthyroidism, and emphysema. • May cause headaches, tremors, or palpitations. • Don't administer with alkaline solutions.
lidocaine ***To treat ventricular ectopy, VT, and VF*** *I.V. push:* 1 to 1.5 mg/kg bolus initially, then boluses of 0.5 to 0.75 mg/kg q 5 to 10 min if necessary to total of 3 mg/kg. *I.V. infusion:* Standard dilution. Administer 30 to 50 mcg/kg/min (2 to 4 mg/min). *Endotracheal:* 2 to 2½ times the I.V. dose	• Don't mix with sodium bicarbonate. • Don't use if patient has high-grade sinoatrial or atrioventricular block. • Discontinue if PR interval or QRS complex widens or if arrhythmias worsen. • May lead to central nervous system toxicity. • Monitor blood levels and reduce dose after 24 hours of infusion if necessary because half-life of lidocaine increases after 24 to 48 hours.

(continued)

Common emergency cardiac drugs *(continued)*

Drug, route, and dosage	Nursing considerations
lidocaine *(continued)*	• Reduce dose by half in elderly patients (>70 years), those with hepatic dysfunction, and those with decreased cardiac output (for example, from acute myocardial infarction, heart failure, or shock).
nitroprusside sodium *To treat heart failure and hypertensive emergencies* *I.V. infusion:* Prepare by adding 50 or 100 mg of drug to 250 ml of D$_5$W or normal saline solution. Administer 0.1 to 5 mcg/kg/min (therapeutic range is 0.5 to 8 mcg/kg/min).	• May cause cyanide or thiocyanate toxicity in patients with hepatic or renal insufficiency. • Wrap solution and tubing in opaque material to prevent deterioration when exposed to light. • Use an infusion pump. • May cause hypotension.
procainamide *To treat life-threatening ventricular arrhythmias* *I.V. infusion:* Give 20 to 30 mg/min, until arrhythmia is suppressed, hypotension occurs, or the QRS complex widens by 50% or 17 mg/kg of drug is given. Maintenance I.V. infusion is 1 to 4 mg/min.	• Too-rapid injection can cause precipitous hypotension. • Avoid use in patients with preexisting QT prolongation and torsades de pointes. • Reduce maintenance dosage in presence of renal failure.
sodium bicarbonate *To treat acidosis during cardiac arrest* *I.V. push:* 1 mEq/kg initially, then a half dose q 10 min.	• Don't mix with epinephrine, dopamine, or dobutamine. • Forms an insoluble precipitate when mixed with calcium salts.

Preparation. Keep in mind that ventricular fibrillation causes cardiac output to drop to zero and leads to unconsciousness. Thus, if the ECG suggests ventricular fibrillation but your patient remains responsive and awake, the ECG is wrong—probably because of electrical interference. No matter what the ECG tells you, *never defibrillate a patient who's alert;* if you do, you could trigger lethal arrhythmias or cardiac standstill.

Upon deciding that defibrillation is necessary, call promptly for help and begin CPR. When the defibrillator arrives, make sure that you or another staff member continue CPR during preparation of the equipment.

If you're preparing the defibrillator, follow these steps:
• Plug the defibrillator in and turn it on.
• Attach the defibrillator's ECG leads to the patient, or apply monitoring defibrillator pads to the chest.
• If you're using hard paddles, apply conductive gel or paste to the paddles or place two gel pads on the patient's bare chest in the appropriate position. If you're using gel or paste, coat the entire surface of the paddles by rubbing them together. Be sure to remove any gel from your hands and the sides of the paddles because any excess will provide a pathway for the electric current and cause burns.
• Select the electric charge on the defibrillator control, following your hospital's policy or the doctor's orders. (The AHA recommends 200 joules for the first attempt at defibrillation; 200 to 300 joules for the second attempt; and 360 joules for the third and all subsequent attempts.)

Procedure. First, check the patient's monitor to be sure that it still indicates ventricular fibrillation or tachycardia. Then stop CPR for 5 to 10 seconds and palpate for a carotid pulse. *If you detect a pulse, don't defibrillate the patient.*

Defibrillation may be done using hard paddles or monitoring/defibrillation self-adhering gel pad electrodes, which free your hands. If the carotid pulse is absent, position the paddles or electrode patches. If you're defibrillating a male patient, put one paddle or electrode beneath the clavicle, to the right of the upper end of his sternum; put the other

CHARTING TIPS

Charting codes effectively

Guidelines established by the American Heart Association direct you to keep a written, chronological account of a patient's condition throughout resuscitation efforts. If you're a designated recorder for a patient's cardiopulmonary arrest record, document therapeutic intervention and the patient's responses to these as they occur. Don't rely on your memory to record the sequence of events.

If a code is called, you'll complete a *code record*. On this form you'll record detailed information about the code including observations, interventions, and any drugs given to the patient.

one on the left lateral wall of his chest, to the left of the cardiac apex. For a female, place the paddles or electrodes at the mid- or anterior-axillary level, not over the breasts.

If you're using *anterior-posterior paddles*, place the flat one (without a discharge button) under the patient, behind the heart and just below the left scapula. Place the other paddle on the chest, directly over the patient's heart.

Once the paddles are properly placed, press them firmly against the patient's skin to ensure good contact. (Be sure to keep the standard paddles at least $3/4''$ [2 cm] apart at all times, to prevent arcing.) Then push the charge button until the display indicates that the proper power level

Performing synchronized cardioversion

Like defibrillation, synchronized cardioversion delivers an electric charge to the heart to correct arrhythmias. However, with cardioversion, much lower energy levels are used (typically 25 to 50 joules), and the burst of electricity is precisely timed to coincide with the peak of the R wave.

You can't use cardioversion to treat ventricular fibrillation because a fibrillating heart doesn't generate an R wave. But it's the treatment of choice for unstable ventricular tachycardia (accompanied by chest pain, dyspnea, and hypotension) and unstable paroxysmal atrial tachycardia that fails to respond to drug therapy.

You may perform synchronized cardioversion as an elective or emergency procedure. In elective cases, the nurse usually assists the doctor, but in an emergency, many hospitals authorize nurses to perform the procedure.

Preparing the patient

For emergency cardioversion, you'll prepare the patient as you would for defibrillation. However, the patient will commonly have adequate cardiac output, so you won't have to initiate cardiopulmonary resuscitation and you'll have a bit more time to work. Sedate the patient, as ordered, unless he's profoundly hypotensive, unconscious, or showing signs of pulmonary edema. If there's time, explain the need for prompt cardioversion.

If you're assisting with elective cardioversion, explain to the patient that food and fluids will be restricted for 12 hours. Make sure that he understands the doctor's explanation of risks and complications. Tell the patient that you'll insert an I.V. line (if one hasn't already been inserted) in case medications are needed and that he'll undergo a 12-lead electrocardiogram (ECG) before cardioversion. If the patient is receiving oxygen, explain that the doctor will discontinue oxygen therapy during the procedure, as a precaution against fire, but will reinstitute it immediately afterward.

Check the patient's medication history. Elective cardioversion is often contraindicated in a patient receiving a digitalis glycoside because of the risk of lethal arrhythmias. If the patient is receiving a digitalis glycoside, make sure that his potassium level is normal because potassium plays a key role in conducting and regulating electric impulses within the heart.

Performing cardioversion

Once you've prepared the patient for cardioversion, follow these steps:
• Take the patient's vital signs and gather emergency resuscitation equipment.
• Connect the patient to the defibrillator's ECG leads and turn on the oscilloscope.
• Turn on the synchronization control and ensure that each R wave is marked. If not marked, increase the gain to create a taller R wave.
• Give sedation or brief-acting amnesic medication through the I.V. line.
• Now set the control to the proper energy level (as indicated by the doctor or hospital protocol).
• Prepare and place the paddles or adhesive gel pad as you would for

Performing synchronized cardioversion *(continued)*

defibrillation, then press them firmly onto the patient's chest and push the charge button until the display indicates that the proper energy level has been reached.
• Say "All clear!" and verify that no one is touching the patient or the bed.
• Hold the discharge button down until the paddles or gel pads discharge. Unlike defibrillation, the paddles will not discharge immediately; there will be a slight delay while the defibrillator synchronizes with the R wave.
• After the paddles discharge, remove them from the patient's chest and evaluate the ECG to determine whether cardioversion was successful. If the arrhythmia wasn't corrected, repeat the procedure using a higher setting.
• After successful cardioversion, check the patient's vital signs every 15 minutes for at least an hour or until precardioversion levels are reached.

has been reached, and in a loud voice say, "All clear!" to warn everyone to step back. *Before operating the defibrillator,* make sure that the area surrounding the patient isn't wet and that no one is touching the bed or the patient. You should be touching only the paddles, not the patient.

Hold down the discharge button to deliver the electric current and then remove the paddles from the patient's chest. Check the ECG and carotid pulse to determine whether defibrillation was successful. If it wasn't, defibrillate the patient again. If the patient still doesn't respond, continue defibrillation and all resuscitation measures until the doctor ends resuscitation or the patient stabilizes. When you've finished, turn off and unplug the defibrillator. Clean the paddles with soap and water.

Monitoring and aftercare. Check the patient's vital signs every 15 minutes for at least an hour, and monitor the ECG continuously. If the cardiac rhythm worsens, notify the doctor immediately. Assess the patient's chest for burns. If burns have occurred, apply the prescribed ointment.

In some cases, the doctor may choose to surgically insert an implantable cardiac defibrillator (ICD), which automatically delivers an electric current to the heart when it senses irregular rhythms. (See *Hightech help for failing hearts,* page 230.) If your patient is scheduled to have an ICD implanted, reinforce the doctor's explanation of the device.

Patient education. Teach the patient to take his pulse for a full minute every day before rising and to notify his doctor immediately if the rate is less than 60 or greater than 100 beats/minute or if he experiences palpitations, dizziness, or fainting. Emphasize that he must keep regular appointments with his doctor for routine ECGs and evaluation of his response to medication.

High-tech help for failing hearts

Like many nurses, you may be seeing an increasing number of patients with a history of ventricular fibrillation. Studies show that these patients are at high risk for further episodes of ventricular tachyarrhythmia, making them good candidates for an implantable cardiac defibrillator (ICD). An ICD can help control ventricular fibrillation even after the patient leaves the hospital; newer ICD models can also convert such arrhythmias as ventricular tachycardia and torsades de pointes.

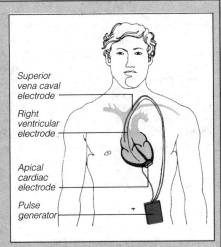

Superior vena caval electrode

Right ventricular electrode

Apical cardiac electrode

Pulse generator

The doctor implants the ICD (which has three defibrillator electrodes attached to its pulse generator) into the patient's abdominal cavity. He inserts the apical cardiac electrode through a left thoracotomy at the fifth intercostal space. Using fluoroscopy, he inserts the second electrode via the superior vena cava, positioning it near the right atrial junction. He positions the third electrode in the right ventricle. Newer devices can be implanted using a transvenous approach. Also, the newer units may combine traditional pacing components with the ICD.

When the ICD senses a ventricular tachyarrhythmia, it discharges a small shock (25 to 30 joules) to defibrillate the heart automatically. If the initial discharge doesn't end the arrhythmia, the ICD can discharge up to four more times, increasing the voltage each time. The unit usually lasts 3 years or for up to 100 discharges.

Nursing care

Your main responsibility for a patient with an ICD involves preoperative and postoperative care and patient teaching. Tell the patient that he'll have small incisions in the left side of his chest, right shoulder, and abdomen and that once the unit is implanted he'll be able to feel it discharge. (Some patients describe the sensation as a sudden blow to the chest.) Warn the patient that if ventricular arrhythmias occur, he'll probably experience sudden faintness or shortness of breath (or both), followed by the discharge and a return to a feeling of well-being. The episode usually lasts less than 30 seconds.

Recommend to the patient's family that they learn to perform cardiopulmonary resuscitation in case the ICD doesn't convert the rhythm after delivering the programmed number of shocks.

If your patient will be getting an ICD, outline the special precautions he'll have to take.

Valsalva's maneuver

Valsalva's maneuver is an easy-to-perform maneuver that can help correct atrial arrhythmias by triggering vagal stimulation of the heart. Instruct the patient to take a deep breath and then to bear down as if defecating. If no syncope, dizziness, or arrhythmias occur, have him continue to hold his breath and bear down for 10 seconds. Then tell him to exhale and breathe quietly. If the maneuver is successful, the patient's heart rate will begin to slow before he exhales.

Initially, the maneuver raises intrathoracic pressure from its normal level of −3 to −4 mm Hg to levels of 60 mm Hg or higher. This increase in pressure is transmitted directly to the great vessels and the heart, causing decreased venous return and stroke volume and lowered systolic pressure. Within seconds, the baroreceptors respond by increasing the heart rate and causing peripheral vasoconstriction.

When the patient exhales at the end of the maneuver, blood pressure begins to rise. But peripheral vasoconstriction is still present, and the combination of rising blood pressure and vasoconstriction causes vagal stimulation, which in turn slows the heart rate.

Because Valsalva's maneuver can cause mobilization of venous thrombi, bleeding, ventricular arrhythmias, and asystole, it's contraindicated for patients with severe CAD, acute MI, or moderate to severe hypovolemia.

Patient preparation. In simple terms, explain Valsalva's maneuver and its purpose to the patient. Describe it as "trying to exhale while holding your breath," and briefly demonstrate it.

Warn your patient that he may feel faint or dizzy, and place him in a supine position. Start an I.V. line if one isn't running already, and take vital signs. Then attach a 12-lead ECG to the patient and gather resuscitation equipment and medications. Monitor the ECG and continue to record it throughout the entire procedure.

Procedure. Instruct the patient to take a deep breath and then to bear down as if defecating. If no syncope, dizziness, or arrhythmias occur, have him hold his breath and bear down for 10 seconds. Tell him to exhale and breathe quietly. If the maneuver is successful, the patient's heart rate will begin to slow before he exhales. (See *Cough CPR: Weapon against ventricular arrhythmias,* page 232.)

Monitoring and aftercare. Assess the patient's ECG and vital signs once he completes the procedure. You'll need to monitor the patient's ECG continuously for at least 12 hours to ensure that arrhythmias don't return. If an atrial arrhythmia doesn't resolve following the maneuver, the doctor will probably order drug therapy.

Cough CPR: Weapon against ventricular arrhythmias

A simple reflex mechanism—the cough—may help convert lethal ventricular arrhythmias to normal sinus rhythm. Researchers have found that continuous, forced coughing spurts, 1 to 3 seconds apart and just before or at the onset of ventricular tachycardia or fibrillation, can help the patient maintain consciousness for up to 30 seconds.

Having the patient perform cough cardiopulmonary resuscitation (CPR) may give you extra time to prepare defibrillation. The patient can perform cough CPR on his own, in any position and on any surface. By taking a breath between each cough, he can maintain cardiac and pulmonary function.

How does cough CPR work? By closing the epiglottis and strongly contracting the respiratory muscles, it greatly increases intrathoracic pressure. A deep breath lowers intrathoracic pressure, promoting venous return to the heart. A deep cough raises intrathoracic pressure, increasing coronary perfusion.

The compressive force of such a pressure increase propels blood forward. Researchers believe increased coronary perfusion, which decreases myocardial ischemia, also occurs during cough CPR, from increased aortic pressure and reflex coronary vasodilation secondary to baroreceptor activation.

For cough CPR to work, the patient must be capable of sustaining an adequate cough. (Many patients have long but ineffective coughing spells.)

Patient education. If Valsalva's maneuver corrects the arrhythmia, teach the patient to do it at home. Tell him that if palpitations or angina occurs after he leaves the hospital, he should lie down (to prevent fainting or dizziness) and perform the maneuver for 10 seconds. Warn him that if the maneuver doesn't relieve his symptoms, he'll need to call his doctor immediately.

Carotid sinus massage

Carotid sinus massage (CSM) is a noninvasive method for evaluating and terminating certain tachyarrhythmias. Patient response to CSM differs, depending on the type of arrhythmia involved. This difference limits CSM's usefulness as a treatment.

• With sinus tachycardia, the heart rate slows gradually when CSM is applied and speeds up again after it's terminated.
• In atrial tachycardia, the response is unpredictable; the arrhythmia may terminate or remain unaffected, or atrioventricular (AV) block may worsen.
• In paroxysmal atrial tachycardia, reversion to sinus rhythm occurs 20% of the time.
• In nonparoxysmal tachycardia and ventricular tachycardia, there's no response.
• In atrial fibrillation or flutter, ventricular rate slows because of increased AV block.

Continuous ECG monitoring during the procedure is essential.

CSM may cause ventricular stand-still, ventricular tachycardia, or ventricular fibrillation. By worsening AV block, CSM can also cause junctional or ventricular escape rhythms.

Another potential complication is cerebral damage from inadequate tissue perfusion. If the carotid artery is totally occluded during CSM, decreased cerebral blood flow may cause a CVA. Also, compression of the carotid sinus may loosen endothelial plaque, which can migrate and cause a CVA.

Don't perform CSM on patients with digitalis toxicity, cerebrovascular disease, or previous carotid surgery. Perform CSM cautiously on elderly patients, on those receiving digitalis glycosides, and on individuals with heart block, hypertension, CAD, diabetes mellitus, or hyperkalemia. Note that some experts recommend against performing CSM on any patient over age 40.

Patient preparation. With the patient in bed, place a pillow behind the scapulae to extend his neck. Insert an I.V. line and gather emergency resuscitation equipment. Turn the patient's head away from the site being massaged; this will make the artery less likely to roll behind the trachea during massage.

Explain the procedure to the patient, and connect him to a cardiac monitor or to an ECG machine. Assess and document his cardiac rhythm and neurologic status and auscultate both carotid arteries for bruits. A bruit close to the jaw line suggests arteriosclerotic plaques in the carotid artery and is an absolute contraindication to CSM.

Procedure. Depending on hospital and unit protocol, a nurse or a doctor may perform CSM. It involves manual stimulation of pressure receptors in the carotid artery, which in turn triggers a parasympathetic response and depresses heart rate and conductivity.

Using the tips of your index and middle fingers, locate the patient's larynx, and then slide your fingers laterally into the groove between the trachea and the neck muscles. You'll know you've found the carotid artery when you feel a strong pulse. Next, follow the carotid artery to the bifurcation—the location of the carotid sinus area—by sliding your fingers to the angle of the mandible. Place four fingers medial to the pulsating artery. Press the artery against the underlying vertebrum and begin massaging it firmly in a head-to-toe direction. Massage for *no longer than 5 seconds* because of the risk of asystole. Release the artery as soon as the ECG shows that the heart rate has begun to slow.

If massage on one side is ineffective, perform CSM on the other side, again massaging for no longer than 5 seconds. Massage only one carotid sinus at a time; never massage both simultaneously.

Monitoring and aftercare. As soon as you finish CSM, check the patient's vital signs, watching especially for hypotension and bradycardia. Continue cardiac monitoring for at least 4 hours to assess the effects of treatment and to alert you to the return of the arrhythmia. Also check your patient's neurologic status every hour for the first 4 hours to detect signs of CVA.

Patient education. Show the patient how to take his radial pulse. Instruct him to take it for a full minute each morning before getting out of bed. He should also take his pulse whenever he experiences chest pain, palpitations, dizziness, or fainting. Warn him that these symptoms, or a heart rate of less than 60 or greater than 100 beats/minute, indicate that he should call his doctor.

Pacemaker insertion

Pacemakers are battery-operated generators that emit timed electrical signals, trigger contraction of the heart muscle, and control the heart rate. Whether temporary or permanent, they're used when the heart's natural pacemaker fails to work properly.

Temporary pacemakers. To pace the heart during CPR or open-heart surgery, after cardiac surgery, and when sinus arrest, symptomatic sinus bradycardia, or complete heart block occurs, a temporary pacemaker is chosen. Temporary pacing may also correct tachyarrhythmias that fail to respond to drug therapy. In emergency situations, the patient may receive a temporary pacemaker if time or his condition doesn't permit or require implantation of a permanent pacemaker. The doctor may also use a temporary pacemaker to observe

pacing's effects on cardiac function so he can select an optimal rate before implantation of a permanent pacemaker. Method of insertion varies, depending on the device.

Temporary pacemakers come in four types: transcutaneous, transvenous, epicardial, and transthoracic. A *transcutaneous* pacemaker is completely noninvasive and easily applied. This pacemaker proves especially useful in an emergency. A *transvenous* pacemaker is a balloon-tipped pacing catheter inserted via the subclavian or jugular vein into the right ventricle. Transvenous pacemakers offer better control of the heartbeat than transcutaneous or transthoracic pacemakers, but electrode insertion takes longer, thus limiting its usefulness in an emergency. *Epicardial* pacemakers are implanted during open-heart surgery. The electrodes permit rapid treatment of postoperative complications. The leads can be attached to a pulse generator when needed. *Transthoracic* pacing involves needle insertion of leads into the heart. Used in emergencies, it rarely stimulates the heart and commonly causes complications.

Permanent pacemakers. The patient may receive a permanent pacemaker when the heart's natural pacemaker becomes irreversibly disrupted. Indications include symptomatic bradycardia, advanced symptomatic AV block, sick sinus syndrome, sinus arrest, sinoatrial block, Stokes-Adams syndrome, tachyarrhythmias, and ectopic rhythms caused by antiarrhythmic drugs.

Permanent pacemaker implantation is a common procedure. More than 300 types of pacemakers exist, and many of them are programmable to perform varied functions. Pacemakers are categorized according to their capabilities. Choice of a pacemaker depends on the patient's age and condition, the doctor's preference and, increasingly, the device's cost, which can be several thousand dollars.

Most doctors use the transvenous endocardial approach to implant a permanent pacemaker. Postoperative monitoring is vital for patients receiving a permanent pacemaker. The patient may develop serous or bloody drainage from the insertion site, swelling, ecchymosis, pain from the incision, and impaired mobility; less common complications include venous thrombosis, embolism, infection, pneumothorax, pectoral or diaphragmatic muscle stimulation from the pacemaker, arrhythmias, cardiac tamponade, HF, and abnormal pacemaker operation with lead dislodgment. Late complications (up to several years) include failure to capture, failure to sense, firing loss, and pacemaker rejection.

Patient preparation. If pacing is done in an emergency, briefly explain the procedure to the patient, if possible.

If the patient is scheduled for permanent implantation, ensure that he and his family understand the doctor's explanation of the need for an artificial pacemaker, the potential complications, and the alternatives. Obtain baseline vital signs and record a 12-lead ECG or rhythm strip. Evaluate radial and dorsalis pedis pulses and assess the patient's mental status.

Restrict food and fluids for 12 hours before the procedure. Explain to the patient that he may receive a sedative before the procedure and will probably have his upper chest shaved and scrubbed with an antiseptic solution. Inform him that when he arrives in the operating room, his hands may be restrained so that they don't inadvertently touch the sterile area, and his chest will be draped with sterile towels. Unless he's scheduled to undergo a thoracotomy, explain that he'll receive a local, rather than a general, anesthetic. Tell him that he'll be in the operating room for about an hour.

Monitoring and aftercare. After pacemaker insertion, provide continuous ECG monitoring. Chart the type of insertion, lead system, pacemaker mode, and pacing guidelines. Take vital signs every 30 minutes until the patient stabilizes, and watch the ECG for signs of pacemaker problems.

Be on guard for signs of a perforated ventricle, with resultant cardiac tamponade. These include persistent hiccups, distant heart sounds, pulsus paradoxus, hypotension accompanied by narrow pulse pressure, increased venous pressure, bulging neck veins, cyanosis, decreased urine output, restlessness, and complaints of fullness in the chest. Report any of these signs immediately and prepare the patient for emergency surgery.

If your patient's condition worsens dramatically and he requires defibrillation, follow these guidelines to avoid damaging the pacemaker:
• Place the paddles at least 4″ (10 cm) from the pulse generator and avoid anterior-posterior paddle placement.
• Have a backup temporary pacemaker available.
• If your patient has an external pacemaker, turn it off.
• Finally, keep the current under 200 joules, if possible.

Assess the area around the incision for swelling, tenderness, and hematoma, but don't remove the occlusive dressing for the first 24 to 72 hours without the doctor's order. When you do remove it, check the wound for drainage, redness, and unusual warmth or tenderness.

After the initial period of immobilization, begin passive ROM exercises for the affected arm, if ordered. Progress to active ROM exercises in 2 weeks.

To avoid arrhythmias, take the following steps:
• Install a fresh battery before each insertion. This will help avoid temporary pacemaker malfunction. Carefully secure the external catheter wires and the pacemaker box. Assess the threshold daily. Watch closely for premature ventricular contractions, a sign of myocardial irritation.
• Restrict the patient's activity after insertion, as ordered. This will also avert permanent pacemaker malfunction. Monitor the pulse rate regularly, and watch for signs of decreased cardiac output.
• Warn the patient about environmental hazards, as indicated by the pacemaker manufacturer. Although hazards may not present a problem, 24-hour Holter monitoring may be helpful in doubtful situations. Tell the patient to report light-headedness or syncope, and stress the importance of regular checkups.

Patient education. Tell the patient to:
• take his pulse every day before getting out of bed. Instruct him to record his heart rate, along with the date and time, to help the doctor determine whether the pacemaker requires adjustment.
• call the doctor immediately if his pulse rate drops below the minimal pacemaker setting or if it exceeds 140 beats/minute.
• check the implantation site each day. Normally, the site bulges slightly. If it reddens, swells, drains, or becomes warm or painful, he should call the doctor.
• report difficulty breathing, dizziness, fainting, swollen hands or feet, or redness, warmth, pain, drainage, foul-smelling odor, or swelling at the insertion site.
• avoid placing excessive pressure over the insertion site, making sudden or jerky movements, or extending his arms over his head for 8 weeks after discharge.
• follow his normal routines, including sexual activity, and to bathe and shower normally. Urge him to follow dietary and exercise instructions. The patient should exercise every day but must not

overdo it, even if he feels like his energy has increased since his pacemaker was inserted. Tell him to avoid rough horseplay or lifting heavy objects and to be especially careful not to stress the muscles near the pacemaker.

• carry his pacemaker identification at all times and to show his card to airline attendants when he travels; the pacemaker will set off metal detectors but won't be harmed.

• take special precautions to prevent disruption of the pacemaker by electrical or electronic devices. For example, he should avoid placing electric hair clippers or shavers directly over the pacemaker and avoid close contact with electric motors and gasoline engines. He should also keep away from automobile antitheft devices and high-voltage electric lines.

• avoid strong magnetic forces such as those from a magnetic resonance imaging (MRI) machine. The patient must tell the doctor of his implanted pacemaker before undergoing MRI.

• keep all scheduled doctor's appointments. Explain to the patient that his pacemaker will need to be checked regularly at the doctor's office or over the telephone to make sure it's in good working order. Pacemaker batteries usually last about 10 years and a brief hospitalization is necessary for replacement.

Checking the pacemaker by telephone. Instruct the patient on how to operate the pacemaker transmitter, which enables the doctor to check pacemaker function by telephone.

• Before using the transmitter for the first time, the patient should check the battery. Tell him he'll need to replace the battery every 2 to 3 months.

• If using chest electrodes, tell the patient to open or take off his shirt and undershirt, so that the transmitter's electrodes rest against his bare skin.

• When ready to transmit the signal, the patient should call his doctor. When the doctor's office is ready to receive the signal, the patient must switch the transmitter's switch to the *ON* position.

• Instruct the patient to hold the telephone's mouthpiece against the transmitter's speaker. He must hold the telephone steady and try to remain still for about 30 seconds.

• The patient should hold the telephone to his ear and listen for further instructions. The doctor may want him to repeat the procedure while holding a special magnet over the pacemaker. If so, the patient must be careful to hold the magnet flat and steady over the pacemaker.

REFERENCES AND READINGS

Baas, L.S., et al. "Pacemaker Electrical Safety in Critical Care and Telemetry Units," *American Journal of Critical Care,* accepted for publication, 1997.

Baas, L.S., et al. "Quality of Life and Self Care in Persons with Heart Failure," *Progress in Cardiovascular Nursing,* accepted for publication, 1997.

Bainger, E.M., and Fernsler, J.I. "Quality of Life Before and After Implantation of an

Internal Cardioverter Defibrillator," *American Journal of Critical Care* 4(1):36-43, January 1995.

Barviere, C.C. "A New Device for Control of Bleeding after Transfemoral Catheterization," *Critical Care Nurse* 15(1):51-53, February 1995.

Braunwald, E. *Heart Disease: A Textbook of Cardiovascular Medicine,* 5th ed. Philadelphia: W.B. Saunders Co., 1996.

Bunbar, S.B., et al. "Mood Disturbance in Patients with Recurrent Ventricular Dysrhythmia Before Insertion of Implantable Cardioverter Defibrillator," *Heart and Lung* 25(4):253-61, July 1996.

Caldwell, C.A., and Quall, S.J. "Intra-aortic Balloon Counterpulsation Timing," *American Journal of Critical Care* 5(4):254-61, July 1996.

Clochesy, J.M., et al. *Critical Care Nursing,* 2nd ed. Philadelphia: W.B. Saunders Co., 1996.

Connors, K.F., and Lamas, G.A. "Postmyocardial Infarction Patients: Experiences from the SAVE Trial," *American Journal of Critical Care* 4(1):23-28, January 1995.

Dolman, S., and Paradiso-Hardy, F. "Intracoronary Urokinase for Restoring Circulation in Occluded Saphenous Vein Grafts," *Critical Care Nurse* 16(6):24-40, December 1996.

Dracup, K., et al. "Rethinking Heart Failure," *American Journal of Nursing* 95(7):22-28, July 1995.

Hurst, J.W., et al. *The Heart,* 8th ed. New York: McGraw-Hill Book Co., 1995.

Jaarsma, T., et al. "Sexual Function in Patients with Heart Failure," *Heart and Lung* 25(4):262-70, July 1996.

Juran, N.B., et al. "Survey of Current Practice Patterns for Percutaneous Transluminal Coronary Angioplasty, *American Journal of Critical Care* 5(6):442-48, November 1996.

Keeling, A., et al. "Reducing Time in Bed After Cardiac Catheterization (TIBS II)," *American Journal of Critical Care* 5(4):277-81, July 1996.

Kinney, et al., eds. *Comprehensive Cardiac Care,* 8th ed. St. Louis: Mosby–Year Book, Inc., 1996.

Nichols, K., and Collins, J. "Update on Implantable Cardioverter Defibrillators: Knowing the Difference in Devices and Their Impact on Patient Care," *AACN Clinical Issues: Advanced Practice in Acute and Critical Care* 6(1):31-43, February 1995.

Nursing98 Drug Handbook. Springhouse, Pa.: Springhouse Corp., 1998.

Professional Guide to Diseases, 5th ed. Springhouse, Pa.: Springhouse Corp., 1995.

Simko, L.C., and Walker, J.H. "Reoperative Antioxidant and Allopurinol Therapy for Reducing Reperfusion-Induced Injury in Patients Undergoing Cardiothoracic Surgery," *Critical Care Nurse* 16(6):69-75, December 1996.

Sparks, S.M., et al. *Nursing Diagnosis Pocket Manual.* Springhouse, Pa.: Springhouse Corp., 1996.

6

NEUROLOGIC CARE

For many nurses, neurologic care poses a formidable challenge. Neurologic assessment, for instance, can take longer than most other assessments and requires sophisticated skills. Because of technologic advances, neurologic tests have become increasingly accurate but also more complex. Treatments and procedures, too, have taken strides forward. Facing challenges like these successfully requires thorough preparation, sound clinical skills, and careful patient preparation and education.

ASSESSMENT

Assessment, the first step of the nursing process, is critical. You can identify neurologic problems while performing a complete assessment or while investigating a complaint. You can evaluate overall neurologic function and detect abnormalities as you assess mental status, the cranial nerves, sensorimotor function, and reflexes.

Physical examination

A complete neurologic assessment provides information about five categories of neurologic function: cerebral function (including level of consciousness [LOC], mental status, and language), cranial nerves, motor system and cerebellar functions, sensory system, and reflexes. Complex and time-consuming, this assessment can take 2 to 3 hours to complete. Unless you work as a nurse practitioner, you probably won't perform a complete neurologic assessment.

Usually, you'll perform a neurologic screening assessment. This type of assessment evaluates some of the key indicators of neurologic function and helps identify areas of dysfunction. A neurologic screening assessment usually includes evaluation of LOC, selected cranial nerve assessment, and motor and sensory screening.

If a screening assessment reveals areas of neurologic dysfunction, you

CHARTING TIPS

Documenting neurologic assessment

When documenting assessment findings you will, of course, always describe the patient's response to the stimulus. But don't forget to document the stimulus used to elicit the response.

Many clinicians use subjective terms to describe level of arousal. However, learn to describe it objectively. For example, describe a lethargic patient's responses this way: "awakened when called loudly, then immediately fell asleep."

A patient's response will vary with the stimulus used, but if you describe the behavior in concrete terms, your documentation will give a more accurate, useful picture of the patient's condition.

must evaluate those areas in more detail.

Finally, you may have to perform a brief neurologic assessment, called a neuro check. This will enable you to make rapid, repeated evaluations of several key indicators of nervous system status: LOC, pupil size and response, verbal responsiveness, extremity strength and movement, and vital signs. After you've established baseline values, regularly reevaluating these key indicators reveals trends in a patient's neurologic function and helps detect transient changes that can be warning signs of problems.

Always begin with an assessment of cerebral function, including

LOC. Because the brain's neurons are extremely sensitive to changes in their internal environment, cerebral dysfunction usually serves as the earliest sign of a developing central nervous system (CNS) disorder.

Cerebral function

Basic assessment of cerebral function includes LOC, communication and, briefly, mental status. Further assessment includes formal evaluation of language skills and a complete mental status evaluation.

Level of consciousness. To assess the patient's consciousness, you'll need to evaluate his level of arousal or wakefulness and orientation to person, place, and time.

Level of arousal (wakefulness). Assess the patient's degree of wakefulness. Decreased arousal commonly precedes disorientation.

Begin by quietly observing the patient's behavior. If the patient is sleeping, try to arouse him by speaking his name in a normal tone of voice. If he doesn't respond, try to arouse him starting with a minimal stimulus, increasing its intensity as necessary.

Next, note the type and intensity of stimulus required to elicit a response. Compare the findings with results of previous assessments. Note any trends or any factors that could affect patient responsiveness such as administration of CNS depressant medications. (See *Documenting neurologic assessment*.)

Using the Glasgow Coma Scale

Originally designed to help predict a patient's survival and recovery after a head injury, the Glasgow Coma Scale assesses level of consciousness (LOC). It minimizes the use of subjective impressions to evaluate LOC by testing and scoring three observations: eye response, motor response, and response to verbal stimuli.

Each response receives a point value. If the patient is alert, can follow simple commands, and is completely oriented to person, place, and time, his score will total 15 points. If the patient is comatose, his score will total 7 or less. A score of 3, the lowest possible score, indicates deep coma and a poor prognosis.

Many hospitals display the Glasgow Coma Scale on neurologic flowsheets to show changes in the patient's LOC over time.

Observation	Response elicited	Score
Eye response	Opens spontaneously	4
	Opens to verbal command	3
	Opens to pain	2
	No response	1
Motor response	Reacts to verbal command	6
	Reacts to painful stimuli:	
	—Identifies localized pain	5
	—Flexes and withdraws	4
	—Assumes flexor posture	3
	—Assumes extensor posture	2
	No response	1
Verbal response	Is oriented and converses	5
	Is disoriented, but converses	4
	Uses inappropriate words	3
	Makes incomprehensible sounds	2
	No response	1

Orientation. To assess orientation, always ask open-ended questions, which require the patient to provide more than a yes-or-no answer. Test orientation to time by asking the patient the time of day, day of the week, date (month and year), and season. If mental status becomes impaired, orientation to time usually vanishes before orientation to place and person.

To minimize the subjectivity of LOC assessment and to establish a greater degree of reliability, you may use the Glasgow Coma Scale. (See *Using the Glasgow Coma Scale.*)

Communication. Assess the patient's ability to comprehend speech, writing, numbers, and gestures. Language skills include learning and recalling words, using grammar, and structuring message content logically. Speech involves neuromuscular actions of the mouth, tongue, and oropharynx.

Verbal responsiveness. During the interview and physical assessment, observe the patient when you ask a question. Note the quality of the patient's speech, the appropriateness of his responses, the words he chooses, his articulation, and his understanding and execution of verbal commands. Increasing language difficulties may indicate deteriorating neurologic status, warranting further evaluation and doctor notification.

Impaired language function occurs in dysphasia or aphasia. Speech problems include articulation difficulties and slurred speech, which may result from facial muscle paralysis.

Formal language skills evaluation. Evaluation of the extent and characteristics of the patient's language deficits is usually performed by a speech pathologist. This may help pinpoint the site of a CNS lesion.

Mental status. Performed by a doctor or specially trained nurse, a complete mental status examination provides information about the patient's cognitive, psychological, and intellectual skills. It's usually only performed on a chronically disoriented patient or a patient with suspected mental status deficits after prescreening.

Mental status screening. To identify the need for more in-depth evaluation, you may perform an abbreviated version of the complete mental status examination. This brief screening proves useful if a patient's responses to interview questions seem unreliable or indicate a possible disturbance of memory or cognitive processes. (See *Mental status screening questions.*)

Cranial nerves

Cranial nerve (CN) assessment provides valuable information about the condition of the CNS, particularly the brain stem. Because of their anatomic locations, some cranial nerves are more vulnerable to the effects of increasing intracranial pressure (ICP). Therefore, a neurologic screening assessment of the cranial nerves focuses on these key nerves: the optic (II), oculomotor (III), trochlear (IV), and abducens (VI). Evaluate the other nerves only if the patient's history or symptoms indicate a potential cranial nerve disorder or when performing a complete nervous system assessment. (See *When cranial nerves function normally,* page 244, and *Evaluating brain stem function,* pages 245 and 246.)

Motor function

This portion of the assessment evaluates the motor function of the cerebral cortex, cerebellum, spinal cord, and the muscles.

A screening assessment always includes examination of the patient's muscle strength (including size and symmetry), arm and leg movement, and gait.

Patients who need a complete neurologic examination or who dis-

Mental status screening questions

As part of a neurologic screening assessment, ask the following questions to help identify patients with disordered thought processes. An incorrect answer to any question may indicate a need for a complete mental status examination.

Question	Function screened
What is your name?	Orientation to person
What is today's date?	Orientation to time
What year is it?	Orientation to time
Where are you now?	Orientation to place
How old are you?	Memory
Where were you born?	Remote memory
What did you have for breakfast?	Recent memory
Who is the U.S. president?	General knowledge
Can you count backwards from 20 to 1?	Attention and calculation skills
Why are you here?	Judgment

play a motor deficit during the screening assessment may undergo a complete motor system assessment. When performing a complete assessment, proceed from head to toe assessing all muscles of the major joints. Then assess the patient's gait and cerebellar functions.

Remain alert for any involuntary movement of the limbs, trunk, or face. Determine whether the movement is proximal or distal and whether it occurs during sleep. Further assess any involuntary movements for rhythm or repetition.

Muscle tone and cerebellar function. Muscle tone represents the muscles' resistance to passive stretching. To test muscle tone, move the patient's extremities through passive range-of-motion (ROM) exercises progressing from the fingers, wrist, elbow, and shoulder to the ankle, knee, and hip. To evaluate cerebellar function, test the patient's balance and coordination. (See *Assessing cerebellar function,* pages 247 and 248.)

Sensory system

The sensory system portion of the assessment evaluates how well the sensory receptors detect a stimulus, how well the afferent nerves carry sensory nerve impulses to the spinal cord, and the ability of the sensory tracts in the spinal cord to carry sensory messages to the brain. You'll also assess the sensory, interpretive, and integrative functions of the cerebral cortex.

Basic screening usually consists of evaluating light-touch sensation in all extremities and comparing arms and legs for symmetry of sensation.

When cranial nerves function normally

Olfactory (CN I)
• Patient can identify a variety of smells.

Optic (CN II)
• Patient has visual acuity and full visual fields.
• Fundoscopic examination reveals no pathology.

Oculomotor (CN III), trochlear (CN IV), and abducens (CN VI)
• Patient follows up to six cardinal positions of gaze.
• Pupils are unremarkable.
• Patient exhibits no nystagmus and no ptosis.

Trigeminal (CN V)
• Patient clenches his teeth with firm bilateral pressure.
• Patient has no lateral jaw deviation with the mouth open.
• Patient feels a cotton wisp touched to the forehead, cheek, and chin.
• Patient differentiates sharp and dull sensations on the face.
• Patient blinks when cotton is touched to each cornea.

Facial (CN VII)
• Patient has facial symmetry.

• Patient can raise the eyebrows symmetrically and grimace.
• Patient can shut eyes tightly.
• Patient can identify sweet and sour on the anterior tongue.

Acoustic (CN VIII)
• Patient can hear a whisper at 1′ to 2′ (0.3 to 0.6 m).
• Patient can hear a watch tick at 1″ to 2″ (2.5 to 5 cm).
(The patient does not lateralize the Weber test.)
• Patient can hear AC better than BC in the Rinne test.

Glossopharyngeal (CN IX) and vagus (CN X)
• Patient speaks and swallows without hoarseness.
• The palate and uvula rise symmetrically when the patient says "ah."
• Patient has a bilateral gag reflex.

Spinal accessory (CN XI)
• Patient demonstrates resistance to head turning and can shrug against resistance.

Hypoglossal (CN XII)
• Patient can stick his tongue out, move it from side to side, and push it strongly against resistance.

Because the sensory system becomes fatigued with repeated stimulation, complete sensory system testing in all dermatomes tends to give unreliable results. A few screening procedures usually can reveal any dysfunctions.

Before beginning, ask the patient about any areas of numbness or unusual sensations. Such areas require special attention. Compare sensations on both sides of the patient's body in the upper arm, back of the hand, thigh, lower leg, and top of the foot. Be alert for complaints of numbness, tingling, or unusual sensations that accompany the tactile stimulus. Also note

Evaluating brain stem function

In an unconscious patient, you can assess brain stem function by testing for the oculocephalic (doll's eyes) reflex and the oculovestibular reflex. Most likely, you'll assist a doctor in performing these techniques. If the patient has a cervical spine injury, expect to use the oculovestibular reflex test as an alternative. The oculovestibular reflex test may also be used to determine the status of the vestibular portion of CN VIII.

Oculocephalic reflex

Before beginning, examine the patient's cervical spine. *Don't perform this procedure if you suspect a cervical spine injury.*

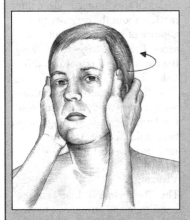

• If the patient has no cervical spine injury, place both hands on either side of his head and use your thumbs to hold open his eyelids gently.
• While watching the patient's eyes, briskly rotate his head from side to side, or briskly flex and extend his neck.
• Observe how the patient's eyes move in relation to head movement. In a normal response, which indicates an intact brain stem, the eyes appear to move opposite to the movement of the head. For example, if the neck flexes, the eyes appear to look upward. If the neck extends, the eyes gaze downward.

In an abnormal (doll's eyes) response, the eyes appear to move passively in the same direction as the head, indicating the absence of an oculocephalic reflex. This suggests a deep coma or severe brain stem damage at the level of the pons or midbrain.

Oculovestibular reflex

To assess the oculovestibular reflex, the doctor must first determine that the patient has an intact tympanic membrane and a clear external ear canal.

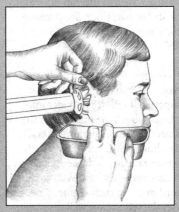

• Elevate the head of the bed 30 degrees.

(continued)

Evaluating brain stem function (continued)

• Using a large syringe with a small catheter on the tip, slowly irrigate the external auditory canal with 20 to 200 ml of cold water or ice water.
• During irrigation, watch the patient's eye movements. In a patient with an intact oculovestibular reflex, the eyes will show nystagmus and will dart away from the stimulat-ed ear. In a normal, conscious individual, as little as 10 ml of ice water will produce such a response and may also cause nausea. In a comatose patient with an intact brain stem, the eyes tonically deviate toward the stimulated ear. Absence of eye movement suggests a brain stem lesion.

the degree of stimulation required to evoke a response. A light, brief touch should be sufficient.

If a localized deficit appears, or if the patient complains of localized numbness or an unpleasant sensation (dysesthesia), perform a complete sensory assessment. Also perform a complete neurologic assessment for a patient with motor or reflex abnormalities or trophic skin changes, such as ulceration, atrophy, or absent sweating. (See *Assessing the sensory system,* pages 249 and 250.)

Reflexes

Assessment of deep tendon and superficial reflexes provides information about the integrity of the sensory receptor organ and evaluates how well afferent nerves relay sensory messages to the spinal cord. It also evaluates how well the spinal cord or brain stem segment mediates the reflex, how well the lower motor neurons transmit messages to the muscles, and how well the muscles respond to the motor message. It's usually reserved for a complete neurologic assessment.

You'll also indirectly glean information about the presence or absence of inhibiting brain messages. These messages travel along the corticospinal tract to modify reflex strength.

Reflexes fall into one of three groups: deep tendon reflexes, superficial reflexes, and pathologic superficial reflexes. (See *Assessing the reflexes,* pages 251 to 253.)

Vital signs

The CNS, primarily by way of the brain stem and autonomic nervous system, controls the body's vital functions: heart rate and rhythm; respiratory rate, depth, and pattern; blood pressure; and body temperature. Note that changes in vital signs—temperature, pulse rate, respiration, and blood pressure—aren't usually early indicators of CNS deterioration.

Temperature. Damage to the hypothalamus or upper brain stem can impair the body's ability to maintain a constant temperature, resulting in profound hypothermia (temperature below 94° F [34.4 ° C]) or

Assessing cerebellar function

To evaluate cerebellar function, you'll test the patient's balance and coordination while he performs heel-to-toe walking, the Romberg test, point-to-point movements, and rapid skilled movements.

Heel-to-toe walking

Ask the patient to walk heel to toe and observe his balance. Although he may be slightly unsteady, he should be able to maintain his balance while walking forward.

on either side of him so that you can support him if he sways to one side. Note whether he loses his balance or sways. If he falls to one side, the Romberg test is positive.

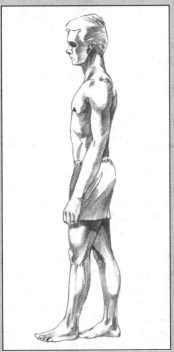

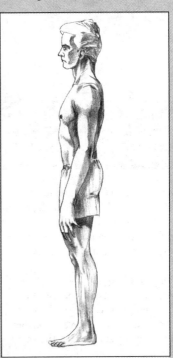

Romberg test

Ask the patient to stand with his feet together, his eyes open, and his arms at his side. Observe his balance, and then ask him to close his eyes. Hold your outstretched arms

Point-to-point movements

Have the patient sit about 2′ (0.6 m) away from you. Hold your index finger up, and ask him to touch the tip of his index finger to the tip of yours and then to touch his nose. Next,

(continued)

Assessing cerebellar function *(continued)*

move your finger to another position and ask him to repeat the maneuver. Have him increase his speed gradually as you repeat the test. Then test his other hand.

ger and then to each of his remaining fingers. Then instruct him to increase his speed. Observe his movements for smoothness and accuracy. Repeat the test on his left hand.

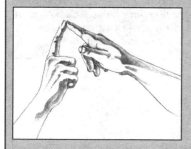

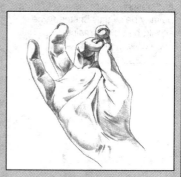

Rapid skilled movements
Ask the patient to touch the thumb of his right hand to his right index fin-

---

hyperthermia (temperature above 106° F [41.1° C]). Such damage can result from petechial hemorrhages in the hypothalamus or brain stem, trauma, or destructive lesions.

Pulse rate. Because the autonomic nervous system controls heart rate and rhythm, pressure on the brain stem and cranial nerves slows the pulse rate by stimulating the vagus nerve.

Bradycardia occurs in the later stages of increasing ICP and usually accompanies a rising systolic blood pressure and widening pulse pressure. The patient commonly has a bounding pulse. Cervical spinal cord injuries can also cause bradycardia.

In a patient with acutely increased ICP or a brain injury,

tachycardia signals decompensation (a condition in which the body has exhausted its compensatory measures for managing ICP), which rapidly leads to death.

Respiration. Respiratory centers in the medulla and pons control the rate, depth, and pattern of respiration. Neurologic dysfunction, particularly when it involves the brain stem or both cerebral hemispheres, commonly alters respirations. Assessment of respiration provides valuable information about a CNS lesion's site and severity.

One of the first signs of a cerebral or upper brain stem disorder is Cheyne-Stokes respiration. However, it may occur normally in an elderly patient during sleep, proba-

Assessing the sensory system

Further evaluate the patient's sensory function by assessing for two-point discrimination, temperature sensation, sense of position (proprioception), and point localization. Also assess number identification, superficial pain, response to vibration, extinction, and the patient's ability to recognize objects by the sense of touch (stereognosis). Perform all sensory testing with the patient's eyes closed.

Two-point discrimination

Alternately touch one or two sharp objects to the patient's skin. First assess whether he can feel one or two points; then assess the smallest distance between the two points at which he can still discriminate the presence of two points. Acuity varies in different body areas. On the finger pads, an area rich in tactile sensory receptors, the average distance necessary for two-point discrimination is less than 5 mm (less than 1/4"). On the back, however, two-point discrimination requires a much wider distance.

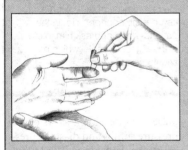

Temperature sensation

First fill two test tubes with water, one hot and the other cold. Alternately touch the patient's skin with the hot and cold tubes, and ask him to differentiate between them. Test and compare distal and proximal portions of all extremities.

Sense of position

Grasp the sides of the patient's great toe between your thumb and forefinger. Move the toe upward or downward, asking the patient to describe the position. Repeat on the other foot, and then perform the same technique on the patient's fingers.

If the patient exhibits an impaired sense of position, proceed to the next joint on the extremity and repeat the procedure. On the leg, progress from the ankle to the knee; on the arm, from the wrist to the elbow.

Point localization

Have the patient close both eyes while you briefly touch a point on his skin. Ask him to open his eyes and point to the place just touched. He should be able to identify the spot.

Number identification

Trace a number on the patient's palm with an object such as the blunt end of a pencil. He should be able to identify the number.

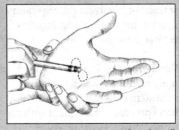

(continued)

Assessing the sensory system *(continued)*

Superficial pain
Lightly touch—but don't puncture—the patient's skin using a sharp object such as a sterile needle. Occasionally alternate sharp and blunt ends. (Remember to discard the sharp object safely after use, and never use the same object on another patient.)

Ask the patient to identify the sensation as sharp or dull. Test and compare the distal and proximal portions of all extremities. If he displays abnormal pain sensation, test for temperature sensation.

Response to vibration
Tap a low-pitched tuning fork (preferably 128 cycles/second) on the heel of your hand, then place the base of the tuning fork firmly on an interphalangeal joint (any of the patient's fingers or his great toe).

Ask the patient to describe the sensation, differentiating between pressure and vibration, and then to state when the feeling stops. Proceed from distal to proximal areas.

If the patient has intact distal vibration sensation, further testing is unnecessary. However, if he suffers from an absence of distal vibration sensation, test the next most proximal bony prominence. When assessing the leg, progress from the medial malleolus to the patella, to the anterior superior iliac spine, to the spinous process of the vertebra. For the arm, progress from the wrist to the elbow to the shoulder.

Extinction
Touch two corresponding parts on the patient (such as the forearms just above the wrist) simultaneously. Ask him to describe the location of the touch. He should sense the touch in both locations.

Stereognosis
Place a familiar object, such as a key, pencil, or paper clip, in the patient's hand and ask him to identify the object by feel—which he should be able to do.

---

bly the result of generalized brain atrophy from aging.

Spinal cord damage above C7 weakens or paralyzes the respiratory muscles, causing varying degrees of respiratory impairment.

Blood pressure. Pressor receptors in the medulla oblongata of the brain stem constantly monitor blood pressure. In a patient with no history of hypertension, rising systolic blood pressure may signal rising ICP. If ICP continues to rise,

pulse pressure widens as systolic pressure climbs and diastolic pressure remains stable or falls. In the late stages of acutely elevated ICP, blood pressure plummets as cerebral perfusion fails, resulting in the patient's death.

Although rare, hypotension accompanying a brain injury is an ominous sign. In addition, cervical spinal cord injuries may interrupt sympathetic nervous system pathways, causing peripheral vasodilation and hypotension.

Assessing the reflexes

Expect to use different procedures for testing each deep tendon, superficial, and pathologic superficial reflex. Reflex assessment helps evaluate the intactness of specific cervical (C), thoracic (T), lumbar (L), or sacral (S) spinal segments. These segments are listed parenthetically after the appropriate reflex.

Deep tendon reflexes

The deep tendon reflexes include the patient's biceps, triceps, brachioradialis, quadriceps, and Achilles reflexes.

Biceps reflex (C5, C6). Have the patient partially flex one arm at the elbow with the palm facing down. Place your thumb or finger over the biceps tendon. Then tap lightly over your finger with the reflex hammer. An impulse from the tapping should travel to the biceps tendon and cause brisk elbow flexion that's visible and palpable.

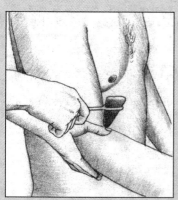

Triceps reflex (C7, C8). Have the patient partially flex one arm at the elbow with the palm facing the body. Support the arm and pull it slightly across the patient's chest. Using a direct blow with the reflex hammer, tap the triceps tendon at its insertion (about 1″ to 2″ [2.5 to 5 cm] above the elbow on the olecranon process of the ulnar bone). Normally, this action causes brisk extension of the elbow with visible and palpable contraction of the triceps muscle.

Brachioradialis (supinator) reflex (C5, C6). Position the patient with one arm flexed at the elbow, palm down, and resting in the lap or, if he's lying down, against the abdomen. Then tap the styloid process of the radius with the reflex hammer, about 1″ to 2″ above the wrist. Normally, this action causes elbow flexion, forearm supination, and finger and hand flexion.

Quadriceps (knee-jerk or patellar) reflex (L2, L3, L4). Seat the patient with one knee flexed and the lower leg dangling over the side of the examination table, or place him in the supine position. (For the supine patient, place your hand under his knee, slightly raising and flexing it.) Then tap the patellar tendon with the reflex hammer. The patient's knee should extend and the quadriceps should contract.

Achilles (ankle-jerk) reflex (S1, S2). First, position the patient with his knee bent and his ankle dorsiflexed. For best results, have him sit with his legs dangling over the side of the examination table. Then tap the

(continued)

Assessing the reflexes *(continued)*

Achilles tendon, which should cause plantar flexion followed by muscle relaxation.

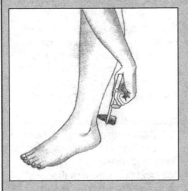

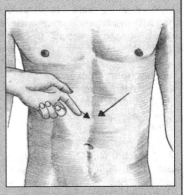

Superficial reflexes

The superficial reflexes include the pharyngeal, abdominal, and cremasteric reflexes as well as the anal and bulbocavernous reflexes. Assess the last two reflexes, known as the perineal reflexes, only in patients with suspected sacral spinal cord or sacral spinal nerve disorders.

Pharyngeal reflex (CN IX, CN X). Have the patient open his mouth wide. Then touch the posterior wall of the pharynx with a tongue blade. Normally, this will cause the patient to gag.

Abdominal reflex (T8, T9, T10). Use a fingernail or the tip of the handle of the reflex hammer to stroke one side, and then the opposite side, of the patient's abdomen above the umbilicus. Repeat on the lower abdomen. Normally, the abdominal muscles contract and the umbilicus deviates toward the stimulated side.

Cremasteric reflex (L1, L2). In a male patient, use a tongue blade to scratch the inner aspect of each thigh gently. This should cause elevation of the testicles.

Anal reflex (S3, S4, S5). Gently scratch the skin at the side of the anus with a blunt instrument, such as a tongue blade or a gloved finger. Look for puckering of the anus, a normal response.

Bulbocavernous reflex (S3, S4). In a male patient, apply direct pressure over the bulbocavernous muscle behind the scrotum and gently pinch the foreskin or glans. This action should cause the bulbocavernous muscle to contract.

Pathologic superficial reflexes

The pathologic superficial reflexes include the grasp, sucking, snout, and Babinski's reflexes. They indicate central nervous system damage.

Assessing the reflexes (continued)

Grasp reflex. Stimulate the palm of the patient's hand with your fingers. (Because a lack of inhibition by the brain can cause the patient to squeeze tightly, avoid finger injury or pain by crossing your middle and index fingers before placing them in his palm.) In a positive grasp reflex, the patient's hand will grasp yours upon stimulation, indicating frontal lobe damage, bilateral thalamic degeneration, or cerebral degeneration or atrophy.

Sucking reflex. Stimulate the patient's lips with a mouth swab. A

sucking movement on stimulation can indicate cerebral degeneration.

Snout reflex. Gently percuss the oral area with your fingers. This action may make the patient's lips pucker, indicating cerebral degeneration or late-stage dementia.

Babinski's reflex. Stroke the lateral aspect of the sole of the patient's foot. A positive Babinski reflex occurs when the toes dorsiflex and fan out, indicating upper motor neuron disease.

DIAGNOSTIC TESTS

Studies used in evaluating the nervous system include laboratory tests, radiographic and angiographic studies, scans, and electrophysiologic studies.

Keep in mind that studies that seem routine to you may frighten your patient. Because anxiety may affect test results, carefully prepare him for all procedures. (See *Diagnostic tests for neurologic disorders,* pages 254 to 258.)

NURSING DIAGNOSES

When caring for patients with neurologic disorders, you'll find that certain nursing diagnoses are commonly used. These diagnoses appear below, along with appropriate nursing interventions and rationales. (Rationales appear in italic type.)

Sensory/perceptual alteration

Related to sensory deprivation, sensory/perceptual alteration is commonly seen in elderly patients who are hospitalized or institutionalized and in patients who are on isolation precautions. It may also be used for patients with cerebrovascular accident (CVA), head injury, or organic brain syndrome.

Expected outcomes
• Patient openly expresses feelings regarding vision (hearing) loss.
• Patient maintains orientation to person, place, and time.
• Patient regains visual (auditory) functioning to the extent possible.
• Patient shows interest in external environment.

(Text continues on page 258.)

Diagnostic tests for neurologic disorders

Test	Purpose	Nursing considerations
Skull X-rays	To help detect fractures, bony tumors or unusual calcifications, pineal displacement, skull or sella turcica erosion, or vascular abnormalities	• Explain the procedure. Tell the patient that his head will be immobilized and several X-rays of his skull will be taken from various angles. • Assure the patient that he won't experience pain during the procedure. • This test requires no restrictions on food or fluid.
Spinal X-rays	To help detect spinal fracture, displacement, and subluxation; destructive lesions; arthritic changes or spondylolisthesis; structural abnormalities; and congenital abnormalities	• Explain the procedure and that the X-rays won't hurt. • Advise the patient that he'll be placed in various positions for the X-ray films. • This test requires no food or fluid restrictions. • Inform him that he must remain as still as possible and hold his breath when required.
Cerebral angiography	To help detect stenosis or occlusion associated with thrombi or spasms; help identify aneurysms and arteriovenous malformations; locate vessel displacement associated with tumors, abscesses, cerebral edema, hematoma, or herniation; and help assess collateral circulation	• Explain the procedure. • Restrict food and fluid for 8 to 10 hours before the test. • Note any allergies to iodine or shellfish. • Explain that following the dye injection the patient may feel warm or flushed. • After the test, keep him on bed rest, as ordered. Monitor vital signs and neurologic status for 24 hours. • Observe for bleeding, check distal pulses, and apply a pressure bandage to the puncture site. • Observe the puncture site for signs of extravasation and apply an ice bag to ease the discomfort and swelling. • Apply pressure to the site if bleeding occurs.
Digital subtraction angiography	To help visualize extracranial and intracranial cerebral blood flow; to detect and evaluate cere-	• Explain the procedure. • Ask about allergies to iodine or shellfish. • Restrict food for 4 hours before the test.

Diagnostic tests for neurologic disorders *(continued)*

Test	Purpose	Nursing considerations
Digital subtraction angiography *(continued)*	brovascular abnormalities	• Instruct the patient that he may feel warm or flushed when the contrast medium is injected. • Caution him to lie still on the X-ray table. • After the test, check the venipuncture site for signs of extravasation, such as redness or swelling. If bleeding occurs, apply firm pressure to the puncture site.
Myelography	To help locate a spinal lesion, a ruptured disk, spinal stenosis, or an abscess through a combination of fluoroscopy and radiography	• Explain the procedure. • Restrict food and fluid for 8 hours before the test. • Check for allergies to iodine or shellfish. • Instruct the patient that he may feel a warm or flush sensation when the contrast dye is injected. • Explain that he may feel some pain from the position he'll assume and from the needle insertion. • After the test, the patient will be positioned flat or with his head slightly elevated for 24 hours depending on the contrast medium used. • Monitor vital signs and neurologic status closely for the first 24 hours. • For several days following the test, observe the patient for signs and symptoms of meningeal irritation: headache, stiff neck, pain on hip flexion, nausea and vomiting, fever, or seizures.
Computed tomography	To help detect brain contusion, brain calcifications, cerebral atrophy, hydrocephalus, inflammation, space-occupying lesions, and vascular changes	• Explain the procedure. • Restrict food and fluids for 4 hours before the test. • Instruct the patient that he may feel a flushed or warm sensation when the contrast medium is injected. • Explain that the scanner will encircle him for 10 to 30 minutes and he must lie still.

(continued)

Diagnostic tests for neurologic disorders (continued)

Test	Purpose	Nursing considerations
Computed tomography (continued)		• After the test, tell the patient that he may resume his usual activities and diet.
Brain scan	To locate and show the size of cerebral lesions; can't specify if the lesion is caused by a tumor, cerebral edema, an infarction, a hematoma, or an abscess	• Explain the procedure. • Withhold medications, such as antihypertensives, vasoconstrictors, and vasodilators, for 24 hours before the test. • Tell the patient that he'll be asked to change positions several times during the test and to keep his hands at his sides.
Magnetic resonance imaging	To detect structural and biochemical abnormalities associated with such conditions as transient ischemic attacks (TIAs), tumors, multiple sclerosis (MS); cerebral edema, and hydrocephalus	• Explain the procedure and that the test will take $1\frac{1}{2}$ hours. • Instruct the patient to remove all jewelry. Emphasize that no metal is permitted in the test room. • Tell him that he'll be asked to lie on a table that slides into an 8' long tunnel. • Instruct him that he should breathe normally but not talk or move during the test. • Tell him that the machinery will be noisy. • Encourage him to relax.
Positron emission tomography	To help detect cerebral dysfunction associated with tumors, seizures, TIAs, head trauma, Alzheimer's disease, Parkinson's disease, or MS	• Explain the procedure and that it exposes the patient to a low level of radiation. • If an I.V. tracer is used, the patient will have an I.V. started. • After the test, observe the venipuncture site for bleeding or redness.
SPECT scan	To measure blood perfusion of brain tissue; useful in demonstrating cerebral blood flow in focal and diffuse cerebral disorders, dementia, trauma, or cerebrovascular disease	• Explain the procedure. • Instruct the patient that he will lie on a stretcher and he must lie still. • Advise him he will undergo venipuncture for the isotope injection and that radiation is minimal. • After the test, observe the venipuncture site for bleeding and redness.

Diagnostic tests for neurologic disorders *(continued)*

Test	Purpose	Nursing considerations
Electroen-cephalogra-phy	To help identify seizure disorders, head injury, intracra-nial lesions, TIAs, cerebrovascular accidents, or brain death	• Explain the procedure and that elec-trodes will be attached to the head and neck. • Have patient wash hair 1 to 2 days before the test. • Warn him that he must remain still throughout the test. • After the test, the electrodes will be removed. The patient may wash his hair and resume usual activities.
Electromyog-raphy	To help distinguish lower motor neuron disorders from mus-cle disorders and help evaluate neuro-muscular disorders	• Explain the procedure and that it takes 1 hour. • Instruct the patient that he may feel some discomfort when the doctor inserts a needle attached to an elec-trode into the muscle. • Tell the patient that he must remain still except when asked to contract or relax a muscle. • After the test, he may resume his usual activities.
Evoked poten-tial studies	To help detect sub-clinical lesions, such as tumors of CN VIII; to help diagnose blindness in infants	• Explain the procedure and tell the patient to wash his hair 1 to 2 days before the test. • Instruct him that he will need to be still during the test. • Tell him that electrodes will be applied to his head and neck and he will be asked to perform various activities such as gazing at a checkerboard pattern. • Advise him that he may also have electrodes placed on an arm and leg and be asked to respond to a tapping sensation. • After the test, the electrodes will be removed. He may wash his hair and resume his usual activites.
Lumbar punc-ture	To obtain a speci-men of cerebro-spinal fluid (CSF); to aid in diagnosis of meningitis, hemor-	• Explain the procedure. • Tell the patient he'll be positioned on the edge of the bed with his knees drawn to chest and chin resting on chest.

(continued)

Diagnostic tests for neurologic disorders *(continued)*

Test	Purpose	Nursing considerations
Lumbar puncture *(continued)*	rhage, tumors, and brain abscesses; and to measure CSF pressure	• Tell him to report any tingling or sharp pain during injection of the local anesthetic. • Advise him to be still. • After the test, he must lie flat for 4 to 24 hours. He may turn from side to side. • Encourage him to increase fluid for the rest of the day.

Nursing interventions and rationales

• Assist or encourage the patient to use glasses, a hearing aid, or other adaptive devices to *help reduce sensory deprivation.*

• Reorient the patient to reality by calling him by name and repeatedly telling him your name. Give background information (time, place, date) throughout the day, and orient him to environment, including sights and sounds. Use large signs as visual cues. If the patient is ambulatory and disoriented, post his photo on the door. *These measures help reduce the patient's sensory deprivation.*

• Arrange the environment to offset deficits. For instance, place the patient in a room with a good view of his surroundings. Encourage family members to bring in personal articles, such as books, cards, and photos. Keep articles in the same place to promote a sense of identity. Use such safety precautions as a night-light when needed. *These measures reduce sensory deprivation.*

• Communicate the patient's response level to his family or friends and to the staff. Record this on the plan of care and update as needed. *The patient's sensory deprivation level can be evaluated by his response to stimuli.*

• Talk to the patient while providing care. Encourage his family or friends to discuss past and present events with him. Arrange to be with the patient at predetermined times during the day to avoid isolation. *Verbal stimuli can improve the patient's orientation to reality.*

• Hold the patient's hand when talking. Discuss interests with the patient and his family. Obtain needed items such as talking books. *Sensory stimuli help reduce the patient's sensory deprivation.*

• Assist the patient and his family in planning short trips outside the health care facility. Educate them about mobility, toileting, feeding, suctioning, and other measures. *Trips help reduce the patient's sensory deprivation.*

Chronic pain

Related to neurologic alteration, chronic pain may occur in patients with migraine or vascular headaches, reflex sympathetic dystrophy, meningitis, trigeminal neuralgia, multiple sclerosis (MS), or herniated disk.

Expected outcomes
- Patient expresses feelings of pain.
- Patient identifies factors that affect occurrence or severity of pain.
- Patient develops pain management program that includes activity and rest, exercise, and medication regimen.
- Patient demonstrates relaxation techniques and performs them at least twice daily.

Nursing interventions and rationales
- Assess the patient's pain symptoms, physical complaints, and activities of daily living (ADLs). Administer analgesics as prescribed. Monitor and record the effectiveness and adverse effects of the medication. (Keep in mind that pain behavior and pain talk may be inconsistent.) *Correlating the patient's pain behavior with activities, time of day, and visits may be useful in modifying tasks.*
- Teach the patient how to use relaxation techniques to relieve pain *as an adjunct to medications and to foster independence.*
- Teach the patient and his family such techniques as massage, use of ice, or exercise *to relieve pain and foster independence.*

- Work closely with staff members and the patient's family *to achieve pain management goals and maximize the patient's cooperation.*
- Use behavior modification—For example, spend time with the patient only if your conversation doesn't include remarks about his pain. Use contingency rewards for refraining from talking about pain. *Such measures help the patient refocus on other matters.*
- Encourage self-care activities. Develop a schedule. *This helps the patient gain a sense of control and reduces dependence on caregivers and society.*
- Establish a specific time to talk with the patient about pain and its psychological and emotional effects *to establish a trusting, supportive relationship encompassing the patient's biopsychosocial, sexual, and financial concerns.*

Impaired physical mobility

Related to neurologic alteration, impaired physical mobility may occur in amyotrophic lateral sclerosis (ALS), cerebral palsy, CVA, MS, muscular dystrophy, myasthenia gravis, Parkinson's disease, poliomyelitis, or spinal cord injury.

Expected outcomes
- Patient maintains muscle strength and joint ROM.
- Patient shows no evidence of complications, such as contractures, venous stasis, thrombus formation, or skin breakdown.
- Patient achieves highest level of mobility.

• Patient, family member, or friend carries out mobility regimen.

Nursing interventions and rationales

• Perform ROM exercises, unless contraindicated, at least once every shift. Progress from passive to active, as tolerated. *This prevents joint contractures and muscular atrophy.*

• Turn and position the patient every 2 hours. Establish a turning schedule for dependent patients; post this schedule at bedside and monitor frequency of turning. *This prevents skin breakdown by relieving pressure.*

• Place joints in functional positions, use a trochanter roll along the thigh, abduct the thighs, use high-top sneakers, and put a small pillow under the patient's head. *These measures maintain joints in a functional position and prevent musculoskeletal deformities.*

• Identify the patient's level of functioning using a functional mobility scale. Communicate the patient's skill level to all staff members *to provide continuity and preserve an identified level of independence.*

• Encourage independence in mobility by assisting the patient in using a trapeze and side rails, in using his unaffected leg to move the affected leg, and in performing self-care activities. *This increases muscle tone and improves the patient's self-esteem.*

• Place items within reach of the patient's unaffected arm if one-sided weakness or paralysis is present *to promote the patient's independence.*

• Monitor and record daily any evidence of immobility complications (such as contractures, venous stasis, thrombus, pneumonia, or urinary tract infection [UTI]). *Patients with a history of neuromuscular disorders or dysfunctions may be more prone to develop complications.*

• Provide progressive mobilization to the limits of the patient's condition (bed mobility to chair mobility to ambulation) *to maintain muscle tone and prevent complications of immobility.*

• Refer the patient to a physical therapist for development of a mobility regimen *to restore functioning.*

• Encourage attendance at physical therapy sessions and support activities on the unit by using the same equipment and technique. Request written mobility plans and use these as references. *All members of the health care team should reinforce learned skills in the same manner.*

• Instruct the patient and his caregivers in ROM exercises, transfers, skin inspection, and the mobility regimen *to help prepare the patient for discharge.*

• Demonstrate the mobility regimen and note the date. Have the patient and his caregivers do a return demonstration and note the date. *This ensures continuity of care and correct completion.*

• Help identify resources to carry out the mobility regimen, such as the Stroke Club International, the United Cerebral Palsy Associations, and the National Multiple Sclerosis

Society. *This helps provide a comprehensive approach to rehabilitation.*

Impaired swallowing

Related to neuromuscular impairment, impaired swallowing may occur in CVA, head injury, maxillofacial trauma, or tracheostomy.

Expected outcomes

• Patient shows no evidence of aspiration pneumonia.
• Patient achieves adequate nutritional intake.
• Patient maintains weight.
• Patient maintains oral hygiene.

Nursing interventions and rationales

• Elevate the head of the bed 90 degrees during mealtimes and for 30 minutes after completion of the meal *to decrease the risk of aspiration.*
• Position the patient on his side when recumbent *to reduce the risk of aspiration.*
• Keep a suction apparatus at bedside; observe and report instances of cyanosis, dyspnea, or choking. *These symptoms indicate there is material in the patient's lungs.*
• Monitor intake and output and daily weight until the patient is stabilized. Establish an intake goal—for example, "patient consumes ____ml of fluid and ____% of solid food." Record and report any deviation from this. *Evaluating calorie and protein intake daily allows any necessary modifications to begin quickly.*
• Consult with the dietitian to modify the patient's diet, and conduct a calorie count as needed *to establish nutritional requirements.*
• Consult with the dysphagia rehabilitation team, if available, *to obtain expert advice.*
• Provide mouth care three times daily *to promote the patient's comfort and enhance his appetite.*
• Keep the oral mucous membranes moist with frequent rinses; use a bulb syringe or suction, if necessary, *to promote comfort.*
• Lubricate the patient's lips *to prevent cracking and blisters.*
• Encourage him to wear properly fitted dentures *to enhance his chewing ability.*
• Remove soiled equipment, control smells, and provide a quiet atmosphere for eating. *A pleasant atmosphere stimulates appetite; food aroma stimulates salivation.*
• Instruct the patient and his caregivers in positioning, dietary requirements, specific feeding techniques including facial exercises (for example, whistling), using a short straw to provide sensory stimulation to the lips, tipping the head forward to decrease aspiration, applying pressure above the lip to stimulate mouth closure and the swallowing reflex, and checking the oral cavity frequently for food particles (remove if present). *These measures allow the patient to take an active role in maintaining health.*

Bowel incontinence

Related to neuromuscular involvement, bowel incontinence may occur in ALS, brain or spinal cord tumor, CVA, diabetic neuropathy, Guillain-Barré syndrome, Huntington's disease, MS, myasthenia gravis, or spinal cord injury.

Expected outcomes
• Patient establishes and maintains a regular pattern of bowel care.
• Patient states an understanding of bowel care routine.
• Patient and caregivers demonstrate increasing skill in carrying out bowel care routine independently.
• Patient or caregiver states an understanding of the need to regulate food or fluids that cause constipation or diarrhea.

Nursing interventions and rationales
If the patient has an upper motor neuron lesion with an intact anal reflex, take the following steps.
• Establish a regular pattern for bowel care. For example, after breakfast every other day, maintain the patient in an upright position after inserting a suppository and allow $1/2$ hour for the suppository to melt and the maximum reflex response to occur. *A regular pattern encourages adaptation and routine physiologic function.*
• Discuss and demonstrate bowel care with the patient and his caregivers and observe return demonstration *to check skills and establish a therapeutic relationship.*
• Establish a date when the patient or caregivers will perform the bowel routine independently, with supportive assistance, *to reassure the patient of dependable care.*
• Instruct the patient and his family on the need to regulate foods and

fluids that cause diarrhea or constipation *to encourage good nutritional habits.*
• Maintain a dietary intake diary *to identify irritating foods;* instruct the patient to avoid these *to prevent painful flatulence.*
• Obtain an order allowing modified bowel preparations for tests and procedures *to avoid interrupting the patient's routine and to encourage regular bowel function.*
• Encourage the patient to use protective padding under his clothing, changing it as necessary *to prevent odor, skin breakdown, or embarrassment.*

DISORDERS

This section discusses the causes, assessment findings, nursing interventions, and evaluation criteria for the most common neurologic disorders. These disorders include paroxysmal disorders, brain and spinal cord disorders, CNS infections, degenerative disorders, and cranial nerve disorders.

Paroxysmal disorders
Paroxysmal disorders include headaches and epilepsy.

Headache
About 90% of the time, headaches result from muscle contraction or vascular abnormalities. Occasionally, though, headaches indicate an underlying intracranial, systemic, or psychological disorder.

Throbbing, vascular headaches called migraine headaches affect up to 10% of Americans. They have a strong familial incidence. (See *Clinical features of migraine headaches*, page 264.)

Causes. Most chronic headaches result from tension, or muscle contraction, which may stem from emotional stress, fatigue, menstruation, or environmental stimuli (such as noise, crowds, and bright lights). Other possible causes include glaucoma; inflammation of the eyes or of the nasal or paranasal sinuses mucosa; diseases of the scalp, teeth, extracranial arteries, or external or middle ear; and muscle spasms of the face, neck, or shoulders. Headaches may also result from vasodilators (such as nitrates, alcohol, or histamine), systemic disease, hypoxia, hypertension, head trauma or tumor, intracranial bleeding, abscess, or aneurysm. The cause of migraine headache remains unknown.

Headache pain may emanate from the pain-sensitive structures of the skin, scalp, muscles, arteries, or veins; from cranial nerves V, VII, IX, and X; and from cervical nerves C1, C2, and C3.

Assessment findings. Initially, migraine headache usually produces unilateral pulsating pain, which later becomes more generalized. A scintillating scotoma, hemianopsia, unilateral paresthesias, or a speech disorder may precede the headache. The patient may experience irritability, anorexia, nausea, vomiting, and photophobia.

Both muscle contraction and traction-inflammatory vascular headaches produce a dull, persistent ache, tender spots on the head and neck, and a feeling of tightness around the head with a characteristic "hatband" distribution. The patient commonly experiences severe, unrelenting pain. If caused by intracranial bleeding, these headaches may result in neurologic deficits, such as paresthesias and muscle weakness; narcotics fail to relieve pain in these cases. The patient with a headache caused by a tumor experiences the severest pain upon awakening.

Question the patient about the following items:
• duration and location of the headache
• time of day the headache usually begins
• nature of the pain (intermittent or throbbing)
• concurrence with other symptoms such as blurred vision
• precipitating factors, such as tension, menstruation, loud noises, menopause, or alcohol use
• medications being taken such as oral contraceptives
• incidence of prolonged fasting.

Examination of the head and neck includes percussion, auscultation for bruits, inspection for signs of infection, and palpation for defects, crepitus, or tender spots (especially after trauma). The patient may also undergo a complete neurologic examination, assessment for other systemic diseases such as hypertension, and a psychosocial evaluation if such factors are suspected.

Clinical features of migraine headaches

Migraine form	Signs and symptoms
Common migraine *(most prevalent, 85%)* Usually occurs on weekends and holidays	• Prodromal signs and symptoms (fatigue, nausea and vomiting, and fluid imbalance), which precede headache by about a day • Sensitivity to light and noise (most prominent feature) • Headache pain (unilateral or bilateral, aching or throbbing) lasting longer than in classic migraine
Classic migraine *(incidence 10%)* Usually occurs in compulsive personalities and within families	• Prodromal signs and symptoms, including visual disturbances, such as zigzag lines and bright lights (most common); sensory disturbances (tingling of face, lips, and hands); or motor disturbances (staggering gait) • Recurrent headaches
Hemiplegic and ophthalmoplegic migraine *(rare)* Usually occurs in young adults	• Severe, unilateral pain • Extraocular muscle palsies (involving third cranial nerve [CN]) and ptosis • With repeated headaches, possible permanent third CN injury • In hemiplegic migraine, neurologic deficits (hemiparesis, hemiplegia) that may persist after headache subsides
Basilar artery migraine Occurs in young women before their menstrual periods	• Prodromal signs and symptoms, which usually include partial vision loss followed by vertigo, ataxia, dysarthria, tinnitus and, sometimes, tingling of fingers and toes, lasting from several minutes to almost an hour • Headache pain, severe occipital throbbing, vomiting

Diagnostic tests. The doctor may order skull X-rays (including cervical spine and sinus), electroencephalogram (EEG), computed tomography (CT) scan, and lumbar puncture.

Treatment. Depending on the type of headache, analgesics—ranging from aspirin to codeine or meperidine—may provide symptomatic relief. A tranquilizer such as diazepam may help during acute attacks. Other measures include identification and elimination of causative factors and, possibly, psychotherapy for headaches caused by emotional stress. Chronic tension headaches may also require muscle relaxants. (See *Reflexotherapy*, page 266.)

For migraine headache, ergotamine alone or with caffeine provides the most effective treatment. These drugs and others, such as metoclopramide or naproxen, work best when taken early in the course of an attack. If nausea and vomiting make oral administration impossible, these drugs may be given as rectal suppositories. Drugs that can help prevent migraine headache include propranolol and calcium channel blockers, such as verapamil and diltiazem.

Nursing interventions. The patient with migraine usually needs to be hospitalized only if nausea and vomiting are severe enough to induce dehydration and possible shock.

Patient education. You'll need to teach the patient to avoid exacerbating factors. Use his history as a guide. Advise him to lie down in a dark, quiet room during an attack and to place ice packs on his forehead or a cold cloth over his eyes.

Instruct the patient to take prescribed medication at the onset of migraine symptoms, to prevent dehydration by drinking plenty of fluids after nausea and vomiting subside, and to use other headache relief measures.

Evaluation. Determine the effectiveness of analgesics, tranquilizers, or muscle relaxants administered and document your findings. Look for the patient to express an understanding of the cause of his headache and its treatment. Note if the patient says he's without pain.

Epilepsy

Patients affected with epilepsy are susceptible to recurrent seizures—paroxysmal events associated with abnormal electrical discharges of neurons in the brain. The sites of the discharges determine the clinical manifestations that occur during the attack. Seizures are among the most commonly observed neurologic dysfunctions in children and can occur with widely varying CNS conditions.

Causes. About one-half of all epilepsy cases are idiopathic. However, idiopathic epilepsy may indicate that genetic factors have in some way altered the seizure threshold to influence neuronal discharge. Seizures may occur as part of congenital defects and some genetic disorders (such as tuberous sclerosis and phenylketonuria). Researchers have detected hereditary EEG abnormalities in some families.

A seizure disorder also can be acquired as a result of birth trauma, perinatal infection, anoxia, infectious diseases (meningitis, encephalitis, or brain abscess), ingestion of toxins (mercury, lead, or carbon monoxide), brain tumors, head injury or trauma, metabolic disorders (such as hypoglycemia or hypoparathyroidism), or CVA.

Assessment findings. Accurate description of seizure activity is a vital part of assessment and can

ALTERNATIVE THERAPY

Reflexotherapy

Reflexotherapy—also known as reflexology—is a bodywork technique similar to acupressure in which hand pressure is applied to specific points on the feet and, less commonly, on the hands or ears.

Reflexology is based on the theory that sensitive nerve endings at reference points on the feet, hands, or ears correspond to all major organs or other parts of the body. Applying pressure to these points facilitates movement of life energy along channels in the body to the corresponding area. Among other things, reflexotherapy is used to treat tension and migraine headaches.

assist in correct classifications. Recurring seizures may be classified as partial or generalized (some patients may be affected by more than one type).

Partial seizures. Seizures in this class arise from a localized area of the brain and cause specific symptoms. In some patients, partial seizure activity may spread to the entire brain, causing a generalized seizure. Partial seizures include jacksonian and complex partial seizures (psychomotor or temporal lobe).

A *jacksonian seizure* begins as a localized motor seizure characterized by the spread of abnormal activity to adjacent areas of the brain. It typically produces a stiffening or jerking in one extremity, accompanied by a tingling sensation in the same area. The patient seldom loses consciousness. A jacksonian seizure may progress to a generalized tonic-clonic seizure.

The symptoms of a *complex partial seizure* will vary but usually include purposeless behavior. This seizure may begin with an aura, a sensation the patient feels immediately before the seizure. An aura represents the beginning of abnormal electrical discharges within a focal area of the brain and may include a pungent smell, GI distress (nausea or indigestion), a rising or sinking feeling in the stomach, a dreamy feeling, an unusual taste, or a visual disturbance. Overt signs of a complex partial seizure include a glassy stare, picking at one's clothes, aimless wandering, lip-smacking or chewing motions, and unintelligible speech. Mental confusion may last several minutes after the seizure.

Generalized seizures. These seizures cause a generalized electrical abnormality within the brain. (See *Distinguishing among types of generalized seizures.*)

Status epilepticus. This term describes a continuous seizure state, which can occur in all seizure types. In the most life-threatening form, generalized tonic-clonic status epilepticus, the patient experiences a continuous generalized tonic-clonic seizure without intervening return of consciousness. Accompanied by respiratory distress, status epilepticus can result from abrupt withdrawal of antiepileptic medica-

Distinguishing among types of generalized seizures

Generalized seizures include absence, myoclonic, generalized tonic-clonic, and akinetic.

Absence seizure

Also called petit mal seizures, absence seizures occur mostly in children, although they may affect adults as well. An absence seizure usually begins with a brief change in level of consciousness, indicated by blinking or rolling of the eyes, a blank stare, and slight mouth movements. The patient retains his posture and continues preseizure activity without difficulty. Typically, each seizure lasts from 1 to 10 seconds. If not properly treated, seizures can recur as often as 100 times a day. Absence seizures may progress to generalized tonic-clonic seizures.

Myoclonic seizure

Also called bilateral massive epileptic myoclonus, a myoclonic seizure is characterized by brief, involuntary muscular jerks of the body or extremities, which may occur in a rhythmic fashion.

Generalized tonic-clonic seizure

Also called a grand mal seizure, a generalized tonic- clonic seizure typ-

ically begins with a loud cry precipitated by air rushing from the lungs through the vocal cords. The patient then falls to the ground, losing consciousness. The body stiffens (tonic phase), then alternates between episodes of muscle spasm and relaxation (clonic phase). Tongue-biting, incontinence, labored breathing, apnea, and subsequent cyanosis may also occur. The seizure stops in 2 to 5 minutes, when abnormal electrical conduction of the neurons is completed. The patient then regains consciousness but is somewhat confused and may have difficulty talking. If he can talk, he may complain of drowsiness, fatigue, headache, muscle soreness, and arm or leg weakness. He may fall into a deep sleep after the seizure.

Akinetic seizure

An akinetic seizure is characterized by a general loss of postural tone and a temporary loss of consciousness. It occurs in young children, and is sometimes called a drop attack because it causes the child to fall.

---

tions, hypoxic encephalopathy, acute head trauma, metabolic encephalopathy, or septicemia secondary to encephalitis or meningitis.

Diagnostic tests. Primary diagnostic tests include CT scan and EEG. A CT scan offers density readings of the brain and may indicate abnormalities in internal structures.

Paroxysmal abnormalities on the EEG confirm the diagnosis of epilepsy by providing evidence of the continuing tendency to have seizures. A normal EEG doesn't rule out epilepsy because the paroxysmal abnormalities occur intermittently. Other helpful tests include serum glucose and calcium studies, lumbar puncture, brain scan, skull X-rays, and cerebral angiography.

Treatment. Typically, treatment consists of drug therapy. The most commonly prescribed drugs include phenytoin, carbamazepine, phenobarbital, or primidone administered individually for generalized tonic-clonic seizures and complex partial seizures. Valproic acid, clonazepam, and ethosuximide are commonly prescribed for absence seizures. New drug therapy treats complex partial, idiopathic, and atypical partial seizures with felbamate and partial or secondary generalized tonic-clonic seizures with gabapentin.

If drug therapy fails, treatment may include surgery to remove a demonstrated focal lesion. Emergency treatment for status epilepticus usually consists of diazepam, phenytoin, or phenobarbital; 50% dextrose I.V. (when seizures are secondary to hypoglycemia); and thiamine I.V. (in chronic alcoholism or withdrawal).

Nursing interventions. A patient taking antiepileptic medications requires constant monitoring for toxic signs and symptoms, such as nystagmus, ataxia, lethargy, dizziness, drowsiness, slurred speech, irritability, nausea, and vomiting. When administering phenytoin I.V., use a large vein, administer slowly (not more than 50 mg/minute), and monitor vital signs often.

Patient education. Encourage the patient and family to express their feelings. Answer their questions,

and dispel some of the misconceptions about epilepsy. Assure them that by following a prescribed regimen of medication most patients control their epilepsy and maintain a normal lifestyle.

Stress the need for compliance with the prescribed drug schedule. Assure the patient that antiepileptic drugs are safe *when taken as ordered.* Reinforce dosage instructions, and find methods to help the patient remember to take medications. Caution him not to run out of medication.

Warn against possible adverse reactions—drowsiness, lethargy, hyperactivity, confusion, visual and sleep disturbances—all of which indicate the need for dosage adjustment. Instruct the patient to report adverse reactions immediately.

Emphasize the importance of having antiepileptic drug blood levels checked at regular intervals, even if the seizures are under control. Also warn the patient against drinking alcoholic beverages.

Generalized tonic-clonic seizures may necessitate first aid. Teach the patient's family how to give such aid correctly; include the following points:
• Avoid restraining the patient during a seizure.
• Help the patient to a lying position, loosen any tight clothing, and place something flat and soft, such as a pillow, jacket, or hand, under his head.
• Clear the area of hard objects.
• *Don't* force anything into the patient's mouth if his teeth are clenched—you could lacerate the

mouth and lips or displace teeth, precipitating respiratory distress. However, if the patient's mouth is open, protect his tongue by placing a soft object (such as a folded cloth) between his teeth.
• Turn his head to provide an open airway.
• After the seizure subsides, reassure the patient that he's all right, orient him to time and place, and inform him that he has had a seizure.

Finally, know which social agencies in your community can help epileptic patients. Refer the patient to the Epilepsy Foundation of America for general information and to the state motor vehicle department for information about his driver's license.

Evaluation. Look for seizure activity to decrease or stop. Note whether the patient, especially if he's a child, has expressed his feelings regarding his illness. Finally, assess whether he remains injury-free.

Brain and spinal cord disorders

Brain and spinal cord disorders include CVA, cerebral aneurysm, arteriovenous malformation, and malignant brain tumors.

Cerebrovascular accident

Also called a stroke, a CVA is a sudden impairment of cerebral circulation in one or more of the blood vessels supplying the brain. A CVA interrupts or diminishes oxygen supply and commonly causes serious damage or necrosis in brain tissues. The sooner circulation returns to normal after a CVA, the better the prognosis.

CVAs are classified by their course of progression. The least severe, a transient ischemic attack (TIA), results from a temporary interruption of blood flow. A progressive CVA, or stroke-in-evolution (thrombus-in-evolution), begins with slight neurologic deficit and worsens in a day or two. It's usually considered a warning sign of an impending thrombotic CVA. In fact, TIAs have been reported in 50% to 80% of patients who've had a cerebral infarction from such thrombosis. In a complete CVA, the patient experiences maximal neurologic deficits at onset.

Causes. CVA usually results from thrombosis. Other causes include embolism and hemorrhage.

Certain risk factors increase the likelihood of CVA, such as atherosclerosis, hypertension, arrhythmias, rheumatic heart disease, diabetes mellitus, gout, postural hypotension, and cardiac hypertrophy. Other risk factors include high serum triglyceride levels, a sedentary lifestyle, use of oral contraceptives, cigarette smoking, and a family history of CVA.

Assessment findings. Clinical features of CVA vary with the artery affected, the severity of damage, and the extent of collateral circulation that develops to help the brain compensate for decreased blood supply. If CVA occurs in the left hemisphere, it produces symptoms on the right side; consequently, the reverse holds true. However, a CVA that causes CN damage produces signs of CN dysfunction on the same side as the hemorrhage. Symptoms are usually classified according to the artery affected. (Symptoms can also be classified as premonitory, generalized, and focal.)

Middle cerebral artery. This type of CVA may cause aphasia, dysphasia, visual field cuts, and hemiparesis on the affected side (more severe in the face and arm than in the leg).

Carotid artery. The patient may experience weakness, paralysis, numbness, sensory changes, visual disturbances on the affected side, altered LOC, bruits, headaches, aphasia, and ptosis.

Vertebrobasilar artery. Signs and symptoms may include weakness on the affected side, numbness around the lips and mouth, visual field cuts, diplopia, poor coordination, dysphagia, slurred speech, dizziness, amnesia, and ataxia.

Anterior cerebral artery. This type of CVA can cause confusion, weakness and numbness (especially in the leg) on the affected side, incontinence, loss of coordination, impaired motor and sensory functions, and personality changes.

Posterior cerebral arteries. The patient may experience visual field cuts, sensory impairment, dyslexia, coma, and cortical blindness; paralysis usually doesn't occur.

TIAs. Distinctive characteristics include the transient duration of neurologic deficits and complete return of normal function. The symptoms easily correlate with the location of the affected artery and include double vision, speech deficits (slurring or thickness), unilateral blindness, staggering or uncoordinated gait, unilateral weakness or numbness, falling because of weakness in the legs, and dizziness.

Diagnostic tests. CT scan shows evidence of thrombotic or hemorrhagic stroke, tumor, or hydrocephalus. Brain scan shows ischemic areas but may not be abnormal for up to 2 weeks after the CVA. Other supporting tests include:
• lumbar puncture—in subarachnoid hemorrhage, cerebrospinal fluid (CSF) may be bloody
• ophthalmoscopy—may show signs of hypertension and atherosclerotic changes in retinal arteries
• angiography—outlines blood vessels and pinpoints the site of occlusion or rupture
• EEG—may help to localize the area of damage.

Other baseline laboratory studies include urinalysis, coagulation studies, complete blood count (CBC), serum osmolality, and electrolyte, glucose, triglyceride, creatinine, and blood urea nitrogen levels.

Treatment. Medical management of CVA commonly includes physical rehabilitation, dietary and drug regimens to help reduce risk factors, possibly surgery, and care measures to help the patient adapt to specific deficits, such as motor impairment and paralysis. Depending on the CVA's cause and extent, the patient may undergo a craniotomy to remove a hematoma, an endarterectomy to remove atherosclerotic plaques from the inner arterial wall, or an extracranial bypass to circumvent an artery that's blocked by occlusion or stenosis. Ventricular shunts may be needed to drain CSF.

Drug therapy for CVA includes:
• anticoagulants, such as aspirin or ticlopidine. Usually, aspirin is contraindicated in hemorrhagic CVA because it increases bleeding tendencies; however, it may be useful in preventing TIAs.
• anticonvulsants, such as phenytoin or phenobarbital
• stool softeners such as dioctyl sodium sulfosuccinate
• corticosteroids such as dexamethasone
• analgesics such as codeine.

Newly approved therapy for ischemic stroke uses a thrombolytic drug such as alteplase—provided that the drug can be administered within 3 hours of symptom onset.

Nursing interventions. *Maintain a patent airway and oxygenation.* Watch for ballooning of the cheek with respiration. The side that balloons is the side affected by the stroke. An unconscious patient may aspirate saliva; keep him in a lateral position to allow secretions to drain naturally, or suction secretions as needed. Insert an artificial airway, and start mechanical ventilation or supplemental oxygen, if necessary.
• *Check vital signs and neurologic status.* Monitor blood pressure, LOC, pupillary changes, motor function (voluntary and involuntary movements), sensory function, speech, skin color, temperature, signs of increased ICP, and nuchal rigidity or flaccidity. Remember, if CVA is impending, blood pressure rises suddenly, pulse is rapid and bounding, and the patient may complain of headache. Also, watch for signs and symptoms of pulmonary emboli, such as chest pains, shortness of breath, dusky color, tachycardia, fever, and changed sensorium. If the patient is unresponsive, monitor his arterial blood gas (ABG) levels often and alert the doctor to increased partial pressure of carbon dioxide ($PaCO_2$) or decreased partial pressure of oxygen (PaO_2) in arterial blood.
• *Maintain fluid and electrolyte balance.* If the patient can take liquids by mouth, offer them as fluid limitations permit. Give I.V. fluids, as ordered; never give large volumes rapidly because this can raise ICP.
• *Ensure adequate nutrition.* Check for gag reflex before offering small oral feedings of semisolid foods. If oral feedings aren't possible, insert a nasogastric (NG) tube.
• *Manage GI problems.* Be alert for signs of straining at stool, as it increases ICP. Modify the diet and administer stool softeners, as ordered. If the patient vomits, keep him positioned on his side to prevent aspiration.
• *Provide careful mouth care.* Clean and irrigate the patient's mouth. Care for his dentures, as needed.
• *Provide meticulous eye care.* Remove secretions and instill eye-

drops, as ordered. Patch the patient's affected eye if he can't close the lid.

• *Position the patient.* Align extremities correctly. Use devices such as a footboard to prevent footdrop and contracture; use convoluted foam, flotation, pulsating mattresses, or sheepskin to avoid pressure sores. To prevent pneumonia, turn the patient at least every 2 hours. Raise the affected hand to control dependent edema, and place it in a functional position.

• *Help the patient exercise.* Perform ROM exercises for both the affected and unaffected sides. Encourage the patient to use his unaffected side to exercise his affected side.

• *Give medications, as ordered.* Watch for and report adverse reactions.

• *Establish rapport and maintain communication with the patient.* If he is aphasic, set up a simple method of communicating. Remember that the unresponsive patient can hear.

• *Provide psychological support.* Set realistic short-term goals. Involve the patient's family in his care when possible, and explain his deficits and strengths.

Patient education. The extent of teaching depends on the degree of neurologic deficit. With the aid of a physical and an occupational therapist, obtain appliances such as walkers, grab bars for the bathtub and toilet, and ramps, as needed. If speech therapy is indicated, encourage the patient to begin as soon as possible, and follow through with the speech pathologist's suggestions.

Involve the patient's family in rehabilitation. With their input, cooperation, and support, devise a realistic discharge plan.

Before discharge, warn the patient or his family to report any premonitory signs of CVA, such as severe headache, drowsiness, confusion, and dizziness. Stress the need for regular follow-up visits.

If aspirin has been prescribed to minimize the risk of embolic CVA, tell the patient to watch for possible GI bleeding. Make sure the patient realizes that he can't substitute acetaminophen for aspirin.

Evaluation. Look for a patent airway, normal breath sounds, adequate mobility, maintenance of or improvement in LOC, and adequate nutritional status. Also, note if the patient has expressed his feelings regarding his condition. (See *Managing nonhemorrhagic cerebrovascular accident,* pages 274 to 279.)

Cerebral aneurysm

Cerebral aneurysm is localized dilation of a cerebral artery that results from a weakness in the arterial wall. Cerebral aneurysms commonly rupture and cause subarachnoid hemorrhage. Sometimes bleeding also spills into brain tissue and subsequently forms a clot. This may result in potentially fatal increased ICP and brain tissue damage.

Causes. Cerebral aneurysm results from a congenital vascular disease, infection, or atherosclerosis.

Assessment findings. Onset of cerebral aneurysm is abrupt and causes sudden severe headache, nausea, vomiting, and possible altered LOC.

Meningeal irritation may cause nuchal rigidity, back and leg pain, fever, restlessness, irritability, occasional seizures, and blurred vision. Bleeding into brain tissue may lead to hemiparesis, unilateral sensory defects, dysphagia, and visual defects. Oculomotor nerve compression may lead to diplopia, ptosis, dilated pupil, and inability to rotate the eyes.

Diagnostic tests. Angiography can confirm an unruptured cerebral aneurysm. Unfortunately, diagnosis usually follows aneurysmal rupture. A CT scan may help detect subarachnoid hemorrhage. Cerebral angiography is still the standard diagnostic test. It provides visualization of all the vessels and their branches and can also detect vasospasm.

Treatment. The doctor may attempt to repair the aneurysm. Usually, surgical repair (by clipping, ligating, or wrapping the aneurysm neck with muscle) takes place within several days after the initial bleed. Surgery performed within 2 days after hemorrhage has proved effective in grades I and II (minimal or mild bleeding).

The patient may receive conservative treatment if surgical correction poses too much risk, if the aneurysm is in a particularly dangerous location, or if vasospasm necessitates a delay in surgery. Treatment may include bed rest in a quiet, darkened room, which may continue for 4 to 6 weeks. The patient must avoid coffee, other stimulants, and aspirin. He may receive codeine or another analgesic, hydralazine or another antihypertensive drug (if he's hypertensive), corticosteroids (to reduce edema), and phenobarbital or another sedative. Nimodipine may be used to limit possible neurologic deficits due to vasospasm.

Nursing interventions. During initial treatment after hemorrhage, establish and maintain a patent airway. Position the patient to promote pulmonary drainage and prevent upper airway obstruction. If he's intubated, preoxygenate with 100% oxygen before suctioning to remove secretions. Provide frequent nose and mouth care.

• Impose aneurysm precautions to minimize the risk of rebleeding and to avoid increased ICP. Such precautions include bed rest in a quiet, darkened room (keep the head of the bed flat or below 30 degrees, as ordered), limited visitors, and avoidance of coffee, other stimulants, and strenuous physical activity. Explain the need for these restrictive measures to the patient and his family.

• Monitor ABG levels, LOC, and vital signs frequently, and accurately measure intake and output. Avoid taking temperature rectally because vagus nerve stimulation may cause cardiac arrest.

(Text continues on page 280.)

Managing nonhemorrhagic cerebrovascular accident

DRG: 14 CVA-nonhemorrhagic
Expected length of stay (LOS): 7 days
Admission date: _____

Discharge date: _____
Actual LOS: _____

Expected outcomes	Key indicators	Date: Emergency care unit	Day 1	Day 2
Expected outcome Patient will receive care from a multidisciplinary health care team. **Diagnosis** Risk for anticipatory grief related to (R/T) loss of function associated with stroke **Expected outcome** Patient will receive spiritual support as necessary.	Consults		□ Neurology □ Stroke team (including physical therapy, occupational therapy (OT), speech, social service (SS), dietary, neuroscience clinical specialist, and pastoral care □ Dysphagia evaluation □ Spiritual needs identification	□ Psychiatry □ Daily pastoral care visit
Diagnosis Potential for alteration in fluid and electrolyte balance **Expected outcome** Patient will have stabilized fluid and electrolyte balance.	Diagnostics	□ Computed tomography (CT) scan of head □ Electrocardiogram (ECG) □ SMA-20 □ Lipid profile □ Prothrombin time (PT), partial thromboplastin time (PTT)	□ Carotid ultrasound □ two-dimensional echocardiogram □ Transcarotid Doppler □ Oculoplethysmography □ PT/PTT □ Magnetic resonance imaging/magnetic resonance angiography (MRI)/(MRA) □ Fasting blood glucose	□ Video swallow □ Arteriogram □ Platelet count →→→→

Day 3	Day 4	Day 5	Day 6	Day 7
□ Vascular surgery □ Psychiatry	□ Smoking cessation			
□ Daily pastoral care visits	→→→→→	→→→→→	→→→→→	→→→→→
□ PT/PTT	→→→→→	→→→→→	→→→→→	

(continued)

Managing nonhemorrhagic cerebrovascular accident *(continued)*

Expected outcomes	Key indicators	Emergency care unit	Day 1	Day 2
	I.V. therapy	□ I.V. fluids	□ I.V. fluids	□ I.V. fluids
Diagnosis Alteration in cerebral tissue perfusion R/T ischemic/thrombotic event **Expected outcome** Patient will maintain/regain nervous system function, stable neuro signs.	Assessment	□ Neuro baseline nursing assessment	□ Initial nursing assessment complete □ Neuro assessments every 2 hr □ Vital signs (VS) every ___ hr	□ Ongoing nursing assessment □ Neuro assessments every ___ □ VS every ___ hr
	Pharmacology	□ Heparin	→→→→→ □ Coumadin □ Aspirin/Ticlid	→→→→→ →→→→→ →→→→→
Diagnosis Potential for alteration in bowel and bladder elimination and nutrition **Expected outcome** Patient will regain bowel and bladder function and nutritional state.	Nutrition/elimination		□ Diet _____ □ Weight _____	□ Diet _____ □ Dysphagia recommendations per speech
		□ Indwelling urinary catheter	→→→→→	□ Indwelling urinary catheter discontinued □ Bladder training begins
			□ Bowel program	→→→→→
Diagnosis Impaired physical mobility R/T neurologic deficit **Expected outcome** Patient will remain free of complications R/T immobility. Patient will maintain or regain function. (Improvement of stroke-related deficit).	Activity/safety		□ Bed rest Head of bed at 30 degrees □ Aspiration precautions □ Fall risk assessment □ Fall prevention	→→→→→ →→→→→ →→→→→ →→→→→
			□ Deep vein thrombosis (DVT) prophylaxis: □ Antiembolism stockings □ Compression boots	□ Physical therapy: □ Physical therapy evaluation □ OT evaluation

Day 3	Day 4	Day 5	Day 6	Day 7
□ I.V. _____	□ I.V. _____	□ I.V. _____	□ I.V. discontinued_____	
□ Ongoing nursing assessments	→→→→	→→→→	→→→→	→→→→
□ Appropriate feeding and swallowing strategies	→→→→	→→→→	□ No signs of aspiration	→→→→
□ Heparin	→→→→	→→→→	□ Heparin discontinued	
□ Coumadin	→→→→	→→→→	→→→→	→→→→
□ Aspirin/Ticlid	→→→→	→→→→	→→→→	→→→→
□ Nutritional assessment	□ Nutritional needs met per dietitian's recommendations.			
□ Advance diet/tube feeding		→→→→	→→→→	→→→→
		□ Patient tolerating diet	□ Optimal diet level	
□ Bowel program	→→→→	→→→→	→→→→	→→→→
□ Out of bed (OOB) as tolerated	→→→→	→→→→	→→→→	→→→→
□ Aspiration precautions	→→→→	→→→→	→→→→	→→→→
Physical therapy:	□ Physical therapist's recommendations for rehab and placement			
□ Maintenance of range-of-motion (ROM)				
□ Strengthening of affected extremities	→→→→	→→→→	→→→→	→→→→
□ Transfer and gait training	→→→→	→→→→	→→→→	→→→→
□ Reeducation of affected extremities				

(continued)

Managing nonhemorrhagic cerebrovascular accident *(continued)*

Expected outcomes	Key indicators	Emergency care unit	Day 1	Day 2
Diagnosis Impaired communication—written or verbal R/T cerebral ischemia or infarct **Expected outcome** Patient will develop functional communication system.	Rehab (physical therapy) Rehab (speech) treatments		☐ Speech therapy: ☐ Speech evaluation	☐ Speech therapy: ☐ _____ ☐ _____
Diagnosis Knowledge deficit R/T disease process, diet, medication, and rehabilitation **Expected outcome** Patient and family will verbalize understanding of disease process, rehabilitation, and home care needs.	Patient/family education		☐ Stroke education package given to patient and family ☐ Assessment of baseline information about disease process	☐ Review/reinforcement of stroke education information by nursing staff and clinical nurse specialist ☐ Review of current care plan (clinical pathway) ☐ Patient and family education about speech disorder and goals
Diagnosis Knowledge deficit R/T disease process **Expected outcome** Patient will access appropriate level of rehabilitation care.	Discharge planning		☐ Social work assessment of post-hospital needs ☐ Contact with family by Social Service	☐ Counsel family or significant other about options available for post-hospital care.
Have the daily outcomes been met?	Yes No	Yes No	Yes No	Yes No
Caregivers' initials and signatures				

Adapted with permission from Sacred Heart Hospital, Allentown, Pa.

Day 3	Day 4	Day 5	Day 6	Day 7
Speech: ☐ ——————— ☐ Dysphagia treatment	☐ ————— →→→→	☐ ———————— →→→→	☐ ———————— →→→→	☐ ————— →→→→
☐ Continue stroke education per clinical pathway ☐ Discussion of anticoagulation meds and provision of patient education material ☐ Patient and family education regarding functional deficit and therapy needs ☐ Patient and family education about swallowing, diet precautions, and feeding techniques	→→→→ →→→→ ☐ Patient and family education about special diet needs ☐ Patient and family demonstration of feeding techniques	☐ Discharge and home education instructions reviewed with patient and family ☐ Patient and family demonstration of transfer assist and follow-up exercise as appropriate →→→→	→→→→ →→→→ ☐ Verification of patient and family understanding of special dietary needs →→→→	☐ Verification of patient and family understanding of discharge instructions →→→→ →→→→ →→→→
☐ Follow-up on discharge options with family and significant other as needed	☐ Family assist in finalizing plans for care ☐ Transfer to acute rehabilitation	→→→→	☐ Arrangements finalized for patient transfer to appropriate level of post-hospital care	☐ Discharge according to plans
Yes No	Yes No	Yes No	Yes No	Yes No
Caregivers' initials and signatures —————————————— ——————————————	——————————————— ———————————————			

• Watch for these danger signals, which may indicate an enlarging aneurysm, rebleeding, intracranial clot, increased ICP, vasospasm, or other complications: decreased LOC, unilateral enlarged pupil, onset or worsening of hemiparesis or motor deficit, increased blood pressure, slowed pulse rate, worsening of headache or sudden onset of a headache, renewed or worsened nuchal rigidity, and renewed or persistent vomiting.

• Give fluids, as ordered, and monitor I.V. infusions to avoid increased ICP.

• If the patient has facial weakness, assist him during meals, placing food in the unaffected side of his mouth. If he can't swallow, insert an NG tube, as ordered, and give all tube feedings slowly. Prevent skin breakdown by taping the tube so it doesn't press against the nostril.

• Provide a high-bulk diet to prevent straining at stool, which can increase ICP. Stool softeners can also be used.

• Administer medications, as ordered, and observe closely for adverse reactions.

• With CN III or facial palsy, administer artificial tears to the affected eye, and tape the eye shut at night to prevent corneal damage.

• Include the patient's family in his care as much as possible. Encourage family members to adopt a positive attitude, but discourage unrealistic goals.

• Before discharge, refer the patient to a home health nurse or a rehabilitation center if necessary.

Patient education. This will depend on the extent of neurologic deficit. If the patient can't speak, establish a simple means of communication, or use cards or a slate. Try to limit conversation to topics that won't frustrate the patient. Instruct his family to speak to him in a normal tone, even if he's unresponsive.

Evaluation. Look for a patent airway, normal breath sounds, maintenance of LOC with no neurologic deficits, adequate hydration and nutrition, absence of injury, and absence of complications related to increased ICP. Note whether the patient has expressed his feelings regarding his condition.

Arteriovenous malformation

In this disorder, a tangled array of dilated vessels forms an abnormal communication network between the arterial and venous systems. Although they may appear in any part of the CNS, arteriovenous malformations (AVMs) usually affect the cerebral hemispheres and may penetrate the lateral ventricles.

AVMs vary from small, focal lesions to large lesions encompassing an entire hemisphere of the brain. They cause shunting of arterial blood directly into the venous system, instead of through the connecting capillary network. As a result, other cerebral areas don't receive adequate perfusion.

Causes. AVMs usually result from congenital defects in capillary development. Recent evidence indicates they may also develop after traumatic injury.

Assessment findings. Hemorrhage and seizures usually provide the first indications of an AVM. In about one-half of the patients hospitalized with this disorder, the AVM has bled sometime before admission.

Seizures initially may be focal or jacksonian but many become generalized. Psychomotor seizures indicate temporal lobe lesions, whereas focal or generalized seizures indicate frontal and parietal lesions.

Patients with AVM commonly will complain of headache; however, the significance of this common symptom may not be readily apparent. Some patients experience migraine-like headaches. Assess for AVM in any patient who complains of both seizures and headache.

Depending on the size and location of the AVM and the thickness of the skull, auscultation may reveal a bruit in a small percentage of patients, especially in a child because of the thinner skull.

Other possible symptoms include transient episodes of syncope, dizziness, motor weakness, sensory deficits or tingling, aphasia, dysarthria, visual deficits (usually hemianopsia), and mental confusion as well as dementia or intellectual impairment.

Diagnostic tests. Cerebral angiography provides the most definitive diagnostic information. Besides localizing the AVM, it permits visualization of large feeding arteries and large drainage veins.

The CT scan, especially with a contrast medium, enables differentiation from a clot or tumor. An EEG may help in localizing an AVM. Skull X-rays and magnetic resonance imaging (MRI) may also aid in diagnosing AVM.

Treatment. The choice of treatment depends on the size and location of the AVM, on the feeder vessels supplying it, and on the age and condition of the patient. Possible methods include conservative medical management, embolization, proton-beam radiation, laser surgery, surgical excision, and a combination of embolization and surgery.

Nursing interventions. If hemorrhage hasn't occurred, expect to focus your efforts on preventing bleeding. This means controlling hypertension, seizure activity, and other activities or stress that could elevate the patient's systemic blood pressure. Expect to provide treatment similar to that for an unruptured cerebral aneurysm.
• Maintain a quiet, therapeutic environment.
• Monitor and control associated hypertension with drug therapy, as ordered.
• Conduct ongoing neurologic assessment.
• Monitor vital signs frequently.
• Assess and monitor characteristics of headache, seizure activity, or bruit, as needed.

If the AVM has ruptured, work to control elevated ICP and intracranial hemorrhage in addition to performing the steps listed above.

The patient with a ruptured AVM may have bleeding into the sub-arachnoid, subdural, or epidural space or into the brain itself, usually causing a concurrent elevation in ICP. Expect to perform measures similar to those used for a ruptured cerebral aneurysm.

Patient education. Provide appropriate preoperative patient instruction. After surgery, focus teaching on helping the patient develop independence.

Evaluation. Look for the patient to maintain an appropriate LOC, temperature, pulse rate, respiratory rate, and blood pressure. He should have no pain or seizures. Note whether the patient has expressed feelings of loss.

Malignant brain tumors

Brain tumors are the most common type of CNS cancer. More than 50% of all brain tumors are malignant but overall brain tumors only account for 1.5% of all cancers in the United States.

Causes. The cause of malignant brain tumors is unknown; however, occupational exposure and radiation to the brain for treatment of other cancers may be a predisposing factor.

Assessment findings. Clinical manifestations vary depending upon the site, size, and expansion of the tumor. They are generally classified into three major types: those related to increased ICP, those related to

movement of brain structures, and those related to focal effects.

Diagnostic tests. CT scan and MRI are used to determine size and location. Positron emission tomography (PET) may be used to biochemically classify the tumor. Cerebral angiography may be used when metastatic tumors are suspected. Biopsy is necessary for definitive diagnosis.

Treatment. Treatment is determined by four criteria: primary site; tumor grade; overall condition of the patient; and tumor type. Surgical excision is usually the initial treatment followed by radiation or chemotherapy or both.

Chemotherapy drugs are delivered by intra-arterial or intraventricular (Ommaya reservoir) routes. Stereotactic radiosurgery may be used.

Nursing interventions. During your first contact with the patient, perform a comprehensive assessment (including a complete neurologic evaluation) to provide baseline data and to help develop your plan of care. Obtain a thorough health history concerning onset of symptoms. Help the patient and his family cope with treatment, potential disabilities, and lifestyle changes resulting from the tumor.

Throughout hospitalization, follow these guidelines:
• Assess neurologic status including LOC every 1 to 4 hours; pupil size, symmetry, and reaction to light; motor and sensory function; and vital signs.

- Maintain airway patency.
- Administer osmotic diuretics, steroids, and antacids as ordered.
- Elevate head of bed 15 to 30 degrees to promote venous drainage.
- Prevent Valsalva's maneuver and isometric movements that may increase intra-abdominal or intrathoracic pressure.
- Implement medical plan to prevent seizures.
- Restrict fluids to 1,500 ml/24 hours. Carefully monitor fluid and electrolyte balance.
- Begin rehabilitation early. Encourage independence in ADLs.

Patient education. Instruct the patient and his family about signs of complications, such as increased ICP and cerebral edema. Inform them that signs and symptoms may increase with radiation before they decrease. Teach them early indications of recurrence. Urge compliance with therapy.

Evaluation. Look for an uneventful recovery from surgery, without complications. The patient should tolerate chemotherapy or radiation treatments. He should understand the medication regimen, adverse effects, and signs and symptoms of increased ICP and the need for immediate medical attention if these occur.

CNS infections

This section covers two disorders caused by CNS infections: meningitis and Guillain-Barré syndrome.

Meningitis

In meningitis, the brain and the spinal meninges become inflamed, usually as a result of bacterial infection. Such inflammation may involve all three meningeal membranes—the dura mater, the arachnoid, and the pia mater.

Causes. Meningitis almost always occurs as a complication of another bacterial infection—bacteremia (especially from pneumonia, empyema, osteomyelitis, or endocarditis), sinusitis, otitis media, encephalitis, myelitis, or brain abscess.

Meningitis may also follow skull fracture, a penetrating head wound, lumbar puncture, or ventricular shunting procedures. Aseptic meningitis may result from a virus or other organism. Sometimes, no causative organism can be identified.

Assessment findings. Findings may include fever, chills, malaise, headache, vomiting, nuchal rigidity, positive Brudzinski's and Kernig's signs, exaggerated and symmetrical deep tendon reflexes, and opisthotonos.

Other possible findings include sinus arrhythmias; irritability; photophobia, diplopia, and other visual problems; delirium, deep stupor, and coma; twitching; and seizures.

Diagnostic tests. Typical CSF findings (and positive Brudzinski's and Kernig's signs) usually establish the diagnosis. Look for elevated CSF pressure, high CSF protein levels and, possibly, low glucose levels. CSF culture and sensitivity tests usually identify the infecting organism unless it's a virus.

Treatment. Treatment includes appropriate antibiotic therapy and vigorous supportive care. Usually, the patient receives I.V. antibiotics for at least 2 weeks, followed by oral antibiotics, such as penicillin G, ampicillin, or nafcillin; if known allergy to penicillin, tetracycline, chloramphenicol, or kanamycin. Other drugs include a digitalis glycoside such as digoxin to control arrhythmias, mannitol to decrease cerebral edema, an I.V. anticonvulsant or a sedative to reduce restlessness, and aspirin or acetaminophen to relieve headache and fever.

Supportive measures include bed rest, hypothermia, and measures to prevent dehydration. Isolation is necessary if nasal cultures are positive.

Nursing interventions. Assess neurologic function often.
• Watch for deterioration. Be especially alert for a temperature increase up to 102° F (38.9° C), deteriorating LOC, onset of seizures, and altered respirations, all of which may signal an impending crisis.
• Monitor fluid balance. Maintain adequate fluid intake but avoid fluid overload because of the danger of cerebral edema. Measure central venous pressure, and record intake and output accurately.
• Position the patient carefully to prevent joint stiffness and neck pain. Turn him often, according to a planned positioning schedule and assist with ROM exercises.
• Maintain adequate nutrition and elimination.
• Maintain a quiet environment. Relieve headache with a nonnarcotic analgesic, such as aspirin or acetaminophen, as ordered. (Narcotics interfere with accurate neurologic assessment.)
• Provide reassurance and support. The patient may be frightened by his illness and frequent lumbar punctures. If he's delirious or confused, attempt to reorient him often. Reassure the family that these behavior changes usually disappear.

Patient education. To help prevent meningitis, teach patients with chronic sinusitis or other chronic infections the importance of proper medical treatment. Follow strict aseptic technique when treating patients with head wounds or skull fractures.

Evaluation. The patient should remain afebrile with no alteration in LOC, and have adequate hydration and nutrition. He should be pain-free and his blood pressure, pulse and respiratory rates should remain within normal limits.

Guillain-Barré syndrome

An acute, rapidly progressive, and potentially fatal form of polyneuritis, Guillain-Barré syndrome causes segmental demyelination of the peripheral nerves. In this disorder, signs of sensory and motor losses occur simultaneously. About 95% of patients experience spontaneous and complete recovery.

Causes. The cause remains unknown, but it may be a cell-mediated immunologic attack on peripheral nerves in response to a virus. Precipitating factors may include mild febrile illness, surgery, rabies or swine influenza vaccination, viral illness, Hodgkin's disease or some other cancer, or systemic lupus erythematosus.

Assessment findings. Along with a history of preceding febrile illness (usually a respiratory tract infection), look for paresthesia and muscle weakness. The major neurologic symptom, muscle weakness usually appears in the legs first (ascending type), then extends to the arms and facial nerves in 24 to 72 hours. It sometimes develops in the arms first (descending type) or in the arms and legs simultaneously. In milder forms of this disease, muscle weakness may be absent.

Other possible features include facial diplegia (possibly with ophthalmoplegia [ocular paralysis]), dysphagia or dysarthria and, less commonly, weakness of the muscles supplied by the 11th cranial (spinal accessory) nerve. Assess also for hypotonia and areflexia.

Diagnostic tests. CSF protein level begins to rise several days after onset of signs and symptoms, peaking in 4 to 6 weeks.

White blood cell count in CSF remains normal, but in severe disease CSF pressure may rise above

normal. The CBC shows leukocytosis and immature forms early in the illness, but blood studies soon return to normal.

Electromyography may show repeated firing of the same motor unit instead of widespread sectional stimulation. In addition, nerve conduction velocities are slowed soon after paralysis develops.

Treatment. Plasma exchange for patients with Guillain-Barré syndrome is now the initial therapy of choice. Otherwise, treatment is primarily supportive, consisting of endotracheal intubation or tracheotomy if the patient has difficulty clearing secretions. The doctor may order a trial dose of prednisone if the course of the disease is relentlessly progressive. If prednisone produces no noticeable improvement after 7 days, the drug is discontinued.

Nursing interventions. Watch for ascending sensory loss, which precedes motor loss. Also, monitor vital signs and LOC.
• Assess and treat respiratory dysfunction. If respiratory muscles are weak, take serial vital capacity recordings. Use a spirometer with a mouthpiece or a face mask for bedside testing.
• Obtain ABG measurements. Because neuromuscular disease results in primary hypoventilation with hypoxemia and hypercapnia, be alert for a PaO_2 below 70 mm Hg, which signals respiratory failure. Also watch for signs of a rising $PaCO_2$ (confusion, tachypnea).

• Auscultate for breath sounds, turn and position the patient, and encourage deep breathing and coughing (if secretions are present). Begin respiratory support at the first sign of dyspnea (in adults, vital capacity less than 800 ml; in children, less than 12 ml/kg of body weight) or a decreasing PaO_2.

• If respiratory failure becomes imminent, establish an emergency airway with an endotracheal tube, as ordered.

• Provide meticulous skin care to prevent skin breakdown and contractures.

• Perform passive ROM exercises within the patient's pain limits. When the patient's condition stabilizes, change to gentle stretching and active assistance exercises.

• To prevent aspiration, test the gag reflex, and elevate the head of the bed before the patient eats. If the gag reflex is absent, give NG feedings until this reflex returns.

• As the patient regains strength and can tolerate a vertical position, be alert for postural hypotension. Monitor blood pressure and pulse rate and, if necessary, apply toe-to-groin elastic bandages or an abdominal binder to prevent postural hypotension.

• Inspect the patient's legs regularly for signs of thrombophlebitis, a common complication. Apply anti-embolism stockings and give prophylactic anticoagulants, as ordered.

• If the patient has facial paralysis, provide eye and mouth care every 4 hours.

• Measure and record intake and output every 8 hours. Encourage adequate fluid intake (2,000 ml/day), unless contraindicated. If urine retention develops, begin intermittent catheterization, as ordered. Because the abdominal muscles are weak, the patient may need manual pressure on the bladder before he can urinate.

• To prevent and relieve constipation, offer prune juice and a high-bulk diet. If necessary, give daily or alternate-day suppositories (glycerin or bisacodyl), or Fleet enemas, as ordered.

• Refer the patient for physical therapy, as needed.

Patient education. Before discharge, teach the patient how to transfer from bed to wheelchair and from wheelchair to toilet or tub and how to walk short distances with a walker or a cane. Teach the family how to help him eat, compensating for facial weakness, and how to help him avoid skin breakdown. Stress the need for a regular bowel and bladder routine.

Evaluation. Look for adequate respiratory function with a patent airway and clear lungs, adequate nutritional status, and optimal activity level. Note also if the patient expresses his feelings of loss to staff, friends, or family.

Degenerative disorders

Degenerative disorders include myasthenia gravis, ALS, MS, Parkinson's disease, and Alzheimer's disease.

Myasthenia gravis

Myasthenia gravis produces sporadic but progressive weakness and abnormal fatigability of striated (skeletal) muscles, which are exacerbated by exercise and repeated movement but improved by anticholinesterase drugs. Usually, myasthenia gravis affects muscles innervated by the CNs (face, lips, tongue, neck, and throat), but it can affect any muscle group. It commonly coexists with immunologic and thyroid disorders.

Myasthenia gravis follows an unpredictable course of recurring exacerbations and periodic remissions and has no known cure. Drug treatment has improved the prognosis and allows patients to lead relatively normal lives, except during exacerbations. When the disease involves the respiratory system, it may be life-threatening.

Causes. Myasthenia gravis is probably an autoimmune disorder that impairs transmission of nerve impulses.

Assessment findings. Cardinal symptoms include gradually progressive skeletal muscle weakness and fatigue. Typically, the patient experiences mild weakness upon awakening that worsens during the day.

Early signs and symptoms may include weak eye closure, ptosis, and diplopia; blank, masklike facies; difficulty chewing and swallowing; hanging jaw; and bobbing head.

Respiratory muscle involvement may lead to symptoms of respiratory failure.

Diagnostic tests. The classic proof of myasthenia gravis, the Tensilon test, shows improved muscle function after an I.V. injection of edrophonium or neostigmine. In myasthenic patients, muscle function improves within 30 to 60 seconds and lasts up to 30 minutes. However, long-standing ocular muscle dysfunction commonly fails to respond to such testing.

The Tensilon test also can differentiate a myasthenic crisis from a cholinergic crisis (caused by acetylcholine overactivity at the neuromuscular junction, possibly from anticholinesterase overdose).

Electromyography, with repeated neural stimulation, may help confirm this diagnosis. Other tests may include nerve conduction studies and a CT scan of the chest.

Treatment. Treatment is symptomatic. Anticholinesterase drugs, such as neostigmine and pyridostigmine, counteract fatigue and muscle weakness and allow about 80% of normal muscle function. These drugs become less effective as the disease worsens. Corticosteroids may help to relieve symptoms.

Some patients may undergo plasmapheresis. Patients with thymomas require thymectomy, which may lead to remission in adult-onset myasthenia.

Acute exacerbations that cause severe respiratory distress necessitate emergency treatment. Tracheotomy, positive-pressure ventilation, and vigorous suctioning to remove secretions usually bring improvement in a few days. Anticholinesterase drugs are discontinued until respiratory function begins to improve. Myasthenic crisis requires immediate hospitalization and vigorous respiratory support.

Nursing interventions. Establish an accurate neurologic and respiratory baseline. Thereafter, monitor tidal volume and vital capacity regularly. The patient may need a ventilator and frequent suctioning to remove accumulating secretions. Keep alert for signs and symptoms of an impending crisis (increased muscle weakness, respiratory distress, and difficulty talking or chewing).

Evenly space administration of drugs. Be prepared to give atropine for anticholinesterase overdose or toxicity.

Plan exercise, meals, patient care, and activities to make the most of energy peaks. For example, give medication 20 to 30 minutes before meals to facilitate chewing or swallowing. Allow the patient to participate in his care.

Patient education. Thorough teaching is essential because myasthenia gravis is usually a lifelong condition. Help the patient plan ADLs to coincide with energy peaks. Stress the need for frequent rest periods. Emphasize that periodic remissions, exacerbations, and day-to-day fluctuations are common.

Teach the patient how to recognize adverse effects and signs and symptoms of anticholinesterase drug toxicity (headaches, weakness, sweating, abdominal cramps, nausea, vomiting, diarrhea, excessive salivation, and bronchospasm) and corticosteroid toxicity. Warn him to avoid strenuous exercise, stress, infection, and needless exposure to the sun or cold weather. All of these things may worsen signs and symptoms.

Advise the patient with diplopia that an eye patch or glasses with one frosted lens may be helpful.

Refer the patient to the Myasthenia Gravis Foundation.

Evaluation. Look for normal vital signs, maintenance of adequate hydration and elimination, maintenance of skin integrity, and achievement of optimal activity level. Note whether the patient has expressed his feelings of loss.

Amyotrophic lateral sclerosis

ALS causes progressive physical degeneration but leaves the patient's mental status intact, enabling him to perceive every change acutely. The most common motor neuron disease of muscular atrophy, ALS results in degeneration of upper motor neurons in the medulla oblongata and lower motor neurons in the spinal cord. Most patients die within 3 to 10 years after onset.

Precipitating factors for acute deterioration include trauma, viral infections, and physical exhaustion. Disorders that must be differentiated from ALS include CNS syphilis, MS, spinal cord tumors, and syringomyelia.

Causes. An individual may acquire ALS through autosomal dominant inheritance, nutritional deficiency of motor neurons related to a disturbance in enzyme metabolism, metabolic interference in nucleic acid production by the nerve fibers, or autoimmune disorders that affect immune complexes in the renal glomerulus and basement membrane.

Individuals whose occupations require strenuous physical labor face the greatest risk of developing noninherited ALS.

Assessment findings. Characteristic clinical features indicate a combination of upper and lower motor neuron involvement without sensory impairment. These features include atrophy and weakness, especially in the muscles of the forearms and the hands; impaired speech; difficulty chewing and swallowing; difficulty breathing; normal mental status; and possible choking and excessive drooling.

Diagnostic tests. Electromyography and muscle biopsy help show nerve rather than muscle disease. Examination of CSF reveals increased protein content in one-third of patients.

Treatment. No effective treatment exists for ALS. Management aims to control symptoms and provide emotional and physical support.

Nursing interventions. ALS challenges the patient's and caregivers' ability to cope. Care begins with a complete neurologic assessment, a baseline for future evaluations of disease progression. Then take the following steps:

• Implement a rehabilitation program designed to maintain independence as long as possible.
• Help the patient obtain equipment, such as a walker and a wheelchair. Arrange for a home health nurse to oversee home care, to provide support, and to teach the family about the illness.
• Depending on the patient's muscular capacity, assist with bathing, personal hygiene, and transfers from wheelchair to bed. Help establish a regular bowel and bladder routine.
• To prevent skin breakdown, provide good skin care when the patient is bedridden. Use sheepskins or pressure-relieving devices.
• If the patient has trouble swallowing, give him soft, solid foods and position him upright during meals. Gastrostomy and NG tube feedings may be necessary if he can no longer swallow. Teach the patient or family how to administer gastrostomy feedings.
• Provide emotional support. Prepare the patient and family for his eventual death, and encourage the start of the grieving process. Patients with ALS may benefit from a hospice program.

Patient education. Teach the patient to suction himself. He should have a suction machine handy at home to reduce fear of choking.

Evaluation. Look for the patient to maintain adequate respiratory function with a patent airway, clear lungs, and adequate results from pulmonary function studies. Seek to maintain an appropriate communication pattern and physical mobility for as long as possible. Note whether the patient has expressed feelings of loss. Skin integrity should be maintained.

Multiple sclerosis

A major cause of chronic disability in young adults, MS results from progressive demyelination of the white matter of the brain and spinal cord; it's characterized by exacerbations and remissions. Sporadic patches of demyelination in the CNS induce widely disseminated and varied neurologic dysfunction. Diagnosis requires evidence of multiple neurologic attacks and characteristic remissions and exacerbations.

MS may be mild with prolonged remissions or progress rapidly, disabling the patient by early adulthood or causing death within months of onset.

Causes. The cause of MS remains uncertain, but current theories suggest a slow-acting viral infection, an autoimmune response of the nervous system, or an allergic response to an infectious agent.

Assessment findings. Accurate diagnosis requires evidence of multiple neurologic attacks and characteristic remissions and exacerbations. Signs and symptoms are extremely variable and include the following:
• visual disturbances, such as optic neuritis, diplopia, ophthalmoplegia, and blurred vision
• sensory impairment such as paresthesias
• muscle dysfunction, such as weakness, paralysis (ranging from monoplegia to quadriplegia), spasticity, hyperreflexia, intention tremor, and gait ataxia
• urinary disturbances, such as incontinence, frequency, urgency, and frequent infections
• emotional lability, such as mood swings, irritability, euphoria, or depression.

Associated signs and symptoms include poorly articulated or scanning speech and dysphagia.

Diagnostic tests. Because of the difficulty inherent in establishing a diagnosis, some patients may undergo years of periodic testing and close observation, depending on the course of the disease.

MRI can aid diagnosis. In one-third of patients, EEG shows abnormalities. Lumbar puncture shows elevated gamma globulin fraction of immunoglobulin G but normal total protein levels in CSF. An elevated CSF gamma globulin level is significant only when serum gamma globulin levels are normal; it reflects hyperactivity of the immune system because of chronic demyelination. Oligoclonal bands of immunoglobulin can be detected when CSF gamma globulin is examined by electrophoresis.

The patient may also undergo psychological testing as well as additional neurologic tests, such as CT scans and evoked potential studies, to rule out other disorders.

Treatment. The aim of treatment is to shorten exacerbations and, if possible, relieve neurologic deficits so that the patient can resume a normal lifestyle. Corticotropin, prednisone, or dexamethasone is used to reduce the associated edema of the myelin sheath during exacerbations. Corticotropin and corticosteroids seem to relieve symptoms and hasten remission but don't prevent future exacerbations.

Other drugs used include chlordiazepoxide to mitigate mood swings, baclofen or dantrolene to relieve spasticity, and bethanechol or oxybutynin to relieve urine retention and minimize frequency and urgency. During acute exacerbation, supportive measures include bed rest, comfort measures such as massages, prevention of fatigue, prevention of pressure sores, bowel and bladder training (if necessary), treatment of bladder infections with antibiotics, physical therapy, and counseling.

Nursing interventions. Appropriate care depends on the severity of the disease and the symptoms.

Assist with physical therapy. Increase patient comfort with massages and relaxing baths. Make sure bathwater is not too hot because hot water may temporarily intensify otherwise subtle symptoms. Assist with active, resistive, and stretching exercises to maintain muscle tone and joint mobility, decrease spasticity, improve coordination, and boost morale.

Promote emotional stability. Help the patient establish a daily routine to maintain optimal functioning. Activity level is regulated by tolerance level. Encourage daily physical exercise and regular rest periods to prevent fatigue. Watch for drug adverse effects.

Patient education. Educate the patient and family concerning the chronic course of MS. Inform the patient that exacerbations are unpredictable. Emphasize the need to avoid stress, infections, and fatigue and to maintain independence by developing new ways of performing ADLs. Tell the patient to avoid exposure to infections. Stress the importance of eating a nutritious, well-balanced diet that contains sufficient roughage to prevent constipation.

Evaluate the need for bowel and bladder training during hospitalization. Encourage adequate fluid intake and regular urination. Eventually, the patient may require urinary drainage by self-catheterization or, in men, condom drainage. Teach the correct use of suppositories to help establish a regular bowel schedule.

Refer the patient to the National Multiple Sclerosis Society.

Evaluation. Treatment seeks to maintain adequate mobility within limitations, to ensure adequate nutritional balance, and to control pain during periods of exacerbation. The patient should maintain adequate urine elimination without complications caused by UTI. As the disease progresses, seek to maintain adequate respiratory function.

Parkinson's disease

A slowly progressive, degenerative neurologic movement disorder, Parkinson's disease is one of the most common cripplers in the United States. The disease is not fatal. Death may result from aspiration pneumonia or some other infection.

Causes. Although the cause of Parkinson's disease remains uncertain, dopamine deficiency prevents affected brain cells from performing their normal inhibitory function within the CNS.

Assessment findings. Signs and symptoms include:
• insidious tremor that begins in the fingers (unilateral pill-rolling tremor), increases during stress or anxiety, and decreases with purposeful movement and sleep
• muscle rigidity causing resistance to passive muscle stretching, which may be uniform (lead-pipe rigidity) or jerky (cogwheel rigidity)
• difficulty walking (gait lacks normal parallel motion)
• high-pitched monotone voice
• drooling
• masklike facial expression with poor blink reflex and wide-open eyes
• loss of positive control (the patient walks with body bent forward)
• slowed, monotonous, slurred speech that may become severely dysarthric
• dysphagia
• oculogyric crises (eyes are fixed upward, with involuntary tonic movements); occasionally, blepharospasm.

Diagnostic tests. Although urinalysis may reveal decreased dopamine levels, laboratory data usually have little value in identifying Parkinson's disease. Consequently, diagnosis depends on the patient's age and history and the characteristic clinical picture. To form a conclusive diagnosis, the doctor must rule out involutional depression, cerebral arteriosclerosis, other causes of tremor and, in patients under age 30, intracranial tumors, Wilson's disease, and phenothiazine or other drug toxicity.

Treatment. Treatment seeks to relieve symptoms and keep the patient functional as long as possible. Treatment consists of drugs, physical therapy and, in severe disease states unresponsive to drugs, stereotactic neurosurgery.

Drug therapy usually includes levodopa, a dopamine replacement that achieves its best effect during early stages. The patient takes the drug in increasing doses until symptoms are relieved or adverse reactions appear. The doctor will usually order levodopa in combination with carbidopa to halt peripheral dopamine synthesis. When levodopa proves ineffective or too toxic, alternative drug therapy includes anticholinergics such as trihexyphenidyl, antihistamines such as diphenhydramine, and amantadine, an antiviral agent.

When drug therapy fails, stereotactic neurosurgery may relieve symptoms. Electrical coagulation, freezing, radioactivity, or ultrasound destroys the ventrolateral nucleus of the thalamus to prevent involuntary movement.

Also, individually planned physical therapy helps maintain normal muscle tone and function. Appropriate physical therapy includes both active and passive ROM exercises, routine ADLs, walking, and baths and massage to help relax muscles.

Nursing interventions. Effectively caring for the patient with Parkinson's disease requires careful monitoring of drug treatment, emphasis on teaching self-reliance, and generous psychological support.

If the patient has had surgery, watch for signs of hemorrhage and increased ICP by frequently checking LOC and vital signs.

Encourage independence. The patient with excessive tremor may achieve partial control of his body by sitting on a chair and using its arms to steady himself. Remember that fatigue may cause him to depend more on others.

Help the patient overcome problems. Help establish a regular bowel routine by encouraging him to drink at least 2,000 ml of liquids daily and eat high-bulk foods. He may need an elevated toilet seat.

Help the patient and family express their feelings about this debilitating disease.

Patient education. Teach the patient and family about the disease, its progressive stages, and drug adverse effects. Show the family how to prevent pressure sores and contractures by proper positioning. Inform them of the dietary restrictions levodopa imposes, and explain household safety measures to prevent accidents.

Establish long- and short-term treatment goals, and be aware of the patient's need for intellectual stimulation and diversion.

Refer the patient and family to the National Parkinson Foundation or the United Parkinson Foundation.

Evaluation. Assess whether the patient can maintain adequate respiratory function as demonstrated by a patent airway, clear lungs, and adequate respiratory excursion. Note whether he can maintain adequate urinary function without complications caused by UTI. The patient should perform ADLs within the limits imposed by his condition. The patient and his family should express an understanding of Parkinson's disease and its treatment.

Alzheimer's disease

Alzheimer's disease is a presenile dementia that accounts for over one-half of all dementias. The brain tissue of patients with primary degenerative dementia has three hallmark features: neurofibrillary tangles, neuritic plaques, and granulovascular degeneration. Unfortunately, the patient with this disorder faces a poor prognosis.

Causes. The cause of Alzheimer's disease remains unknown. Several factors are thought to be implicated. These include neurochemical factors, such as deficiencies in the neurotransmitters acetylcholine, somatostatin, substance P, and norepinephrine; environmental factors, such as aluminum and manganese; viral factors such as slow-growing CNS viruses; trauma; and genetic immunologic factors.

Assessment findings. Onset is insidious. Initial changes are almost imperceptible, but they gradually progress to serious problems.

Initial signs and symptoms include forgetfulness, recent memory loss, difficulty learning and remembering new information, deterioration in personal hygiene and appearance, and inability to concentrate.

Later signs and symptoms consist of difficulty with abstract thinking and activities that require judgment; progressive difficulty communicating; severe deterioration in memory, language, and motor function, resulting in coordination loss and an inability to speak or write; repetitive actions or perseveration (a key sign); personality changes, such as restlessness and irritability; nocturnal awakenings; and disorientation. Urinary or fecal incontinence is common in final stages, and the patient may develop twitching and seizures. Death commonly results from an increased susceptibility to infection.

Diagnostic tests. Psychometric testing and neurologic examination can help establish the diagnosis. PET scan measures the metabolic activity of the cerebral cortex and may help confirm an early diagnosis.

EEG, CT scan, and MRI may help diagnose later stages of Alzheimer's disease. Additional tests may help rule out other causes of dementia.

Treatment. No cure or definitive treatment for Alzheimer's exists. Therapy may consist of cerebral vasodilators, such as ergoloid mesylates, isoxsuprine, and cyclandelate to enhance the brain's circulation; hyperbaric oxygen to increase oxygen supply to the brain; psychostimulators such as methylphenidate to enhance the patient's mood; and antidepressants if depression seems to exacerbate the patient's dementia. Most drug therapies currently being used are experimental. These include choline salts, lecithin, physostigmine, deanol, enkephalins, and naloxone, which may slow the disease process. Another approach to treatment includes avoiding use of antacids, aluminum cooking utensils, and aluminum-containing antiperspirants to help decrease aluminum intake.

Nursing interventions. Establish an effective communication system with the patient and family to help them adjust to the patient's altered cognitive abilities.
- Provide emotional support.
- Protect the patient from injury by providing a safe, structured environment.

• Encourage the patient to exercise, as ordered, to help maintain mobility.

• Set up an appointment with a social services agency, which will help the family assess its needs.

Patient education. Teach the patient's family about the disease, and listen to their concerns. Refer the family to support groups. To locate groups in your area, contact the Alzheimer's Disease and Related Disorders Association.

Evaluation. Treatment seeks to maintain the patient's orientation for as long as possible and to keep him free from injury. Note if the patient has established an adequate sleep pattern and if he can maintain adequate nutrition. Assess whether the family has a sufficient support system to cope with this crisis; both the patient and the family need to express their feelings of loss.

Cranial nerve disorders

A malfunctioning CN can cause painful trigeminal neuralgia and disorders of shorter duration such as Bell's palsy.

Trigeminal neuralgia

Also called tic douloureux, this disorder affects one or more branches of the fifth cranial (trigeminal) nerve. Upon simulation of a trigger zone, the patient experiences paroxysmal attacks of excruciating facial pain. Trigeminal neuralgia can subside spontaneously, with remissions lasting from several months to years. It occurs on the right side of the face more commonly than the left.

Causes. The cause is unknown.

Assessment findings. The patient's pain history forms the basis for diagnosis. Characteristically, the patient experiences searing or burning jabs of pain lasting from 1 to 15 minutes (usually 1 to 2 minutes), localized in an area innervated by one of the divisions of the trigeminal nerve and initiated by a light touch to a hypersensitive area, such as the tip of the nose, the cheeks, or the gums.

Diagnostic tests. To rule out sinus or tooth infections, and tumors, the patient may undergo skull X-rays or a CT scan.

Treatment. Oral administration of carbamazepine or phenytoin may temporarily relieve or prevent pain. Narcotics may prove helpful during the pain episode.

When these medical measures fail or attacks become increasingly frequent or severe, neurosurgical procedures may provide permanent relief. The preferred procedure is percutaneous electrocoagulation of nerve rootlets under local anesthesia. Percutaneous radiofrequency trigeminal gangliolysis and percutaneous retrogasserian glycerol rhizotomy also relieve pain. Microsurgery can treat vascular decompression of the trigeminal nerve.

Nursing interventions. Observe and record the characteristics of each attack, including the patient's protective mechanisms. Provide emotional support, and encourage the patient to express his fear and anxiety. Promote independence through self-care and maximum physical activity. Reinforce natural avoidance of stimulation (air, heat, and cold) of trigger zones (lips, cheeks, and gums).

Provide adequate nutrition in small, frequent meals at room temperature. After surgical decompression of the root or partial nerve dissection, check neurologic and vital signs frequently.

Patient education. Warn the patient receiving carbamazepine to immediately report fever, sore throat, mouth ulcers, easy bruising, or petechial or purpuric hemorrhage because these symptoms may signal thrombocytopenia or aplastic anemia and may require discontinuation of drug therapy.

After resection of the first branch of the trigeminal nerve, tell the patient to avoid rubbing his eyes and using aerosol sprays. Advise him to wear glasses or goggles outdoors and to blink often.

After surgery to sever the second or third branch, tell the patient to avoid hot foods and drinks, which could burn his mouth, and to chew carefully to avoid biting his mouth. Advise him to place food in the unaffected side of his mouth when chewing, to brush his teeth and rinse his mouth often, and to see the dentist twice a year to detect cavities. (Cavities in the area of the severed nerve will not cause pain.)

Evaluation. Assess the effectiveness of medications. Is the patient's pain controlled during acute attacks? Also note if the patient has expressed feelings of loss or fear.

TREATMENTS

This section discusses ongoing advances in treating neurologic dysfunction, including drug therapy, surgery, and related treatments to provide effective nursing care.

Drug therapy

Drugs are critical to the treatment of many neurologic disorders. Anticonvulsants such as carbamazepine, clonazepam, mephenytoin, felbamate, and gabapentin help control seizures. Beta-adrenergic blockers such as propranolol prevent migraine headache, whereas ergot alkaloids such as dihydroergotamine and ergotamine tartrate can relieve it. Corticosteroids such as prednisone help lower ICP. Narcotic and opioid analgesics, such as codeine phosphate, morphine sulfate, and meperidine, can be used for mild to moderate pain. Cholinergics—such as ambenonium chloride and prostigmine bromide—are useful in the treatment of myasthenia gravis, whereas antiparkinsonian agents—such as benztropine, biperiden hydrochloride, and levodopa—are useful in treating Parkinson's disease. Skeletal muscle relaxants, such as baclofen and dantrolene, help relieve the spasticity found in MS.

When caring for a patient undergoing drug therapy, you'll need to be alert for severe adverse reactions and for interactions with other drugs. Some drugs such as the barbiturates also carry a high risk for toxicity and dependence.

Keep in mind that therapy's success hinges on the patient's strict adherence to his medication schedule. Compliance is especially critical for drugs that require steady-state blood levels for therapeutic effectiveness (such as anticonvulsants) or for drugs used prophylactically (such as beta-adrenergic blockers).

Surgery

Life-threatening neurologic disorders usually call for emergency surgery. For example, an epidural hematoma typically requires immediate aspiration. A cerebral aneurysm requires correction through clipping or another technique. These and other surgeries often involve a craniotomy, a procedure that opens the skull and exposes the brain.

Prepare to be responsible for the patient's preoperative assessment and postoperative care. You'll also have to answer questions raised by the patient and his family and provide appropriate education—whether it involves ventricular shunt care or cosmetic care after craniotomy. And because the prospect of surgery usually provokes fear and anxiety, you'll need to provide ongoing emotional support.

Craniotomy

Craniotomy involves creation of a surgical incision into the skull,

thereby exposing the brain for any number of treatments. These treatments may include ventricular shunting, excision of a tumor or abscess, hematoma aspiration, and aneurysm clipping. Craniotomy has many potential complications, including infection, hemorrhage, respiratory compromise, and increased ICP; the degree of risk depends largely on the patient's condition and the surgery's complexity.

After the patient receives a general anesthetic, the surgeon cuts through the scalp, cuts out a bone flap with a small saw, and exposes the brain. He then proceeds with the surgery. Afterward, he reverses the incision procedure and covers the site with a sterile dressing. Then the patient is taken to the intensive care unit (ICU) for recovery.

Patient preparation. Help the patient and family cope with the surgery by clarifying the doctor's explanation and by encouraging them to ask questions. (See *Cranial surgery*, page 298.)

Explain preoperative procedures. Tell the patient that his hair will be washed on the night before surgery. In the operating room, his head will be shaved, and he'll receive steroids to reduce postoperative inflammation. His legs may also be wrapped with elastic bandages to improve venous return and reduce the risk of thrombophlebitis. He may also have a urinary catheter inserted.

Also prepare the patient for postoperative recovery. Explain that he'll awaken from surgery with a

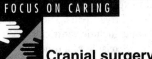

Cranial surgery

Because cranial surgery can be an overwhelming procedure, spending time with the patient and family preoperatively, especially if the diagnosis is a tumor, will help to reduce anxiety. Answer the patient and family's questions honestly. Reassure them and try to instill a level of confidence.

Provide the family with written reminders such as:
• the expected length of surgery
• where to wait until the surgery is over
• phone number for the intensive care unit and visiting times if appropriate.

Provide the patient with a cap or a turban that he can wear postoperatively to decrease anxiety about appearance and enhance self-esteem.

large dressing on his head to protect the incision. He may have a surgical drain implanted in his skull for a few days and will be receiving prophylactic antibiotics. Warn him to expect a headache and facial swelling for 2 to 3 days after surgery, and reassure him that he'll receive pain medication. Explain that, if all goes well, he should be ambulatory 2 to 3 days after surgery. The surgeon will usually remove the sutures within 7 days.

Before surgery, perform a complete neurologic assessment. Carefully record your assessment data to use as a baseline for postoperative evaluation.

Arrange a preoperative visit to the ICU for the patient and his family. Explain the equipment and introduce them to the staff.

Monitoring and aftercare. After surgery, carefully monitor the patient's vital signs and neurologic status. Check him every 15 minutes for the first 4 hours, then once every 30 to 60 minutes for the next 24 to 48 hours.

To help prevent increased ICP, position the patient on his side. Elevate his head 15 to 30 degrees. With another nurse's help, turn him carefully every 2 hours.

Throughout postoperative care, observe the patient closely for signs of increased ICP. Immediately notify the doctor if you note worsening mental status, pupillary changes, or focal signs, such as increasing weakness in an extremity.

Closely observe the patient's respiratory status, noting rate and pattern. Immediately report any abnormalities. Encourage him to deepbreathe and cough, but warn him not to do this too strenuously. Suction gently, as ordered.

Carefully monitor fluid and electrolyte balance. The doctor may restrict fluid intake to minimize cerebral edema and prevent increased ICP. Monitor and record intake and output, check urine specific gravity every 2 hours, and weigh the patient, as ordered. Check serum electrolyte levels every 24 hours and watch the patient for signs of imbalance. Because fluid and electrolyte imbalance can precipitate seizures, report confusion, stupor, weakness, or lethargy immediately.

Provide good wound care. Make sure the dressing stays dry and in place, and that it's not too tight. Excessive dressing tightness may indicate swelling—a sign of increased ICP. If the patient has a closed drainage system, periodically check drain patency and note and document the amount and characteristics of any discharge. Notify the doctor of excessive bloody drainage, possibly indicating cerebral hemorrhage, or of clear or yellow drainage, which may indicate a CSF leak. Also monitor the patient for signs of wound infection, such as fever and purulent drainage.

Finally, provide supportive care. Ensure a quiet, calm environment to help lower ICP. Administer anticonvulsants, as ordered, and maintain seizure precautions. Provide other ordered medications, such as steroids to prevent or reduce cerebral edema, stool softeners to prevent increased ICP from straining, and analgesics to relieve pain.

Patient education. Before discharge, teach the patient proper wound care techniques. Tell him to keep the suture line dry and to regularly clean the incision according to the doctor's instructions. Instruct him to evaluate the incision regularly for redness, warmth, or tenderness and to report any of these findings to the doctor.

If the patient is self-conscious about hair loss, suggest a hat, wig, or scarf. As hair begins to grow back, advise the patient to apply a lanolin-based lotion to keep his scalp supple and decrease itching. However, tell him not to apply lotion to the suture line.

Remind the patient to continue taking prescribed anticonvulsant medications to minimize the risk of seizures. Depending on the type of surgery performed, he may need to continue anticonvulsant therapy for up to 12 months after surgery. Also remind him to report any adverse drug reactions, such as excessive drowsiness or confusion.

Cerebral aneurysm repair

Surgical treatment represents the only sure method to prevent initial rupture or rebleeding of a cerebral aneurysm. The surgeon can choose among several techniques, depending on the shape and location of the aneurysm. He may clamp the affected artery, wrap the aneurysm wall with a biological or synthetic material, or clip or ligate the aneurysm.

After cerebral angiography has ruled out vasospasm, the surgeon performs a craniotomy—usually in the suboccipital or subfrontal areas—to expose the aneurysm.

Then the surgeon wraps the aneurysm with a biological or synthetic material. Or, he opens a small, spring-loaded clip and slips it over the neck of the aneurysm or over its feeder vessel. Then he releases it, letting it close to block blood flow to the aneurysm. He then ligates and removes the sac of the aneurysm.

Finally, the surgeon reverses the craniotomy procedure to close the incision.

Patient preparation. Explain the purpose of the surgery to the patient. Tell him he'll receive a general anesthetic and then undergo a craniotomy to open the skull and expose the aneurysm.

Before the operation, frequently monitor the patient's neurologic status, checking his pupillary response, LOC, and motor function. Record your assessment data to use as a baseline for your postoperative evaluation.

Because stress and activity elevate arterial pressure, which in turn can cause the aneurysm to rupture or rebleed, enforce bed rest and encourage the patient to rest and sleep as much as possible. Provide him with a darkened, quiet environment and try to anticipate all of his physiologic needs. Restrict his activities and limit visitors. Explain the reasons for these precautions and restrictions to the patient and his family, and enlist the family's help in enforcing them.

Despite these restrictions, the patient needs some activity to prevent skin breakdown and reduce the risk of pulmonary complications. Encourage him to deep-breathe, but warn him that coughing and sneezing may cause problems. If you need to suction the patient, do so gently. Carefully turn the patient every 2 hours. As appropriate, encourage him to perform ROM exercises every 2 hours. (If the patient can't perform active exercises, provide passive exercise for his legs more often than every 2 hours to help prevent thrombus formation.) To also help prevent thrombus formation, apply antiembolism stockings, elastic bandages, or automatic compression boots.

Administer medications, as ordered. These may include anticonvulsants to prevent seizures, corticosteroids to prevent cerebral edema, stool softeners to prevent increased ICP from straining, and analgesics to relieve headache. If the patient is receiving I.V. fluids, carefully monitor and record his fluid intake and output.

The aneurysm can rupture at any time, so watch for and immediately report any early signs and symptoms of it: a new or worsening headache, renewed or increased nuchal rigidity, or decreasing LOC. Also notify the doctor of signs of increased ICP, including pupillary changes and focal neurologic deficits such as increasing weakness in an extremity.

If the patient is awaiting surgery for an already-ruptured aneurysm, observe him for signs of rebleeding and elevated ICP.

Monitoring and aftercare. Monitor the patient for vasospasm, the constriction of intracranial blood vessels from smooth-muscle contraction. It may occur suddenly and without warning, and usually begins in the vessel adjacent to the aneurysm. Depending on its intensity, it can spread through the major cerebral vessels, causing ischemia and possible infarction of involved areas with corresponding loss of neuromuscular function. Call the doctor immediately if you note hemiparesis, worsening of an existing motor deficit, visual disturbances, seizures, or altered LOC.

After surgery, explain to the patient that he can gradually resume his normal activities. Focus on measures to promote healing of the craniotomy site.

Keep in mind that a patient with a cerebral aneurysm may be left with neurologic deficits that frustrate and possibly embarrass him and his family. Your positive, caring attitude and support can help them cope.

Patient education. Emphasize the importance of returning for scheduled follow-up examinations and tests. For additional instructions, see "Craniotomy," page 297.

Intracranial hematoma aspiration

An intracranial hematoma usually requires lifesaving surgery to lower ICP. Even if the patient doesn't face an immediate threat to his life, he usually must undergo surgery to prevent irreversible damage from cerebral or brain stem ischemia.

For a solid clot or a liquid one that can't be completely aspirated through burr holes, the surgeon performs a craniotomy and aspirates the hematoma with a small suction tip. He also may use saline irrigation. He then ligates any bleeding vessels in the hematoma cavity and closes the bone and scalp flaps. (If cerebral edema is severe, he

may leave the craniotomy site exposed until edema subsides.) Usually, he places a drain in the surgical site.

If the hematoma is fluid, the surgeon may use a twist drill to bore holes through the skull. Once he reaches the clot, he inserts a small suction tip into the holes to aspirate it. He then inserts drains, which usually remain in place for 24 hours.

Hematoma aspiration carries the risk of severe infection and seizures as well as the physiologic problems associated with immobility during the prolonged recovery period. Even if hematoma removal proves successful, associated head injuries and complications such as cerebral edema can produce permanent neurologic deficits, coma, or even death.

Patient preparation. If emergency aspiration is necessary, briefly explain the procedure to the patient, if possible. If you have more time, clarify the surgeon's explanation and encourage the patient to ask questions. Then prepare the patient as you would for a craniotomy.

Monitoring and aftercare. After surgery, take the following steps:
• Perform a complete neurologic assessment and compare your findings to preoperative results.
• As ordered, give analgesics to relieve pain, antibiotics to prevent infection, and anticonvulsants to prevent seizures.
• Carefully monitor the patient's vital signs and watch for signs or

symptoms of elevated ICP—headache, altered respirations, deteriorating LOC, and visual disturbances. Keep resuscitation equipment on hand.

Take steps to prevent increased ICP, especially if the patient's hematoma was aspirated through the holes. As ordered, and if the patient's condition permits, keep his head elevated about 30 degrees to promote venous drainage from the brain. Also as ordered, maintain fluid restrictions and give osmotic diuretics or corticosteroids to decrease cerebral edema. Accurately record fluid intake and output.

Regularly check the surgical dressing and the surrounding area for excessive bleeding or drainage. Evaluate drain patency by noting the amount of drainage. Although the doctor may set specific guidelines, drainage usually shouldn't exceed 100 ml during the first 8 hours after surgery, 75 ml during the following 8 hours, and 50 ml over the next 8 hours. Report any abnormal drainage. Also ensure that the drainage is tested for glucose to detect any leakage of CSF.

If the patient is on bed rest for a prolonged period, turn the patient frequently and perform passive ROM exercises for all extremities.

Patient education. Teach the patient and his family to perform proper suture care techniques. Tell them to observe the suture line for signs of infection, such as redness and swelling, and to report any such signs immediately. Also advise them to watch for and report any neurologic symptoms, such as altered LOC and sudden weakness.

Instruct the patient to continue taking prescribed anticonvulsant medications, as ordered, to minimize the risk of seizures. Have him report any adverse reactions, such as drowsiness or confusion.

Advise him to wear a wig, hat, or scarf until hair grows back. Tell him to use a lanolin-based lotion to help keep the scalp supple and decrease itching. Caution against applying lotion to the suture line.

Instruct him to take acetaminophen or another mild nonnarcotic analgesic for headaches, if needed.

Cerebellar stimulator implantation

Cerebellar stimulator implantation uses electrical impulses to regulate uncoordinated neuromuscular activity. This device is used to prevent seizures in patients who don't respond to drug therapy and may also provide better neuromuscular control in those with cerebral palsy. Possible benefits for such patients include reduced spasticity and abnormal movements, improved muscle and sphincter control, clearer speech, and decreased seizure activity. However, not all patients realize these benefits. And, in those who do, improvement may occur gradually over several months or even years.

The cerebellar stimulator consists of two surgically implanted cerebellar electrodes attached to either an internal or an external power source and pulse generator.

This device stimulates the fibers of the cerebellar cortex.

The surgeon makes a small scalp incision and drill hole in the right occipital area to help relieve postoperative intracranial hematoma or excessive edema. Then he drills two burr holes in the suboccipital area and carefully places an electrode pad on the surface of each lobe of the cerebellum. Using X-rays, he checks electrode placement.

The surgeon creates a subcutaneous pocket in the infraclavicular area or the right lower abdominal quadrant and implants the pulse generator and power source of the monophasic internal system. He then makes a subcutaneous tunnel running from the scalp incision down the side of the neck to the pocket. Through this tunnel he threads the electrode leads and lead connectors. He then supervises the necessary hookups and testing of the unit's function and the patient's response.

Patient preparation. Tailor your explanation to the patient's age and level of understanding. Explain that the device regulates the brain's muscle control center much like a pacemaker regulates the heart, providing regularly timed electrical impulses that stimulate the muscles to function normally.

Explain the various components and how they work, stressing that the device's low-voltage electrical current can't harm him. Briefly describe the implantation procedure. Explain that after he receives a general anesthetic, his head will be shaved and placed in a special headrest for the operation. Then the surgeon will make four incisions for implanting the electrodes and other system components: two on the head, one on the neck, and one on the abdomen. Tell him that when he wakes he'll feel the most pain from the neck incision but will receive pain medication.

Discuss postoperative care measures, such as activity and fluid restrictions, progressive ambulation, and antibiotic therapy. Mention that you'll monitor him carefully to evaluate the device.

Before surgery, perform a complete neuromuscular evaluation to serve as a baseline.

Monitoring and aftercare. After surgery, carefully assess the patient's neurologic status and vital signs every hour for the first 24 hours, then once every 2 hours for the next few days. Watch for developing complications, such as increased ICP, infection, fluid imbalance, and aspiration pneumonia. Provide I.V. fluids, as ordered, if the patient experiences excessive nausea and vomiting because of cerebellar manipulation. Also observe for and record any seizure activity or spasticity to help the doctor evaluate the device.

Maintain the patient on bed rest until the second day after surgery. Keep his head elevated 15 to 30 degrees and turn him every 2 hours. Slowly increase his activities but be sure he avoids overexertion. Excessive activity can cause pooling of serous fluid or CSF in the subcutaneous pocket, possibly damaging the equipment.

Regularly check the patient's dressings for excessive bleeding or drainage, and change them as necessary. Assess suture lines for signs of infection and provide wound care. Administer antibiotics and analgesics, as ordered, but don't give the patient sedatives for sleep; they may skew neurologic findings.

Patient education. Explain that the patient can gradually resume his normal routine, but advise against excessive physical activity.

Teach him and his family how to change a dressing. Tell them to change it about once every 2 days until the surgeon removes the sutures (usually about 2 weeks after surgery). Instruct them in proper wound care techniques for the suture lines.

Tell the patient to watch for and report early signs of infection, such as fever and swelling or redness at the suture lines or subcutaneous pouches. Instruct him to record the time, type, and duration of any seizures. Explain that this record will help the doctor evaluate the effectiveness of the cerebellar stimulator.

Finally, explain that the patient should keep regular follow-up appointments to check on his condition and the unit's function.

Ventricular shunting

Ventricular shunting for hydrocephalus involves insertion of a catheter into the ventricular system to drain CSF into another body space (usually the peritoneal sac) for absorption. The shunt extends from the cerebral ventricle to the scalp, where it's tunneled under the skin to the appropriate cavity.

Ventricular shunts treat hydrocephalus. By draining excessive CSF or relieving blockage of CSF flow, shunting can lower ICP and prevent brain damage caused by persistently elevated ICP.

To implant a shunt, the surgeon performs a craniotomy to gain access to the implantation site. He then inserts a catheter into the ventricular system. Shunts may be ventriculoperitoneal, ventriculoatrial, or ventriculocisternal.

Patient preparation. Tell the patient or his family that this procedure lowers ICP and helps prevent brain damage. Prepare the patient as you would for a craniotomy. Explain that he'll have dressings on his head and, depending on the site of drainage, on his abdomen or chest.

Carefully monitor the patient's vital signs and neurologic status and watch for signs and symptoms of increased ICP, such as headache, vomiting, irritability, visual disturbances, and decreased LOC.

Monitoring and aftercare. Carefully monitor for signs of infection and use strict aseptic technique when providing shunt and suture care. You may also be called upon to pump the shunt and check for any malfunction.

Besides infection, ventricular shunting carries a risk of ventricular collapse from improper catheter placement or faulty pumping techniques. The shunt can become blocked or kinked resulting in elevated ICP.

Provide postoperative care as you would for a patient recovering from craniotomy. However, rather than elevate the patient's head after surgery, gradually raise his head in stages, about 20 degrees at a time. This will help him adjust to lowered ICP. During this period, carefully check vital signs and neurologic status every 2 hours. Immediately report any signs of elevated ICP, which may indicate a blocked or malfunctioning shunt.

Check for and report any signs or symptoms of infection, such as fever, headache, nuchal rigidity, and local pain and inflammation. If infection occurs, the doctor will probably order I.V. antibiotics. If the infection doesn't subside within 1 to 2 weeks, he'll remove and replace the shunt.

To avoid placing pressure on the shunt suture lines, position the patient on the nonoperative side. This will protect against suture abrasion and prevent local dependent edema.

If ordered, pump the shunt. Use proper technique to avoid excessive CSF drainage from the ventricular system, which can abruptly reduce ICP and lead to ventricular collapse or blood vessel rupture. While pumping, watch for signs of rapidly rising ICP, which may indicate ventricular collapse.

Patient education. Teach the patient's family about proper suture line care. Demonstrate how to mix a 1:1 hydrogen peroxide and saline solution and how to use sterile technique when cleaning the suture line. Tell them to report signs of infection or increased ICP immediately.

Advise the patient's family to make sure the patient doesn't lie over the catheter's course for a prolonged period.

Teach the patient and his family how to pump the shunt. As ordered, teach them to locate the pump by feeling for the soft center of the device under the skin behind the ear and to depress the center of the pump with a forefinger and then slowly release it. Advise the patient to pump only as many times as the doctor has ordered (usually between 25 and 50 times, once or twice a day). Caution that excessive pumping can lead to serious complications.

After shunt insertion, the doctor may order a 6- to 12-month course of anticonvulsant drug therapy. If so, reinforce the importance of complying with the medication schedule to prevent seizures. Also discuss possible drug adverse effects—especially those affecting the CNS and cardiovascular system—and the need to inform the doctor of any adverse reactions.

Other neurologic treatments

Additional treatments include a noninvasive technique for correcting an AVM, barbiturate coma, and plasmapheresis.

AVM embolization

AVM embolization is a noninvasive technique that allows treatment of an AVM when surgical excision proves unsafe or impossible. The neuroradiologist, guided by cerebral angiography, injects or inserts silicone beads or polymer material to occlude blood flow to the AVM.

Although it rarely destroys the AVM, embolization may shrink the defect and usually decreases the risk of rupture and hemorrhage. It may also reduce pressure on adjacent brain tissue, possibly relieving existing neurologic abnormalities caused by the AVM.

Patient preparation. Explain to the patient that this procedure will shrink his AVM and decrease the risk of cerebral hemorrhage. Briefly describe the steps of this 2-hour procedure.

Tell the patient that he'll be placed on an X-ray table with his head immobilized and he'll be asked to lie still. Tell him that he'll receive either a local or a general anesthetic at the catheter insertion site. Caution him that he'll probably feel a transient burning sensation during injection of the contrast medium and that he may feel flushed and warm and experience nausea or vomiting, headache, and a salty taste in his mouth after injection. Reassure him that the injection is painless.

Check the patient's history for hypersensitivity to iodine, iodine-containing foods such as shellfish, or other radiographic contrast media. Notify the doctor of any such hypersensitivities; he may need to order prophylactic medications or may choose not to perform the procedure.

Instruct the patient to fast for 8 to 10 hours before the procedure and to void just before it starts. Tell him to put on a hospital gown and to remove all jewelry, dentures, hairpins, and other radiopaque objects in the X-ray field. If ordered, administer a sedative and an anticholinergic 30 to 45 minutes before the procedure.

Monitoring and aftercare. Before AVM embolization, monitor the patient closely for any developing complications, including headache, focal or generalized tonic-clonic seizures, increased ICP, and focal neurologic signs, such as twitching or tremors.

During contrast medium injection, keep emergency resuscitation equipment readily available. Monitor the patient for early signs or symptoms of hypersensitivity, such as erythema, pruritus, thready pulse, sweating, and anxiety. If you detect any of these, inform the surgeon immediately; he will stop the injection and, if necessary, begin emergency treatment.

After catheter removal, take the following steps:
• Enforce bed rest. Monitor the patient's vital signs and neurologic status every hour for the first 4 hours and then every 4 hours for the next 20 hours. Apply an ice bag to relieve pain and reduce swelling, and keep the site immobilized.

• Check the insertion site for redness and swelling, indicating extravasation.

• Control any bleeding with firm pressure.

• If catheterization was done in the femoral artery, keep the affected leg still for 12 hours after the procedure. Watch for possible thrombus or hematoma formation by regularly checking all pulses distal to the insertion site and assessing the affected leg's temperature, color, and sensation.

• If a carotid artery was used for catheterization, observe the patient for dysphagia and respiratory distress, which can result from extravasation. Also watch for signs or symptoms of thrombosis, hematoma, or arterial spasm, such as disorientation and weakness or numbness in the extremities. Immediately notify the doctor if any of these develop.

• Provide a quiet, softly lit environment and limit visitors. This will help reduce the risk of AVM bleeding after embolization.

• Administer analgesics and sedatives, as ordered, and provide a soft, high-fiber diet with stool softeners, as needed.

Patient education. Instruct the patient and his family to immediately report any abnormal symptoms, such as severe headache, weakness in the extremities, or deteriorating LOC. Explain that these symptoms require immediate medical evaluation.

Barbiturate coma

When conventional treatments, such as fluid restriction, diuretic or corticosteroid therapy, or ventricular shunting, fail to correct sustained or acute episodes of increased ICP, the doctor may order barbiturate coma. In this treatment, the patient receives high I.V. doses of a short-acting barbiturate (such as pentobarbital or phenobarbital) to produce coma. The drug reduces the patient's metabolic rate and cerebral blood flow, possibly relieving increased ICP and protecting cerebral tissue.

Barbiturate coma offers a last resort for patients with acute ICP elevation above 40 mm Hg, persistent elevation above 20 mm Hg, or rapidly deteriorating neurologic status that's unresponsive to other treatments. If this treatment proves unsuccessful in lowering ICP, the prognosis for recovery is poor.

Besides having only a marginal degree of effectiveness, barbiturate coma carries some serious risks. The most serious risk results from the small margin between therapeutic and toxic doses. On the one hand, a high dose is needed to induce coma; on the other, toxicity can produce severe, possibly fatal, CNS and respiratory depression. Even a therapeutic dose can cause complications, such as hypotension and arrhythmias. Overly abrupt withdrawal of barbiturates may produce convulsions or delirium.

Before inducing barbiturate coma, the doctor orders an EEG and possibly brain stem auditory-evoked response testing to establish a neurologic baseline. He also orders the patient placed on mechanical ventilation, ICP monitoring, cardiac and intra-arterial pressure monitoring, and pulmonary artery pressure monitoring.

The doctor then administers a loading dose of barbiturate, 3 to 5 mg/kg via I.V. push, and watches the ICP monitor for a pressure decrease of at least 10 mm Hg within 10 minutes. If this drop doesn't occur, he may administer a second dose 2 hours later.

Once the loading dose lowers ICP significantly, he orders hourly maintenance doses of 1 to 3 mg/kg or amounts sufficient to achieve a steady-state serum level of 2 to 4 mg/dl.

After the doctor determines that the patient's ICP has stabilized within acceptable limits (between 4 and 15 mm Hg), he discontinues therapy. He'll also order discontinuation if therapy proves unsuccessful at lowering ICP or if the patient shows signs of progressive neurologic impairment. To prevent adverse effects of abrupt withdrawal (including seizures and hallucinations), expect to withdraw barbiturates gradually, at a rate based on the patient's condition and the doses administered during therapy.

Patient preparation. Expect to focus your attention on the patient's family. They'll probably be frightened by the patient's condition and apprehensive about the treatment. Provide clear explanations of the procedure and its effects, and encourage them to ask questions. Convey a sense of optimism but provide no guarantee of the treatment's success. Because barbiturate coma represents a last-ditch effort to reduce ICP and save the patient's life, prepare them for the possibility that the patient may die or have permanent neurologic impairment.

Also prepare the family for observable—and, to them, quite disturbing—changes in the patient's status during therapy, such as decreased respirations, hypotension, and loss of muscle tone and reflexes. Reassure them that despite the patient's disturbing appearance, he's being carefully monitored and provided with the necessary supportive care to ensure safe treatment. Briefly explain the various monitoring and supportive measures used during therapy.

Monitoring and aftercare. During barbiturate coma, closely monitor the patient's ICP, electrocardiogram (ECG), and vital signs. Notify the doctor of increased ICP, arrhythmias, or hypotension. Check serum barbiturate levels frequently, as ordered.

Because you may not be able to evaluate a patient's neurologic function while he's in a drug-induced coma, provide respiratory and nutritional support and direct your care to preventing complications such as respiratory depression.

After discontinuation of therapy, and as the patient emerges from coma, watch him for signs of returning neurologic function. Begin by checking his gag reflex and assessing his response to painful stimuli, then work up to a full neurologic evaluation. Remember, however, that only after withdrawal is complete and the

CRITICAL THINKING

Identifying a problem with barbiturate coma therapy

Your patient has been receiving several days of barbiturate coma treatment and up until today, the therapy has been successful and your patient's intracranial pressure (ICP) has been decreasing. However, today you note a sudden rise in the patient's ICP reading. You find no stimulation at the patient's bedside that would increase the ICP. Upon further investigation you note that both the patient's pupils are dilated and unresponsive to light.

You check the chart. The patient is also receiving a smooth-muscle relaxant called pancuronium (Pavulon). You take the patient's vital signs. Suddenly the blood pressure is higher than baseline readings and the patient is also newly tachycardiac. While assessing the patient further, you repeat the ICP reading and the vital signs. You note that they've now returned to baseline; however, the pupils still remain extremely dilated and unresponsive to light. What is happening to your patient?

Suggested response

Most likely, your patient is having a seizure. Phenobarbital, which was used to institute the barbiturate coma, decreases the action of the phenytoin that he's receiving. The seizure cannot be visualized because Pavulon masks muscle activity.

patient is fully conscious can you begin to determine the full extent of any neurologic impairment.

When easing the patient off of barbiturates, watch for sporadic elevations in ICP and for adverse effects of barbiturate withdrawal. If you note tremors, agitation, delirium, hallucinations, incoordination, or seizures, notify the doctor; place the patient in a quiet, darkened room; and keep him still. Take seizure precautions, such as padding the bed rails and keeping emergency equipment available.

Finally, don't neglect to consider the patient's family; they'll probably have many fears and doubts about this treatment and will benefit greatly from your clear explanations and ongoing emotional support.

For a test of your critical thinking skills, see *Identifying a problem with barbiturate coma therapy*.

Patient education. Tailor your instructions to the patient's specific neurologic impairments. For patients with preexisting neurologic dysfunction, remind the family that the elevated ICP may have caused additional impairment and that they should prepare to adjust the patient's care accordingly.

Plasmapheresis

Plasmapheresis consists of a therapeutic removal of plasma from withdrawn blood and the reinfusion of formed blood elements. Blood removed from the patient flows into a cell separator, where it's divided into plasma and formed elements. The plasma is collected in a container for disposal, while the formed elements are mixed with a plasma replacement solution and returned to the patient through a vein. In a newer method of plasmapheresis, the plasma is separated out, filtered to remove a specific disease mediator, and then returned to the patient.

The procedure, done under a doctor's supervision, requires a specially trained technician or nurse to operate the cell separator and a primary nurse to monitor the patient and provide supportive care.

By removing and replacing the plasma, plasmapheresis cleans the blood of harmful substances such as toxins and of disease mediators, such as immune complexes and autoantibodies. Consequently, plasmapheresis has several neurologic applications, such as in Guillain-Barré syndrome, MS, and especially myasthenia gravis. In myasthenia gravis, plasmapheresis removes circulating antiacetylcholine receptor antibodies. If successful, treatment may relieve symptoms for months; however, results vary. Used most commonly in patients with long-standing neuromuscular disease, plasmapheresis may also treat acute exacerbations. Acutely ill patients may undergo this procedure as often as four times a week; others about once every 2 weeks.

Plasmapheresis risks several possible complications: a hypersensitivity reaction to the ingredients of the replacement solution and hypocalcemia from excessive binding of circulating calcium to the citrate solution used as an anticoagulant in the replacement solution. Hypomagnesemia can follow repeated plasmapheresis, producing severe muscle cramps and tetany. And, the patient risks hypotension and other complications of low blood volume.

Patient preparation. Briefly discuss the treatment and its purpose with the patient. Tell him that a needle will be inserted into one or both arms and that his blood will be pumped through a filtering machine, cleaned of harmful substances, then returned to his body. Explain that the procedure may take up to 5 hours. Inform him that, during treatment, frequent blood samples will be taken to monitor calcium and potassium levels, and his blood pressure and heart rate will be checked regularly. Instruct him to report any paresthesias.

Advise the patient to eat lightly before treatment and to drink milk before and during treatment to help reduce the risk of hypocalcemia. Tell the patient to urinate before the procedure.

Before treatment, take vital signs for a baseline. As ordered, apply ECG leads to monitor heart rate. Also as ordered, draw blood samples for tests to determine baseline levels of hemoglobin, hematocrit, and other blood substances. If possible, give medications after treatment instead of before, to prevent their removal from the blood.

Monitoring and aftercare. As plasmapheresis begins, observe the patient for signs of hypersensitivity, such as respiratory distress, hives, diaphoresis, hypotension, or thready pulse. If any such signs occur, immediately notify the doctor, who will stop the procedure and provide emergency treatment.

During treatment, monitor vital signs every 30 minutes. (Don't take blood pressure readings in the arm being used for blood withdrawal and reinfusion.) Pay particular attention to temperature; reinfusion of blood that has cooled while in the cell separator can produce hypothermia.

Report any serious arrhythmias. Because arrhythmias can result from electrolyte imbalance or volume depletion, monitor blood levels of calcium and potassium and replace electrolytes, as ordered. Monitor intake and output to ensure adequate hydration. Also watch for signs of circulatory compromise. Compare levels of hematocrit, hemoglobin, electrolytes, antibody titers, and immune complexes with pretreatment levels.

If the patient is undergoing plasmapheresis for unstable myasthenia gravis, keep emergency equipment on hand and monitor blood pressure and pulse rate. Observe for signs or symptoms of myasthenic crisis (dysphagia, ptosis, and diplopia), which this treatment can precipitate.

After completion of treatment and removal of needles, apply direct pressure on the puncture sites, then apply pressure dressings. Periodically assess the dressings for drainage and the puncture sites for signs of extravasation.

Patient education. Tell the patient he may feel tired for a day or two after plasmapheresis. (If he's undergoing repeated treatments, he may develop chronic fatigue.) Advise him to rest frequently during this period and to avoid strenuous activities. Unless contraindicated, instruct him to maintain a high-protein diet and to take a multivitamin with iron daily.

Inform the patient undergoing repeated treatments that he may require transfusions of fresh-frozen plasma to replace normal clotting factors lost in removed plasma.

Because plasmapheresis can cause immunosuppression, warn him to avoid contact with persons with colds or other contagious viruses. Also instruct him to watch for and report any signs of hepatitis.

REFERENCES AND READINGS

Cochran, I., et al. "Stroke Care: Piecing Together the Long-term Picture," *Nursing94* 23(5):34-41, 1994.

Dolan, J. *Critical Care Nursing: Clinical Management Through the Nursing Process*, 2nd ed. Philadelphia: F.A. Davis Co., 1996.

Fischbach, F.A. *A Manual of Laboratory and Diagnostic Tests*, 5th ed. Philadelphia: Lippincott-Raven Pubs., 1996.

Guyton, A. *Textbook of Medical Physiology*, 9th ed. Philadelphia: W.B. Saunders Co., 1995.

Hackler, W., et al. "Intravenous Thrombolysis with Recombinant Tissue Plasminogen Activator for Acute Hemispheric Stroke," *JAMA* 274(13):1017-25.

Hickey, J.V. *Clinical Practice of Neurological and Neurosurgical Nursing*, 4th ed. Philadelphia: Lippincott-Raven Pubs., 1997.

Illustrated Guide to Diagnostic Tests, 2nd ed. Springhouse, Pa.: Springhouse Corp., 1997.

Jordam, K.G. "Neurophysiologic Monitoring in the Neuroscience ICU," *Neurologic Clinics* 13(3):579-626, 1995.

McCafferty, M., and Beebe, A. *Pain: A Clinical Manual for Nursing Practice*. St. Louis: Mosby–Year Book, Inc., 1994.

Nursing98 Drug Handbook. Springhouse, Pa.: Springhouse Corp., 1998.

Professional Guide to Diseases, 5th ed. Springhouse, Pa.: Springhouse Corp., 1995.

Rakel, R.E., ed. *Conn's Current Therapy 1996*. Philadelphia: W.B. Saunders Co., 1996.

Shepard, J.T., and Fox, S.W. "Assessment and Management of Hypertension in Acute Ischemic Stroke Patients," *Journal of Neuroscience Nursing* 28(1):5-12, 1996.

Sparks, S.M., et al. *Nursing Diagnosis Pocket Manual*, Springhouse, Pa.: Springhouse Corp., 1996.

Wilberger, J.E., and Cantella, D. "High-dose Barbiturates for Intracranial Pressure Control," *New Horizons* 3(3):469-73, 1995.

Wilson, J.D., et al., eds. *Harrison's Principles of Internal Medicine*, 13th ed. New York: McGraw-Hill Book Co., 1994.

7

MUSCULOSKELETAL CARE

Be prepared to call on the full range of your nursing skills when providing musculoskeletal care. Fractures, dislocations, and other musculoskeletal injuries are some of the most common problems you'll see. Osteoarthritis and other disorders commonly debilitate the muscles, bones, and joints of elderly patients.

This chapter will help you refine the many clinical skills needed for this diverse patient population.

ASSESSMENT

When the patient's health history or physical findings suggest musculoskeletal involvement, you'll need to perform a complete assessment of this system, beginning with a thorough history.

Evaluate the patient's body symmetry, posture, gait, and muscle and joint function as well as his general appearance. You may need to check neurovascular status, including motion, sensation, and circulation.

Because joint or bone pain symptoms commonly indicate a systemic disease, the patient may require a complete physical examination.

Physical examination

Perform a head-to-toe assessment, simultaneously evaluating muscle and joint function of each body area in turn. You'll need to observe the patient's posture, gait, and coordination, and inspect and palpate his muscles, joints, and bones.

Preparing for the examination

Gather the necessary equipment, including a tape measure and a goniometer or protractor for measuring angles. Position the examination table to allow full range of motion (ROM) for the patient and easy access for the assessment.

Observing posture, gait, and coordination

Assessment begins the instant you see the patient. Observe muscle strength, facial muscle movement, body symmetry, and obvious physical or functional deformities or abnormalities.

Assess the patient's overall body symmetry as he moves. Note marked dissimilarities in side-to-side size, shape, and motion.

Posture. Evaluating posture includes inspecting spinal curvature and knee positioning.

Spinal curvature. Instruct the patient to stand as straight as possible. Standing to the patient's side, back, and front, respectively, inspect the spine for alignment and the shoulders, iliac crests, and scapulae for symmetry of position and height. Then have the patient bend forward from the waist with arms relaxed and dangling. Standing behind him, inspect the straightness of the spine, noting flank and thorax position and symmetry. Normally, convex curvature characterizes the thoracic spine and concave curvature characterizes the lumbar spine in a standing patient.

Other normal findings include a midline spine without lateral curvatures, a concave lumbar curvature that changes to a convex curvature in the flexed position, and iliac crests, shoulders, and scapulae at the same horizontal level.

Knee positioning. Have the patient stand with his feet together. Note the relation of one knee to the other. They should be bilaterally symmetrical and located at the same height in a forward-facing position. Normally, the knees are less than 1″ (2.5 cm) apart and the medial malleoli (ankle bones) are less than 1⅛″ (3 cm) apart.

Gait. Direct the patient to walk away, turn around, and walk back. Observe and evaluate his posture, movement (such as pace and length of stride), foot position, coordination, and balance. During the *stance phase,* the foot on the floor should flatten completely and be able to bear the weight of the body. As he pushes off, the toes should be flexed. In the *swing phase,* the foot in midswing should clear the floor and pass the opposite leg in its stance phase. When the swing phase ends, he should be able to control the swing as it stops, as the foot again contacts the floor.

Other normal findings include smooth, coordinated movements, the head leading the body when turning, and erect posture with approximately 2″ to 4″ (5 to 10 cm) of space between the feet. Be sure to remain close to an elderly or infirm patient and ready to help if he should stumble or start to fall.

Coordination. Evaluate how well a patient's muscles produce movement. Coordination results from neuromuscular integrity; a lack of muscular or nervous system integrity, or both, impairs the ability to make voluntary and productive movements.

Assess gross motor skills by having the patient perform any body action involving the muscles and joints in natural directional movements, such as lifting the arm to the side or other ROM exercises. Assess fine motor coordination by asking him to pick up a small object.

Inspecting and palpating muscles

Expect to perform inspection and palpation simultaneously during the musculoskeletal assessment. You will evaluate muscle tone, mass, and strength. Palpate the muscles gently, never forcing movement when the patient reports pain or when you feel resistance. Watch his face and body language for signs of discomfort; a patient may suffer silently.

Tone and mass. Assess muscle tone by palpating a muscle at rest and during passive ROM. Palpate a muscle at rest from the muscle attachment at the bone to the edge of the muscle. Normally, a relaxed muscle should feel soft, pliable, and nontender; a contracted muscle, firm.

Muscle mass is the actual size of a muscle. Assessment of muscle mass usually involves measuring the circumference of the thigh, the calf, and the upper arm. When measuring, establish landmarks to ensure measurement at the same location on each area.

Strength and joint ROM. Assessing joint ROM tests the joint function; assessing muscle strength against resistance tests the function of the muscles. (See *Assessing muscle strength and joint range of motion*, page 316.)

Inspecting and palpating joints and bones

Expect to measure the patient's height and the length of the extremities (arms and legs), and evaluate joint and bone characteristics and joint ROM.

Never force joint movement if you feel resistance or if the patient complains of pain. General deviations from normal include pain, swelling, stiffness, deformities, altered ROM, crepitation (a grating sound or sensation accompanying joint movement), ankylosis (joint fusion or fixation), and contracture (muscle shortening).

Length of the extremities. Place the patient in the supine position on a flat surface with his arms and legs fully extended and his shoulders and hips adducted. Measure each arm from the acromial process to the tip of the middle finger. Measure each leg from the anterior superior iliac spine to the medial malleolus with the tape crossing at the medial side of the knee.

Cervical spine. Inspect the cervical spine from behind, from the side, and from the front of the patient as he sits or stands. Observe the alignment of the head with the body. The nose should be in line with the midsternum and extend beyond the shoulders when viewed from the side. The head should align with the shoulders. Normally, the seventh cervical and first thoracic vertebrae appear more prominent than the others.

Clavicles. Inspect and palpate the length of the clavicles, including the sternoclavicular and acromioclavicular joints. Normal findings include firm, smooth, and continuous bones.

(Text continues on page 324.)

Assessing muscle strength and joint range of motion

To evaluate muscle strength, have the patient perform active range-of-motion (ROM) movements as you apply resistance. Normally, the patient can move joints a certain distance (measured in degrees) and can easily resist pressure applied against movement. If the muscle group is weak, lessen the resistance to permit a more accurate assessment. Note that strength is normally symmetrical.

To assess joint ROM, ask the patient to move specific joints through normal ROM. If he can't do so, perform passive ROM. Use a goniometer to measure the angle achieved.

On the following pages, you'll find descriptions and diagrams of tests for muscle strength and ROM, including the expected degree of motion for each joint tested.

Grading muscle strength

When evaluating muscle strength, use the scale at right. Column 1 describes the possible muscle response and its significance. Column 2 grades the response.

Muscle response and significance	Grade rating
No visible or palpable contraction • Paralysis	0
Slightly palpable contraction • Paresis, severe weakness	1
Passive ROM maneuvers when gravity is removed • Paresis, moderate weakness	2
Active ROM against gravity alone or against light resistance • Mild weakness	3 to 4
Active ROM against full resistance • Normal	5

CERVICAL SPINE AND NECK
Muscle strength

To assess muscles responsible for flexion of the cervical spine, place your hand on the patient's forehead, applying pressure. Ask him to bend his head forward and touch his chin to his chest. (Perform this maneuver only after cervical spine injury has been ruled out.)

To assess muscles responsible for cervical spine rotation, place your hand along the jaw. Ask the patient to push laterally against your hand while you attempt to prevent movement. At the same time, palpate the sternocleidomastoid on the opposite side. Repeat on the other side.

To assess muscles responsible for extension of the cervical spine, apply pressure with your hand on the patient's occipital bone. Ask him to bend his head backward as far as possible.

Range of motion

Ask the patient to flex his neck, attempting to touch his chin to his

Assessing muscle strength and joint range of motion *(continued)*

chest, and to extend his neck, bending his head backward.

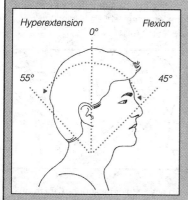

Next, ask him to bend laterally, touching his ears to his shoulders.

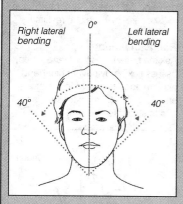

Then, ask him to rotate his head from side to side.

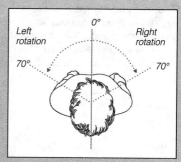

SHOULDER
Muscle strength
Test the trapezius muscles (of the shoulder and upper back) simultaneously. Ask the patient to shrug his shoulders freely, then again as you press down on them.

Range of motion
Observe and measure ROM as the patient demonstrates forward flexion, with the arms straight in front, and backward extension, with the arms straight and extended backward.

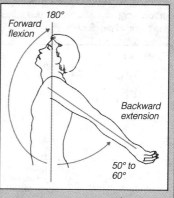

(continued)

Assessing muscle strength and joint range of motion (continued)

To assess abduction, ask the patient to raise his straightened arm out to the side; to assess adduction, ask him to move his straightened arm to midline.

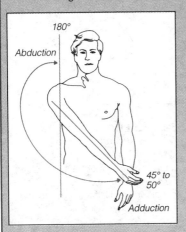

To assess external rotation, ask the patient to abduct his arm with his elbow bent, placing his hand behind his head.

To assess internal rotation, ask the patient to abduct his arm with his elbow bent, placing his hand behind the small of his back.

UPPER ARM AND ELBOW
Muscle strength

To test triceps strength, try to flex the patient's arm while she tries to extend it (as shown).

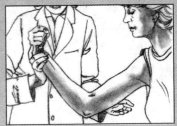

To assess biceps strength, try to pull the patient's flexed arm into extension while she resists.

To test deltoid strength, push down on the patient's arm (abducted to 90 degrees) while she resists.

Range of motion

Ask the patient to sit or stand. Then, assess flexion by having him bend his arm and attempt to touch the shoulder. To assess extension, ask him to straighten his arm.

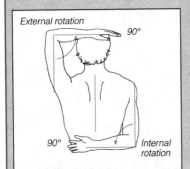

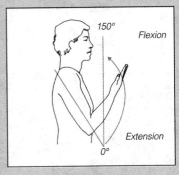

Assessing muscle strength and joint range of motion (continued)

Assess pronation by holding the patient's elbow in a flexed position while he rotates the arm until the palm faces the floor.

Assess supination by holding the patient's elbow in a flexed position while he rotates the arm until the palm faces upward.

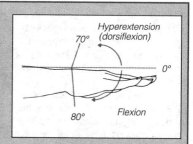

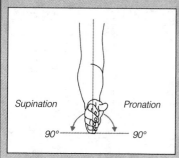

WRIST AND HAND
Muscle strength

Test muscle strength and movement of both hands simultaneously by having the patient squeeze the first two fingers of your hand, make a fist, resist your efforts to straighten a flexed wrist, and resist your efforts to flex a straightened wrist. (Normally, the dominant hand may be slightly stronger.)

Range of motion

To assess flexion, ask the patient to bend his wrist downward; assess extension by having him straighten his wrist. To assess hyperextension or dorsiflexion, ask him to bend his wrist upward.

To assess the metacarpophalangeal joints, ask the patient to hyperextend (dorsiflex), extend (straighten), and flex (make a fist) the fingers.

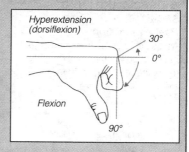

Assess radial deviation by asking the patient to move his hand toward the radial side; assess ulnar deviation by asking him to move his hand toward the ulnar side.

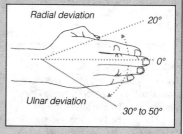

(continued)

Assessing muscle strength and joint range of motion *(continued)*

Also ask the patient to straighten the fingers, then spread them (abduct) and bring them together (adduct). Abduction should be 20 degrees between fingers; adduction, the fingers touch.

To assess palmar adduction, ask the patient to bring the thumb to the index finger; assess palmar abduction by asking the patient to move the thumb away from the palm. Assess opposition by having the patient touch the thumb to each fingertip.

THORACIC AND LUMBAR SPINE
Range of motion

Assess rotation by first stabilizing the patient's pelvis, then asking him to rotate the upper body from side to side.

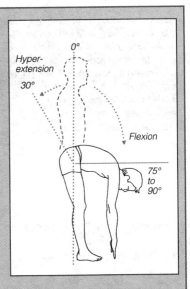

Ask the patient to bend to each side (lateral bending).

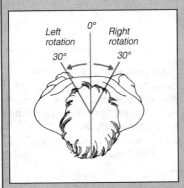

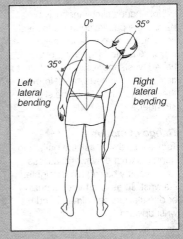

With the patient standing, observe and evaluate spinal ROM as he demonstrates hyperextension by bending backward from the waist and flexion by bending to touch the floor with the knees slightly bent.

Assessing muscle strength and joint range of motion *(continued)*

HIP AND PELVIS
Muscle strength

With the patient lying (prone and, later, supine), then sitting, evaluate muscle strength and palpate muscles as you carry out the following tests.

To assess hip extensors, ask the prone patient to hyperextend her leg backward (toward the ceiling) as you try to push her leg downward.

To assess hip flexors, ask the patient to sit and raise her knee to her chest as you apply downward pressure proximal to the knee.

To assess hip abductors, ask the side-lying patient to move her straightened leg away from midline as you try to push it toward midline.

To assess hip adductors, ask the side-lying patient to move her leg toward midline as you try to pull it away from midline (as shown).

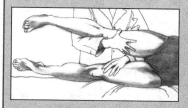

Range of motion

With the patient prone or standing, observe and evaluate ROM as the patient demonstrates flexion by bending the knee to the chest with the back straight. *Caution:* Don't perform this movement without the surgeon's permission on a patient who has undergone total hip replacement because the motion can cause the prosthesis to dislocate.

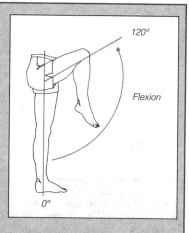

120°

Flexion

0°

Evaluate extension by asking the patient to straighten his knee, and hyperextension by asking him to extend his leg backward with his knee straight. *Note:* This motion can be performed with the patient prone or standing.

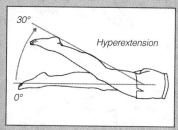

30°

Hyperextension

0°

To assess abduction, have the patient move his straightened leg away from midline; assess adduction by having him move his straightened leg toward midline. *Caution:* This motion can displace a hip prosthesis.

(continued)

Assessing muscle strength and joint range of motion *(continued)*

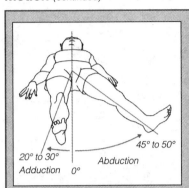

20° to 30° Adduction 0°   Abduction   45° to 50°

Finally, assess internal and external rotation by asking the patient to bend his knee and turn the leg inward and outward, respectively.

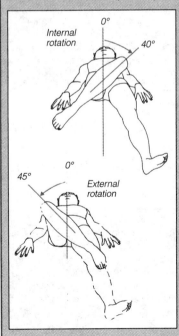

0°
Internal rotation   40°

0°
45°   External rotation

KNEE
Muscle strength

To assess knee extensors, ask the patient to sit or lie supine and extend his leg as you attempt to flex it.

To assess knee flexors, ask the patient to sit or lie supine while you try to extend his leg as he flexes his knee.

Range of motion

With the patient sitting or standing, observe and measure ROM as the patient demonstrates extension by straightening his leg at the knee. With the patient standing, have him demonstrate flexion by bending his leg at the knee and bringing his foot up to touch his buttock.

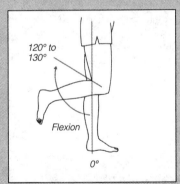

120° to 130°

Flexion

0°

ANKLE AND FOOT
Muscle strength

To assess dorsiflexion of the ankle joint, apply pressure with your hand to the dorsal surface of the patient's foot as he attempts to bend his foot up.

Assessing muscle strength and joint range of motion *(continued)*

To assess plantar flexion, apply pressure with your hand to the plantar surface of the patient's foot as he attempts to bend his foot down.

To assess inversion, apply pressure with your hand to the medial surface of the patient's first metatarsal bone as he attempts to move his toes inward. Assess eversion by placing your hand on the lateral surface of the 5th metatarsal bone and applying pressure as he attempts to move his toes outward.

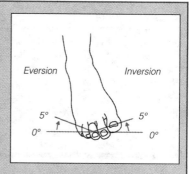

Eversion   *Inversion*

5°   5°

0°   0°

Range of motion

Ask the patient who is sitting, lying, or standing to demonstrate plantar

To assess forefoot adduction and abduction, stabilize the patient's heel while he turns his forefoot inward and outward, respectively.

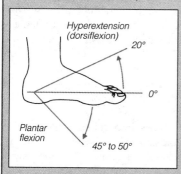

Hyperextension (dorsiflexion)

20°

0°

Plantar flexion

45° to 50°

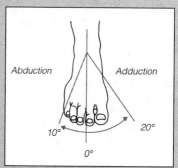

Abduction   *Adduction*

10°   20°

0°

flexion by bending his foot downward and dorsiflexion by bending his foot upward.

Then ask him to invert his foot by pointing the toes and turning the foot inward and to evert the foot by pointing the toes and turning the foot outward.

TOES
Muscle strength

To assess flexion, apply pressure with your finger to the plantar surface of the patient's toes as he attempts to bend his toes downward.

To assess extension, apply pressure with your finger to the dorsal surface of the patient's toes as he attempts to point his toes upward.

(continued)

Assessing muscle strength and joint range of motion *(continued)*

Range of motion

To assess the metatarsophalangeal joints, ask the patient to extend (straighten) and flex (curl) the toes. Then, ask him to hyperextend his toes by straightening and pointing them upward.

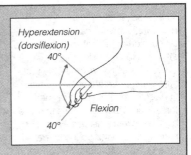

Hyperextension (dorsiflexion) 40°

Flexion 40°

Scapulae. To inspect and palpate the scapulae, sit directly behind the patient as he sits with his shoulders thrust backward. Normally, the scapulae are located over thoracic ribs two through seven. Check for an equal distance from the medial scapular edges to the midspinal line.

Ribs. After assessing the scapulae, inspect the ribs for visual abnormalities and palpate the surfaces of the ribs. Normal findings include firm, smooth, continuous bones.

Shoulders. Palpate the moving joints for crepitus. Inspect the skin overlying the shoulder joints for erythema, masses, or swelling.

Next, palpate the acromioclavicular joint and the area over the greater humeral tuberosity. Ask the patient to hold his arm at his side; then have him move his arm across his chest (adduction). Next, place your thumb on the anterior portion of the patient's shoulder joint and your fingers on the posterior portion of the joint. Ask the patient to abduct his arm, and palpate the shoulder joint as he does so.

Now stand behind the patient. With your fingertips placed over the greater humeral tuberosity, instruct him to rotate his shoulder internally by moving the arm behind the back. This allows you to palpate a portion of the musculotendinous rotator cuff as well as the bony structures of the shoulder joint.

Elbows. Inspect joint contour and the skin over each elbow. Palpate the elbows at rest and during movement.

Wrists. Inspect the wrists for masses, erythema, skeletal deformities, and swelling. Palpate the wrist at rest and during movement by gently grasping it between your thumb and fingers.

Fingers and thumbs. On each hand, inspect the fingers and thumb for nodules, erythema, spacing, length, and skeletal deformities. Palpate fingers and thumb at rest and during movement.

Thoracic and lumbar spine. You'll need to palpate the length of the spine for tenderness and vertebral alignment. To check for tenderness, percuss each spinous process with the ulnar side of your fist.

Note whether the patient is able to move with a full ROM, while maintaining balance, smoothness, and coordination.

Hips and pelvis. Inspect and palpate over the bony prominences: iliac crests, symphysis pubis, anterior spine, ischial tuberosities, and greater trochanters. Palpate the hip at rest and during movement.

Knees. Inspect the knees with the patient seated. Palpate the knee at rest and during movement. Inspect and palpate the popliteal spaces. Knee movements should be smooth. Palpate the joint line. If pain is elicited, you may be exacerbating a torn meniscus.

Ankles and feet. Inspect and palpate the ankles and feet at rest and during movement.

Toes. The patient may be sitting or lying supine for toe assessment. Inspect all toe surfaces. Palpate toes at rest and during movement.

DIAGNOSTIC TESTS

Expect the doctor to order any of the following diagnostic studies to confirm the diagnosis and to help identify the underlying cause: blood, urine, and synovial fluid tests; radiographic and imaging studies; arthroscopy;

and arthrocentesis. (See *Diagnostic tests for musculoskeletal disorders,* pages 326 to 328.)

NURSING DIAGNOSES

When caring for patients with musculoskeletal disorders, you'll find that several nursing diagnoses are commonly used. These diagnoses appear below, along with appropriate nursing interventions and rationales. (Rationales appear in italic type.)

Pain

The nursing diagnosis of pain can be related to joint inflammation, surgical intervention, or traction. Expect to help patients with musculoskeletal problems cope with both local and widespread pain.

Expected outcomes
- Patient describes level and characteristic of pain.
- Patient rates pain on a scale of 1 to 10.
- Patient describes factors that intensify pain.
- Patient tries nonpharmacologic methods for pain relief.
- Patient expresses a feeling of comfort and relief from pain.
- Patient describes appropriate interventions for pain relief.

Nursing interventions and rationales
- Assess the patient's perception of pain, including its characteristics and methods to alleviate it. *This provides a baseline from which to plan and evaluate interventions.*

(Text continues on page 328.)

Diagnostic tests for musculoskeletal disorders

Test	Purpose	Nursing considerations
Bone marrow aspiration	To help diagnose rheumatoid arthritis, tuberculosis, amyloidosis, syphilis, bacterial or viral infections, tumors, and hematologic problems	• Explain the procedure and that the patient will feel pressure as the doctor inserts the needle and that the aspiration may hurt. • Tell him the procedure lasts about 10 minutes and that he'll be sedated and given a local anesthetic. • After the test, observe the aspiration site for bleeding and signs of infection.
Arthrocentesis	To help assess infection and distinguish forms of arthritis	• Explain the 10-minute procedure. • Explain that he'll be asked to assume a position and remain still. • After the test, apply cold packs to the puncture site. • Advise the patient not to use the joint excessively and to report any increased pain, tenderness, swelling, warmth, redness, or fever.
Skeletal X-rays	To help diagnose fractures, dislocations, bone diseases, and joint diseases	• Make sure the patient removes all jewelry. • Advise him that he may be placed in various positions as X-ray films are taken. • Instruct him to remain as still as possible and to hold his breath when required.
Bone scan	To help detect abnormal skeletal pathology	• Restrict food and fluid for 4 hours before the test if contrast medium is to be used. • Administer prescribed analgesics. • Note any hypersensitivity to contrast medium. • Advise the patient he is required to drink 4 to 6 glasses of water or tea in the interval between injection of the tracer and the actual scanning. • Assure him that the test is painless. • Instruct patient to void immediately before the test. • After the test, observe the venipuncture site for bleeding or hematoma. • Encourage him to increase his fluids for 1 to 3 hours following the test.

Diagnostic tests for musculoskeletal disorders *(continued)*

Test	Purpose	Nursing considerations
Computed tomography	To visualize bones and joints	• Restrict food for 4 hours before the test if contrast medium is to be used. • Note any hypersensitivity to contrast medium. • Inform the patient that he may experience transient adverse reactions such as flushing, metallic taste and headache following the injection of the contrast meidum. • Instruct the patient to remove any metal objects before the test. • After the test, inform the patient that he may resume his usual diet if restricted before the test.
Magnetic resonance imaging	To assess bone, soft tissue, and joints	• Explain that the test isn't painful. • Ask patient if he suffers from claustrophobia. If so, he may require sedation. • Tell him that he'll hear the scanner clicking, whirring, and thumping as it moves inside the housing. • Reassure him that he'll be able to communicate with the technician at all times. • Instruct him to remove all metal objects before the test.
Arthroscopy	To help assess joint problems and document pathology	• Explain that the procedure is done in the operating room under general or local anesthesia. • Instruct the patient to fast after midnight. • Advise him that the area around the joint will be cleaned and shaved. • After the test, advise him against excessive use of the joint for a few days. • Monitor the site for signs of infection or hemarthrosis or a synovial cyst.
Serum calcium	To aid diagnosis of neuromuscular, skeletal, and endocrine disorders	• Explain the procedure, including venipuncture. • After the test, observe the venipuncture site for bleeding.

(continued)

Diagnostic tests for musculoskeletal disorders *(continued)*

Test	Purpose	Nursing considerations
Serum phosphorous	To detect endocrine, skeletal, and calcium disorders	• Explain the procedure, including venipuncture. • Have venipuncture performed without using a tourniquet, if possible, because this may cause venous stasis, which can alter the results. • After the test, observe the venipuncture site for bleeding or hematoma.
Rheumatoid factor	To confirm rheumatoid arthritis when clinical diagnosis is doubtful	• Explain the procedure, including venipuncture. • After the test, keep venipuncture site covered and dry for 24 hours. Observe the site for bleeding or hematoma.

• Give analgesics as needed and prescribed. *This promotes rest and enhances healing.*
• Teach the patient pain-control techniques, such as distraction, imagery, meditation, hot and cold applications, and transcutaneous electrical nerve stimulation (TENS). *This gives the patient options for dealing with pain.*
• Assess effectiveness of each intervention *to identify need for change.*
• Use behavior modification techniques to help a patient with chronic pain: Establish specific times when he may talk about his pain and discourage such talk at other times. *This prevents the patient from dwelling on pain.*

Self-care deficit

Related to musculoskeletal impairment, the self-care deficit diagnosis may be used for patients who have difficulty with feeding themselves, bathing and hygiene, dressing and grooming, and toileting. This nursing diagnosis may be associated with such disorders as fractures, multiple trauma, muscular dystrophy, rheumatoid arthritis, and any other condition in which musculoskeletal impairment is severe.

Expected outcomes
• Patient's self-care needs are met.
• Patient appears appropriately dressed and groomed.
• Patient's diet is tailored to include food that he can handle easily.
• Assistive devices are made readily available, if necessary.
• Patient, family member, or caregiver carries out a toileting program daily.

Nursing interventions and rationales

• Observe patient's functional level every shift; document and report any changes. *This allows adjustment of actions when needed.*

• Perform prescribed treatment for underlying musculoskeletal impairment. Monitor progress, reporting favorable and adverse responses to treatment. *Therapy must be consistently applied to aid independence.*

• Encourage the patient to voice feelings and concerns about self-care deficits *to help achieve his highest functional level.*

• Provide supportive measures, as indicated.

If the patient has difficulty with feeding:

• Determine the types of food best handled by patient—for example, finger foods or a soft or liquid diet *to encourage independence.*

• Place patient in high Fowler's position (if not contraindicated) *to reduce swallowing difficulty.*

• Wash patient's face and hands before each meal *to prevent infection.*

• Support weakened extremities. Provide assistive devices, as needed, at each meal; instruct patient on their use. *These allow independence.*

• Supervise or assist at each meal—for example, cut food into small pieces and provide for patient's preferences in food seasonings. *This reduces the risk of choking.*

• Don't rush feeding. *Rushing causes stress, reducing digestive activity and producing intestinal spasms.*

• Keep suction equipment at bedside *to remove aspirated foods.*

• Instruct the patient or family member in feeding techniques and use of equipment. Have one of them give a return demonstration. *This increases compliance.*

If the patient has difficulty with bathing and hygiene:

• Monitor completion of bathing and hygiene daily. *Reinforcement may encourage daily activities.*

• Provide assistive devices, as needed, for bathing and hygiene care. Instruct on their use. *Appropriate devices promote independence.*

• Assist with or perform bathing and hygiene daily only when patient has difficulty *to promote a feeling of independence.*

• Instruct patient or family member in bathing and hygiene techniques. Have one of them give a return demonstration. *Return demonstration identifies problem areas.*

If the patient has trouble with dressing and grooming:

• Provide enough time for patient to perform dressing and grooming. *Rushing promotes failure.*

• Monitor patient's abilities for dressing and grooming daily. *This identifies problem areas early.*

• Encourage family to provide clothing easily managed by patient. *Clothing slightly larger than regular size may make dressing easier.*

• Provide assistive devices, such as a toothbrush and a comb or brush, *to encourage independence.*

• Assist with or perform dressing and grooming: Brush teeth, comb hair, and clean nails. Provide help only when patient has difficulty *to promote a feeling of independence.*

• Instruct patient or family member in dressing and grooming techniques. Have one of them demonstrate these techniques under supervision. *Return demonstration identifies any problem areas.*

If the patient experiences difficulty with toileting:

• Monitor intake and output and skin condition; record episodes of incontinence. *Accurate intake and output records can identify potential imbalances.*

• Teach and incorporate pelvic floor (Kegel) exercises into the plan of care for the incontinent patient. *Regularly performed exercises may lead to continence.*

• Use assistive devices as needed, such as external catheter at night, bedpan or urinal every 2 hours during day, and adaptive equipment for bowel care. Instruct on their use. As control improves, reduce use of assistive devices. *Assisting at appropriate level aids self-esteem.*

• Assist with toileting if needed. *Allow patient to perform independently as much as possible.*

• Perform urinary and bowel care if needed. Follow urinary or bowel elimination plans. *Monitoring success or failure of toileting plans helps identify and resolve problem areas.*

• Instruct patient or family member in toileting routine (in writing if necessary). Have one of them demonstrate toileting routine under supervision. *Return demonstration identifies any problem areas.*

• Refer patient, as needed, to psychiatric liaison nurse, support group, home health care agency, or a community agency such as Meals On Wheels.

Activity intolerance

Related to impaired physical mobility, the diagnosis of activity intolerance may be associated with pain or edema. The patient's activity may be severely restricted by such conditions as fractures requiring skeletal traction, rheumatoid arthritis, vertebral fractures, neurogenic arthropathy, Paget's disease, muscular dystrophy, and other disorders.

Expected outcomes

• Patient uses assistive devices to carry out activities.

• Patient develops a plan to incorporate meaningful activities into his daily routine.

• Patient participates in activities to the extent possible.

• Patient modifies activities to adjust to decreased activity tolerance.

• Patient's pulse, respirations, and blood pressure remain within established parameters during activity.

Nursing interventions and rationales

• Perform active or passive ROM exercises to all extremities every 2 to 4 hours. *These exercises foster muscle strength and tone, maintain joint mobility, and prevent contractures.*

• Turn and reposition the patient every 2 hours. Establish a turning schedule for the dependent patient. Post schedule at bedside and monitor frequency. *Turning and repositioning prevents skin breakdown and improves breathing.*

• Maintain proper body alignment at all times *to avoid contractures and maintain optimal musculoskeletal balance and physiologic function.*

• Encourage active exercise. Provide a trapeze or other assistive device whenever possible. *Such devices simplify moving and turning for many patients and also allow them to strengthen some upper-body muscles.*

• Teach isometric exercises *to allow patient to maintain or increase muscle tone and joint mobility.*

• Have patient perform self-care activities. Begin slowly and increase daily, as tolerated. *Activities will help patient regain health.*

• Involve patient in care-related planning and decision making *to improve compliance.*

• Monitor physiologic responses to increased activity level, including respirations, heart rate and rhythm, and blood pressure, *to ensure they return to normal within a few minutes after exercising.*

• Teach caregivers to assist patient with self-care activities in a way that maximizes patient's potential. *This enables caregivers to participate.*

• Place needed objects within reach *to encourage independence.*

• Explain the importance of following prescribed medical and physical therapy regimens. *When the patient's understanding of his condition improves, his compliance increases.*

Body image disturbance

Related to physical disability or deformity, the diagnosis of body image disturbance may be associated with clubfoot, muscular dystrophy, rheumatoid arthritis, osteoporosis, Paget's disease, kyphosis, and scoliosis.

Nursing interventions and rationales

• Encourage patient to express feelings about physical changes and their effect on his life. *Active listening is the most basic therapeutic skill.*

• Allow a specific amount of uninterrupted, non-care-related time to engage patient in conversation. *This encourages the patient to express his feelings at his own pace.*

• Assess the patient's mental status through interview and observation at least once daily. *This helps detect abnormal feelings and behaviors.*

• Assess the patient's emotional readiness to make major decisions. *This will avoid forcing him into premature decision making.*

• Arrange situations to encourage social interaction. *Improving social environment helps restore confidence.*

• Make appropriate referrals for community agency help or counseling. *This gives the patient options when he can't manage by himself.*

DISORDERS

When caring for patients with musculoskeletal problems, expect to encounter a wide range of underlying causes: trauma, heredity, autoimmunity, or the normal aging process. Musculoskeletal disorders primarily affect joints, bones, or connective tissue.

Joint disorders

Arthritic disorders are among the most common chronic conditions you'll encounter. Painful and disabling, joint disorders call for a team approach that emphasizes patient participation. Arthritic disorders discussed in this section include rheumatoid arthritis, osteoarthritis, septic arthritis, and gout. This section also discusses herniated disks.

Rheumatoid arthritis

Rheumatoid arthritis (RA) is a chronic, systemic inflammatory disease that primarily attacks peripheral joints and surrounding muscles, tendons, ligaments, and blood vessels. Spontaneous remissions and unpredictable exacerbations mark the course of RA. Potentially crippling, RA usually requires lifelong treatment and sometimes surgery. In most patients, the disease follows an intermittent course and allows normal activity, although 10% suffer total disability. Prognosis worsens with the development of nodules, vasculitis, and high titers of rheumatoid factor (RF).

Causes. RA is currently believed to have an autoimmune basis, though the cause remains unknown.

Assessment findings. Initial symptoms may include fatigue, malaise, anorexia, persistent low-grade fever, weight loss, and lymphadenopathy.

Later, the patient may develop joint pain, tenderness, warmth, and swelling. Usually, joint symptoms occur bilaterally and symmetrically. Other symptoms may include morning stiffness, paresthesias in hands and feet, and stiff, weak, or painful muscles. The patient may also develop rheumatoid nodules—subcutaneous, round or oval, nontender masses, usually on pressure areas such as the elbow.

Advanced signs include joint deformities and diminished joint function.

Diagnostic tests. In early stages, X-rays show bone demineralization and soft-tissue swelling. Later, X-rays show loss of cartilage and narrowing of joint spaces. In more advanced stages of illness, they show cartilage and bone destruction, and erosion, subluxations, and deformities.

Laboratory studies may provide the following results:
• Positive RF test, as indicated by a titer of 1:160 or higher.
• Elevated serum globulins, as revealed by serum protein electrophoresis.
• Elevated erythrocyte sedimentation rate (ESR). This test may be useful in monitoring response to therapy because elevation commonly parallels disease activity.

In addition, synovial fluid analysis usually shows increased volume and turbidity but decreased viscosity and complement (C3 and C4) levels, white blood cell (WBC) count is commonly more than 10,000/mm^3, and complete blood count usually shows moderate anemia and slight leukocytosis.

Treatments. Salicylates, particularly aspirin, provide the mainstay of RA therapy because they decrease inflammation and relieve joint pain. Other useful medications include nonsteroidal anti-inflammatory agents (such as indomethacin, ketorolac, and ibuprofen), anti-malarials (chloroquine and hydroxychloroquine), gold salts, penicillamine, and corticosteroids (prednisone). Immunosuppressives, such as cyclophosphamide and azathioprine, are also therapeutic.

Supportive measures include 8 to 10 hours of sleep every night, frequent rest periods between daily activities, and splinting to rest inflamed joints. A physical therapy program, including ROM exercises and individualized therapeutic exercises, forestalls loss of joint function. Application of heat relaxes muscles and relieves pain. Moist heat (hot soaks, paraffin baths, whirlpool) usually works best for patients with chronic disease. Ice packs are effective during acute episodes.

Advanced disease may require synovectomy, joint reconstruction, or total joint arthroplasty.

Nursing interventions. Assess all joints carefully. Look for deformities, contractures, immobility, and inability to perform everyday activities.
• Monitor vital signs, and note weight changes, sensory disturbances, and level of pain. Give analgesics, as ordered, and watch for adverse effects.
• Provide meticulous skin care. Use lotion not soap, for dry skin.

• Explain all diagnostic tests and procedures. Tell the patient to expect multiple blood samples.
• Monitor the duration, not the intensity, of morning stiffness because duration more accurately reflects the severity of the disease. Encourage the patient to take hot showers or baths to reduce the need for pain medication.
• Apply splints carefully. Observe for pressure sores if the patient is in traction or wearing splints.
• Make sure the patient and his family understand that RA is a chronic disease that requires major changes in lifestyle. Emphasize that no miracle cures exist.
• Encourage a balanced diet, but make sure the patient understands that special diets won't cure RA. Emphasize the need for weight control because obesity stresses joints.
• Urge the patient to perform activities of daily living (ADLs) such as dressing and feeding himself (supply easy-to-open cartons, lightweight cups, and unpackaged silverware).
• Encourage the patient to discuss his fears concerning dependency, sexuality, body image, and self-esteem. Refer him to an appropriate social service agency, as needed.
• Discuss sexual aids: alternative positions, pain medication, and moist heat to increase mobility.
• Before discharge, make sure the patient knows how and when to take prescribed medication and how to recognize possible adverse effects.

Patient education. Teach the patient how to stand, walk, and sit upright and erect. Tell him to sit in chairs with high seats and armrests because it's easier to get up from a chair if his knees are lower than his hips. Suggest an elevated toilet seat.

Instruct the patient to pace daily activities, resting for 5 to 10 minutes out of each hour and alternating sitting and standing tasks. Adequate sleep and correct sleeping posture are important. He should sleep on his back on a firm mattress and should not place a pillow under his knees, to prevent flexion deformity.

Counsel the patient to avoid putting undue stress on joints and to use the largest joint available for a given task. Enlist the aid of the occupational therapist to teach how to protect arthritic joints.

Suggest dressing aids—a long-handled shoehorn, a reacher, elastic shoelaces, a zipper pull, and a buttonhook—and helpful household items, such as easy-to-open drawers, a handheld shower nozzle, handrails, and grab bars. Finally, refer the patient to the Arthritis Foundation for more information.

Evaluation. Note whether compliance with exercise and dietary regimen slows debilitation. Has the patient maintained or improved his ability to perform ADLs? Does he use effective pain-control interventions? Finally, assess whether the patient obtains and uses appropriate assistive devices.

Osteoarthritis

The most common form of arthritis, osteoarthritis is a chronic condition that causes deterioration of the joint cartilage and formation of reactive new bone at the margins and subchondral areas of the joints. Degeneration occurs from a breakdown of chondrocytes, most commonly in the hips and knees (weight-bearing joints). A thorough physical examination confirms typical symptoms, and lack of systemic symptoms rules out an inflammatory joint disorder such as RA.

Disability depends on the site and severity of involvement and can range from minor limitation of the fingers to severe disability in people with hip or knee involvement. The rate of progression varies, and joints may remain stable for years in an early stage of deterioration.

Causes. The exact cause of osteoarthritis is unknown. Primary osteoarthritis, a normal part of aging, results from many things, including metabolic, genetic, chemical, and mechanical factors. Secondary osteoarthritis usually follows trauma or congenital deformity.

Assessment findings. The severity of the following signs and symptoms increases with poor posture, obesity, and occupational stress:
• joint pain (the most common symptom) that occurs after exercise or weight bearing and that is usually relieved by rest
• stiffness in the morning and after exercise that is usually relieved by rest
• aching during changes in weather
• "grating" of the joint during motion
• limited movement.

In addition, irreversible changes in the distal joints (Heberden's nodes) and proximal joints (Bouchard's nodes) occur in osteoarthritis of the interphalangeal joints. Nodes may be painless at first but eventually become red, swollen, and tender, causing numbness and loss of dexterity.

Diagnostic tests. X-rays of the affected joint help confirm diagnosis of osteoarthritis. X-rays may include posterior, anterior, lateral, and oblique views and typically show narrowing of joint space or margin, cystlike bony deposits in joint space and margins, joint deformity from degeneration or articular damage, and bony growths at weight-bearing areas (hips, knees).

Treatments. Most measures are palliative. Medications for relief of pain and joint inflammation include aspirin (or other nonnarcotic analgesics), phenylbutazone, indomethacin, ketorolac, ibuprofen, propoxyphene, and intra-articular injections of corticosteroids. Such injections may delay the development of nodes in the hands.

Effective treatment also reduces joint stress by supporting or stabilizing the joint with crutches, braces, a cane, a walker, a cervical collar, or traction. Other supportive measures include massage, moist heat, paraffin dips for hands, protective techniques, adequate rest (particularly after activity) and, occasionally, exercise when the knees are affected.

Patients who have severe osteoarthritis with disability or uncontrol-lable pain may undergo one or more of the following surgical procedures:
• arthroplasty (partial or total)—replacement of a deteriorated joint or part with a prosthetic appliance
• arthrodesis—surgical fusion of bones; used primarily in the spine (laminectomy)
• osteoplasty—scraping of deteriorated bone from a joint
• osteotomy—excision of bone to change alignment and relieve stress.

Nursing interventions. Promote adequate rest, particularly after activity. Plan rest periods during the day, and provide for adequate sleep at night. Teach the patient to pace daily activities.

Assist with physical therapy, and encourage the patient to perform gentle ROM exercises. Provide emotional support to help cope with limited mobility. Explain that osteoarthritis is *not* a systemic disease.

If the patient needs surgery, provide appropriate preoperative and postoperative care.

Other specific nursing measures depend on the affected joint:

Hand. Apply hot soaks and paraffin dips to relieve pain, as ordered.

Spine (lumbar and sacral). Recommend a firm mattress (or bed board) to decrease morning pain.

Spine (cervical). Check cervical collar for constriction; watch for redness with prolonged use.

Hip. Use moist heat pads to relieve pain and administer antispasmodic drugs, as ordered. Assist with ROM and strengthening exercises, always making sure the patient gets the proper rest afterward.

Check crutches, cane, braces, and walker for proper fit, and teach the patient to use them correctly. For example, the patient with unilateral joint involvement should use a cane or walker on the unaffected side. Advise use of cushions when sitting, and suggest an elevated toilet seat.

Knee. Twice daily, assist with prescribed ROM exercises, exercises to maintain muscle tone, and progressive resistance exercises to increase muscle strength. Provide elastic supports or braces if needed.

Patient education. Teach the patient to follow these guidelines:
• Plan for adequate rest during the day, after exertion, and at night.
• Take medication as prescribed, and report adverse effects immediately.
• Avoid overexertion. Take care to stand and walk correctly, to minimize weight-bearing activities, and to be especially careful when stooping or picking up objects.
• Always wear well-fitting supportive shoes; don't allow the heels to become too worn down.
• Use assistive devices as necessary.
• Install safety devices at home such as handrails in the bathroom.
• Do gentle ROM exercises.
• Maintain proper body weight to lessen joint stress.

Evaluation. Assess whether compliance with exercise regimen slows down the debilitating effects of osteoarthritis. Look for the patient to maintain or improve his ability to perform ADLs and to obtain and use appropriate assistive devices. Note whether he understands and uses pain control interventions for involved joints.

Septic arthritis

A medical emergency, septic arthritis occurs when bacteria invade a joint, resulting in inflammation of the synovial lining. If the organisms enter the joint cavity, effusion and pyogenesis follow, with eventual destruction of bone and cartilage. Septic arthritis can lead to ankylosis and even fatal septicemia. Prompt antibiotic therapy and joint aspiration or drainage cure most patients.

Causes. In most cases, bacteria spread from a primary site of infection, usually in adjacent bone or soft tissue. Common infecting organisms include four strains of gram-positive cocci: *Staphylococcus aureus, Streptococcus pyogenes, Streptococcus pneumoniae,* and *Streptococcus viridans;* two strains of gram-negative cocci: *Neisseria gonorrhoeae* and *Haemophilus influenzae;* and various gram-negative bacilli: *Escherichia coli, Salmonella,* and *Pseudomonas,* for example. Anaerobic organisms such as gram-positive cocci usually infect adults and children over age 2. *H. influenzae* most commonly infects children under age 2.

Various factors can predispose a person to septic arthritis. Any concurrent bacterial infection or serious chronic illness (such as malignancy, renal failure, RA, systemic lupus erythematosus, diabetes, or cirrhosis) heightens susceptibility. Immunodeficiency diseases or prior immunosuppressive therapy increase susceptibility. Intravenous drug abuse can also cause septic arthritis. Other predisposing factors include recent articular trauma, joint surgery, intra-articular injections, and local joint abnormalities.

Assessment findings. Acute septic arthritis begins abruptly, causing intense pain, inflammation, and swelling of the affected joint, with low-grade fever. It usually affects a single joint, most commonly, a large joint, but it can strike any joint, including the spine and small peripheral joints. Systemic signs of inflammation may not appear in some patients. Migratory polyarthritis sometimes precedes localization of the infection. If the bacteria invade the hip, pain may occur in the groin, upper thigh, or buttock or may be referred to the knee.

Diagnostic tests. Identifying the causative organism in a Gram stain or culture of synovial fluid or a biopsy of synovial membrane confirms septic arthritis. Joint fluid analysis shows gross pus or watery, cloudy fluid of decreased viscosity usually with 50,000/mm³ or more WBCs containing primarily neutrophils. When synovial fluid culture is negative, positive blood culture may confirm the diagnosis. In many cases, synovial fluid glucose is compared with a simultaneous 6-hour postprandial blood sugar.

Other diagnostic measures include the following:
• X-rays can show typical changes as early as 1 week after initial infection—distention of joint capsules, for example, followed by narrowing of joint space (indicating cartilage damage) and erosions of bone (joint destruction).
• Radioisotope joint scan for less accessible joints (such as spinal articulations) may help detect infection or inflammation.
• Two sets of positive culture and Gram stain smears of skin exudates, sputum, urethral discharge, stools, urine, or nasopharyngeal smear confirm septic arthritis.

Treatments. Antibiotic therapy should begin promptly; it may be modified when sensitivity results become available. Penicillin G is effective against infections caused by *S. aureus, S. pyogenes , S. pneumoniae , S. viridans ,* and *N. gonorrhoeae.* A penicillinase-resistant penicillin such as nafcillin is recommended for penicillin G–resistant strains of *S. aureus;* ampicillin, for *H. influenzae;* gentamicin, for gram-negative bacilli. Medication selection requires drug sensitivity studies of the infecting organism. Bioassays or bactericidal assays of synovial fluid and bioassays of blood may confirm clearing of the infection.

Treatment of septic arthritis requires monitoring of progress through frequent analysis of joint fluid cultures, synovial fluid leukocyte counts, and glucose determinations. Codeine or propoxyphene can be given for pain, if needed. (Aspirin causes a misleading reduction in swelling, hindering accurate monitoring of progress.) The affected joint can be immobilized with a splint or put into traction until movement can be tolerated.

Arthrocentesis to remove purulent joint fluid should be repeated daily until fluid appears normal. If excessive fluid is aspirated or the leukocyte count remains elevated, open surgical drainage (usually arthrotomy with lavage of the joint) may be necessary for resistant infection or chronic septic arthritis.

Late reconstructive surgery is warranted only for severe joint damage and only after all signs of active infection have disappeared, which usually takes several months. In some cases, the recommended procedure may be arthroplasty or joint fusion. Prosthetic replacement remains controversial, but it has helped patients with damaged femoral heads or acetabula.

Nursing interventions. Practice strict aseptic technique with all procedures. Wash hands carefully before and after giving care. Dispose of soiled linens and dressings properly. Prevent contact between immunosuppressed patients and infected patients.

Watch for signs and symptoms of joint inflammation: heat, redness, swelling, pain, or drainage. Monitor vital signs and fever pattern. Remember that corticosteroids mask signs and symptoms of infection.

Check splints or traction regularly. Keep the joint in proper alignment, but avoid prolonged immobilization. Start passive ROM exercises immediately, and progress to active exercises as soon as the patient can move the affected joint and put weight on it.

Monitor pain levels and medicate accordingly, especially before exercise, remembering that the pain of septic arthritis is easy to underestimate. Give analgesics and narcotics for acute pain, and heat or ice packs for moderate pain.

Patient education. Explain all diagnostic tests and procedures. Warn the patient before the first aspiration that it will be *extremely* painful. Discuss all prescribed medications with the patient. Explain why therapy must be carefully monitored.

Evaluation. Assess whether compliance with exercise regimen slows down the debilitating effects of septic arthritis. Look for the patient to maintain or improve his ability to perform ADLs and to obtain and use appropriate assistive devices. Assess whether he understands and uses pain-control interventions.

Gout

In gout, urate deposits lead to painfully arthritic joints. Gout can strike any joint but favors those in the feet and legs. Gout follows an intermittent course and leaves many patients free from symptoms for years between attacks. Gout can lead to chronic disability or incapacitation and, rarely, severe hypertension and progressive renal disease.

Causes. Although the cause of primary gout remains unknown, it seems linked to a genetic defect in purine metabolism, which causes overproduction of uric acid (hyperuricemia), retention of uric acid, or both. In secondary gout, which develops during the course of another disease (such as obesity, diabetes mellitus, hypertension, polycythemia, leukemia, myeloma, sickle cell anemia, and renal disease), hyperuricemia results from the breakdown of nucleic acid. Secondary gout can also follow drug therapy, especially after hydrochlorothiazide or pyrazinamide, which interferes with urate excretion. Increased concentration of uric acid leads to urate deposits, called tophi, in joints or tissues, causing local necrosis or fibrosis.

Assessment findings. Gout develops in four stages: asymptomatic, acute, intercritical, and chronic.

In *asymptomatic* gout, serum urate levels rise but produce no symptoms. As the disease progresses, it may cause hypertension or nephrolithiasis, with severe back pain.

The first *acute* attack strikes suddenly and peaks quickly. Although it usually involves only one or a few joints, this initial attack is extremely painful. Affected joints appear hot, tender, inflamed, dusky red, or cyanotic. The metatarsophalangeal joint of the great toe usually becomes inflamed first (podagra), then the instep, ankle, heel, knee, or wrist joints. A low-grade fever may be present. Mild acute attacks may subside quickly but tend to recur at irregular intervals. Severe attacks may persist for days or weeks.

Intercritical periods are the symptom-free intervals between gout attacks. Most patients have a second attack within 6 months to 2 years, but in some the second attack is delayed for 5 to 10 years. Delayed attacks are more common in those who are untreated and tend to be longer and severer than initial attacks. Such attacks are also polyarticular, invariably affecting joints in the feet and legs, and are sometimes accompanied by fever. A migratory attack sequentially strikes various joints and the Achilles tendon and is associated with either subdeltoid or olecranon bursitis.

Eventually, *chronic* polyarticular gout sets in. This final, unremitting stage (chronic or tophaceous gout) is marked by persistent painful polyarthritis, with large, subcutaneous tophi in cartilage, synovial membranes, tendons, and soft tissue. Tophi form in fingers, hands, knees, feet, ulnar sides of the forearms, helix of the ear, Achilles tendons and, rarely, in internal organs, such as the kidneys and myocardium. The skin over the tophus may ulcerate and release a chalky, white exudate or pus. Chronic inflammation and tophaceous deposits precipitate secondary joint degeneration, with eventual erosions, deformity, and disability. Kidney involvement, with associated tubular damage, leads to chronic renal dysfunction. Hypertension and albuminuria occur in some patients; urolithiasis is common.

Pseudogout also causes abrupt joint pain and swelling but results from an accumulation of calcium pyrophosphate in periarticular joint structures. (See *What is pseudogout?* page 341.)

Diagnostic tests. The presence of monosodium urate monohydrate crystals in synovial fluid taken from an inflamed joint or tophus establishes the diagnosis. Aspiration of synovial fluid (arthrocentesis) or of tophaceous material reveals intracellular crystals of sodium urate.

Although hyperuricemia isn't specifically diagnostic of gout, tests reveal above-normal serum uric acid levels. Urine uric acid levels are usually higher in secondary gout than in primary gout.

Initially, X-ray examinations are normal. However, in chronic gout, X-rays show a punched-out look, as urate acids replace bony structures. As the disorder destroys cartilage, the joint space narrows and degenerative changes become evident. Outward displacement of the overhanging margin from the bone contour characterizes gout.

Treatments. Treatment for the patient with acute gout consists of bed rest; immobilization and protection of the inflamed, painful joints; and local application of heat or cold. Analgesics such as acetaminophen relieve the pain associated with mild attacks, but acute inflammation requires concomitant treatment with oral or I.V. colchicine every hour for 8 hours, until the pain subsides or nausea, vomiting, cramping, or diarrhea develops. Phenylbutazone or indomethacin in therapeutic doses may be used instead but is less specific. Resistant inflammation may require corticosteroids or corticotropin (I.V. drip or I.M.), or joint aspiration and an intra-articular corticosteroid injection.

Treatment for chronic gout aims to decrease serum uric acid levels. The doctor may order continuing maintenance dosage of allopurinol to suppress uric acid formation or control uric acid levels, thereby preventing further attacks. However, use this drug cautiously in patients with renal failure. Colchicine prevents recurrent acute attacks until uric acid returns to its normal level but doesn't affect the acid level. Uricosuric agents—probenecid and sulfinpyrazone—promote uric acid excretion and inhibit accumulation of uric acid, but their value is limited in patients with renal impairment. Don't give these drugs to patients with calculi.

Adjunctive therapy emphasizes a few dietary restrictions, primarily the avoidance of alcohol and purine-rich foods. Obese patients should try to lose weight to relieve stress on painful joints.

Surgery may be necessary to improve joint function or correct deformities. Infected or ulcerated tophi must be excised and drained. Tophi can also be excised to prevent ulceration, improve the patient's appearance, or make it easier for him to wear shoes or gloves.

Nursing interventions. Encourage bed rest, but use a bed cradle to keep covers off extremely sensitive, inflamed joints. Give pain medication, as needed, especially during acute attacks. Apply hot or cold packs to inflamed joints. Administer medication, as ordered. Watch for adverse effects. Be alert for GI disturbances with colchicine.

Urge the patient to drink plenty of fluids (up to 2 qt [2 L] a day) to prevent calculi formation. When forcing fluids, record intake and output accurately. Be sure to monitor serum uric acid levels regularly. Alkalinize urine with sodium bicarbonate or other agent, if ordered.

Watch for acute gout attacks that may occur 24 to 96 hours after surgery. Even minor surgery can precipitate an attack. Before and after surgery, give colchicine to help prevent gout attacks, as ordered.

Patient education. Make sure the patient understands the importance of checking serum uric acid levels periodically. Counsel him to avoid high-purine foods, such as anchovies, liver, sardines, kidneys, sweetbreads, lentils, and alcoholic beverages—especially beer and wine—that raise the urate level. Explain the principles of a gradual weight reduction diet to obese patients. Such a diet features foods containing moderate amounts of protein and little fat.

Advise the patient receiving allopurinol, probenecid, and other drugs to report any adverse effects immediately. (Adverse effects include drowsiness, dizziness, nausea, vomiting, urinary frequency, and dermatitis.) Warn the patient taking probenecid or sulfinpyrazone to avoid aspirin or other salicylates.

Inform the patient that long-term colchicine therapy is essential during the first 3 to 6 months of

What is pseudogout?

Also called calcium pyrophosphate disease, pseudogout results when calcium pyrophosphate crystals collect in periarticular joint structures. Without treatment, it leads to permanent joint damage in about one-half of the patients it affects, most of whom are elderly.

Like gout, pseudogout causes abrupt joint pain and swelling— most commonly affecting the knee, wrist, ankle, and other peripheral joints. These recurrent, self-limiting attacks may be triggered by stress, trauma, surgery, severe dieting, thiazide therapy, and alcohol abuse. Associated symptoms are similar to those of rheumatoid arthritis.

Diagnosis of pseudogout depends on joint aspirations and synovial biopsy to detect calcium pyrophosphate crystals. X-rays reveal calcific densities in the fibrocartilage and linear markings along bone ends. Blood tests may detect an underlying endocrine or metabolic disorder.

Effective treatment of pseudogout may include joint aspiration to relieve fluid pressure; instillation of steroids; administration of analgesics, phenylbutazone, salicylates, or other nonsteroidal antiinflammatories; and, if appropriate, treatment of the underlying endocrine or metabolic disorder.

treatment with uricosuric drugs or allopurinol.

Evaluation. Note whether the patient achieves pain relief or control, complies with drug therapy and dietary regimen to maintain normal serum urate levels, and avoids recurrence of acute episodes.

Herniated disk

Herniated disk occurs when all or part of the nucleus pulposus—the soft, gelatinous, central portion of an intervertebral disk—forces through the weakened or torn outer ring (anulus fibrosus). The extruded disk may impinge on spinal nerve roots as they exit from the spinal canal or on the spinal cord itself, resulting in back pain. Most herniation occurs in the lumbar and lumbosacral regions.

Causes. Herniated disk may result from severe trauma or strain or from intervertebral joint degeneration.

Assessment findings. The overriding symptom of lumbar herniated disk is severe low back pain that radiates to the buttocks, legs, and feet (usually unilaterally) and intensifies with Valsalva's maneuver, coughing, sneezing, or bending.

The patient may also experience motor and sensory loss in the area innervated by the compressed spinal nerve root and, in later stages, weakness and atrophy of leg muscles.

Diagnostic tests. The straight-leg-raising test and its variants are perhaps the best tests to determine herniated disk. For the straight-leg-raising test, the patient lies supine while the examiner places one hand on the patient's ilium (to stabilize the pelvis) and the other hand

under the ankle. The examiner then slowly raises the patient's leg. The test is positive only if the patient complains of posterior leg (sciatic) pain, not back pain. In LeSegue's test, the patient lies flat while the thigh and knee are flexed to a 90-degree angle. Resistance and pain as well as absent or decreased ankle or knee deep tendon reflexes indicate spinal root compression.

While essential to rule out other abnormalities, X-rays of the spine may not diagnose herniated disk because marked disk herniation can escape detection. Myelography, computed tomography scan, and magnetic resonance imaging provide the most specific diagnostic information, showing spinal compression by the herniated disk.

Treatments. The patient initially undergoes conservative treatment, consisting of several days of bed rest (possibly with pelvic traction), heat applications, and an exercise program. Aspirin reduces inflammation and edema at the site of injury. The patient may also benefit from muscle relaxants, especially diazepam, methocarbamol, or hydrocodone (an analgesic).

A herniated disk that fails to respond to conservative treatment may necessitate surgery. The most common procedure, laminectomy, involves excision of a portion of the lamina and removal of the protruding disk. If laminectomy doesn't alleviate pain and disability, a spinal fusion may be necessary to overcome segmental instability. Sometimes a surgeon will perform laminectomy and spinal fusion concurrently to stabilize the spine.

Nursing interventions. During conservative treatment, watch for any deterioration in neurologic status (especially during the first 24 hours after admission), which may indicate an urgent need for surgery.
• Use antiembolism stockings or a sequential pressure device (stockings), as prescribed, and encourage the patient to move his legs, as allowed. Provide high-topped sneakers to prevent footdrop.
• Work closely with the physical therapy department to ensure a consistent regimen of leg- and back-strengthening exercises.
• Give plenty of fluids to prevent renal stasis and constipation, and remind the patient to cough, deep-breathe, and use an incentive spirometer.
• Provide good skin care.
• After laminectomy, diskectomy, or spinal fusion, enforce bed rest, as ordered. Monitor vital signs, and check for bowel sounds and abdominal distention. Use logroll technique to turn the patient.
• If a blood drainage system (such as Hemovac) is in use, check the tubing frequently for kinks and a secure vacuum. Empty the Hemovac at the end of each shift, as ordered, and record the amount and color of drainage.
• Report colorless moisture on dressings (possible cerebrospinal fluid [CSF] leakage) or excessive drainage immediately. Observe neurovascular status of legs (color, motion, temperature, and sensation).
• Give analgesics, as ordered, especially 30 minutes before initial attempts at sitting or walking. Assist the patient during his first attempt to walk. Provide a straight-backed chair for limited sitting.
• Assure the patient of his progress, and offer encouragement.

Patient education. Teach the patient who has undergone spinal fusion how to wear a brace, if ordered. Assist with straight-leg-raising and toe-pointing exercises, as ordered. Before discharge, teach proper body mechanics—bending at the knees and hips (never at the waist), standing straight, and carrying objects close to the body. Advise the patient to lie down when tired and to sleep on his side (never on his abdomen) on an extra-firm mattress or a bed board. Urge maintenance of proper weight.

Tell the patient who must receive a muscle relaxant of possible adverse effects, especially drowsiness. Warn him to avoid activities that require alertness until he has built up a tolerance to the drug's sedative effects.

Evaluation. Look for absence of pain, ability to maintain adequate mobility, and ability to perform ADLs. The patient should understand treatments and any lifestyle adjustments.

Bone disorders

This section addresses disorders of bone structure and function. You will find information on osteoporosis, scoliosis, osteomyelitis, Paget's disease, and hallux valgus.

Osteoporosis

Osteoporosis is a metabolic bone disorder in which the rate of bone resorption accelerates while the rate of bone formation slows down, causing a loss of bone mass. Bones lose calcium and phosphate salts and thus become porous, brittle, and abnormally vulnerable to fracture. Osteoporosis may be primary or secondary to an underlying disease. Primary osteoporosis most commonly develops in postmenopausal women. Senile osteoporosis refers to onset between ages 70 and 85. Risk factors include inadequate intake or absorption of calcium, estrogen deficiency, and sedentary lifestyle.

Osteoporosis primarily affects the weight-bearing vertebrae, ribs, femurs, and wrist bones. Vertebral and wrist fractures are common.

Causes. The cause of primary osteoporosis is unknown. Secondary osteoporosis may result from prolonged therapy with steroids, heparin, anticonvulsants, or thyroid preparations or from aluminum-containing antacids or total immobility or disuse of a bone. It's also linked to alcoholism, malnutrition, malabsorption, scurvy, lactose intolerance, hyperthyroidism, osteogenesis imperfecta, and Sudeck's atrophy (localized to hands and feet, with recurring attacks).

Assessment findings. Although osteoporosis develops insidiously, discovery of the disease usually occurs suddenly. Many elderly persons become aware of the disorder when they bend to lift something, hear a snapping sound, then feel a sudden pain in the lower back. Any movement or jarring aggravates the backache. Other signs and symptoms include pain in the lower back that radiates around the trunk, deformity, kyphosis, loss of height, and a markedly aged appearance.

Diagnostic tests. X-rays, laboratory tests, and bone mass quantification tests such as dual photon energy X-ray may aid diagnosis. X-rays show typical degeneration in the lower thoracic and lumbar vertebrae. The vertebral bodies may appear flattened, with varying degrees of collapse and wedging, and may look denser than normal. Loss of bone mineral is evident in later stages.

Serum calcium, phosphorus, and alkaline phosphatase levels are all within normal limits, but the parathyroid hormone level may be elevated.

Treatments. The patient receives symptomatic treatment to prevent additional fractures and to control pain. Measures include a physical therapy program, emphasizing gentle exercise and activity. The doctor may order estrogen to decrease the rate of bone resorption and calcium and vitamin D to support normal bone metabolism. Drug therapy merely arrests osteoporosis; it does not cure it. Weakened vertebrae should be supported, usually with a back brace. Surgery can correct pathologic fractures of the femur by open reduction and internal fixation. Colles' fracture requires reduction followed by plaster-cast immobilization for 4 to 10 weeks.

Nursing interventions. Your plan of care should focus on the patient's fragility, stressing careful positioning, ambulation, prescribed exercises, and injury prevention strategies.

Check the patient's skin daily for redness, warmth, and new sites of pain, which may indicate new fractures. Encourage activity; help the patient walk several times daily. As appropriate, perform passive ROM exercises or encourage the patient to perform active exercises. Make sure the patient regularly attends scheduled physical therapy sessions.

Provide a balanced diet high in nutrients that support skeletal metabolism: vitamin D, calcium, and protein. Give analgesics, as needed. Apply heat to relieve pain. Finally, impose safety precautions.

Patient education. Thoroughly explain osteoporosis to the patient and her family. If they don't understand the disease, they may feel guilty. Explain how easily an osteoporotic patient's bones can fracture.

Before discharge, make sure the patient and her family understand the prescribed drug regimen. The patient should also report any new pain sites immediately, especially after trauma, no matter how slight. Advise the patient to sleep on a firm mattress and avoid excessive bed rest. Make sure she knows how to wear her back brace.

Teach the patient good body mechanics—to stoop before lifting anything and to avoid twisting and prolonged bending.

If a female patient is taking estrogen, emphasize the need for routine gynecologic checkups, including Papanicolaou tests, and tell her to report any abnormal vaginal bleeding. Also instruct her in the proper technique for self-examination of the breasts. Tell her to examine her breasts monthly and to report any lumps immediately.

Evaluation. Assess whether adherence to prescribed regimen of medication, exercise, and dietary intake of calcium, vitamin D, and protein prevents progression of the disease. Note if the patient demonstrates good body mechanics and if she can identify and avoid activities that increase the risk of fracture.

Scoliosis

A lateral curvature of the spine, scoliosis may occur in the thoracic, lumbar, or thoracolumbar spinal segment. The curve may be convex to the right or to the left. Rotation of the vertebral column around its axis occurs and may cause rib cage deformity. The two types of scoliosis—*functional* (postural) and *structural*—are both commonly associated with kyphosis (humpback) and lordosis (swayback).

Causes. *Functional scoliosis* results from poor posture or a discrepancy in leg lengths.

Structural scoliosis involves deformity of the vertebral bodies. It may be congenital, paralytic, or idiopathic. Congenital scoliosis is usually related to an inherited defect, such as wedge vertebrae, fused ribs or vertebrae, or hemivertebrae. Paralytic or musculoskeletal scoliosis develops after asymmetrical paralysis of the trunk muscles from polio, cerebral palsy, or muscular dystrophy. Idiopathic scoliosis, the most common form, may be transmitted as an autosomal dominant or multifactorial trait. It appears in a previously straight spine during the growing years.

Assessment findings. The most common curve in functional or structural scoliosis arises in the thoracic segment, with convexity to the right, and compensatory curves (S curves) in the cervical segment above and the lumbar segment below, both with convexity to the left. Once the disease becomes well established, backache, fatigue, and dyspnea may occur.

Physical examination reveals unequal shoulder heights, elbow levels, and heights of the iliac crests. Muscles on the convex side of the curve may be rounded; those on the concave side, flattened, producing asymmetry of paraspinal muscles.

Diagnostic tests. Anterior, posterior, and lateral spinal X-rays, taken with the patient standing upright and bending, confirm scoliosis and determine the degree of curvature and flexibility of the spine.

Treatments. The severity of the deformity and potential spine growth determine appropriate treatment. Interventions include close observation, exercise, a brace (for example, a Milwaukee brace), surgery, or a combination of these. Treatment should begin early, when spinal deformity is still subtle.

A mild curve (less than 25 degrees) can be monitored by X-rays and an examination every 3 months. An exercise program may strengthen torso muscles and prevent curve progression. A heel lift may help.

A curve of 25 to 40 degrees requires spinal exercises and a brace. Alternatively, the patient may undergo TENS. A brace halts progression in most patients but does not reverse established curvature.

A curve of 40 degrees or more requires surgery (spinal fusion, usually with instrumentation) because a lateral curve progresses 1 degree a year, even after skeletal maturity. Preoperative preparation may include Cotrel dynamic traction for 7 to 10 days. Postoperative care commonly requires immobilization in a localizer cast (Risser cast) for 3 to 6 months. Periodic checkups follow for several months to monitor stability of the correction. (For more information, see "Laminectomy and spinal fusion," page 361.)

Nursing interventions. The patient with scoliosis will need emotional support, meticulous skin and cast care, and thorough teaching. Scoliosis commonly affects adolescent girls; be especially sensitive to these patients.

If the patient needs traction or a cast before surgery, check the skin around the cast edge daily. Keep the cast clean and dry and the edges of the cast "petaled" (padded). Warn the patient not to insert anything or let anything get under the cast and to immediately report cracks in the cast, pain, burning, skin breakdown, numbness, or odor. Watch for skin breakdown and symptoms of cast syndrome (nausea with abdominal pressure and pain).

Patient education. If the patient needs a brace, follow these guidelines:
• Enlist the help of a physical therapist, a social worker, and an orthotist (orthopedic appliance specialist). Explain what the brace does and how to care for it.
• Tell the patient to wear the brace 23 hours a day and to remove it only for bathing and exercise. While she is still adjusting to the brace, tell her to lie down and rest several times a day.
• To prevent skin breakdown, advise the patient not to use lotions, ointments, or powders on areas where the brace contacts the skin. Suggest she use rubbing alcohol or tincture of benzoin to toughen the skin. Tell her to keep the skin dry and clean and to wear a snug T-shirt under the brace.
• Advise the patient to increase activities gradually and avoid vigorous sports. Stress the importance of conscientiously performing prescribed exercises. Recommend swimming during the hour out of the brace, but strongly warn against diving.
• Instruct the patient to turn her whole body, instead of just her head, when looking to the side.

If the patient needs traction or a cast before surgery, explain these procedures to her and her family. Because a body cast is applied on a special frame and the patient's head and face are covered throughout the procedure, it can be traumatic.

Evaluation. Make sure that the patient doesn't sustain neurovascular deficit or loss of skin integrity because of bracing, traction, or surgery. Is the patient able to maintain an activity level normal for his age and developmental level? Evaluate the results of surgery, if appropriate: Pain should be absent or controlled; lung sounds, skin color and turgor, elimination patterns, and arterial blood gas (ABG) levels should be normal; and shoulders and hips should be more horizontally aligned.

Osteomyelitis

A pyogenic bone infection, osteomyelitis may be chronic or acute. The infection causes tissue necrosis, breakdown of bone structure, and decalcification. Although it may remain localized, osteomyelitis can spread through the bone to the marrow, cortex, and periosteum. Usually a blood-borne disease, acute osteomyelitis most commonly affects rapidly growing children.

Chronic osteomyelitis (rare) is characterized by multiple draining sinus tracts and metastatic lesions.

In children, the most common sites of infection include the lower end of the femur and the upper end of the tibia, humerus, and radius. In adults, the most common sites are the pelvis and vertebrae, usually the result of contamination associated with surgery or trauma. Patient history, physical examination, and blood tests help to confirm osteomyelitis. With prompt treatment, the prognosis for acute osteomyelitis is good. Chronic osteomyelitis carries a poor prognosis.

Causes. Osteomyelitis commonly results from a combination of local trauma—usually quite trivial but resulting in hematoma formation—and an acute infection originating elsewhere in the body. The most common pyogenic organism in osteomyelitis is *Staphylococcus aureus;* others include *Streptococcus pyogenes, Pneumococcus, Pseudomonas aeruginosa, Escherichia coli,* and *Proteus vulgaris.*

Assessment findings. The clinical signs for chronic and acute osteomyelitis are similar. Chronic infection, however, can persist intermittently for years, flaring up spontaneously after minor trauma. The only sign may be persistent drainage of pus from an old pocket in a sinus tract. Acute osteomyelitis usually has a rapid onset.

Local signs and symptoms include sudden pain in the affected bone; tenderness, heat, and swelling over the affected area; and restricted movement.

Diagnostic tests. Relevant tests include laboratory studies, X-rays, and bone scans. The WBC count shows leukocytosis, and the patient has an elevated ESR. Blood culture results enable the doctor to identify the causative organisms. X-rays may not show bone involvement until the disease has been active for some time, usually 2 to 3 weeks. Bone scans may enable the doctor to detect infection early.

Treatments. To prevent further bone damage, interventions against acute osteomyelitis may begin before definitive diagnosis. Measures include administration of large doses of antibiotics I.V. (usually a penicillinase-resistant penicillin, such as nafcillin or oxacillin) after blood cultures are taken; early surgical drainage to relieve pressure buildup and sequestrum formation; immobilization of the affected bone by plaster cast, traction, or bed rest; and supportive treatment, such as analgesics and I.V. fluids.

If an abscess forms, treatment includes incision and drainage, followed by a culture of the drainage matter. Antibiotic therapy to control infection includes administration of systemic antibiotics, intracavitary instillation of antibiotics through closed-system continuous irrigation with low intermittent suction, limited irrigation with blood drainage system with suction (Hemovac), and local application of packed, wet, antibiotic-soaked dressings.

In addition, chronic osteomyelitis usually requires surgery to remove dead bone and to promote drainage. Even after surgery, the prognosis remains poor. Many patients feel great pain and require prolonged hospitalization. Therapy-resistant chronic osteomyelitis in an arm or leg may necessitate amputation.

Nursing interventions. Follow these guidelines:
• Use strict aseptic technique when changing dressings and irrigating wounds. If the patient is in skeletal traction for compound fractures, cover insertion points of pin tracks with small, dry dressings, and tell him not to touch the skin around the pins and wires.
• Administer I.V. fluids, as needed. Provide a diet high in protein and vitamin C.
• Assess vital signs every 4 hours; also assess wound appearance, and new sites of pain, which may indicate secondary infection, daily.
• Support the affected limb with firm pillows. Keep the limb level with the body. Don't let it sag. Provide good skin care. Turn the patient gently every 2 hours and watch for signs of developing decubitus ulcers.
• Provide good cast care. Support the cast with firm pillows and "petal" the edges with pieces of adhesive tape or moleskin to smooth rough edges. Check circulation and drainage every 4 hours for the first 24 hours postoperatively. Promptly report excessive drainage or signs of neurovascular deficits.

• Protect the patient from mishaps, such as jerky movements and falls that may threaten bone integrity. Report sudden pain, crepitus, or deformity immediately. Watch for any sudden malposition of the limb, which may indicate fracture.
• Provide emotional support. Offer the patient appropriate diversions.

Patient education. Before discharge, counsel the patient on how to protect and clean his wound and, most important, how to recognize signs of recurring infection (increased body temperature, redness, localized heat, and swelling). Stress the need for follow-up examinations. Urge the patient to seek prompt treatment for possible sources of recurrence—blisters, boils, sties, and impetigo.

Evaluation. Note whether the patient has sustained any neurovascular deficit. The patient should achieve pain relief or control; new areas of pain, possibly indicating secondary infection, should not appear. Assess whether the patient pursues activities that avoid risk of fracture. Following therapeutic interventions, look for normal body temperature, absence of pain and edema, and full ROM.

Paget's disease

Paget's disease is a slowly progressive metabolic bone disease. An initial phase of excessive bone resorption (osteoclastic phase) is followed by a reactive phase of excessive abnormal bone formation (osteoblastic phase). Chaotic, fragile, and weak, the new bone structure causes painful deformities. Paget's disease usually localizes in one or several areas of the skeleton (most commonly the lower torso); occasionally, widely distributed skeletal deformity occurs. It can be fatal, particularly if associated with heart failure, bone sarcoma, or giant cell tumors.

Causes. The cause remains unknown, but one theory holds that early viral infection causes a dormant skeletal infection that erupts years later as Paget's disease.

Assessment findings. Asymptomatic in early stages, Paget's disease eventually produces severe, persistent pain that intensifies with weight bearing and that may impair movement. Characteristic cranial enlargement occurs over frontal and occipital areas (hat size may increase). Headaches also occur with skull involvement. Bony infringement on cranial nerves may impair hearing and visual acuity. Other signs may include kyphosis, barrel chest, and asymmetrical bowing of the tibia and femur. The pagetic sites may be warm and tender, with slow and incomplete healing of fractures. The patient may walk with a waddling gait and experience increased susceptibility to pathologic fractures.

Diagnostic tests. Diagnosis may require X-rays, a bone scan, a bone biopsy, and laboratory tests. Before symptoms develop, X-rays may show increased bone expansion and density. A bone scan shows early pagetic lesions (radioisotope con-

centrates in areas of active disease). A bone biopsy reveals the characteristic mosaic pattern.

Blood tests reveal anemia and an elevated serum alkaline phosphatase level. (Routine biochemical screens make early diagnosis more common.) In the 24-hour urine test, hydroxyproline (amino acid excreted by kidneys and index of osteoclastic hyperactivity) is elevated.

Treatments. Drug therapy includes calcitonin (a hormone, given subcutaneously or I.M.) and etidronate (by mouth) or plicamycin, a cytotoxic antibiotic.

Calcitonin and etidronate retard bone resorption and reduce serum alkaline phosphate levels and urinary hydroxyproline secretion. Although calcitonin requires long-term maintenance therapy, improvement is noticeable after the first few weeks of treatment. Etidronate produces improvement after 1 to 3 months.

Plicamycin produces remission of symptoms within 2 weeks and biochemical improvement in 1 to 2 months. However, it may destroy platelets or compromise renal function.

Self-administration of calcitonin and etidronate helps patients with Paget's disease lead near-normal lives. Nevertheless, these patients may need surgery to reduce or prevent pathologic fractures, correct secondary deformities, and relieve neurologic impairment. To decrease the risk of excessive bleeding from hypervascular bone, drug therapy with calcitonin and etidronate or plicamycin must precede surgery.

Joint replacement is difficult if bonding material (methyl methacrylate) is used because it doesn't set properly on pagetic bone.

Other treatment is symptomatic and supportive. Aspirin, indomethacin, or ibuprofen usually controls pain.

Nursing interventions. To evaluate the effectiveness of analgesics, assess the patient's level of pain daily. Watch for new areas of pain or restricted movement—which may indicate new fracture sites—and sensory or motor disturbances, such as difficulty in hearing, seeing, or walking.

In addition, you should monitor the patient's serum calcium and alkaline phosphatase levels as well as his intake and output. Encourage adequate fluid intake to minimize renal calculi formation.

If the patient is on prolonged bed rest, prevent decubitus ulcers by providing good skin care. Reposition the patient frequently, and use a flotation mattress. Provide high-topped sneakers to prevent footdrop.

Patient education. Your discussions should cover self-administration of medications, potential adverse effects, and steps the patient can take to adjust to lifestyle changes.

Demonstrate how to inject calcitonin and rotate injection sites. Warn the patient that adverse effects may occur (nausea, vomiting, local inflammation at injection site, facial flushing, itching of hands, and fever), but reassure him that they're usually mild and infrequent. Warn against imprudent use of analgesics.

Tell the patient receiving etidronate to take this medication with fruit juice 2 hours before or after meals (milk or other high-calcium fluids impair absorption), to divide daily dosage to minimize adverse effects, and to watch for and report stomach cramps, diarrhea, fractures, and increasing or new bone pain.

Tell the patient receiving plicamycin to watch for signs of infection, easy bruising, bleeding, and fever and to report for regular follow-up laboratory tests.

Teach the patient how to pace activities and, if necessary, how to use assistive devices. Encourage him to follow a recommended exercise program—avoiding both immobility and excessive activity. Suggest a firm mattress or a bed board to minimize spinal deformities. To prevent falls at home, advise removing throw rugs and other small obstacles. Finally, emphasize the importance of regular checkups, including the eyes and ears.

Evaluation. Assess whether the patient avoids activities that increase risk of fracture and whether he maintains ROM. Note any neurologic deficits and whether treatment has prevented disease progression.

Hallux valgus

Hallux valgus is a lateral deviation of the great toe at the metatarsophalangeal joint. It occurs with medial enlargement of the first metatarsal head and bunion formation.

Causes. Hallux valgus may be congenital or familial but is commonly acquired from degenerative arthritis or from prolonged pressure, especially from narrow-toed, high-heeled shoes that compress the forefoot.

Assessment findings. This disorder first appears as a red, tender bunion. The patient may develop angulation of the great toe away from the midline of the body toward the other toes. In advanced stages of the disorder, he may develop a flat, splayed forefoot, severely curled toes (hammertoes), and a small bunion on the fifth metatarsal. (See *Understanding hammertoe.*)

Diagnostic tests. X-rays confirm diagnosis by showing medial deviation of the first metatarsal and lateral deviation of the great toe.

Treatments. In early stages of acquired hallux valgus, good foot care and proper shoes may eliminate the need for further treatment. Other useful measures for early management include felt pads to protect the bunion, foam pads or other devices to separate the first and second toes at night, and a supportive pad and exercises to strengthen the metatarsal arch. Early treatment is vital in patients predisposed to foot problems, such as those with RA or diabetes mellitus. If the disease progresses to severe deformity with disabling pain, the doctor may order a bunionectomy.

Nursing interventions. Before bunionectomy, obtain a patient history and assess the neurovascular status of the foot (temperature, color, sensation, and blanching). If necessary, teach the patient how to walk with crutches.

After bunionectomy, follow these guidelines.
• Apply ice to reduce swelling. Increase negative venous pressure and reduce edema by supporting the foot with pillows, elevating the foot of the bed, or putting the bed in a Trendelenburg position.
• Record the neurovascular status of the toes, including the patient's ability to move them (dressing may inhibit movement), every hour for the first 24 hours, then every 4 hours. Report any change in neurovascular status to the surgeon immediately.
• Prepare the patient for walking by having him dangle his foot over the side of the bed for a short time before he gets up, allowing a gradual increase in venous pressure. If crutches are needed, make sure he masters this skill before discharge. The patient also should have a proper cast shoe or boot to protect the cast or dressing.

Patient education. Before discharge, instruct the patient to limit activities, to rest frequently with his feet elevated, to elevate his feet when he feels pain or has edema, and to wear wide-toed shoes and sandals after the dressings are removed.

Review proper foot care, such as cleanliness and cutting toenails

Understanding hammertoe

In hammertoe, the patient's toe assumes a clawlike pose from hyperextension of the metatarsophalangeal joint, flexion of the proximal interphalangeal joint, and hyperextension of the distal interphalangeal joint.

Hammertoe usually occurs under pressure from hallux valgus displacement. This causes a painful corn on the top of the interphalangeal joint and on the bone end, and a callus on the sole of the foot, both of which make walking painful. Hammertoe may be mild or severe and can affect one toe or all five, as in clawfoot (which also causes a very high arch).

Causes

Hammertoe can be congenital (and familial) or acquired from constantly wearing short, narrow shoes, which put pressure on the end of the long toe. Acquired hammertoe is commonly bilateral and often develops in children who rapidly outgrow shoes and socks.

Treatment

In young children, or adults with early deformity, repeated foot manipulation and splinting of the affected toe relieve discomfort and may correct the deformity. Other treatment includes protection of protruding joints with felt pads, corrective footwear (open-toed shoes and sandals, or special shoes that conform to the shape of the foot), the use of a metatarsal arch support, and exercises such as passive manual stretching of the proximal interphalangeal joint. Severe deformity requires surgical fusion of the proximal interphalangeal joint in a straight position.

---

straight across to prevent ingrown nails and infection. Suggest exercises to strengthen foot muscles such as standing at the edge of a step on the heel then raising and inverting the top of the foot.

Finally, stress the importance of follow-up care and prompt medical attention for painful bunions, corns, and calluses.

Evaluation. Assess whether the use of properly fitting shoes, felt or foam pads, and general foot care have decreased irritation and inflammation and prevented further disability. Following surgical intervention, evaluate whether the patient has sustained any neurovascular deficits or loss of skin integrity. Once the patient resumes ambulation, he should be free from pain and deformity in the great toe.

Muscle and connective tissue disorders

This section covers tendinitis and bursitis, carpal tunnel syndrome, and polymyositis and dermatomyositis.

Tendinitis and bursitis

Tendinitis is a painful inflammation of tendons and of tendon-muscle attachments to bone, usually in the shoulder rotator cuff, hip, Achilles tendon, or hamstring. A form of tendinitis, calcific dendritis produces proximal weakness. Bursitis is a painful inflammation of one or more of the bursae—closed sacs that contain small amounts of synovial fluid and facilitate the motion of muscles and tendons over bony prominences. Bursitis usually occurs in the subdeltoid, olecranon, trochanteric, calcaneal, or prepatellar bursae. Bursitis may be septic, calcific, acute, or chronic.

Causes. Tendinitis results from trauma; musculoskeletal disorders, such as rheumatic diseases and congenital defects; postural misalignment; abnormal body development; or hypermobility.

Acute and chronic bursitis follows recurring joint trauma or inflammatory joint disease (RA, gout). Septic bursitis follows wound infection or bacterial invasion of skin over the bursa.

Assessment findings. Tendinitis indications include restricted shoulder movement, especially abduction, swelling, and localized pain that is intensified rather than relieved by heat. Typically, this is severest at night. The signs and symptoms of calcific tendinitis include proximal weakness and, possibly, acute calcific bursitis. Indications of bursitis include irritation and inflammation at the site, pain, and limited movement.

Diagnostic tests. In tendinitis, X-rays may show bony fragments, osteophyte sclerosis, or calcium deposits. Arthrography may show occasional small irregularities on the undersurface of the tendon. In bursitis, X-rays may show calcium deposits in calcific bursitis.

Treatments. Treatment to relieve pain includes resting the joint (by immobilization with a sling, splint, or cast), systemic analgesics, application of cold or heat, ultrasound, or local injection of an anesthetic and corticosteroids to reduce inflammation. A mixture of a corticosteroid and an anesthetic such as lidocaine usually relieves pain immediately. Extended-release injections of a corticosteroid, such as triamcinolone or prednisolone, offer longer pain relief. Until the patient is free from pain and able to perform ROM exercises easily, treatment also includes oral anti-inflammatory agents, such as sulindac and indomethacin. Short-term analgesics include codeine, propoxyphene, acetaminophen with codeine and, occasionally, oxycodone.

Supplementary treatment includes fluid removal by aspiration, physical therapy to preserve motion and prevent frozen joints (improvement usually follows in 1 to 4 weeks), and heat therapy (for calcific tendinitis, ice packs). Rarely, calcific tendinitis requires surgical removal of calcium deposits. Long-term control of chronic bursitis and tendinitis may require changes in lifestyle to prevent recurring joint irritation.

Nursing interventions. Assess the severity of pain and the ROM to determine effectiveness of the treatment. Before injecting corticosteroids or local anesthetics, ask the patient about drug allergies.

Assist with intra-articular injection. Scrub the patient's skin thoroughly with povidone-iodine or a comparable solution. After the injection, massage the area to ensure penetration through the tissue and joint space. Apply ice intermittently for about 4 hours to minimize pain. Avoid applying heat to the area for 2 days.

Patient education. Tell the patient to take anti-inflammatory agents with milk to minimize GI distress and report any signs of distress immediately.

Teach the patient to wear a triangular sling during the first few days of an attack of subdeltoid bursitis or tendinitis to support the arm and protect the shoulder, particularly at night. Demonstrate how to wear the sling so it will not put too much weight on the shoulder. Instruct the patient's family how to pin the sling or how to tie a square knot that will lie flat on the back of the patient's neck. To protect the shoulder during sleep, the patient may wear a splint instead of a sling. Instruct him to remove the splint during the day.

Teach him how to maintain joint mobility and prevent muscle atrophy by performing exercises or physical therapy when he is free from pain. Advise him to avoid activities that aggravate the injured joint.

Evaluation. The patient should identify and use effective pain-control interventions for involved joints and tendons. He should maintain normal ROM.

Carpal tunnel syndrome

The most common nerve entrapment syndrome, carpal tunnel syndrome results from compression of the median nerve at the wrist, within the carpal tunnel (formed by the carpal bones and the transverse carpal ligament). Compression neuropathy causes sensory and motor changes in the median distribution of the hand.

Carpal tunnel syndrome poses a serious occupational health problem. Assembly-line workers, packers, and keyboard users are most at risk. Any strenuous use of the hands aggravates this condition. (See *Viewing the carpal tunnel*, page 356.)

Causes. Many conditions can cause the contents or structure of the carpal tunnel to swell and press the median nerve against the transverse carpal ligament. Such conditions include RA, flexor tenosynovitis (associated with rheumatic disease), nerve compression, pregnancy, renal failure, menopause, diabetes mellitus, acromegaly, edema following Colles' fracture, hypothyroidism, amyloidosis, myxedema, benign tumors, tuberculosis, and other granulomatous diseases. Dislocation or acute sprain of the wrist can also damage the median nerve.

Assessment findings. Symptoms of carpal tunnel syndrome include weakness, pain, burning, numbness, or tingling in one or both hands. This paresthesia affects the thumb,

Viewing the carpal tunnel

You can clearly see the carpal tunnel in this palmar view and cross section of a right hand. Note the median nerve, flexor tendons of fingers, and blood vessels passing through the tunnel on their way from the forearm to the hand.

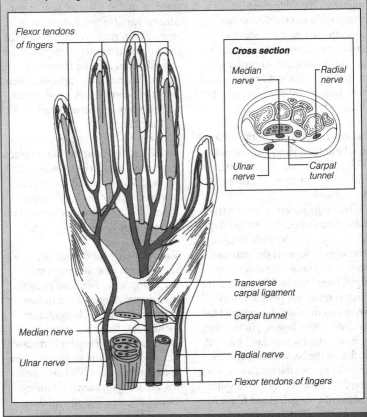

Flexor tendons of fingers

Cross section

Median nerve

Radial nerve

Ulnar nerve

Carpal tunnel

Transverse carpal ligament

Carpal tunnel

Median nerve

Radial nerve

Ulnar nerve

Flexor tendons of fingers

forefinger, middle finger, and one-half of the fourth finger. Other indications include decreased sensation to light touch or pinpricks in the affected fingers; an inability to clench the hand into a fist; nail atrophy; dry, shiny skin; and pain, possibly spreading to the forearm and, in severe cases, as far as the shoulder.

Diagnostic tests. Tinel's sign (tingling over the median nerve on light percussion) is present. The patient has a positive response to Phalen's wrist-flexion test (holding the forearms vertically and allowing both hands to drop into complete flexion at the wrists for 1 minute), reproducing symptoms of carpal tunnel syndrome.

A compression test also supports the diagnosis: A blood pressure cuff inflated above systolic pressure on the forearm for 1 to 2 minutes provokes pain and paresthesia along the distribution of the median nerve. Electromyography detects a median nerve motor conduction delay of more than 5 msec. Other laboratory tests may identify underlying disease.

Treatments. Conservative treatment includes resting the hands by splinting the wrist in neutral extension for 1 to 2 weeks. If the patient's occupation is responsible, he may have to seek other work. Effective treatment may also require correction of an underlying disorder. When conservative treatment fails, the only alternative is surgical decompression of the nerve by sectioning the entire transverse carpal tunnel ligament. Neurolysis (freeing of the nerve fibers) may also be necessary.

Nursing interventions. Give mild analgesics, as needed. Encourage the patient to use his hands as much as possible; however, if the condition has impaired the dominant hand, you may have to help with eating and bathing.

After surgery, monitor vital signs, and regularly check the color, sensation, and motion of the affected hand. Suggest occupational counseling for the patient who has to change jobs because of carpal tunnel syndrome.

Patient education. Teach the patient how to apply a splint. Tell him not to make it too tight. Show him how to remove the splint to perform gentle ROM exercises, which should be done daily. Make sure the patient knows how to do these exercises before discharge.

Advise the patient to exercise his hands occasionally in warm water. If the arm is in a sling, tell him to remove the sling several times a day to do exercises for his elbow and shoulder.

Evaluation. Muscle strength and normal ROM in the affected hand and wrist should progressively return. The patient should experience no pain or paresthesias in the affected hand.

Polymyositis and dermatomyositis

Diffuse, inflammatory myopathies of unknown cause, polymyositis and dermatomyositis produce symmetrical weakness of striated muscle—primarily the proximal muscles of the shoulder and pelvic girdles, neck, and pharynx. In dermatomyositis, muscle weakness is accompanied by pronounced skin changes. These diseases usually progress slowly, with frequent exacerbations and remissions.

Usually, the prognosis worsens with age. The 7-year survival rate for adults is approximately 60%. If properly treated, 80% to 90% of affected children regain normal function. If untreated, however, childhood dermatomyositis may progress rapidly to disabling contractures and muscular atrophy.

Causes. Although the causes of these disorders are unknown, scientists think they may result from autoimmunity, perhaps combined with defective T-cell function.

Assessment findings. Polymyositis signs and symptoms include muscle weakness, tenderness, and discomfort that affects proximal muscles (shoulder, pelvic girdle) more commonly than distal muscles; an inability to move against resistance; dysphagia; and dysphonia.

Dermatomyositis signs and symptoms include an erythematous rash (usually erupts on the face, neck, upper back, chest, and arms and around the nail beds); a heliotropic rash (appears on the eyelids, accompanied by periorbital edema); and violet, flat-topped lesions on the interphalangeal joints.

Diagnostic tests. A muscle biopsy that shows necrosis, degeneration, regeneration, and interstitial chronic lymphocytic infiltration confirms the diagnosis. ESR, WBC count, and muscle enzyme levels (creatine kinase, aldolase, and aspartate aminotransferase) are increased. Urine creatinine level is increased or decreased. Electromyography shows polyphasic short-duration potentials, fibrillation (positive-spike waves), and bizarre, high-frequency, repetitive changes. Antinuclear antibodies are present.

Treatments. High-dose corticosteroid therapy relieves inflammation and lowers muscle enzyme levels. Within 2 to 6 weeks after treatment, serum muscle enzyme levels usually return to normal and muscle strength improves, permitting a gradual tapering of corticosteroid dosage. If the patient responds poorly to corticosteroids, treatment may include cytotoxic or immunosuppressive drugs, such as cyclophosphamide, intermittent I.V. or daily by mouth Supportive therapy includes bed rest during the acute phase, ROM exercises to prevent contractures, analgesics and application of heat to relieve painful muscle spasms, and diphenhydramine to relieve itching. Patients over age 40 need thorough assessment for coexisting cancer.

Nursing interventions. Assess level of pain, muscle weakness, and ROM daily. Give analgesics, as needed. If the patient is bedridden, prevent decubitus ulcers by giving good skin care. To prevent footdrop and contractures, provide high-topped sneakers, and assist with passive ROM exercises at least four times daily. Teach the patient's family how to perform these exercises with the patient.

When you assist with muscle biopsy, make sure the biopsy is not taken from an area of recent needle insertion, such as an injection or electromyography site.

If the patient has a rash, warn him that scratching may cause infection. If antipruritic medication doesn't relieve severe itching, apply tepid sponges or compresses.

Encourage the patient to feed and dress himself but to ask for help when needed. Advise him to pace his activities to counteract muscle weakness. Reassure him that muscle weakness is probably temporary, but allow him to express anxiety.

Patient education. Explain the disease to the patient and his family. Prepare them for diagnostic procedures and possible adverse effects of corticosteroid therapy (weight gain, hirsutism, hypertension, edema, amenorrhea, purplish striae, glycosuria, acne, and easy bruising). Emphatically warn against abruptly discontinuing corticosteroids. Advise a low-sodium diet to prevent fluid retention. Reassure the patient that steroid-induced weight gain will diminish when the drug is discontinued.

Evaluation. The patient should understand signs, symptoms, and course of disease. He should sustain no loss of skin integrity, neurovascular deficits, or contractures. He should perform ROM exercises regularly and ADLs independently as long as possible. The disease's progression should stop or slow.

TREATMENTS

To provide effective care, you'll need a working knowledge of current drug therapy, surgery, and nonsurgical treatments. This section covers these treatments and the use of mobility aids.

Drug therapy

Besides salicylates, the front-line defense against arthropathies, drug therapy may include nonsteroidal anti-inflammatory drugs such as etodolac, ibuprofen, and indomethacin; corticosteroids such as prednisone; skeletal muscle relaxants such as baclofen and carisoprodol; gold compounds such as auranofin and gold sodium thiomalate; and immunosuppressants such as methotrexate and azathioprine.

Surgery

For some patients with musculoskeletal disorders, surgery can offer a bright alternative to a life of chronic pain and disability. To treat degenerative joint changes in osteoarthritis, for example, the surgeon may perform arthrodesis, debridement, osteotomy, or joint replacement. Surgery can also treat joint dislocation and musculoskeletal trauma. For example, the surgeon may perform closed or open reduction for congenital hip dysplasia, or laminectomy or arthrodesis for herniated nucleus pulposus.

For other patients, surgery such as amputation may be palliative but may also have a dramatic impact on self-image. As a result, you'll need to focus on helping the patient come to terms with altered mobility and body image. You'll also need to do considerable teaching, both before and after surgery.

In this section, you'll find out more about your responsibilities in arthroscopy, open reduction, and internal fixation and amputation. You'll also learn about the specific nursing care measures in laminectomy and spinal fusion and joint replacement.

Arthroscopic surgery

During arthroscopy, the surgeon can visually examine and operate on internal joint structures through a fiber-optic scope.

Patient preparation. Explain the type of anesthetic—local or general—that the surgeon will use. If the patient will be receiving a general anesthetic, instruct him not to eat after midnight. Also tell him he may receive a sedative an hour before surgery. Mention that after surgery, he'll briefly have an I.V. line in place. Describe the dressing that he can expect over the site. After knee arthroscopy, review prescribed exercises and ambulation with a cane or crutches, as needed.

Patient education. Tell the patient to watch for signs and symptoms of infection, effusion, or hemarthrosis—unusual drainage, redness, joint swelling, or a "mushy" feeling in the joint. Instruct him to call the doctor if pain, swelling, or stiffness persists for more than a week.

Open reduction and internal fixation

During open reduction, the surgeon restores the normal position and alignment of fracture fragments or dislocated joints. He then inserts internal fixation devices—such as pins, screws, wires, nails, rods, and plates—to maintain alignment until healing can occur.

Patient preparation. Instruct the patient not to eat after midnight. Note that he'll receive a sedative and antibiotics before going to the operating room. Describe the bulky dressing and surgical drain that he'll have in place for several days postoperatively. Tell him that he may need a cast or splint for support when the drain is removed and swelling subsides.

Patient education. Teach the patient how to apply (if appropriate) and care for the device. Tell him to check his skin regularly under and around the device, if possible, for irritation and breakdown. Also instruct the patient to watch for signs of incisional infection. Advise him to exercise and place weight on the affected joint only as the doctor instructs.

Amputation

Perhaps more than any other surgery, amputation can dramatically change a patient's life. Your role includes providing support and detailed instruction in postoperative care.

Patient preparation. Before surgery, reinforce the surgeon's explanation of the procedure and clear up any misconceptions the patient may have. Support the patient as he confronts the loss of a limb.

Explain that after surgery, the surgeon will apply a cast or elastic wrap around the stump. This will help control swelling, minimize pain, and mold the stump so that it fits comfortably into a prosthesis. As appropriate, instruct the patient to report any drainage through the cast, warmth, tenderness, or a foul smell. Tell him that if the cast slips off as swelling subsides, he should immediately wrap the stump. (See *Helping the patient with stump care,* pages 362 and 363.) Or show him how to slip on a custom-fitted elastic stump-shrinker.

Patient education. Emphasize that proper home care of the stump can speed healing. Tell the patient to inspect the stump carefully each day, using a mirror. Instruct him to call the doctor if the incision appears to be opening, looks red or swollen, feels warm, is painful to touch, or is seeping drainage. Teach him to clean the stump daily with mild soap and water, and then rinse and dry it thoroughly.

Instruct the patient to rub the stump with alcohol daily to toughen the skin. Have him avoid applying powder or lotion, which may soften or irritate the skin. Tell him to massage the stump *toward the suture line* to mobilize the scar and prevent its adherence to bone. Advise him to avoid exposing the skin around the stump to excessive perspiration, which can be irritating. He may need to change his elastic bandages or stump socks during the day to avoid this.

As stump muscles adjust to amputation, tell the patient he may have twitching and spasms, or phantom limb pain. Teach him to decrease these symptoms by using heat, massage, or gentle pressure. If his stump is sensitive to touch, tell him to rub it with a dry washcloth for 4 minutes three times a day.

Stress the importance of performing prescribed exercises to help minimize complications, maintain muscle strength and tone, prevent contractures, and promote independence. If appropriate, teach the patient triceps-strengthening exercises for crutch walking, such as push-ups and flexion and extension of the arms using traction weights.

Also stress proper positioning to prevent contractures. If the patient has had a partial arm amputation, tell him to keep his elbow extended and shoulder abducted. If he's had a leg amputation, tell him not to prop his stump on a pillow to avoid hip flexion contracture. After a below-the-knee amputation, have him keep his knee extended to avoid hamstring contracture. After leg amputation, also advise him to lie prone for 4 hours each day to help stretch flexor muscles and to prevent hip flexion contracture. To prevent leg abduction, tell him to keep his legs close together.

To prepare the stump for a prosthesis, teach progressive resistance maneuvers. Begin by telling the patient to push his stump gently against a soft pillow. Have him progress to pushing it against a firm pillow, a padded chair and, finally, a hard chair.

Laminectomy and spinal fusion

In laminectomy, the surgeon removes one or more of the bony laminae that cover the vertebrae. Most commonly performed to relieve pressure on the spinal cord or spinal nerve roots resulting from a herniated disk, laminectomy also may be done to treat compression fracture or dislocation of vertebrae or a spinal cord tumor.

Helping the patient with stump care

When wrapping the stump, tell the patient to follow these steps so that the bandage doesn't slip off.

1. Gather the necessary supplies for wound and skin care. Also get two 3″ elastic bandages, one 4″ elastic bandage, and adhesive tape, safety pins, or clips. Now perform routine wound and skin care. Hold the end of a 3″ bandage at the top of the thigh. Bring the bandage's opposite end downward over the stump and to the back of the leg, as shown.

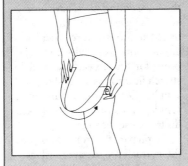

2. Make three turns back and forth to adequately cover the ends of the stump. Hold the bandage ends as shown.

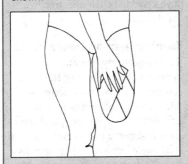

3. Using the other 3″ bandage, make figure-eight turns around the leg to secure the first bandage.

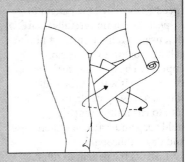

4. Be sure to include the roll of flesh in the groin area. Use even pressure wrapping the stump, keeping it narrow toward the end for a more comfortable fit in the prosthesis. Secure the bandage with clips, safety pins, or adhesive tape.

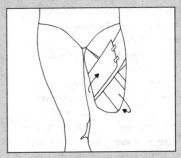

5. Use the 4″ bandage to anchor the stump bandage around the waist. For a below-the-knee amputation,

Helping the patient with stump care *(continued)*

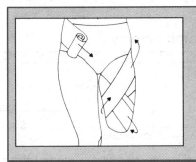

use the knee to anchor the bandage in place.

6. Secure the bandage with clips, safety pins, or adhesive tape. Check the stump bandage regularly. Rewrap it if it bunches at the end.

After removal of several laminae, spinal fusion—grafting of bone chips between vertebral spaces—is commonly performed to stabilize the spine. It also may be done apart from laminectomy in some patients with vertebrae seriously weakened by trauma or disease. Usually, spinal fusion is done only when more conservative treatments—including prolonged bed rest, traction, or the use of a back brace—prove ineffective.

Patient preparation. The patient may be frightened of the scheduled surgery. Try to ease his fears by answering his questions clearly and matter-of-factly. Also try to anticipate questions he's reluctant to ask.

Discuss postoperative recovery and rehabilitation. Point out that surgery won't relieve back pain immediately and that pain may even worsen after the operation. Explain that relief will come only after chronic nerve irritation and swelling subside, which may take up to several weeks. Reassure him that analgesics and muscle relaxants will be available during recovery.

Tell the patient that he'll return from surgery with a dressing over the incision and that he'll be kept on bed rest for the duration prescribed by the surgeon. Explain that he'll be turned often to prevent pressure sores and pulmonary complications. Show him the logroll method of turning, and explain that he'll use this method later to get in and out of bed by himself.

Just before surgery, perform a baseline assessment of motor function and sensation in the patient's lower trunk, legs, and feet. Carefully document the results for comparison with postoperative findings. (See *Managing lumbar laminectomy,* pages 364 to 367.)

Monitoring and aftercare. After surgery, keep the head of the patient's bed flat for at least 24 hours. Urge the patient to remain in the supine position for the prescribed period to prevent any strain on the involved vertebrae. When he's able to assume a side-lying position, make sure he keeps his

(Text continues on page 366.)

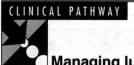

Managing lumbar laminectomy

DRG #215 Lumbar laminectomy
Expected length of stay (LOS): 3.5 days
Admission date:

Discharge date:
Actual LOS:

Expected outcomes	Date	
	Key indicators	Preadmission
Expected outcome Patient will receive care from a multidisciplinary health care team.	Consults	• Medical
Diagnosis Risk for fluid volume deficit related to surgical procedure Risk for postoperative hemorrhage **Expected outcome** Maintain normal hemodynamics.	Diagnostics	• Prothombin time (PT)/partial thromboplastin time (PTT) • Blood chemistry • Complete blood count (CBC) • Electrocardiogram (ECG) • Chest X-ray • Type and screen (T&S)
	I.V. therapy	
Diagnosis Risk for alteration of neurovascular state **Expected outcome** Patient will maintain or regain function; stable neurologic signs.	Assessment	• Initiate assessment. • Initiate neurovascular assessment.
Diagnosis Alteration in comfort, pain related to surgery **Expected outcome** Patient will verbalize a decrease in pain following administration of pain medication.	Pharmacology	

O.R. Day 1	Postop Day 1/Day 2	Postop Day 2/ Day 3	Postop Day 3/ Day 4
→→→→ • Anesthesia	→→→→		
• I.V. fluids:_____ • Cap I.V. when patient tolerating oral (P.O.) fluids.	• Discontinue I.V. after last dose of antibiotics.		
• Admission assessment • Neurovascular assessment • Vital signs (VS) • Dressing assessment	• Ongoing assessment • Ongoing neurovascular assessment • VS • Incision site assessment	• Ongoing assessment	
• Anti-inflammatory: _____ • Muscle relaxant: _____ • Pericolace twice a day • Analgesics: • I.M.: _____ • P.O.: _____ • P.O.: _____ • Prophylactic antibiotic × 3 doses: _____ • Antiemetic: _____	→→→→ →→→→ →→→→ →→→→ →→→→ →→→→ • Discontinue after 3rd dose.		*(continued)*

Managing lumbar laminectomy (continued)

Expected outcomes	Key indicators	Preadmission
Diagnosis Risk for alteration in nutrition state and bowel and bladder function **Expected outcome** Patient will maintain nutritional status and have or establish bowel and bladder function.	Nutrition/elimination	• Instruct patient on nothing-by-mouth (NPO) status for day of surgery.
Diagnosis Risk for activity intolerance related to postoperative pain and limitations **Expected outcome** Patient will increase activity safely and without discomfort postoperatively.	Activity/safety	
Diagnosis Risk for complication related to surgery **Expected outcome** Clean, dry, healing surgical site	Treatments/wound care	
Diagnosis Knowledge deficit related to disease process or surgical procedure **Expected outcome** Patient will verbalize understanding of physical limitations and home care issues.	Patient education	• Laminectomy information booklet from doctor's office • Preadmission interview, follow-up questions regarding expectations answered
Expected outcome Patient will be discharged with appropriate services and follow-up plan.	Discharge plan	• Initiate discharge plan.
Have daily outcomes been met? (If not, complete database sheet.)		Yes No

Adapted with permission from Sacred Heart Hospital, Allentown, Pa.

spine straight with his knees flexed and drawn up toward his chest. Insert a pillow between his knees to relieve pressure on the spine from hip adduction.

Inspect the dressing frequently for bleeding or CSF leakage; report

O.R. Day 1	Postop Day 1/Day 2	Postop Day 2/ Day 3	Postop Day 3/ Day 4
• Assess bowel sounds, abdominal distention, and voiding pattern. • NPO preoperative • Clear liquid postoperative diet • Diet: _____	→→→→ • Diet: _____ _____ _____	• Diet	
• Antiembolism stockings • To bathroom with assistance	• Allow ambulation with assistance—or alone as tolerated. • Encourage activity.	• Allow ambulation alone as tolerated. • Allow shower.	
• If drainage on dressing increases by 50%, change using aseptic technique.	• Clean site with betadine and leave open to air. OR • Change air strip dressing daily.	• Clean site with betadine and leave open to air. OR • Redress with air strip.	
• Teach patient to push with arms when moving from lying to standing. • Teach patient to lie with knees slightly bent.	• Review discharge instruction sheet with patient. • Instruct patient on medications. • Review good body mechanics.	• Review discharge instruction sheet with patient.	
• Plan for discharge follow-up care.	• Discharge.	• Discharge.	
Yes No	Yes No	Yes No	

either immediately. The surgeon will probably perform the initial dressing change himself; you may be asked to perform subsequent changes.

Assess motor and neurologic function in the patient's trunk and lower extremities and compare the results with baseline findings. Also evaluate circulation in his legs and feet and report any abnormalities. Give analgesics and muscle relaxants, as ordered.

Every 2 to 4 hours, assess urine output and auscultate for the return of bowel sounds. If the patient doesn't void within 8 to 12 hours after surgery, notify the doctor and prepare to insert a catheter to relieve retention. If the patient can void normally, assist him in getting on and off a bedpan while maintaining proper alignment.

Patient education. Teach the patient and his caregiver proper incision-care measures. Tell them to check the incision site often for signs and symptoms of infection— increased pain and tenderness, redness, swelling, and changes in the amount and character of drainage— and to report any such signs and symptoms immediately. Instruct the patient to avoid soaking his incision in a tub bath until healing is complete. Also advise him to shower with his back facing away from the stream of water.

Make sure the patient understands the importance of resuming activity gradually after surgery. As ordered, instruct him to start with short walks and to slowly progress to longer distances. Review any prescribed exercises, such as pelvic tilts, leg raises, and toe pointing. Advise him to rest frequently and avoid overexertion.

Review any prescribed activity restrictions. Usually, the doctor will prohibit sitting for prolonged periods, lifting heavy objects or bending over, and climbing long flights of stairs. He may also impose other restrictions, depending on the patient's condition.

Teach the patient proper body mechanics to lessen strain and pressure on his spine. Instruct him to lie on his back, with his knees propped up with pillows, or on his side with his knees drawn up and a pillow placed between his legs. Warn him against lying on his stomach or on his back with legs flat. When sitting, he should place his feet on a low stool to elevate his knees above hip level. He should use a firm, straight-backed chair and sit up straight with his lower back pressed flat against the chair back. When standing for prolonged periods, he should alternate placing each foot on a low stool to straighten his lower back and relieve strain. When bending, he should keep his spine straight and bend at his knees and hips rather than at his waist.

If a back brace is prescribed, teach the patient how to apply it. Also instruct him how to assess his skin integrity.

Instruct the patient to sleep only on a firm mattress. If necessary, advise him to purchase a new one or to insert a bed board between his mattress and box spring.

Joint replacement

Total or partial replacement of a joint with a synthetic prosthesis restores mobility and stability and relieves pain. Joint replacement is now a common treatment for patients with severe chronic arthritis, degenerative joint disorders, and extensive joint trauma. All joints except the spine can be replaced with a prosthesis; hip and knee replacements are the most common. (See *Reconstruction alternatives.*)

Patient preparation. Because of joint replacement's complexity, patient preparation begins long before surgery with extensive tests and studies.

Discuss postoperative recovery with the patient and his family. As appropriate, show him ROM exercises or demonstrate the continuous passive motion device he'll use during recovery from total knee replacement. Say that most likely he will be out of bed the following day. Explain the use of a Hemovac to drain excess blood from the wound. Mention that an anticoagulant will be given after surgery to prevent blood clots.

Point out that he may not experience pain relief immediately after surgery and that pain may actually worsen for several weeks. Reassure him that pain will diminish dramatically once edema subsides and that analgesics will be available as needed.

Ensure that the patient or a responsible family member has signed a consent form.

Monitoring and aftercare. After surgery, keep the patient on bed rest for the prescribed period. Maintain the affected joint in proper alignment. If traction is used, periodically check the weights and other equipment.

Assess the patient's level of pain and provide analgesics, as ordered. If you're giving narcotic analgesics,

Reconstruction alternatives

Arthroplasty is a surgical technique intended to restore motion to a stiffened joint. Joint replacement is one option. Other options include *joint resection* or *interpositional reconstruction.*

Joint resection

This technique involves careful excision of bone portions, creating a 2-cm gap in one or both bone surfaces of the joint. Fibrous scar tissue eventually fills in the gap. Although this surgery restores mobility and relieves pain, it decreases joint stability.

Interpositional reconstruction

In this technique, the surgeon reshapes the joint and places a prosthetic disk between the reshaped bony ends. The prosthesis used for this procedure may be composed of metal, plastic, fascia, or skin. However, with repeated injury and surgical reshaping, total joint replacement may be necessary.

be alert for signs of toxicity or oversedation.

During recovery, monitor for complications of joint replacement, particularly hypovolemic shock from blood loss during surgery. Assess the patient's vital signs frequently, and report hypotension, narrowed pulse pressure, tachycardia, decreased level of consciousness (LOC), rapid and shallow respirations, or cold, pale, clammy skin. Watch for signs of fat embolism, a potentially fatal complication caused by release of fat molecules in response to increased intermedullary canal pressure from the prosthesis. Fat embolism usually develops within 72 hours after surgery and is characterized by apprehension, diaphoresis, fever, dyspnea, pulmonary effusion, tachycardia, cyanosis, seizures, decreased LOC, and a petechial rash on the chest and shoulders.

Inspect the incision frequently for signs of infection. Change the dressing as necessary, maintaining strict aseptic technique. Periodically assess neurovascular and motor status distal to the joint replacement site. Immediately report any abnormalities or complications such as a dislocated total hip replacement (signs and symptoms of this are sudden, severe pain, shortening, or internal or external rotation of the involved leg).

Reposition the patient often to enhance comfort and prevent pressure sores. Encourage coughing and deep breathing to prevent pulmonary complications, and adequate fluid intake to avert urinary stasis and constipation.

Have the patient begin exercising the affected joint as ordered, perhaps even on the day of surgery. The doctor may prescribe continuous passive motion (using a machine or a system of suspended ropes and pulleys) or a series of active or passive ROM exercises.

Before the patient with a knee or hip replacement is discharged, make sure that he has a properly sized pair of crutches and knows how to use them.

Patient education. Reinforce the doctor's and physical therapist's instructions for the patient's exercise regimen. Remind him to closely adhere to the prescribed schedule and not to rush rehabilitation, no matter how good he feels.

Review prescribed limitations on activity. The doctor may order the patient to avoid bending or lifting, extensive stair climbing, or sitting for prolonged periods (including long car trips or plane flights). He will caution against overusing the joint—especially weight-bearing joints.

If the patient has undergone hip replacement, instruct him to keep his hips abducted and not to cross his legs when sitting, to reduce the risk of dislocating the prosthesis. Tell him to avoid flexing his hips more than 90 degrees when rising from a bed or chair. Encourage him to sit in chairs with high arms and a firm seat and to sleep only on a firm mattress.

Caution the patient to promptly report signs and symptoms of possible infection, such as persistent fever and increased pain, tenderness, and stiffness in the joint and surrounding area. Remind him that infection may develop even several months after joint replacement. Tell the patient to report a sudden increase of pain, which may indicate dislodgment of the prosthesis. Also teach him the signs and symptoms of deep vein thrombosis and pulmonary embolism and tell him to report them immediately.

Nonsurgical treatments

Some patients with musculoskeletal disorders require nonsurgical treat-

Looking at external fixation devices

The illustrations below will help you understand how some common external fixation devices work. The doctor's selection of a device will depend on the severity of the patient's fracture and on the type of bone alignment needed.

Universal day frame

The universal day frame is used to manage tibial fractures.

Features

The frame allows readjustment of the position of bony fragments by angulation and rotation. The compression/distraction device allows compression and distraction of bony fragments.

Portsmouth external fixation bar

The Portsmouth external fixation bar device is used to manage complicated tibial fractures.

Features

The locking nut adjustment on the mobile carriage only allows bone compression, so the doctor must accurately reduce bony fragments before applying the device.

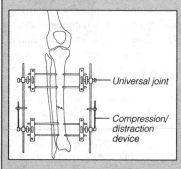

Universal joint

Compression/
distraction
device

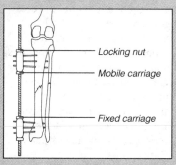

Locking nut

Mobile carriage

Fixed carriage

ment. Such treatment may include closed reduction of a fracture or immobilization.

Closed reduction

Closed reduction involves external manipulation of fracture fragments or dislocated joints to restore their normal position and alignment. It may be done under local, regional, or general anesthesia. (See *Looking at external fixation devices.*)

Patient preparation. If the patient will be receiving a general anesthet-

ic, instruct him not to eat after midnight. Tell him he'll receive a sedative before the surgery. If appropriate, explain how traction can reduce pain, relieve muscle spasms, and maintain alignment while he awaits surgery. Mention that he'll need to wear a bandage, sling, splint, or cast postoperatively.

Patient education. Before discharge, teach the patient how to apply (if appropriate) and care for the immobilization device. Tell him to regularly check his skin under and around the device for irritation and breakdown. Stress the importance of following prescribed exercises.

Immobilization

Used to maintain alignment and limit movement, immobilization devices also relieve pressure and pain. These devices include plaster and synthetic *casts* applied after closed or open reduction of fractures or after other severe injuries; *splints* to immobilize fractures, dislocations, or subluxations; *slings* to support and immobilize an injured arm, wrist, or hand or to support the weight of a splint or hold dressings in place; *skin or skeletal traction*, using a system of weights and pulleys to reduce fractures, treat dislocations, correct deformities, or decrease muscle spasms; *braces* to support weakened or deformed joints; and *cervical collars* to immobilize the cervical spine, decrease muscle spasms, and relieve pain.

Patient preparation. Explain the purpose of the immobilization device the doctor has chosen. If possible, show the patient the device before application and demonstrate how it works. Tell him approximately how long the device will remain in place. Explain that he can anticipate discomfort initially, but reassure him that this will resolve as he becomes accustomed to the device.

Give analgesics and muscle relaxants for pain, as ordered.

Monitoring and aftercare. Take steps to prevent complications of immobility. Reposition the patient frequently to enhance comfort and prevent pressure sores. As ordered, assist with active or passive ROM exercises to maintain muscle tone and prevent contractures. Encourage regular coughing and deep breathing and adequate fluid intake.

Encourage ambulation, and provide assistance as necessary. Encourage the bedridden patient to engage in diversionary activities.

Provide analgesics, as ordered. If you're giving narcotics, watch for signs of toxicity or oversedation.

Patient education. Instruct the patient to promptly report signs and symptoms of complications, including increased pain, drainage, or swelling in the involved area. Stress the need for strict compliance with activity restrictions while the immobilization device is in place.

If the patient has been given crutches to use while a leg or ankle cast, splint, or knee immobilizer is in place, make sure he understands how to use them. If the patient has a removable device such as a knee immobilizer, make sure he knows how to apply it correctly.

Stress the need to keep scheduled appointments to evaluate healing.

Mobility aids

While recuperating from surgery, some patients may need to use mobility aids, such as canes, walkers, or crutches. These devices are also indicated for patients who suffer from weakness, injury, occasional loss of balance, or increased joint pressure.

Canes

Indicated for the patient with one-sided weakness or injury, occasional loss of balance, or increased joint pressure, the cane provides balance and support for walking and reduces fatigue and strain on weight-bearing joints. Available in various sizes, the cane should extend from the greater trochanter to the floor and have a rubber tip.

Although wooden canes are available, three types of aluminum canes are used most commonly. The *standard aluminum cane*—used by the patient requiring only slight assistance to walk—provides the least support; its half-circle handle allows it to be hooked over chairs. The *T-handle cane*—used by the patient with hand weakness—has a straight, shaped handle with grips and a bent shaft. It provides greater stability than the standard cane. The *quadripod (broad-based) cane*—used by the patient with poor balance or the cerebrovascular accident patient with one-sided weakness and inability to hold onto a walker with both hands—has a base with four additional supports in a rectangular array. It provides greater stability than a standard cane but considerably less than a walker.

Patient preparation. Ask the patient to hold the cane on the uninvolved side 4″ to 6″ (10 to 15 cm) from the base of the little toe. If the cane is made of aluminum, adjust its height by pushing in the metal button on the shaft and raising or lowering the shaft; if it's wooden, the rubber tip is removed

and the excess is sawed off. At the correct height, the handle of the cane is level with the greater trochanter and allows approximately 15-degree flexion at the elbow.

Explain the mechanics of cane-walking to the patient. Tell him to hold the cane on the uninvolved side to promote a reciprocal gait pattern and to distribute weight away from the involved side. Instruct the patient to hold the cane close to the body to prevent leaning and to move the cane and the involved leg simultaneously, followed by the uninvolved leg.

Encourage the patient to keep the stride length of each leg and the timing of each step equal. He should always use a railing, if present, when negotiating stairs. Tell him to hold the cane with the other hand or to keep it in the hand grasping the railing. To ascend stairs, the patient should lead with the uninvolved leg and follow with the involved leg; to descend, he should lead with the involved leg and follow with the uninvolved one. Help the patient remember by telling him to use this mnemonic device: The good goes up, and the bad goes down.

To negotiate stairs without a railing, the patient should use the walking technique to ascend and descend the stairs, but move the cane just before the involved leg. To ascend stairs, the patient should hold the cane on the uninvolved side, step with the uninvolved leg, advance the cane, then the involved leg. To descend, he should hold the cane on the uninvolved side, lead with the cane, then the involved leg, and finally the uninvolved leg.

Procedure. After instructing the patient, demonstrate correct cane walking. Then, have him practice in front of you before allowing him to walk alone. When he's ready to climb stairs, advise him that he'll need considerable practice (in the physical therapy department).

Guard the patient carefully by standing behind him slightly to his stronger side and putting one foot between his feet and your other foot to the outside of the uninvolved leg. If necessary, use a walking belt. Decrease your guarding as the patient gains competence.

Walkers

A walker provides greater stability and security than other ambulatory aids. Attachments for standard walkers and modified walkers help meet special needs.

The *standard walker*—used by the patient with unilateral or bilateral weakness or inability to bear weight on one leg—requires arm strength and balance.

The patient who must negotiate stairs without bilateral handrails uses the *stair walker*. It requires arm strength and balance. Its extra set of handles extends toward the patient on the open side. The *rolling walker*—used by the patient with very weak legs—has four wheels and a seat. The *reciprocal walker*—used by the patient with very weak arms—allows one side to be advanced ahead of the other.

Patient preparation. Obtain the appropriate walker. Adjust it to the patient's height, so that it is waist-high. His elbows should be flexed at a 15-degree angle when standing comfortably within the walker with his hands placed on the grips. To adjust the walker, turn it upside down, and change leg length by pushing in the button on each shaft and releasing it when the leg is in the correct position. Make sure the walker is level before the patient attempts to use it.

Procedure. Help the patient stand within the walker, and instruct him to hold the handgrips firmly and equally. If the patient has one-sided leg weakness, tell him to advance the walker 6″ to 8″ (15 to 20.5 cm) and to step forward with the involved leg, supporting himself on the arms, and to follow with the uninvolved leg. If he has equal strength in both legs, instruct him to advance the walker 6″ to 8″ and to step forward with either leg. If he can't use one leg, tell him to advance the walker 6″ to 8″ and to swing onto it, supporting his weight on the hands.

If the patient is using a reciprocal walker, teach him the two-point or four-point gait. If he is using a wheeled standard walker or a stair walker, reinforce the physical therapist's instructions. Stress the need for caution when using a stair walker.

When the patient first practices with the walker, stand behind him, closer to the involved leg. Encourage him to take equal strides, overcoming the tendency to favor the involved leg by taking longer steps with it than with the uninvolved leg. If he starts to fall, support the hips and shoulders to help maintain an upright position, if possible.

Crutches

Crutches remove weight from one or both legs, enabling the patient to support himself with the hands and arms. Successful use requires balance, stamina, and upper-body strength. Crutch selection depends on the patient's condition.

Three types of crutches are commonly used: *standard* (for short-term use) and *forearm and platform crutches* (for long-term use). *Standard aluminum or wooden crutches* aid the patient with a sprain, strain, cast, or pinning. They require stamina and upper-body strength. *Forearm, or aluminum Lofstrand, crutches* assist the paraplegic or other patient using the swing-through gait. These crutches use a collar that fits around the forearm and a horizontal handgrip that provides support. *Platform crutches* aid the arthritic patient with an upper-extremity deficit that prevents weight bearing through the wrist; they're padded for comfort.

Patient preparation. After choosing the appropriate crutches, adjust their height with the patient standing or, if necessary, recumbent. Position the crutches so they extend from a point 4″ to 6″ (10 to 15 cm) to the side and 4″ to 6″ in front of the patient's feet to ¹/₂″ to 2″ (1.3 to 5 cm), or 1 to 2 fingerbreadths, below the axillae. Then, adjust the handgrips so the patient's elbows

are flexed at a 15-degree angle when he's standing with the crutches in resting position.

Consult the doctor and physical therapist to coordinate rehabilitation orders and teaching. Explain your choice of gait, and then teach it.

Procedure. Place a walking belt around the patient's waist, if necessary, to help prevent falls. Tell the patient to position the crutches and to shift his weight from side to side. Then, place him in front of a full-length mirror to aid learning and coordination. (See *Charting falls*, page 376.)

Teach the four-point gait to the patient who can bear some weight on both legs. Although this is the safest gait because three points are always in contact with the floor, it requires greater coordination than others because of its constant shifting of weight. Use the sequence "right crutch, left foot, left crutch, right foot." Suggest counting to help develop rhythm, and make sure each short step is of equal length. If the patient gains proficiency at this gait, teach the faster two-point gait.

Teach the two-point gait to the patient with weak legs but good coordination and arm strength. The most natural crutch-walking gait, it mimics walking, with alternating swings of the arms and legs. Tell the patient to advance the right crutch and left foot simultaneously, followed by the left crutch and the right foot.

Teach the three-point gait to those who can bear only partial or no weight on one leg. Have the patient advance both crutches 6″ to

Charting falls

If a patient falls despite precautions, be sure to chart the event and file an incident report. Check the patient for bruises, lacerations, or abrasions. Document any pain or deformity in the extremities, particularly the hip, arm, leg, or lumbar spine. Assess and record blood pressure while the patient is lying down and sitting up. Look for a drop of 20 to 30 mm Hg in the systolic reading, which may indicate orthostatic hypotension.

Perform a neurologic assessment. Check for slurred speech, a weakness in the extremities, or a change in mental status. Notify the doctor and chart the time.

8″ (15 to 20.5 cm) along with the involved leg. Then have him bring the uninvolved leg forward, bearing most weight on the crutches but some of it on the involved leg. Stress the need to take steps of equal length and duration, without pause.

Teach the swing-to or swing-through gaits—the fastest ones—to the patient with complete paralysis of the hips and legs. When used with chronic conditions, these gaits can lead to atrophy of the hips and legs if appropriate therapeutic exercises are not performed routinely. Instruct the patient to advance both crutches simultaneously and to swing the legs parallel to (swing-to) or beyond the crutches (swing-through).

To get up from a chair, the patient should hold both crutches in one hand, with the tips resting firmly on the floor. Then, instruct him to push up from the chair with his free hand, supporting himself with the crutches. To sit down, the patient supports himself with the crutches in one hand and lowers himself with the other.

To teach the patient to ascend stairs using the three-point gait, tell him to lead with the uninvolved leg and to follow with both the crutches and the involved leg. To descend stairs, he should lead with the crutches and the involved leg and follow with the uninvolved leg.

REFERENCES AND READINGS

Folcik, M.A., et al. *Traction: Assessment and Management.* St. Louis: Mosby–Year Book, Inc., 1994.

Isselbacher, K., et al., eds. *Harrison's Principles of Internal Medicine,* 13th ed. New York: McGraw-Hill Book Co., 1995.

Mader, J.T., et al. "Long-Bone Osteomyelitis: Diagnosis and Management," *Hospital Practice* 29(10): 71-79, October 15, 1994.

Nursing98 Drug Handbook. Springhouse, Pa.: Springhouse Corp., 1998.

Rakel, R.E., ed. *Conn's Current Therapy 1996.* Philadelphia: W.B. Saunders Co., 1996.

Sparks, S.M., et al. *Nursing Diagnosis Pocket Manual.* Springhouse, Pa.: Springhouse Corp., 1996.

Tierney, L., et al. *Current Medical Diagnosis and Treatment 1995.* East Norwalk, Conn.: Appleton & Lange, 1995.

Zupan, A., et al. "Long-Lasting Effects of Electrical Stimulation upon Muscles of Patients Suffering from Progressive Muscular Dystrophy," *Clinical Rehabilitation* 9(2):102-09, May 1995.

8

RENAL AND
UROLOGIC
CARE

The urinary system and the kidneys retain useful materials and excrete foreign or excessive materials and waste. Through this basic function, the kidneys profoundly affect other body systems and the patient's overall health. Assessing the renal and urologic system may uncover clues to possible problems in any body system.

Physical examination

Begin the physical examination by documenting baseline vital signs and weighing the patient. Comparing subsequent weight measurements to this baseline may reveal a developing problem, such as dehydration or fluid retention. Because the urinary system affects many body functions, a thorough assessment includes examination of multiple related body systems in addition to using inspection, auscultation, percussion, and palpation techniques.

Ask the patient to urinate into a specimen cup. Assess the sample for color, odor, and clarity. Give the patient a gown and drapes, have him undress, and proceed with a systematic physical examination.

Inspection

Urinary system inspection includes examination of the abdomen and urethral meatus.

Abdomen. Help the patient assume a supine position with his arms relaxed at his sides. Make sure he's comfortable and draped appropriately. Expose the patient's abdomen from the xiphoid process to the symphysis pubis, and inspect the abdomen for gross enlargements or fullness by comparing the left and right sides, noting any asymmetrical areas. In a normal adult, the abdomen is smooth, flat or scaphoid (concave), and symmetrical. Abdominal skin should be free from scars, lesions, bruises, and discolorations.

Extremely prominent veins may accompany other vascular signs associated with renal dysfunction, such as hypertension and renal artery bruits. Distention, skin tightness and glistening, and striae (streaks or linear scars caused by rapidly developing skin tension) may signal fluid retention. If you suspect ascites, perform the fluid wave test. Ascites may suggest nephrotic syndrome.

Urethral meatus. Help the patient feel more at ease during your inspection by examining the urethral meatus last and by explaining beforehand how you'll assess this area. Be sure to wear gloves.

Urethral meatus inspection may reveal several abnormalities. In a male patient, a meatus deviating from the normal central location may represent a congenital defect. In any patient, inflammation and discharge may signal urethral infection. Ulceration usually indicates a sexually transmitted disease.

Auscultation

Auscultate the renal arteries in the left and right upper abdominal quadrants by pressing the stethoscope bell lightly against the abdomen and telling the patient to exhale deeply. Begin auscultating at the midline and work to the left. Then return to the midline and work to the right. Systolic bruits (whooshing sounds) or other unusual sounds are potentially significant abnormalities. For example, in a patient with hypertension, systolic bruits suggest renal artery stenosis.

Percussion

After auscultating the renal arteries, percuss the patient's kidneys to detect any tenderness or pain, and percuss the bladder to evaluate its position and contents. Abnormal kidney percussion findings include tenderness and pain, suggesting glomerulonephritis or glomerulonephrosis. A dull sound heard on percussion in a patient who has just urinated may indicate urine retention, reflecting bladder dysfunction or infection.

Palpation

Palpation of the kidneys and bladder is the next step in the physical examination. (See *Palpating the urinary organs.*) Through palpation, you can detect any lumps, masses, or tenderness. To achieve optimal results, have the patient relax his abdomen by taking deep breaths through his mouth.

Abnormal kidney and bladder palpation findings may signify various problems. (For some common abnormal assessment findings, see *Interpreting renal and urologic assessment findings,* pages 381 and 382.)

DIAGNOSTIC TESTS

With the help of advanced technology, including improved computer processing and imaging techniques, renal and urologic problems that were previously detectable only by invasive techniques can now be evaluated. (See *Diagnostic tests for renal and urologic disorders,* pages 383 to 389.)

Palpating the urinary organs

In the normal adult, the kidneys usually can't be palpated because they're located deep within the abdomen. However, they may be palpable in a thin patient or in one with reduced abdominal muscle mass. (Because the right kidney is slightly lower than the left, it may be easier to palpate.) Keep in mind that both kidneys descend with deep inhalation.

If palpable, the bladder normally feels firm and relatively smooth. However, remember that an adult's bladder may not be palpable.

Using bimanual manipulation, begin on the patient's right side and proceed as follows.

Kidney palpation

1. Help the patient to a normal supine position, and expose the abdomen from the xiphoid process to the symphysis pubis. Standing at the right side, place your left hand under the back, midway between the lower costal margin and the iliac crest.

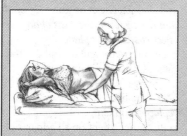

2. Next, place your right hand on the patient's abdomen, directly above your left hand. Angle this hand slightly toward the costal margin. To palpate the right lower edge of the right kidney, press your right fingertips about ½″ (1.3 cm) above the right iliac crest at the midinguinal line; press your fingertips upward into the right costovertebral angle.

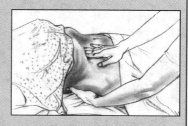

3. Instruct the patient to inhale deeply so that the lower portion of the right kidney can move down between your hands. If it does, note its shape and size. Normally, it feels smooth, solid, and firm, yet elastic. Ask the patient if palpation causes tenderness. (*Note:* avoid using excessive pressure to palpate the kidney because this may cause intense pain.)

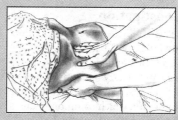

4. To assess the left kidney, move to the patient's left side and position your hands as described above, but with this change: Place your right hand 2″ (5 cm) above the iliac crest. Then apply pressure with both hands as the patient inhales. If the

(continued)

Palpating the urinary organs *(continued)*

left kidney can be palpated, compare it with the right kidney; it should be the same size.

Bladder palpation
Before palpating the bladder, make sure the patient has voided. Then locate the edge of the bladder by pressing deeply in the midline about 1″ to 2″ (2.5 to 5 cm) above the symphysis pubis. As the bladder is palpated, note its size and location and check for lumps, masses, and tenderness. The bladder normally feels firm and relatively smooth. During deep palpation, the patient may report the urge to urinate—a normal response.

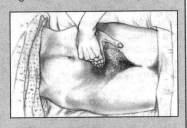

NURSING DIAGNOSES

When caring for patients with renal or urologic disorders, you'll find that several nursing diagnoses are commonly used. These diagnoses appear below, along with appropriate nursing interventions and rationales. (Rationales appear in italic type.)

Constipation

Related to inadequate intake of fluid and bulk, constipation may be caused by prolonged immobility, fluid and dietary restrictions, and use of phosphate binders containing aluminum, which commonly causes serious constipation in dialysis patients.

Expected outcomes
• Patient's fluid and fiber intake is assessed.
• Patient uses bedside commode or walks to toilet facilities.
• Patient participates in development of a bowel program.
• Patient describes measures that help to eliminate constipation.
• Patient reports easy and complete evacuation of stool.
• Patient increases activity level.
• Patient maintains elimination pattern within normal limits.

Nursing interventions and rationales
• Monitor and record frequency and characteristics of stool. *Careful monitoring forms the basis of an effective treatment plan.*
• Record intake and output accurately. Unless contraindicated, encourage fluid intake of 2½ qt (2.5 L) daily *to ensure correct fluid replacement therapy.*
• Place the patient on a bedpan or commode at specific time(s) daily, as close to usual evacuation time (if known) as possible, *to aid adaptation to routine physiologic function.*
• Administer laxative or enema, as ordered, *to promote elimination.* Monitor effectiveness.

Interpreting renal and urologic assessment findings

After completing your assessment, you're ready to form a diagnostic impression of the patient's condition. This chart will help you form such an impression by grouping significant signs and symptoms, related findings you may discover during the health history and physical assessment, and the possible cause indicated by a cluster of these findings.

Key signs and symptoms	Related findings	Possible cause
• Oliguria possibly progressing to anuria • Hematuria or smoky- or coffee-colored urine	• Poststreptococcal throat or skin infection • Systemic lupus erythematosus, vasculitis, or scleroderma • Pregnancy • Elevated blood pressure • Periorbital edema progressing to dependent edema • Ascites • Pleural effusion	Acute glomerulonephritis
• Oliguria • Dark, smoky-colored urine • Anorexia and vomiting	• Crush injury or illness associated with shock such as burns • Muscle necrosis • Exposure to nephrotoxic agent such as lead • I.V. pyelography using dye injection • Recent aminoglycoside therapy • Oliguria progressing to anuria • Dyspnea • Bibasilar crackles • Dependent edema	Acute tubular necrosis
• Proteinuria, hematuria, vomiting, pruritus (patient may be asymptomatic until advanced disease stage)	• Primary renal disorder, such as membranoproliferative glomerulonephritis or focal glomerular sclerosis • Elevated blood pressure • Ascites and dependent edema • Dyspnea • Bibasilar crackles	Chronic glomerulonephritis
• Urinary frequency and urgency • Burning sensation on urination • Nocturia, cloudy hematuria, dysuria • Low back or flank pain	• Female patient • Recurrent urinary tract infection • Recent chemotherapy or systemic antibiotic therapy • Recent vigorous sexual activity • Suprapubic pain on palpation • Fever • Inflamed perineal area	Cystitis

(continued)

Interpreting renal and urologic assessment findings (continued)

Key signs and symptoms	Related findings	Possible cause
• Severe radiating pain from costovertebral angle to flank, suprapubic region, and external genitalia • Nausea and vomiting • Hematuria	• Strenuous physical activity in hot environment • Previous renal calculi • Recent kidney infection • Fever and chills • Poor skin turgor, concentrated urine, and dry mucous membranes	Nephrolithiasis
• Abdominal or flank pain • Gross hematuria	• Youth (especially under age 7) • Congenital anomalies • Firm, smooth, palpable abdominal mass in enlarged abdomen • Fever • Elevated blood pressure • Urine retention	Wilms' tumor

• Teach the patient to gently massage along the transverse and descending colon *to stimulate the bowel and aid stool passage.*

• Instruct the patient and his family in the relation of diet, exercise, and fluid intake to constipation. Develop a plan and provide for mild exercise periods. These measures *promote muscle tone and circulation.*

Fluid volume deficit

Related to actual loss, fluid volume deficit can be associated with dialysis, ingestion of large amounts of diuretics, renal failure, or metabolic acidosis.

Expected outcomes

• Patient's vital signs remain stable.
• Skin color and temperature are normal.

• Electrolyte levels stay within normal range.
• Fluid volume remains adequate.
• Patient produces adequate urine volume.
• Patient has normal skin turgor and moist mucous membranes.
• Urine specific gravity remains between 1.005 and 1.010.
• Patient's fluid and blood volume return to normal.
• Patient understands factors that caused fluid volume deficit.

Nursing interventions and rationales

• Monitor and record vital signs every 2 hours or as often as necessary until stable. Then monitor and record vital signs every 4 hours. *Tachycardia, dyspnea, or hypotension*

(Text continues on page 389.)

Diagnostic tests for renal and urologic disorders

Test	Purpose	Nursing considerations
Urine tests		
Routine urinalysis	To screen urine for renal or urinary tract disease, and to help detect metabolic or systemic diseases unrelated to renal disorders	• Explain the procedure. • Check the patient's history for drugs that may influence results. • Collect a random urine sample of at least 15 ml and the first-voided morning specimen, if possible.
Urine osmolality	To evaluate the diluting and concentrating ability of the kidneys	• Explain the procedure. • Collect a random sample of urine, preferably the first-voided morning specimen.
Blood tests		
Blood urea nitrogen (BUN)	To evaluate renal function, diagnose renal disease, and aid assessment of hydration	• Explain the procedure. • Tell the patient to avoid a diet high in meat. • Check history for drugs that influence BUN results. • After the test, observe venipuncture site for bleeding.
Creatinine clearance	To determine how efficiently the kidneys clear creatinine from the blood	• Explain the procedure. • Inform the patient not to eat an excessive amount of meat before the test. • Tell him the test requires a timed urine specimen and at least one blood sample. • Collect a timed urine specimen in a bottle containing a preservative. • Refrigerate urine specimen or keep it on ice during the collection period. • After the test, observe the venipuncture site for bleeding. • Resume diet, medications, and activity as ordered.
Electrolytes	To aid in diagnosis of renal disease	• Explain the procedure. • No food or fluid restrictions are required. • After the test, observe the venipuncture site for bleeding.

(continued)

Diagnostic tests for renal and urologic disorders *(continued)*

Test	Purpose	Nursing considerations
Blood tests *(continued)*		
Serum creatinine	To measure renal damage	• Explain the procedure. • Instruct the patient to fast for 8 hours before the test. • Check history for drugs that may interfere with test results. • After the test, observe venipuncture site for bleeding.
Serum proteins	To help detect nephritis or nephrosis	• Explain the procedure. • Check patient's history for drugs that may influence levels. • After the test, observe venipuncture site for bleeding.
Urea clearance	To asess total renal function	• Explain the procedure and that it includes two timed urine specimens and one blood sample. • Instruct the patient to fast from midnight before the test and to abstain from exercise. • Check history for drugs that may influence urea clearance. • Instruct him to empty bladder and discard urine. Then give him water to drink to assure adequate urine output. • Collect two urine specimens one hour apart and obtain a blood sample. • After the test, observe the venipuncture site for bleeding. • Resume diet, medications, and activity as ordered.
Structural tests		
Cystourethroscopy	To allow visualization of both the bladder and urethra	• Explain the procedure. • If a general anesthetic has been ordered, inform the patient that he must fast for 8 hours before the test. • Monitor vital signs during and after the test. • After the test, instruct him to drink plenty of fluids and to take prescribed analgesics.

Diagnostic tests for renal and urologic disorders *(continued)*

Test	Purpose	Nursing considerations
Structural tests *(continued)*		
Cystourethros-copy *(continued)*		• Notify doctor if patient doesn't void within 8 hours of the test or if hematuria persists after third voiding.
Kidney-ureter-bladder radiography	To show kidney size, position, and structure	• Explain the procedure. • No food or fluid restrictions are required.
Magnetic resonance imaging	To visualize and stage kidney, bladder, and prostate tumors	• Explain the procedure. • Instruct the patient to remove all metal objects. • Tell him he must remain still throughout the test. • If he's claustrophobic, reassure him and provide emotional support. Sedation may be necessary. • After the test, he may resume his usual activity.
Nephrotomog-raphy	To help identify renal cysts and tumors and assess renal lacerations	• Explain the procedure. • Instruct the patient to fast for 8 hours before the test. • Check history for hypersensitivity to iodine, shellfish, or contrast medium. Warn him of possible adverse reactions. • After the test, observe venipuncture site for bleeding. • Monitor vital signs and urine output for 24 hours after the test. • Observe for signs of posttest allergic reaction.
Renal computed tomography	To detect and evaluate renal pathology and abnormal fluid accumulation around the kidneys and help evaluate the retroperitoneum	• Explain the procedure. • If contrast enhancement will be performed, instruct the patient to fast for 4 hours before the test. Check history for hypersensitivity to iodine, shellfish, or contrast medium. Warn of possible adverse reactions. • After the test, he may resume usual diet. Observe for posttest allergic reaction.

(continued)

Diagnostic tests for renal and urologic disorders (continued)

Test	Purpose	Nursing considerations
Structural tests (continued)		
Retrograde cystography	To help diagnose bladder rupture	• Explain the procedure. • Inform patient that he may experience some discomfort when the catheter is inserted and when the contrast medium is instilled through the catheter. • Check for hypersensitivity to iodine, shellfish, or contrast medium. Warn of possible adverse reactions. • After the test, monitor vital signs as ordered. • Record urine output including time, color, and volume. Report any hematuria that persists after the third voiding. • Watch for signs and symptoms of urinary tract sepsis from urinary tract infection.
Retrograde ureteropyelography	To visualize the renal pelvis, calyces, and ureter when I.V. contrast isn't suitable or when intravenous pyelography visualization is inadequate	• Explain the procedure. • If a general anesthetic is ordered, instruct the patient to fast for 8 hours before the test. • If the patient will be awake, tell him he may feel pressure as the instrument is passed and a pressure sensation in the kidney area when the contrast media is introduced. • After the test, monitor vital signs as ordered. • Monitor fluid intake and urine output for 24 hours. Report gross hematuria or hematuria that persists after third voiding. • Watch for dysuria, which commonly occurs after this test. If catheter is present, observe for inadequate output, which may indicate obstruction and may require irrigation. • Watch for signs of sepsis.
Ultrasonography	To help detect kidney abnormalities	• Explain the procedure. • Inform the patient that he may be asked to breathe deeply during the test. • Tell him he may feel mild pressure as the transducer is passed over the skin. • After the test, remove lubricating jelly from patient's skin.

Diagnostic tests for renal and urologic disorders *(continued)*

Test	Purpose	Nursing considerations
Structural and functional tests		
Intravenous pyelography or excretory urography	To evaluate structure and excretory function of the kidneys, ureters, and bladder	• Explain the procedure. • Be sure the patient is well hydrated. Then instruct him to fast for 8 hours before the test. • Check history for hypersensitivity to iodine, shellfish, or contrast medium. Observe for reactions during test. • Administer a laxative, if ordered, the night before the test. • After the test, observe for delayed reaction to contrast medium and observe for bleeding at venipuncture site. • Resume usual diet and encourage fluid.
Radionuclide renal scan	To assess renal blood flow, nephron and collecting system function, and renal structure	• Explain the procedure. • Inform the patient that he will receive an injection of radionuclide and may experience transient flushing and nausea. • Withhold antihypertensive medications if ordered. • After the test, resume withheld medications.
Renal angiography	To demonstrate the configuration of renal vasculature before surgery, evaluate chronic renal disease or failure, investigate renal masses and renal trauma, and detect complications following renal transplantation	• Explain the procedure. • Instruct the patient to fast for 8 hours before the test. • Check history for hypersensitivity to iodine, shellfish, and contrast medium. Warn him of possible adverse reactions. • Instruct patient to void before the test. • After the test, keep him flat for 6 hours. • Monitor vital signs until stable and monitor popliteal and dorsalis pedis pulses for adequate perfusion at least every 4 hours. • Watch for bleeding and hematoma at injection site. Keep pressure dressing in place. If bleeding occurs, apply pressure immediately.
Biopsy		
Percutaneous renal biopsy	To help differentiate renal disease, assess	• Explain the procedure. • Instruct the patient to restrict food and *(continued)*

Diagnostic tests for renal and urologic disorders *(continued)*

Test	Purpose	Nursing considerations
Biopsy *(continued)*		
Percutaneous renal biopsy *(continued)*	effectiveness of therapy, and reveal renal tumors	fluid for 8 hours before the test. • Inform him that he'll receive a mild sedative. • After the test, monitor vital signs and pressure dressing as ordered. • Instruct him to lie flat on his back for at least 12 hours.
Urodynamic tests		
Cystometry	To assess the bladder's neuromuscular function	• Explain the procedure and that the patient will be catheterized during the test. • After the test, if no more tests are needed, the catheter will be removed. • Warn the patient that after the test, he may experience transient urinary burning or frequency, but that a sitz bath may help alleviate discomfort. • Monitor fluid intake and output for 24 hours. Notify doctor if hematuria persists after the third voiding or if fever and chills develop.
Uroflometry	To evaluate lower urinary tract function and demonstrate bladder outlet obstruction	• Explain the procedure. • Advise the patient not to urinate for several hours before the test and to increase his fluid intake so that he'll have a full bladder and a strong urge to void. • Tell him that he'll void into a special commode chair with a funnel that measures his urine flow rate and the amount of time it takes to void. • Assure him he will have complete privacy. • Instruct him to remain as still as possible while voiding.
Voiding cystourethrography	To assess bladder and urethra	• Explain the procedure. • Inform the patient that a catheter will be placed into his bladder. • Check for hypersensitivity to iodine, shellfish, or contrast medium. Warn him of possible adverse reactions.

Diagnostic tests for renal and urologic disorders *(continued)*

Test	Purpose	Nursing considerations
Urodynamic tests *(continued)*		
Voiding cystourethrography *(continued)*		• During the test he will be asked to assume various positions. • After the test, observe and record patient's voiding. Report hematuria if it persists after the third voiding. • Encourage fluids after the test. • Monitor for chills and fever related to extravasation of contrast medium and urinary sepsis.

may indicate fluid volume deficit or electrolyte imbalance.

• Cover patient lightly. *Overheating can result in vasodilation and reduced circulating blood volume.*

• Measure intake and output every 1 to 4 hours. Record and report significant changes. Include urine, stool, vomitus, wound drainage, and any other output. *Low urine output and high specific gravity indicate hypovolemia.*

• Administer fluids, blood or blood products, or plasma expanders *to replace fluids and whole blood loss.* Monitor and record effectiveness and any adverse reactions.

• Weigh patient at the same time daily to give more accurate and consistent data. *Weight is a good indicator of fluid status.*

• Assess skin turgor and oral mucous membranes every 8 hours to check for dehydration. Give mouth care every 4 hours *to avoid dehydrating mucous membranes.*

• Test urine specific gravity every 8 hours. *Elevated specific gravity may indicate dehydration.*

• Don't allow patient to sit or stand until circulation improves *to avoid orthostatic hypotension.*

• Measure abdominal girth every shift *to monitor ascites and third space shift.* Report changes.

• Administer and monitor medications *to prevent further fluid loss.*

Fluid volume excess

Related to compromised regulatory mechanisms, fluid volume excess can be associated with acute glomerulonephritis, acute or chronic renal failure, pyelonephritis, or other renal diseases.

Expected outcomes

• Patient's blood pressure remains within specified limits.

• Patient demonstrates no signs of hyperkalemia on electrocardiogram (ECG).

- Patient maintains fluid intake and output within prescribed limits.
- Hematocrit stays above the target level. Blood urea nitrogen (BUN), creatinine, sodium, and potassium levels stay within acceptable limits.
- Patient plans 24-hour fluid intake as prescribed.
- Patient's skin remains intact and infection-free.
- Patient describes signs and symptoms that require medical treatment.

Nursing interventions and rationales

- Monitor blood pressure, pulse rate, cardiac rhythm, temperature, and breath sounds at least every 4 hours. Record and report changes, *which may indicate altered fluid or electrolyte status.*
- Monitor BUN, creatinine, electrolyte, and hemoglobin levels and hematocrit. *BUN and creatinine levels indicate renal function; electrolyte, and hemoglobin levels and hematocrit help to indicate fluid status.*
- Weigh patient daily before breakfast, as ordered, *to provide consistent readings.* Check for signs of fluid retention, such as dependent edema, sacral edema, and ascites.
- Give fluids as ordered. Monitor I.V. flow rate carefully *to prevent fluid overload.*
- If oral fluids are allowed, help patient make a schedule for fluid intake. *Patient involvement encourages compliance.*
- Explain the reasons for fluid and dietary restriction *to enhance the patient's understanding.*

- Provide mouth care every 4 hours. Keep mucous membranes moist with water-soluble lubricant *to prevent them from dehydrating.*
- Provide skin care every 4 hours, and change the patient's position at least every 2 hours. Elevate edematous extremities. *These measures enhance venous return, reduce edema, and prevent skin breakdown.*
- Examine skin daily for signs of bruising or other discoloration. *Edema may cause tissue perfusion with skin changes.*
- Increase patient's activity level as tolerated; for example, increase self-care measures performed by patient. *Gradually increasing activity helps body adjust.*
- Apply antiembolism stockings *to increase venous return.* Remove them for 1 hour every 8 hours or according to hospital policy.
- Assess skin turgor *to monitor for dehydration.*
- Measure abdominal girth every shift *to monitor for ascites.*
- Have dietitian see patient *to teach or reinforce dietary restrictions.*

DISORDERS

This section discusses the most common renal and urologic disorders.

Congenital disorders

Two common renal-urologic congenital disorders are medullary sponge kidney and polycystic kidney disease.

Medullary sponge kidney

In medullary sponge kidney, the collecting ducts in the renal pyramids dilate, and cavities, clefts, and cysts form in the medulla. This disorder may affect only a single pyramid in one kidney or all pyramids in both kidneys. The kidneys are usually somewhat enlarged but may be of normal size.

Causes. Most nephrologists consider medullary sponge kidney to be a congenital anomaly and related to polycystic kidney disease.

Assessment findings. Symptoms usually appear only as a result of complications and are seldom present before adulthood. Such complications include formation of calcium phosphate stones, which lodge in the dilated cystic collecting ducts or pass through a ureter, and infection secondary to dilation of the ducts. These complications are likely to produce severe colic, hematuria, lower urinary tract infection (UTI), and pyelonephritis.

Diagnostic tests. Intravenous pyelography (IVP) is usually the key to diagnosis, commonly showing a characteristic flowerlike appearance of the pyramidal cavities when they fill with contrast material.

Urinalysis is usually normal unless complications develop; it may show a slight reduction in concentrating ability or hypercalciuria.

Treatment. Therapy focuses on preventing or treating complications caused by calculi and infection. Specific measures include increasing fluid intake and monitoring renal function and urine output. New

symptoms necessitate immediate evaluation.

Because medullary sponge kidney is a benign condition, surgery is seldom necessary, except to remove calculi during acute obstruction. Serious, uncontrollable infection or hemorrhage requires nephrectomy.

Nursing interventions. When the patient is hospitalized for a stone, strain all urine, administer analgesics freely, and force fluids. Before discharge, tell the patient to watch for and report any signs of stone passage and UTI. Emphasize the need for fluids.

Patient education. Explain that the disorder is benign and the prognosis good.

Evaluation. The patient should understand the disorder. He should be free from infection and calculi.

Polycystic kidney disease

An inherited disorder, polycystic kidney disease is characterized by multiple, bilateral, grapelike clusters of fluid-filled cysts that grossly enlarge the kidneys, compressing and eventually replacing functioning renal tissue. This disorder appears in two distinct forms. The infantile form causes stillbirth or early neonatal death. A few infants with this disease survive for 2 years and then develop fatal renal, heart, liver, or respiratory failure. Onset of the adult form is insidious but commonly becomes obvious between ages 30 and 50. Renal deterioration in the adult form of this disorder commonly leads to renal failure.

Causes. The infantile form appears to be inherited as an autosomal recessive trait. The adult form appears to be inherited as an autosomal dominant trait.

Assessment findings. Signs of infantile polycystic disease include pronounced epicanthal folds, pointed nose, small chin, huge bilateral masses on the flanks, and floppy, low-set ears (Potter facies). These are symmetrical and tense.

Nonspecific early effects of adult polycystic disease include hypertension, polyuria, and symptoms of UTI. Later signs and symptoms include lumbar pain, widening girth, and swollen or tender abdomen. Advanced problems may include recurrent hematuria, life-threatening retroperitoneal bleeding, proteinuria, and colicky abdominal pain. Both kidneys are grossly enlarged and palpable.

Diagnostic tests. The patient may have polycystic kidney disease if I.V. or retrograde pyelography reveals enlarged kidneys, with elongation of the pelvis, flattening of the calyces, and indentations caused by cysts; IVP of the neonate shows poor excretion of contrast medium; ultrasound and computed tomography (CT) scans show kidney enlargement and the presence of cysts; CT scan demonstrates many areas of cystic damage; and urinalysis and creatinine clearance tests indicate abnormalities.

Treatment. Although polycystic kidney disease can't be cured, careful management of associated UTIs and secondary hypertension may prolong life.

Adult polycystic kidney disease discovered in the asymptomatic stage requires careful monitoring, including urine cultures and creatinine clearance tests. When urine culture detects infection, prompt and vigorous antibiotic treatment is necessary even for asymptomatic infection. As renal impairment progresses, selected patients may undergo dialysis, transplantation, or both. Cystic abscess or retroperitoneal bleeding may require surgical drainage. However, because this disease is bilateral, nephrectomy usually is recommended only for severe infection or bleeding.

Nursing interventions. Carefully assess the patient's lifestyle and his physical and mental state; determine how rapidly the disease is progressing. Provide supportive care to minimize any associated symptoms.

Refer the young adult patient or parents of infants with this disorder for genetic counseling.

Patient education. Explain all diagnostic procedures to the patient or his family. Stress to the patient the need to take medication exactly as prescribed, even if symptoms are minimal or absent. Explain that cystoscopic procedures pose a serious risk of infection and that he should avoid them.

Evaluation. The adult patient should have received genetic counseling, should understand diagnostic procedures, and should be free from UTI.

Acute renal disorders

Acute renal disorders include acute renal failure (ARF), acute pyelonephritis, and acute poststreptococcal glomerulonephritis.

Acute renal failure

ARF is the sudden interruption of kidney function from obstruction, reduced circulation, or renal parenchymal disease. It's usually reversible with treatment. Otherwise, it can progress to end-stage renal disease, hemolytic uremic syndrome, and death.

Causes. *Prerenal failure* is associated with diminished blood flow to the kidneys. Its causes include hypovolemia, shock, embolism, blood loss, sepsis, pooling of blood in ascites or burns, heart failure (HF), arrhythmias, and tamponade.

Intrinsic renal failure may result from acute tubular necrosis (the most common cause), acute poststreptococcal glomerulonephritis, systemic lupus erythematosus, periarteritis nodosa, vasculitis, sickle cell disease, bilateral renal vein thrombosis, the use of nephrotoxins, ischemia, renal myeloma, or acute pyelonephritis.

Postrenal failure is associated with bilateral obstruction of urinary outflow. Its causes include renal calculi, blood clots, tumors, benign prostatic hyperplasia, strictures, urethral edema from catheterization, and papillae from papillary necrosis.

Assessment findings. Signs and symptoms of acute renal failure include oliguria (usually the earliest sign), anorexia, nausea, vomiting, diarrhea or constipation, stomatitis, GI bleeding, hematemesis, dry mucous membranes, uremic breath, headache, drowsiness, irritability, confusion, peripheral neuropathy, convulsions, coma, skin dryness, pruritus, pallor, and purpura. Hypotension appears early in the disease.

Later assessment findings include hypertension, arrhythmias, symptoms of fluid overload, HF, systemic edema, anemia, and altered clotting mechanisms. Pulmonary edema and Kussmaul's respirations may also be evident.

Diagnostic tests. Blood tests show elevated BUN, creatinine, and potassium levels, and low pH, hematocrit, and bicarbonate and hemoglobin levels. Urine samples show casts, cellular debris, decreased specific gravity and, in glomerular diseases, proteinuria and urine osmolality close to serum osmolality. Urine sodium level is less than 20 mEq/L if oliguria results from decreased perfusion; greater than 40 mEq/L if it results from an intrinsic problem. Other studies include ultrasonography of the kidneys; plain films of the abdomen and the kidneys, ureters, and bladder; IVP; renal scan; retrograde pyelography; and nephrotomography.

Treatment. The major goals are to reestablish effective renal function, if possible, and to maintain the constancy of the internal environment despite transient renal failure.

Supportive measures include a diet high in calories and low in protein, sodium, and potassium, with supplemental vitamins and restricted fluids. Meticulous electrolyte monitoring is essential to detect hyperkalemia.

If these measures fail to control uremic symptoms, hemodialysis or peritoneal dialysis may be needed.

Nursing interventions. Measure and record intake and output. Weigh the patient daily. Assess hematocrit and hemoglobin level and replace blood components, as ordered. *Don't* use whole blood if the patient is prone to HF and can't tolerate extra fluid volume. Packed red blood cells (RBCs) can be given in "pedipacks" to decrease the volume administered within a given time frame to an acceptable level. Monitor vital signs. Watch for and report any signs or symptoms of pericarditis (pleuritic chest pain, tachycardia, and pericardial friction rub), inadequate renal perfusion (hypotension), or acidosis.

Provide a high-calorie, low-protein, low-sodium, and low-potassium diet, with vitamin supplements. Give the anorectic patient small, frequent meals. Maintain electrolyte balance. Strictly monitor potassium levels. Watch for symptoms of hyperkalemia (malaise, anorexia, paresthesia, and muscle weakness) and ECG changes (tall, peaked T waves, widening QRS complex, and disappearing P waves), and report them immediately. Avoid giving medications containing potassium.

Because the patient is highly susceptible to infection, use aseptic technique. Prevent complications of immobility. Provide good mouth care frequently. Use appropriate safety measures because the patient with central nervous system involvement may be dizzy.

Monitor for GI bleeding by guaiac testing all stools for blood.

Patient education. Provide emotional support. Clearly and fully explain all procedures.

Evaluation. The patient should have no weight gain, have stable vital signs, exhibit no complications or signs of infection, talk openly about his illness, and have normal blood values. He should be prepared to follow his diet and possibly a medical regimen.

Acute pyelonephritis

A sudden bacterial inflammation, acute pyelonephritis, primarily affects the interstitial area and the renal pelvis and, less commonly, the renal tubules. With treatment and continued follow-up care, the prognosis is good.

Causes. Pyelonephritis most commonly results from an ascending infection, less commonly from hematogenous or lymphatic spread. The most common infecting organism is *Escherichia coli*. Others are *Klebsiella, Proteus, Pseudomonas,*

Staphylococcus aureus, Serratia, and *Streptococcus faecalis (Enterococcus).* Risk factors can include diagnostic and therapeutic use of instruments, as in catheterization, cystoscopy, or urologic surgery. Inability to empty the bladder (for example, in patients with neurogenic bladder), calculi, and urinary obstruction from tumors, strictures, or benign prostatic hyperplasia can also lead to pyelonephritis.

Other risk factors include sexual activity in women (intercourse increases the risk of bacterial contamination), pregnancy, diabetes, and other renal diseases.

Assessment findings. Signs and symptoms of pyelonephritis include urinary urgency and frequency, burning during urination, dysuria, nocturia, hematuria, possibly cloudy urine with an ammoniacal or fishy odor, temperature of 102° F (38.9° C) or higher, shaking chills, flank pain, anorexia, and general fatigue.

Diagnostic tests. Urinalysis reveals pyuria and possibly a few RBCs, low specific gravity and osmolality, slightly alkaline pH, and possibly proteinuria, glycosuria, and ketonuria. Urine culture reveals more than 100,000 organisms/mm³ of urine. Kidney-ureter-bladder (KUB) radiography may reveal calculi, tumors, or cysts in the kidneys and the urinary tract. IVP may show asymmetrical kidneys.

Treatment. Therapy centers on antibiotic therapy following urine culture and sensitivity studies.

When the infecting organism can't be identified, therapy usually consists of a broad-spectrum antibiotic. If the patient is pregnant, antibiotics must be prescribed cautiously. Urinary analgesics such as phenazopyridine are also appropriate.

In infection from obstruction or vesicoureteral reflux, antibiotics may be less effective. Surgery may be needed to relieve the obstruction or correct the anomaly. Patients at high risk for recurring urinary tract and kidney infections—such as those using an indwelling urinary catheter for a prolonged period—require long-term follow-up care.

Nursing interventions. Administer antipyretics for fever. Force fluids to achieve a urine output of more than 2,000 ml/day. Don't encourage intake of more than 2 to 3 qt (2 to 3 L) because this may decrease the effectiveness of antibiotics.

Patient education. Teach proper technique for collecting a clean-catch urine specimen. Encourage long-term follow-up care for high-risk patients.

Evaluation. The recovering patient has a normal temperature, has no urinary discomfort or flank pain, forces fluids, and takes antibiotics as prescribed.

Acute poststreptococcal glomerulonephritis

Acute poststreptococcal glomerulonephritis is a relatively common bilateral inflammation of the glomeruli that follows a streptococcal infection of the respiratory tract or, less commonly, a skin infection such as impetigo.

Causes. This disorder results from the entrapment and collection of antigen–antibody complexes (produced in response to streptococcal infection) in the glomerular capillary membranes, inducing inflammatory damage and impeding glomerular function.

Assessment findings. Typically, this disorder begins within 1 to 3 weeks after untreated pharyngitis. The most common signs and symptoms are mild to moderate facial edema, azotemia, hematuria (smoky- or coffee-colored urine), oliguria (less than 400 ml/day), fatigue, mild to severe hypertension, sodium or water retention, headache, mild fever, and costovertebral tenderness.

Diagnostic tests. Diagnosis requires a detailed patient history and assessment of clinical symptoms and laboratory tests. Blood values (elevated electrolyte, BUN, and creatinine levels) and urine values (RBCs, white blood cells [WBCs], mixed cell casts, and protein) indicate renal failure. Elevated antistreptolysin-O titers (in 80% of patients), elevated streptozyme and anti-DNase B titers, and low serum complement levels verify recent streptococcal infection. A throat culture may also show group A beta-hemolytic streptococci. KUB X-rays show bilateral kidney enlargement. A renal biopsy may be necessary to confirm diagnosis or assess renal tissue status.

Treatment. Vigorous supportive care includes bed rest, fluid and dietary sodium restrictions, and correction of electrolyte imbalances. Therapy may include diuretics, such as metolazone or furosemide, to reduce extracellular fluid overload and an antihypertensive such as hydralazine. The use of antibiotics to prevent secondary infection or transmission to others is controversial.

Nursing interventions. Patient care is primarily supportive.

Patient education. If the patient is on dialysis, explain the procedure fully. Tell the patient that follow-up examinations are necessary to detect chronic renal failure. After the disorder resolves, hematuria may recur during nonspecific viral infections; abnormal urinary findings may persist for years.

Advise the patient with a history of chronic upper respiratory tract infections to immediately report signs of infection.

Evaluation. The patient should have normal serum creatinine and BUN levels and a normal urine creatinine clearance, and be free from complications. He should follow a diet high in calories and low in protein and obtain the necessary follow-up examinations.

Chronic renal disorders

The most common chronic renal disorders include nephrotic syndrome, chronic glomerulonephritis, hydronephrosis, renal tubular acidosis, and chronic renal failure.

Nephrotic syndrome

Nephrotic syndrome (NS) is a condition characterized by marked proteinuria, hypoalbuminemia, hyperlipidemia, and edema. Although NS is not a disease itself, it results from a specific glomerular defect and indicates renal damage.

Causes. Primary (idiopathic) glomerulonephritis (affecting children and adults) causes 75% of the cases. Other causes include metabolic diseases such as diabetes mellitus; collagen vascular disorders, such as systemic lupus erythematosus and periarteritis nodosa; circulatory diseases, such as HF, sickle cell anemia, and renal vein thrombosis; nephrotoxins, such as mercury, gold, and bismuth; allergic reactions; and infections, such as tuberculosis and enteritis.

Pregnancy, hereditary nephritis, multiple myeloma, and other neoplastic diseases may also cause NS.

Assessment findings. The dominant clinical feature is mild to severe dependent edema of the ankles or sacrum, or periorbital edema, especially in children. It may lead to ascites, pleural effusion, and swollen external genitalia. Other signs and symptoms are orthostatic hypotension, lethargy, anorexia, depression, and pallor.

Diagnostic tests. Urine testing that reveals consistent proteinuria in excess of 3.5 g/day; increased number of hyaline, granular, and waxy, fatty casts; and oval fat bodies strongly suggests NS. Blood values show increased cholesterol, phospholipid, and triglyceride levels and decreased albumin levels. Histologic identification of the lesion requires kidney biopsy.

Treatment. Treatment requires correction of the underlying cause if possible. Supportive treatment consists of protein replacement with a diet of 1.5 g protein/kg of body weight and restricted sodium intake, diuretics for edema, and antibiotics for infection. Some patients respond to an 8-week course of corticosteroid therapy (such as prednisone), followed by a maintenance dose. Others need a combination course of prednisone and azathioprine or cyclophosphamide.

Nursing interventions. Frequently check urine for protein. (Urine that contains protein appears frothy.) Measure blood pressure with the patient in supine and erect positions.

After kidney biopsy, watch for bleeding and shock. Monitor intake and output and check weight at the same time each morning. Ask the dietitian to plan a high-protein, low-sodium diet.

Provide good skin care. Patients on steroidal therapy may be more prone to shearing skin injuries.

Patient education. Watch for and teach the patient and family how to recognize drug therapy adverse effects, such as bone marrow toxicity from cytotoxic immunosuppressants and cushingoid symptoms from long-term steroid therapy.

Evaluation. The patient should follow dietary and medical regimens, have no proteinuria, and have no complications.

Chronic glomerulonephritis

A slowly progressive, noninfectious disease, chronic glomerulonephritis is characterized by inflammation of the renal glomeruli. It remains subclinical until the progressive phase begins. By the time it produces symptoms, it's usually irreversible. It results in eventual renal failure.

Causes. Primary renal causes include membranoproliferative glomerulonephritis, membranous glomerulopathy, focal glomerular sclerosis, and poststreptococcal glomerulonephritis.

Systemic causes include lupus erythematosus, Goodpasture's syndrome, and hemolytic-uremic syndrome.

Assessment findings. This disease usually develops insidiously and asymptomatically, commonly over many years. At any time, however, it may suddenly become progressive.

The initial stage includes NS, hypertension, proteinuria, and hematuria. Late-stage findings include azotemia, nausea, vomiting, pruritus, dyspnea, malaise, fatigability, anemia, and severe hypertension, which may cause cardiac hypertrophy, leading to HF.

Diagnostic tests. With this disease, urinalysis reveals proteinuria, hematuria, cylindruria, and RBC casts. Blood tests reveal rising BUN and serum creatinine levels, indicating advanced renal insufficiency. X-ray or ultrasound examination shows small kidneys. Kidney biopsy identifies the underlying disease.

Treatment. The goals of treatment are to control hypertension, to correct fluid and electrolyte imbalances, to reduce edema with diuretics such as furosemide, and to prevent HF.

Nursing interventions. Patient care is primarily supportive, focusing on continual observation and sound patient education.

Patient education. Instruct the patient to continue taking prescribed antihypertensives as scheduled, even if he's feeling better, and to report any adverse reactions. Teach him how to assess ankle edema.

Warn the patient to report signs of infection, particularly UTI, and to avoid contact with people who have infections. Urge follow-up examinations.

Evaluation. The patient should have normal vital signs and have no weight gain.

Hydronephrosis

An abnormal dilation of the renal pelvis and the calyces of one or both kidneys, hydronephrosis results from a genitourinary obstruction. Although partial obstruction and hydronephrosis may not produce symptoms initially, increased pressure behind the obstruction eventually results in symptomatic renal dysfunction. With a complete obstruction, irreversible renal damage may occur in as little as 7 days.

Cause. Any type of obstructive uropathy—most commonly, benign prostatic hyperplasia, urethral strictures, and calculi—can cause hydronephrosis.

Assessment findings. Clinical features of hydronephrosis vary with the cause of the obstruction. The patient may be asymptomatic, or he may have mild pain and slightly decreased urine flow; severe, colicky renal pain; or dull flank pain that may radiate to the groin. Other signs and symptoms include hematuria, pyuria, dysuria, alternating oliguria and polyuria, complete anuria, nausea and vomiting, abdominal fullness, pain on urination, dribbling, or hesitancy.

Diagnostic tests. IVP, retrograde pyelography, renal ultrasonography, and renal function studies are necessary to confirm the diagnosis.

Treatment. Treatment includes surgical removal of the obstruction, such as dilatation for a urethral stricture or prostatectomy for benign prostatic hyperplasia. If renal function has already been affected, therapy may include a diet low in protein, sodium, and potassium to stop the progression of renal failure before surgery. Inoperable obstructions may require decompression and drainage of the kidney, using a nephrostomy tube.

Nursing interventions. Postoperatively, closely monitor intake and output, vital signs, and fluid and electrolyte status. Watch for a rising pulse rate and cold, clammy skin, which indicate possible impending hemorrhage and shock. Monitor renal function studies daily.

If a nephrostomy tube has been inserted, check it frequently for bleeding and patency. Irrigate the tube only as ordered, and don't clamp it.

Patient education. Explain hydronephrosis as well as the purpose of diagnostic procedures. If the patient is to be discharged with a nephrostomy tube in place, teach him how to care for it properly. Teach him to report symptoms of hydronephrosis or UTI.

Evaluation. The recovering patient verbalizes an understanding of hydronephrosis and diagnostic procedures, is pain-free, and exhibits no signs of complications.

Renal tubular acidosis

Renal tubular acidosis (RTA)—a syndrome of persistent dehydration, hyperchloremia, hypokalemia, metabolic acidosis, and nephrocalcinosis—results from the kidneys' inability to conserve bicarbonate. This disorder occurs as distal RTA (type I, classic RTA) or proximal RTA (type II).

Causes. Primary distal RTA may be a hereditary defect. Causes of secondary distal RTA include starvation, malnutrition, cirrhosis, several genetically transmitted disorders, and possibly other renal or systemic disorders. Primary proximal RTA is idiopathic. Proximal tubular cell damage in disease causes secondary proximal RTA.

Assessment findings. The patient, especially a child, may experience anorexia, vomiting, occasional fever, polyuria, dehydration, growth retardation, apathy and weakness, tissue wasting, or constipation.

Diagnostic tests. The patient has decreased serum bicarbonate, pH, potassium, and phosphorus levels, but increased serum chloride and alkaline phosphatase levels. Urine tests show alkalinity with low titratable acids and ammonium content, increased bicarbonate and potassium levels, and low specific gravity. X-rays may show nephrocalcinosis in later stages.

Treatment. Supportive treatment for patients with RTA requires replacement of those substances being abnormally excreted, especially bicarbonate, and may include sodium bicarbonate tablets or Shohl's solution to control acidosis, potassium by mouth for dangerously low potassium levels, and vitamin D for bone disease.

Nursing interventions. Monitor laboratory values, especially potassium to detect hypokalemia. Test urine for pH, and strain it for calculi. If rickets develops, explain the condition and its treatment to the patient and his family.

Patient education. Teach the patient how to recognize signs and symptoms of calculi (hematuria and low abdominal or flank pain). Advise him to immediately report any such signs and symptoms. Instruct the patient with low potassium levels to eat foods with a high potassium content, such as bananas and baked potatoes.

Urge compliance with all medication instructions. Inform the patient and his family that the prognosis for RTA and bone lesion healing is directly related to the adequacy of treatment. Because RTA may be caused by a genetic defect, encourage family members to seek genetic counseling.

Evaluation. The patient should follow his medical regimen at home, exhibit no signs of complications, have his family members obtain genetic counseling, and be able to name foods high in potassium.

Chronic renal failure

Typically the result of a gradually progressive loss of renal function, chronic renal failure occasionally results from a rapidly progressive disease of sudden onset. Few symptoms develop until after more than 75% of glomerular filtration is lost. Then the remaining normal parenchyma deteriorate progressively, and symptoms worsen as renal function decreases. If this condition continues unchecked, uremic toxins accumulate and produce potentially fatal physiologic changes in all major organ systems.

Causes. Causes of chronic renal failure include chronic glomerular disease such as glomerulonephritis, congenital anomalies such as polycystic kidney disease, and chronic infections, such as chronic pyelonephritis or tuberculosis. Chronic renal failure may also stem from acute renal failure that fails to respond to treatment, obstructive processes such as calculi, collagen diseases such as systemic lupus erythematosus, nephrotoxic agents such as long-term aminoglycoside therapy, endocrine diseases such as diabetic neuropathy, and vascular diseases, such as renal nephrosclerosis or hypertension.

Assessment findings. The degree of renal failure partly determines the frequency and severity of clinical manifestations. (See *Chronic renal failure's effects on body systems,* pages 402 and 403.)

Diagnostic tests. Creatinine clearance tests can identify the stage of chronic renal failure. Reduced renal reserve occurs when the creatinine clearance glomerular filtration rate (GFR) is 40 to 70 ml/minute. Renal insufficiency occurs at a GFR of 20 to 40 ml/minute, renal failure at a GFR of 10 to 20 ml/minute, and end-stage renal disease at a GFR of less than 10 ml/minute.

Blood studies show elevated BUN, creatinine, and potassium levels; decreased arterial pH and bicarbonate levels; and low hemoglobin level and hematocrit. Urine specific gravity becomes fixed at 1.010; urinalysis may show proteinuria, glycosuria, erythrocytes, leukocytes, and casts, depending on the cause. X-ray studies include KUB films, IVP, nephrotomography, renal scan, and renal arteriography. Kidney biopsy allows histologic identification of the underlying abnormality.

Treatment. Conservative measures include a low-protein diet, which reduces the production of end products of protein metabolism that the kidneys cannot excrete. However, a patient receiving continuous peritoneal dialysis should have a high-protein diet. A high-calorie diet prevents ketoacidosis and the negative nitrogen balance that results in catabolism and tissue atrophy. Such a diet also restricts sodium and potassium.

Maintaining fluid balance requires careful monitoring of vital signs, weight changes, and urine volume (if present).

Treatment may also include regular stool analysis (guaiac test) to detect occult blood. Anemia necessitates iron and folate supplements; severe anemia requires infusion of fresh frozen packed cells or washed packed cells. However, transfusions relieve anemia only temporarily. Recombinant human erythropoietin (r-hepo or Epogen), a glycoprotein, stimulates bone marrow production of RBCs and is commonly used.

Drug therapy may relieve associated symptoms, but dosages may need to be adjusted in medications excreted by the kidneys.

Monitor serum potassium levels carefully to detect hyperkalemia. Emergency treatment for severe hyperkalemia includes dialysis thera-

Chronic renal failure's effects on body systems

Clinical features of chronic renal failure in different body systems include the following.

Renal and urologic system

Initially, salt-wasting and consequent hyponatremia produce hypotension, dry mouth, loss of skin turgor, listlessness, fatigue, and nausea. Later, somnolence and confusion develop. As the number of functioning nephrons decreases, so does the kidneys' capacity to excrete sodium, resulting in salt retention and overload. Accumulation of potassium causes muscle irritability, then weakness as the potassium level continues to rise. Fluid overload and metabolic acidosis also occur. Urine output decreases; urine is dilute and contains casts and crystals.

Cardiovascular system

Renal failure leads to hypertension, arrhythmias (including life-threatening ventricular tachycardia or fibrillation), cardiomyopathy, uremic pericarditis, pericardial effusion with possible cardiac tamponade, heart failure, and peripheral edema.

Respiratory system

Pulmonary changes include reduced pulmonary macrophage activity with increased susceptibility to infection, pulmonary edema, pleuritic pain, pleural friction rub and effusions, uremic pleuritis and uremic lung (or uremic pneumonitis), dyspnea from heart failure, and Kussmaul's respirations as a result of acidosis.

GI system

Inflammation and ulceration of GI mucosa cause stomatitis, gum ulceration and bleeding, and possibly parotitis, esophagitis, gastritis, duodenal ulcers, lesions on the small and large bowel, uremic colitis, pancreatitis, and proctitis. Other GI symptoms include a metallic taste in the mouth, uremic fetor (ammonia smell on breath), anorexia, nausea, and vomiting.

Skin

Typically, the skin is pallid, yellowish bronze, dry, and scaly. Other cutaneous symptoms include severe itching, purpura, ecchymoses, petechiae, uremic frost (mostly in critically ill or terminal patients), thin brittle fingernails with characteristic lines, and dry, brittle hair that may change color and fall out easily.

Neurologic system

Restless leg syndrome, one of the first signs of peripheral neuropathy, causes pain, burning, and itching in the legs and feet, which may be relieved by voluntarily shaking, moving, or rocking them. Eventually, this condition progresses to paresthesia and motor nerve dysfunction (usually bilateral footdrop) unless dialysis is initiated. Other signs and symptoms include muscle cramping and twitching, shortened memory and attention span, apathy, drowsiness, irritability, confusion, coma, and convulsions. EEG changes indicate metabolic encephalopathy.

Chronic renal failure's effects on body systems *(continued)*

Endocrine system
Common abnormalities include stunted growth patterns in children (even with elevated growth hormone levels), infertility and decreased libido in both sexes, amenorrhea and cessation of menses in women, impotence and decreased sperm production in men, increased aldosterone secretion and impaired carbohydrate metabolism.

Hematopoietic system
Anemia, decreased red blood cell survival time, blood loss from dialysis and GI bleeding, mild thrombocytopenia, and platelet defects occur.

Other problems include increased bleeding and clotting disorders, demonstrated by purpura, hemorrhage from body orifices, easy bruising, ecchymoses, and petechiae.

Musculoskeletal system
Calcium-phosphorus imbalance and consequent parathyroid hormone imbalances cause muscle and bone pain, skeletal demineralization, pathologic fractures, and calcifications in the brain, eyes, gums, joints, myocardium, and blood vessels. Arterial calcification may produce coronary artery disease. In children, renal osteodystrophy may develop.

---

py and administration of 50% hypertonic glucose I.V., regular insulin, calcium gluconate I.V., sodium bicarbonate I.V., and cation-exchange resins such as sodium polystyrene sulfonate.

Arterial blood gas measurements may show acidosis; intensive dialysis and thoracentesis can relieve pulmonary edema and pleural effusions. If the GFR falls below 10 ml/minute, hemodialysis or peritoneal dialysis is needed.

Hemodialysis or peritoneal dialysis can help control most manifestations of end-stage renal disease; altering dialyzing bath fluids can correct fluid and electrolyte disturbances. However, anemia, peripheral neuropathy, cardiopulmonary and GI complications, sexual dysfunction, and skeletal defects may persist.

Nursing interventions. Watch for hyperkalemia. Observe for diarrhea and for cramping of the legs and abdomen. As potassium levels rise, watch for muscle irritability and a weak pulse rate. Monitor ECGs for tall, peaked T waves, widening QRS complex, prolonged PR interval, and disappearance of P waves, indicating hyperkalemia.

Assess hydration status carefully. Check for jugular vein distention, and auscultate the lungs for crackles. Measure daily intake and output carefully. Record daily weight and the presence or absence of thirst, axillary sweat, dry tongue, hypertension, and peripheral edema.

Monitor for bone or joint complications. Give medications, as ordered, on schedule. Maintain strict aseptic technique. Use a micropore filter during I.V. therapy.

Observe and document seizure activity. Infuse sodium bicarbonate for acidosis, and sedatives or anticonvulsants for seizures, as ordered. Pad the side rails and keep an oral airway and suction setup at the bedside. Assess neurologic status periodically, and check for Chvostek's and Trousseau's signs.

Patient education. Instruct the outpatient to avoid high-sodium and high-potassium foods. Encourage adherence to fluid and protein restrictions. Stress the need for exercise and sufficient dietary bulk.

Observe for signs of bleeding. Report signs and symptoms of pericarditis, such as pericardial friction rub and chest pain. Also, watch for the disappearance of friction rub, with a drop of 15 to 20 mm Hg in blood pressure during inspiration (paradoxical pulse)—an early sign of pericardial tamponade.

Evaluation. The patient should understand the disease process and medical regimen, have no complications, and have his symptoms controlled by dialysis or transplantation. He should have normal BUN, creatinine, and electrolyte levels and maintain a satisfactory diet with normal bowel function.

Lower urinary tract disorders

The most common lower urinary tract disorders are infections, vesicoureteral reflux, neurogenic bladder, and bladder cancer.

Lower urinary tract infections

Cystitis and urethritis constitute the two types of UTI. An inflammation of the bladder, cystitis usually results from an ascending infection. Urethritis is an inflammation of the urethra. UTIs commonly respond readily to treatment, but recurrence and resistant bacterial flare-up during therapy are possible.

Causes. Most UTIs result from infection by gram-negative enteric bacteria. Other causes include simultaneous infection with multiple pathogens in a patient with neurogenic bladder, an indwelling urinary catheter, or a fistula between the intestine and bladder; and *Chlamydia trachomatis* and *Neisseria gonorrhoeae*.

Assessment findings. Characteristic signs and symptoms include urgency, frequency, dysuria, bladder cramps or spasms, itching, feeling of warmth during urination, nocturia, and possibly hematuria, fever, and urethral discharge in males. Other features include low back pain, malaise, nausea, vomiting, abdominal pain or tenderness over the bladder, chills, and flank pain.

Diagnostic tests. Microscopic urinalysis showing RBC and WBC levels greater than 10/high-power field points to UTI. A clean midstream urine specimen revealing a bacterial count of more than 100,000/ml confirms it. Sensitivity testing suggests the appropriate antibiotic. A blood test or stained smear rules out venereal disease. Voiding cystourethrography (VCUG) or IVP may detect congenital anomalies.

Treatment. A 7- to 10-day course of an appropriate antibiotic is usually the treatment of choice for initial lower UTI. Single-dose antibiotic therapy with co-trimoxazole or amoxicillin may be effective in women with acute noncomplicated UTI.

Recurrent infections caused by infected renal calculi, chronic prostatitis, or a structural abnormality may require surgery. Otherwise, long-term, low-dose antibiotic therapy is preferred.

Nursing interventions. The plan of care should include patient education, supportive measures, and proper specimen collection.

Patient education. Explain the nature and purpose of antibiotic therapy. Emphasize the importance of completing the prescribed course of therapy or, with long-term prophylaxis, of adhering strictly to the ordered dosage. Urge the patient to drink plenty of water.

Teach the female patient how to clean the perineum properly and keep the labia separated during voiding when collecting a urine sample. A noncontaminated midstream specimen is essential for accurate diagnosis. To prevent recurrent UTIs in men, urge prompt treatment of predisposing conditions.

Evaluation. The patient should understand hygiene practices to prevent UTI and have completed the prescribed course of antibiotic therapy.

Vesicoureteral reflux

In patients with vesicoureteral reflux, incompetence of the ureterovesical junction allows backflow of urine into the ureters when the bladder contracts during voiding. Eventually, this backflow empties into the renal pelvis or the parenchyma. UTI can result, possibly leading to acute or chronic pyelonephritis and renal damage.

Causes. Ureterovesical junction incompetence can result from congenital anomalies of the ureters or bladder. Other causes of incompetence include ureteral ectopia lateralis; cystitis, with inflammation of the intravesical ureter; a gaping or golf-hole ureteral orifice; inadequate detrusor muscle buttress in the bladder, stemming from congenital paraureteral bladder diverticulum; acquired diverticulum from outlet obstruction; and high intravesical pressure from outlet obstruction or other cause.

Assessment findings. Signs and symptoms of UTI may indicate vesicoureteral reflux. These include frequency, urgency, burning on urination, hematuria, strong-smelling and, in infants, dark, concentrated urine. With upper urinary tract involvement, expect high fever, chills, flank pain, vomiting, and malaise.

In male infants, the bladder may be hard and thickened on palpation. In children, fever, nonspecific abdominal pain, and diarrhea may be the only clinical effects.

Diagnostic tests. A clean-catch urine specimen shows a bacterial count greater than 100,000/mm³. Microscopic examination may reveal WBCs, RBCs, and an elevated urine pH if infection is present. Specific gravity less than 1.010 demonstrates inability to concentrate urine.

Elevated creatinine (greater than 1.2 mg/dl) and BUN (greater than 18 mg/dl) levels demonstrate advanced renal dysfunction. IVP may show a dilated lower ureter, a ureter visible for its entire length, hydronephrosis, calyceal distortion, and renal scarring.

VCUG identifies and determines the degree of reflux and shows when reflux occurs. It may also pinpoint the causative anomaly. Radioisotope scanning and renal ultrasonography may also be used to detect reflux. Catheterization of the bladder after the patient voids determines the amount of residual urine.

Treatment. Antibiotic therapy is usually effective for reflux secondary to infection, reflux related to neurogenic bladder and, in children, reflux related to a short intravesical ureter (which abates spontaneously with growth). Of girls with vesicoureteral reflux, 80% will have recurrent UTIs within a year, requiring long-term prophylactic antibiotic therapy.

UTI that recurs despite adequate prophylactic antibiotic therapy requires vesicoureteral reimplantation.

Nursing interventions. Postoperatively, closely monitor fluid intake and output. Make sure the catheters are patent and draining well. Watch for fever, chills, and flank pain, which suggest a blocked catheter.

Patient education. To ensure complete emptying of the bladder, teach the patient with vesicoureteral reflux to double-void (void once and then try to void again in a few minutes). Also, because his urge to urinate may be impaired, advise him to void every 2 to 3 hours routinely. Teach him to monitor his bowel habits closely because constipation can cause an increase in pelvic pressure.

If surgery is necessary, explain postoperative care: suprapubic catheter in the male, indwelling urinary catheter in the female and, in both, one or two ureteral catheters or splints brought out of the bladder through a small abdominal incision. The suprapubic or indwelling urinary catheter keeps the bladder empty and prevents pressure from stressing the surgical wound; ureteral catheters drain urine directly from the renal pelvis. After complicated reimplantations, all catheters remain in place for 7 to 10 days. As a child may be discharged while the catheters are still in place, parents must be taught proper catheter care. Explain that the child can move and walk with the catheters but must take care not to dislodge them.

Instruct parents to watch for and report recurring signs of UTI. Emphasize to them the importance of compliance with prescribed antibiotic therapy.

Evaluation. The patient should know how to double-void. The patient's parents should understand diagnostic tests.

Neurogenic bladder

Neurogenic bladder refers to any bladder dysfunction caused by an interruption of normal bladder innervation. It can be *spastic*, caused by an upper motor neuron lesion; *flaccid*, caused by a lower motor neuron lesion; or *mixed*, the result of cortical damage from some disorder or trauma.

Causes. Neurogenic bladder stems from a host of underlying conditions, including cerebral disorders, such as cerebrovascular accident, brain tumor (meningioma and glioma), Parkinson's disease, multiple sclerosis (MS), dementia, and incontinence from aging; spinal cord disease or trauma, such as spinal stenosis or arachnoiditis, cervical spondylosis, myelopathies from hereditary disorders or nutritional deficiencies; and disorders of peripheral innervation, including autonomic neuropathies resulting from endocrine disturbances such as diabetes mellitus (most common). It may also result from metabolic disturbances such as hypothyroidism, acute infectious diseases such as Guillain-Barré syndrome, heavy metal toxicity, chronic alcoholism, collagen diseases such as lupus erythematosus, vascular diseases such as atherosclerosis, and distant effects of cancer such as primary oat cell carcinoma of the lung, and herpes zoster.

Assessment findings. Neurogenic bladder produces a wide range of clinical effects. All types of neurogenic bladder are associated with some degree of incontinence, changes in initiation or interruption of micturition, and an inability to empty the bladder completely. Vesicoureteral reflux, deterioration or infection in the upper urinary tract, and hydroureteral nephrosis may also result.

Spastic neurogenic bladder symptoms depend on the site and extent of the spinal cord lesion. They may include involuntary, frequent scant urination without a feeling of bladder fullness; spontaneous spasms of the arms and legs; increased anal sphincter tone; possible voiding and spontaneous contractions of the arms and legs with tactile stimulation of the abdomen, thighs, or genitalia; and possibly severe hypertension, bradycardia, and headaches, with bladder distention if cord lesions are in the upper thoracic (cervical) level.

Clinical features of flaccid neurogenic bladder include overflow incontinence, diminished anal sphincter tone, and greatly distended bladder without the accompanying feeling of bladder fullness because of sensory impairment.

Symptoms of mixed neurogenic bladder include dulled perception of bladder fullness and a diminished ability to empty the bladder. Because this condition reduces sensation and control, the patient usually feels urgency to void but cannot control the urgency.

Diagnostic tests. Because the causes of neurogenic bladder vary, diagnosis includes a variety of tests. Cerebrospinal fluid analysis, showing increased protein levels, may indicate cord tumor; increased gamma globulin levels may indicate MS.

Skull and vertebral column X-rays show fracture, dislocation, congenital anomalies, or metastasis. Magnetic resonance imaging (MRI) and myelography may show spinal cord compression. EEG may be abnormal if a brain tumor exists. Electromyelography confirms peripheral neuropathy. Brain and CT scans localize and identify brain masses.

Other tests assess bladder function. Cystometry evaluates bladder nerve supply and detrusor muscle tone. A urethral pressure profile determines urethral function. A urine flow study (uroflometry) shows diminished or impaired urine flow. Retrograde urethrography reveals strictures and diverticula. VCUG evaluates bladder neck function and continence, and any vesicoureteral reflux.

Treatment. Techniques of bladder evacuation include Credé's method, Valsalva's maneuver, and intermittent self-catheterization. Credé's method promotes complete emptying of the bladder. After appropriate instruction, most patients can perform this maneuver themselves. Credé's method may not eliminate the need for catheterization. It's contraindicated in cases of vesicoureteral reflux.

Intermittent self-catheterization is more effective than Credé's

method and Valsalva's maneuver in treating neurogenic bladder. Combined with a bladder-retraining program, it can help patients with flaccid neurogenic bladder.

Drug therapy may include terazosin or doxazosin, both adrenergic antagonizers, whose action is at the bladder neck to decrease outlet resistance. When it fails, structural impairment may be repaired through transurethral resection of the bladder neck, urethral dilatation, external sphincterotomy, or urinary diversion procedures. An artificial urinary sphincter may be implanted if permanent incontinence follows surgery.

Nursing interventions. Care for patients with neurogenic bladder varies according to the underlying cause. Watch for signs of infection. If prolonged use of a catheter is necessary, a suprapubic catheter is preferred to decrease the chance of infection.

Patient education. Assure the patient that the lengthy diagnostic process helps identify the most effective treatment plan. Explain the treatment plan to the patient in detail, and teach him and his family bladder evacuation techniques.

Evaluation. The patient should be free from infection, should be continent, and should understand his condition and the treatment techniques.

Bladder cancer

Tumors can develop on the surface of the bladder wall as benign or malignant papillomas or grow within the bladder wall to quickly invade underlying muscles. Almost all bladder cancers are of the transitional cell type arising from the epithelium. Other types include adenocarcinomas and squamous cell carcinomas.

Causes. The cause of bladder cancer is unknown. Well-established risk factors include exposure to environmental carcinogens, such as tobacco, 2-naphthylamine, benzidine, and nitrates, which are known to predispose to transitional cell tumors. Members of certain industrial groups, such as rubber workers, cable workers, weavers, aniline dye workers, hairdressers, petroleum workers, spray painters, and leather finishers are at high risk for developing these tumors. Living in geographic areas where schistosomiasis is endemic (such as Egypt) increases the risk.

Assessment findings. Early-stage bladder cancer is asymptomatic in about one-fourth of patients. Gross, painless, intermittent hematuria is commonly the first sign. Other clinical effects include bladder irritability, urinary frequency, nocturia, and dribbling. Suprapubic pain after voiding occurs in patients with invasive lesions.

Diagnostic tests. IVP can identify a large, early-stage tumor or an infiltrating tumor as well as reveal functional problems in the upper urinary tract. IVP or cystoscopy can detect ureteral obstruction or rigid deformity of the bladder wall.

Cytology is a simple diagnostic test that looks for cancer cells in the urine. Cystoscopy and biopsy confirm bladder cancer and should be performed when hematuria first appears. When these procedures are performed under anesthesia, bimanual examination is usually done to determine if the bladder is fixed to the pelvic wall.

CT scan, transurethral ultrasound, and MRI demonstrate the thickness of the involved bladder wall and detect enlarged retroperitoneal lymph nodes.

Treatment. Transurethral (cystoscopic) resection and fulguration (electrical destruction) or laser therapy are used to remove superficial low-grade bladder tumors. This procedure is adequate when the tumor hasn't invaded the muscle. Intravesical chemotherapy after resection is commonly used because of the high risk of recurrence. Drugs most commonly used for this are thiotepa, mitomycin C, Epody 1, doxorubicin, teniposide (VM-26) and Calmette-Guériné bacillus.

Tumors that are diffuse and unresectable require segmental bladder resection to remove a full-thickness section of the bladder. This procedure is feasible only if the tumor isn't near the bladder neck or ureteral orifices.

For an invasive bladder tumor, radical cystectomy or definitive irradiation, or a combination of preoperative radiation and surgery are used. During cystectomy the surgeon forms a urinary diversion, usually an ileal conduit.

Radical cystectomy and urethrectomy previously caused impotence in males because such resection damaged the sympathetic and parasympathetic nerves that control erection and ejaculation. Nerve-sparing surgical procedures preserve erectile function in 80% of young men.

Treatment for patients with advanced bladder cancer includes cystectomy to remove the tumor, radiation therapy, and systemic combination chemotherapy, such as cisplatin, methotrexate, vinblastine, and doxorubicin.

Nursing interventions. Provide psychological support and patient education.

Patient education. This should include thorough instruction on urinary conduit care. All individuals at high risk for bladder cancer should have periodic cytologic examinations and should know about the danger of significant exposure to irritants, toxins, and carcinogens.

Evaluation. The patient should know how to reduce the risk of bladder cancer. He should follow the treatment regimen and know how to care for his urinary diversion.

Prostate and testicular disorders

Prostate and testicular disorders include prostatitis, epididymitis, and prostatic and testicular cancer.

Prostatitis

An inflammation of the prostate gland, prostatitis may be acute or chronic. Acute prostatitis most often results from gram-negative bacteria and is easy to recognize and treat. However, chronic prostatitis, the most common cause of recurrent UTI in men, isn't easily recognizable.

Causes. Prostatitis results primarily from infection by *E. coli.* It also results from infection by *Klebsiella, Enterobacter, Proteus, Pseudomonas, Streptococcus,* or *Staphylococcus.*

Assessment findings. Signs and symptoms of acute prostatitis include sudden fever, chills, low back pain, myalgia, perineal fullness, arthralgia, urgency, possibly dysuria, nocturia, some degree of urinary obstruction, and cloudy urine. Rectal palpation of the prostate reveals tenderness, induration, swelling, firmness, and warmth.

Chronic prostatitis may be asymptomatic, or it may involve less severe forms of the signs or symptoms of acute prostatitis. These include painful ejaculation, hemospermia, persistent urethral discharge, and sexual dysfunction.

Diagnostic tests. With prostatitis, urine culture can often identify the infecting organism.

Treatment. Systemic antibiotic therapy is the treatment of choice for acute prostatitis. Usually treatment lasts at least 6 weeks.

Supportive therapy may include bed rest, adequate hydration, and use of analgesics and anti-inflammatory agents (indomethacin, ibuprofen), antipyretics, anticholinergics (oxybutynin) and stool softeners, as necessary. If drug therapy fails, treatment may include transurethral prostate resection (TURP)—not usually performed on young men because it leads to sterility. Total prostatectomy may cause sexual impotence and incontinence.

Nursing interventions. Ensure bed rest and adequate hydration; provide stool softeners and give sitz baths, as ordered. As needed, prepare to assist with suprapubic needle aspiration of the bladder or a suprapubic cystostomy.

Patient education. Emphasize the need for strict adherence to the prescribed drug regimen. Instruct the patient to drink at least eight glasses of water a day.

Evaluation. The recovering patient has normal bowel function, is free from infection, drinks plenty of water, and adheres to the prescribed drug regimen.

Epididymitis

Epididymitis—an infection of the epididymis, the cordlike excretory duct of the testis—is one of the most common infections of the male reproductive tract. Usually, the causative organisms spread from established UTI or prostatitis.

Causes. Epididymitis usually results from pyogenic organisms, such as staphylococci, *E. coli,* and streptococci. Other causes include gonorrhea, syphilis, chlamydial infection, trauma (which may reactivate a dormant infection or initiate a new one), and prostatectomy.

Assessment findings. Key signs and symptoms include pain, extreme tenderness, and swelling in the groin and scrotum. Other clinical effects include high fever, malaise, and a characteristic waddle (an attempt to protect the groin and scrotum when walking). Symptoms may follow severe physical strain or considerable sexual excitement.

Diagnostic tests. Three laboratory tests establish the diagnosis. Urinalysis indicates infection through an increased WBC count. Urine culture and sensitivity findings may identify the causative organism. A serum WBC count greater than 10,000/µl indicates infection.

Treatment. The goal of treatment is to reduce pain and swelling and combat infection. Therapy must begin immediately, particularly in the patient with bilateral epididymitis, to prevent sterility.

During the acute phase, treatment consists of bed rest, scrotal elevation with towel rolls or adhesive strapping, broad-spectrum antibiotics, and analgesics. An ice bag applied to the area may reduce swelling and relieve pain.

When epididymitis is refractory to antibiotic therapy, epididymectomy under local anesthesia is necessary.

Nursing interventions. Watch closely for abscess formation or extension of the infection into the testes. Closely monitor the patient's temperature, and ensure adequate fluid intake.

Patient education. If the patient faces the possibility of sterility, suggest counseling, as necessary.

Evaluation. The patient should have normal urinalysis results and a negative urine culture, verbalize the importance of completing the prescribed antibiotic therapy, and be free from pain, infection, and abscesses.

Prostatic cancer

Prostate cancer is the second most common cancer in men over age 50 and is the second leading cause of cancer death among males. It occurs mostly between the ages of 60 and 70.

Cause. Although the cause of prostatic cancer is unknown, age, infectious agents, diet, family history and endocrine function may all play a role.

Assessment findings. Signs and symptoms of prostatic cancer may appear only in the advanced stages of the disease. Clinical effects include difficult urination, dribbling, urine retention, unexplained cystitis, and back pain. A hard nodule may be palpated on rectal examination. This nodule may be felt before symptoms develop.

Diagnostic tests. Screening for prostatic cancer in asymptomatic men is a matter of debate. In general, screening involves a digital rectal examination and prostate-specific antigen testing, although neither is diagnostic. Transrectal prostatic ultrasonography will detect a mass. Biopsy confirms this diagnosis. CT scanning and MRI may also be used.

Serum acid phosphatase is elevated in 80% of patients with metastasized prostatic cancer. Successful therapy restores a normal enzyme level; a subsequent rise points to recurrence.

Treatment. Therapy for prostatic cancer must be chosen carefully because the disease usually affects older men, who frequently have serious coexisting disorders.

Treatments vary but generally include radiation, surgery, chemotherapy, and endocrine or hormone manipulation. Radical prostatectomy is usually effective for localized lesions with no evidence of metastasis. Internal beam radiation focuses radiation on the prostate while minimizing exposure of surrounding tissue. Hormone manipulation may be accomplished through surgical castration, medical castration (using diethylstilbestrol [DES], luteinizing hormone-releasing hormone analogs such as leuprolide [Lupron], and goserelin [Zoladex]), adrenal suppression (surgical or medical), or antiandrogens (flutamide, Anadron,

Casodex).

If hormone or radiation therapy and surgery can't be done or don't work, chemotherapy (using various combinations of cyclophosphamide, vinblastine, doxorubicin, mitomycin C, and 5-fluorouracil) may be tried.

Nursing interventions. When a patient receives radiation or hormonal therapy, watch for and treat nausea, vomiting, dry skin, and alopecia. Also watch for adverse effects of DES (gynecomastia, fluid retention, nausea, and vomiting). Keep in mind that thrombophlebitis (pain, tenderness, swelling, warmth, and redness in calf) is always a possibility in patients receiving DES.

Patient education. Review the treatment regimen with the patient. Explain adverse reactions that require immediate medical attention (such as thrombophlebitis).

Evaluation. Note whether the patient understands the treatment regimen. Also note whether the patient has expressed his feelings about potential sexual dysfunction.

Testicular cancer

Testicular cancer is the leading cause of death from solid tumors in men between the ages of 15 and 34.

Causes. Whites and men with a history of cryptorchidism with surgical correction performed after the age of 5 are at increased risk for testicular cancer, as are male children born to women given exogenous estrogens (birth control pills or DES), but its cause is unknown.

Assessment findings. Clinical features of testicular cancer include a firm, painless, smooth testicular mass and testicular enlargement and heaviness. In later stages, ureteral obstruction, abdominal mass, cough, hemoptysis, shortness of breath, weight loss, fatigue, pallor, and lethargy, with lymph node involvement and distant metastases are possible.

Diagnostic tests. Used together, the following tests may confirm diagnosis: radical inguinal orchiectomy (as biopsy), IVP (detects ureteral deviation resulting from para-aortic node involvement), lymphangiography and abdominal CT, and hematologic workup to include tumor markers alpha-fetoprotein and beta human chorionic gonadotropin. Routine needle biopsy isn't recommended.

Treatment. Combinations of surgery, radiation, and chemotherapy are used, depending on tumor cell type and staging. Surgery includes orchiectomy and possibly retroperitoneal node dissection. Most surgeons remove the testis but preserve the scrotum for a possible low prosthetic testicular implant later.

Seminomas are treated with postoperative radiation to the retroperitoneal and homolateral iliac nodes and, in patients with retroperitoneal extension, prophylactic radiation to the mediastinal and supraclavicular nodes. In nonseminomas, treatment includes postoperative chemotherapy using cisplatin, etoposide (VP-16), and bleomycin.

Chemotherapy is essential in patients with large abdominal or mediastinal nodes and frank distant metastases or in others at high risk for developing metastases. Combinations of cyclophosphamide, ifosfamide, vinblastine, doxorubicin, bleomycin, cisplatin, etoposide, and vincristine have been used.

Nursing interventions. The patient with testicular cancer faces difficult treatment and fears sexual impairment and disfigurement. Your plan of care should focus on providing emotional support, preventing postoperative complications, and minimizing and controlling the adverse effects of radiation and chemotherapy.

Patient education. Reassure the patient that unilateral orchiectomy doesn't cause sterility and impotence, however sperm count may be affected. Therefore, young men considering fathering a child should be counseled about sperm banking *before* surgery.

Explain the testicular self-examination and mention the availability of American Cancer Society literature on sexual concerns of cancer patients.

Evaluation. The patient should resolve concerns about possible sexual disfigurement. He should understand testicular self-examination and the importance of complying with the treatment regimen.

TREATMENTS

If uncorrected, renal and urologic disorders can adversely affect virtually every body system. Treatments for these disorders include drug therapy, surgery, dialysis, and various noninvasive procedures.

Drug therapy

Because renal disorders alter the chemical composition of body fluids and the pharmacokinetic properties of many drugs, standard regimens of some drugs may require adjustment.

Drug therapy for renal and urologic disorders can include antibiotics, urinary tract antiseptics, electrolytes and replacements, and other agents.

Surgery

Surgery is commonplace for many renal and urologic disorders. It may be needed to sustain life such as kidney transplantation in renal failure or to correct a medical problem that can prove devastating to a patient's self-image.

Surgery may be necessary when conservative treatments fail to control the patient's disorder.

Kidney transplantation

Kidney transplantation is an alternative to dialysis for many patients with otherwise unmanageable end-stage renal disease. It also may be necessary to sustain life in a patient who has suffered traumatic loss of kidney function or for whom dialysis is contraindicated. The few absolute contraindications to kidney transplantation include the patient having malignant disease or active infection, including acquired immunodeficiency syndrome.

Careful tissue matching between donor and recipient decreases the risk of organ rejection. Blood relatives make the most compatible donors. Most transplanted kidneys, however, come from cadavers.

Patient preparation. Describe the routine preoperative measures, such as a thorough physical examination and a battery of laboratory tests to detect any infection (followed by antibiotic therapy to clear it up), electrolyte studies, abdominal X-rays, an ECG, a cleansing enema, and shaving of the operative area. Tell the patient he'll undergo dialysis the day before surgery to clean his blood of unwanted fluid and electrolytes. Also point out that he may need dialysis for a few days after surgery.

Discuss the immunosuppressant drugs he'll be taking and explain their possible adverse effects. Point out that he'll be kept temporarily isolated after surgery, either in his hospital room or in a reverse-isolation unit. Explain that he'll have to take these drugs for the rest of his life or at least for as long as he has a functioning kidney transplant. As ordered, begin giving immunosuppressant drugs, such as muromonab-CD3 (orthoclone OKT3), lymphocyte immune globulin, and tacrolimus.

Monitoring and aftercare. First, you need to take special precautions to reduce the risk of infection. Use strict aseptic technique when changing dressings and performing catheter care. Also, limit the patient's contact with staff, other patients, and visitors, and have all people in the patient's room wear surgical masks for the first 2 weeks after surgery. Monitor the patient's WBC count; if it drops precipitously, notify the doctor, who may order isolation.

Throughout the recovery period, watch for signs and symptoms of tissue rejection. Observe the transplantation site for redness, tenderness, and swelling. Does the patient have a fever or an elevated WBC count? Decreased urine output with increased proteinuria? Sudden weight gain or hypertension? Elevated serum creatinine and BUN levels? Report any of these immediately.

Carefully monitor urine output; promptly report output of less than 100 ml/hour. A sudden decrease in urine output could indicate thrombus formation at the renal artery anastomosis site. Prompt surgical intervention here may prevent loss of the transplant. In a living donor transplant, urine flow may begin immediately after revascularization and connection of the ureter to the recipient's bladder. In a cadaver kidney transplant, anuria may persist for 2 days to 2 weeks; dialysis will be necessary during this period. Observe his urine color; it should be slightly blood-tinged for several days and then should gradually clear. Irrigate the catheter, as ordered, using strict aseptic technique.

Assess the patient's fluid and electrolyte balance. Watch for signs and symptoms of hyperkalemia, such as weakness and pulse irregularities. If they develop, notify the doctor. Weigh the patient daily and report any rapid gain, a possible sign of fluid retention.

Patient education. Instruct the patient to carefully measure and record intake and output to monitor kidney function. Teach him how to collect 24-hour urine samples, and tell him to notify the doctor if output falls below 20 oz (600 ml) during any 24-hour period. Tell him to drink at least 1 qt (1 L) of fluid a day unless the doctor orders otherwise.

Have the patient weigh himself at least twice a week and report any rapid gain. Direct him to watch for and promptly report any signs and symptoms of infection or transplant rejection.

Urinary diversion

A urinary diversion provides an alternative route for urine excretion when a disorder or an abnormality impedes normal flow through the bladder. Several types of urinary diversion surgery can be performed. The two most common are continent vesicostomy (or continent cutaneous urinary diversion) and ileal conduit. In ureterostomy, one or both ureters are dissected from the bladder and brought to the skin surface on the flank or the anterior abdominal wall to form one or two stomas.

Cutaneous ureterostomy offers several advantages over other urinary diversion surgeries. Besides being a shorter and easier-to-perform surgery, it can be done successfully on chronically dilated, thick-walled ureters. It is most commonly used on children when a vesicostomy doesn't relieve the obstructed ureter, when the child is acutely ill and presents an anesthesia risk, or when entering the peritoneum is contraindicated. Unlike an ileal conduit, it doesn't involve intestinal anastomoses and thus carries little risk of peritoneal and intestinal complications caused by intestinal absorption of urinary constituents.

Ileal conduit, the most common urinary diversion, involves anastomosis of the ureters to a small portion of the ileum (or colon) excised especially for the procedure, followed by the creation of a stoma from one end of the ileal segment. Because use of the ileum allows for a much larger stoma than can be created from a ureter, an ileal conduit is usually easier to care for than a ureterostomy.

In an orthotopic bladder replacement, a portion of bowel is used to form a reservoir. These constructed bladders allow the patient to void through the urethra using a Valsalva maneuver, without the need for an appliance or stoma. Catheterizations are done when the patient can't empty the bladder by straining and for daily bladder irrigation to eliminate mucous plugs.

Regardless of the type of surgery performed, urinary diversion demands ongoing patient cooperation to ensure its success. Because urine flow is constant, the patient must wear an external collection device at all times, emptying and reapplying it regularly, using the proper technique. What's more, the patient must practice meticulous stoma and peristomal care to help prevent stomal stenosis and skin excoriation.(See *Urinary diversion*, page 418.)

Patient preparation. Review the planned surgery with the patient, reinforcing the doctor's explanations as necessary. Try using a simple anatomic diagram to enhance your discussion, and provide printed information from the United Ostomy Association or other sources if possible. Explain to the patient that he'll receive a general anesthetic and have a nasogastric tube (NG) in place after surgery.

Prepare the patient for the appearance and general location of the stoma. If he's scheduled for an ileal conduit, explain that the stoma will be located somewhere in the lower abdomen, probably below the waistline. If he's scheduled for a cutaneous ureterostomy, explain that the exact stoma site commonly is chosen during surgery, based on the length of patent ureter available.

Before surgery, prepare the bowel to reduce the risk of postoperative infection from intestinal flora. As ordered, maintain a low-residue or clear liquid diet and administer a cleansing enema and an antimicrobial drug. Other measures may include total parenteral nutrition (TPN) or fluid replacement therapy for debilitated patients and prophylactic I.V. antibiotics.

Monitoring and aftercare. After the patient returns from surgery, monitor his vital signs every hour until they're stable. Carefully check and record urine output. Report any decrease, which could indicate obstruction from postoperative edema or ureteral stenosis. Observe urine drainage for pus and blood. Urine is often blood-tinged initially but should clear rapidly.

Record the amount, color, and consistency of drainage from the incision and the NG tube. Notify the doctor of any urine leakage from the drain or suture line. Such leakage may point to developing complications, such as anastomotic leak at the ureter-bowel site. Watch for signs of peritonitis.

Check dressings frequently and change them at least once each shift. The doctor will probably perform the first dressing change.

Ureteral stents are removed after a stentogram determines the absence of anastomotic leaks. Pouchograms are done in 3 weeks. If no leaks or reflux appear, the catheter is removed.

Perform routine ostomy maintenance. Make sure the collection device fits tightly around the stoma; allow no more than a $1/8''$ (3 mm) margin of skin between the stoma and the device's faceplate. Regularly check the appearance of the stoma and peristomal skin. Remember that the main cause of irritation is urine leakage around the edges of the collection device's faceplate. If

CRITICAL THINKING

Urinary diversion

At the age of 23, Marcia Koo developed a neurologic bladder following a spinal cord injury. For years Marcia had been performing clean intermittent catheterization without difficulty. Recently, however, she has been experiencing increasing episodes of incontinence.

Problem—or not?

She had just returned to college and was discouraged with the effect of incontinence on her lifestyle. After videourodynamic testing, a trial dose of anticholinergic medication proved ineffective. It was suggested that Marcia undergo an augmentation enteroplasty with an appendiceal stoma for easier catheterization. Marcia did well after her surgery and was back to college in 3 months.

But during the fourth month, Marcia developed flulike symptoms. She had nausea and vomiting, an interruption in bowel habits, high fever, abdominal cramps, and a distended abdomen for 24 hours. She tried to catheterize the stoma but was un-

successful in obtaining urine. After notifying her urologist, she was transported to the local emergency department (ED). In the ED, a #12 indwelling urinary catheter was inserted into the stoma. Despite attempts at irrigation, no urine is obtained. Why not?

Suggested response

The bowel used to create the lower intravesical pressure and larger capacity bladder will continue to secrete mucus. In cases of dehydration, the mucus becomes thicker and more difficult to pass through the opening of a catheter. Use a larger-sized catheter temporarily to evacuate the mucus and urine.

you detect leakage, change the device, taking care to properly apply the skin sealer to ensure a tight fit.

If skin breakdown occurs, clean the area with warm water and pat it dry, then apply a light dusting of karaya powder and a thin layer of protective dressing. Notify the doctor of severe excoriation.

Patient education. Make sure the patient and his family can properly perform stoma care and change the ostomy pouch. Instruct them to

watch for and report signs and symptoms of complications, such as fever, chills, flank or abdominal pain, and pus or blood in the urine.

Patients with an orthotopic bladder replacement are taught intermittent catheterization and pelvic floor–strengthening exercises. For the patient with a continent pouch diversion, review the catheterization procedure before surgery and encourage the patient to perform irrigations prior to discharge.

Stress the importance of keeping scheduled follow-up appointments with the doctor and enterostomal therapist to evaluate stoma care and make any necessary changes in equipment. For instance, stoma shrinkage, which usually occurs within 8 weeks after surgery, may require a change in pouch size to ensure a tight fit. (See *Stoma care*.)

Transurethral resection of the bladder

A relatively quick and simple procedure, transurethral resection of the bladder (TURB) involves insertion of a resectoscope through the urethra and into the bladder to remove lesions. It can also be performed using a YAG laser. Most commonly performed to treat superficial and early bladder carcinoma, TURB also may be used to remove benign papillomas or to relieve fibrosis of the bladder neck. This treatment isn't indicated for large or infiltrating tumors or for metastatic bladder cancer. (See *What happens in TURB*, page 420.)

When used to remove superficial tumors, TURB may need to be performed a dozen or more times. A typical schedule might involve treatment every 3 months for the first 2 years, then every 6 months for the next 3 years.

Patient preparation. Briefly explain the procedure. Tell the patient that he'll receive a local anesthetic and be awake during treatment. Reassure him that he should experience little or no discomfort and that hematuria and a burning sensation

FOCUS ON CARING

Stoma care

When treating difficult skin problems, consistency of care is very important. Keep in mind that the patient needs your reassurance because of the stress that results from dealing with changes in body image.

By making an extra effort to see the person and not just the problem, you'll develop good rapport with the patient and help him feel more secure and confident. An enterostomal therapy nurse can advise the patient about various appliances and offer important timesaving suggestions about his stoma care routine. This will help him accomplish his activities of daily living as soon as possible.

during urination should quickly subside. Reassure him that analgesics will be available. Also explain that TURB won't interfere with normal genitourinary function.

Patients receiving warfarin therapy must have prothrombin times within normal range before biopsies are taken. Heparin drips are discontinued 6 hours prior to the procedure and partial thromboplastin time is monitored. The heparin is resumed within 6 hours, and coumadin therapy is continued.

As ordered, prepare the patient for IVP to evaluate renal function and rule out tumors elsewhere in the urinary tract; cystoscopy and biopsy to evaluate the location and

What happens in TURB

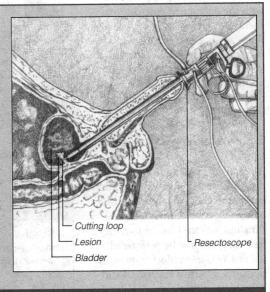

In transurethral resection of the bladder (TURB), the doctor inserts a resectoscope through the urethra into the bladder to remove small, superficial lesions.

— Cutting loop
— Lesion
— Bladder
— Resectoscope

size of the lesion and the stage and grade of the tumor; and a CT scan of the abdomen and a bone scan to detect any metastasis.

Monitoring and aftercare. Maintain adequate fluid intake and provide meticulous catheter care, including frequent irrigation. (The doctor may prescribe continuous or intermittent irrigation, especially if the removal of a large vascular lesion has compromised hemostasis.) Check urine output and assess for abdominal pain or distention, looking for signs of catheter obstruction from blood clots. If you can't clear an obstruction promptly, notify the doctor.

Observe urine drainage for blood. Remember that slight hematuria usually occurs directly after TURB. However, notify the doctor immediately of any frank bleeding. If hematuria seems excessive, observe the patient for signs of hypovolemic shock.

Assess for signs and symptoms of bladder perforation: abdominal pain and rigidity, decreased urine output, and fever. If you suspect perforation, notify the doctor and hold all fluids. Don't irrigate the catheter. Carefully assess the level and location of pain to help detect its source. Try to distinguish among the pain of bladder spasms, catheter irritation (intermittent, spasmodic pain in the urethra), and obstruction (severe, persistent pain in the suprapubic area). As ordered, give antispasmodics for bladder spasm and analgesics for pain from any source.

Patient education. Tell the patient to expect slight, intermittent hematuria for several weeks after TURB. However, he should promptly report bleeding or hematuria that lasts longer than several weeks. Instruct him to report fever, chills, or flank pain.

Cystectomy

Partial or total removal of the urinary bladder and surrounding structures may be necessary to treat advanced bladder cancer. Cystectomy may be partial, simple, or radical. *Partial,* or segmental, cystectomy involves resection of cancerous bladder tissue. *Simple,* or total, cystectomy involves resection of the entire bladder, with preservation of surrounding structures.

Radical cystectomy typically produces impotence in men and sterility in women. A permanent urinary diversion is needed in both radical and simple cystectomy.

Patient preparation. Review the surgery with the patient and his family if appropriate. If the patient will be undergoing simple or radical cystectomy, reassure him that such diversion needn't interfere with his normal activities, and arrange for a visit by an enterostomal therapist.

Explain to the patient that he'll awaken in an intensive care unit after surgery. Mention that he'll have an NG tube, a central venous catheter, and an indwelling urinary catheter in place and a drain at the surgical site.

Tell him that he won't be able to eat or drink until his bowel function returns and that he'll be given I.V. fluids during this period. After that, he can resume oral fluids and eventually progress to solids.

About 4 days before surgery, begin full bowel preparation to help prevent infection. Maintain a low-residue diet for 3 days and then infuse high-calorie fluids on the fourth day. As ordered, give antibiotics—usually erythromycin and neomycin—for 24 hours before surgery. On the night before surgery, administer an enema to clear fecal matter from the bowel.

Monitoring and aftercare. After the patient returns from surgery, monitor the amount and character of urine drainage every hour. If output is low, check the patency of the indwelling urinary catheter or stoma, and irrigate as ordered.

Monitor vital signs closely. Watch especially for signs of hypovolemic shock. Also be alert for hemorrhage if the doctor has ordered anticoagulant therapy to reduce the risk of pulmonary embolism. Periodically inspect the stoma and incision for bleeding, and observe urine drainage for frank hematuria and clots. Slight hematuria usually occurs for several days after surgery but should clear thereafter. Test all drainage from the NG tube, abdominal drains, indwelling urinary catheter, and urine collection appliance for blood, and notify the doctor of positive findings.

Observe the wound site and all drainage for signs or symptoms of infection. Change abdominal dressings frequently. Periodically ask the patient about pain at the incision site and, if he has had a partial cystectomy, ask about bladder spasms, too. Provide analgesics, as ordered. You also may be asked to administer an antispasmodic, such as oxybutynin or propantheline.

Provide scrupulous stoma care and teach the patient or a family member proper management techniques.

Patient education. Instruct the patient to watch for and report any signs or symptoms of UTI. Also tell him to report persistent hematuria.

Make sure the patient understands where to obtain needed stoma supplies. You also may want to refer the patient to a support group such as a local chapter of the United Ostomy Association.

Cystostomy

Cystostomy involves transcutaneous insertion of a catheter through the suprapubic area into the bladder, with connection of the device to a closed drainage system. Typically, cystostomy provides temporary urinary diversion after certain gynecologic procedures, bladder surgery, or prostatectomy and relieves obstruction from calculi, severe urethral strictures or fistulas, or pelvic trauma. Less commonly, it may be used to create a permanent urinary diversion, thereby relieving obstruction from an inoperable tumor. It's commonly useful in infants and young children, whose narrow urethras may hinder insertion of an indwelling urinary catheter.

Patient preparation. Tell the patient (or his parents) that the doctor will insert a soft plastic tube through the skin of the abdomen and into the bladder, then connect the tube to an external collection bag. Explain that the procedure is done under local anesthesia, that it causes little or no discomfort, and that it takes 15 to 45 minutes.

Monitoring and aftercare. Monitor vital signs, intake and output, and fluid status and encourage coughing, deep breathing, and early ambulation. To ensure adequate drainage and tube patency, check the cystostomy tube at least hourly for the first 24 hours after insertion. Carefully document the color and amount of drainage from the tube; note particularly any color changes. Assess tube patency by checking the amount of urine in the drainage bag and by palpating for bladder distention. Make sure the collection bag is below bladder level to enhance drainage and prevent backflow.

As ordered, perform a voiding trial by closing the stopcock (or clamping the tube) for 4 hours, asking the patient to attempt urination, then reopening the tube and measuring residual urine.

To prevent kinks in the tube, curve it gently but don't bend it. Tape the tube securely in place on the abdominal skin to reduce tension and prevent dislodgment. However, if the tube becomes dislodged, immediately notify the doctor; he may be able to reinsert it through the original tract. Irrigate the cystostomy tube as ordered, using the same technique as you would for irrigating an indwelling urinary catheter. Check the tube frequently for kinks or obstruction. If a blood clot or mucus blocks the tube, try milking it to restore patency. However, if you can't clear the obstruction promptly, notify the doctor.

Check dressings often and change them at least once a day or as ordered. Observe the skin around the insertion site for signs of infection and encrustation.

Patient education. Teach the patient about postoperative care of the catheter, collection bag, and surrounding skin. If possible, arrange for a visit by an enterostomal therapist. Encourage the patient to drink plenty of fluids.

Tell the patient or his family to notify the doctor promptly of signs of infection or encrustation at the tube insertion site.

Prostatectomy

When chronic prostatitis, benign prostatic hyperplasia, or prostate cancer fails to respond to drug therapy or other treatments, total or partial prostatectomy may be necessary to remove diseased or obstructive tissue and restore urine flow through the urethra. Depending on the disease, one of four approaches is used. Transurethral resection of the prostate (TURP), the most common approach, involves insertion of a resectoscope into the urethra. Open surgical approaches include supra-

pubic, retropubic, and radical perineal or retropubic prostatectomy.

Prostatectomy can also be performed by transurethral incision of the prostate, transurethral balloon dilatation, stents and coils, and hyperthermia. The advantages of transurethral laser prostatectomy include minimal bleeding, shorter hospitalization with decreased risk of bladder neck stricture and incidence of retrograde ejaculation. Disadvantages include postoperative urine retention and lack of tissue samples for pathology.

Patient preparation. Review the planned surgery with the patient. Before surgery, as ordered, shave and clean the surgical site (unless the patient is scheduled for TURP) and administer a cleansing enema. Explain to the patient that a catheter will remain in place for several days after surgery to ensure proper urine drainage.

Monitoring and aftercare. After prostatectomy, nursing care focuses on preventing or promptly detecting complications, which may include hemorrhage, infection, and urine retention. (See *Managing radical retropubic prostatectomy*, pages 424 to 427.)

Carefully observe the patient for complications. Monitor his vital signs closely, looking for indications of possible hemorrhage and shock. Watch for signs and symptoms of dilutional hyponatremia, characterized by altered mental status, muscle twitching, and seizures. If these

(Text continues on page 426.)

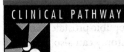

Managing radical retropubic prostatectomy

This partial clinical path focuses on postoperative care. The complete path includes 1 day each of preoperative and operative care.

Length of stay: 3 days

	Postop day 1
Daily outcomes	• Patient tolerating clear liquids • Patient out of bed (OOB) • Minimal Jackson-Pratt (JP) drainage
Diagnostic tests	• Complete blood count (CBC) • SMA-6
Consults	
Assessments	• Regular room: Vital signs (VS) check every shift • Physical assessment every shift • Antiembolism stockings
Treatments/procedures	• Clear liquids as tolerated • JP self-suction • Indwelling urinary catheter to straight drainage (leg bag) • Antiembolism stockings • Hemovac discontinued if total output <20 ml
Medications/I.V.s	• I.V. rate decreased to 75 ml/hr • Stool softener • Pain medication
Activity/rehabilitation	• OOB to chair • Ambulation with assistance
Discharge planning	• Refer for unexpected complications
Patient/family education	• Provide written handouts of: —post-prostatectomy guidelines —care of an indwelling catheter at home. • Teach leg bag and night drainage bag usage and routine.

Postop day 2	Postop day 3	Discharge outcomes
• Patient ambulating halls independently • Patient demonstrating appropriate technique for leg bag care • Patient tolerating regular diet		
• CBC		
• VS every shift • Physical assessment every shift		
• Regular diet as tolerated • Antiembolism stockings discontinued • I.V. discontinued if oral intake is adequate • JP discontinued if total output <20 to 30 ml/shift	• Indwelling urinary catheter discontinued to leg bag	• Regular diet
• Oral pain medication		
• Patient ambulating as desired		• Activity per baseline • No heavy lifting or yard work
• Discuss discharge plan with patient/family. • Refer to Visiting Nurse service, if necessary. • Give supplies.	• Follow-up appointment with doctor for possible staple removal 2 weeks after discharge	
• Reinforce leg bag and night drainage bag usage and routine. • Observe patient skill using leg bag and night drainage bag.	• Inform patient/family of need to call for follow-up appointment with doctor for staple removal.	• Patient able to perform self-care of catheter and wound *(continued)*

Managing radical retropubic prostatectomy (continued)

	Postop day 1
Patient/family education (continued)	• Teach use of catheter holder. • Teach meatal care.
Potential variance	• Unable to eat • Unable to get OOB

Adapted with permission from New York University Medical Center

occur, raise the side rails of the patient's bed to prevent injury. Then notify the doctor, draw blood for serum sodium determination, and prepare hypertonic saline solution for possible I.V. infusion. Frequently check the incision site (unless the patient underwent TURP) for signs of infection, and change dressings as necessary. Also watch for and report signs and symptoms of epididymitis: fever, chills, groin pain, and a tender, swollen epididymis.

Check and record the amount and nature of urine drainage. Maintain catheter patency through intermittent or continuous irrigation, as ordered. Watch for catheter blockage from kinking or clot formation, and correct as necessary. Maintain the patency of the suprapubic tube, if inserted, and monitor the amount and character of drainage. Drainage should be amber or slightly blood-tinged; report any abnormalities. Keep the collection container below the level of the patient's bladder to promote drainage. Keep the skin around the tube insertion site clean and dry.

Expect and report frank bleeding the first day after surgery. If bleeding is venous, the doctor may order increased traction on the catheter or increased pressure in the catheter's balloon end. However, if bleeding is arterial (bright red with numerous clots and increased viscosity), the doctor may need to control it surgically.

Patient education. Tell the patient to drink 10 glasses of water a day, to void at least every 2 hours, and to notify the doctor promptly if he has trouble voiding. Explain that he may experience transient urinary frequency and dribbling after catheter removal.

Reassure the patient that slightly blood-tinged urine usually occurs for the first few weeks after surgery. Instruct him to report bright-red urine or persistent hematuria, however. Tell him to watch for and immediately report any signs and symptoms of infection.

Postop day 2	Postop day 3	Discharge outcomes
• Teach wound care, shower, and pat dry techniques.		
• JP drainage increased • Unable to take oral medications		

Dialysis

Depending on the patient's condition and, at times, his preference, dialysis may take the form of hemodialysis or peritoneal dialysis. Occasionally, hemodynamically unstable patients may be treated with either continuous arteriovenous ultrafiltration or continuous arteriovenous hemofiltration.

Hemodialysis

Hemodialysis removes toxic wastes and other impurities from the blood of a patient with renal failure. In this technique, the blood is removed from the body through a surgically created access site, pumped through a dialyzing unit to remove toxins, and then returned to the body. The extracorporeal dialyzer works through a combination of osmosis, diffusion, and filtration. By extracting urea and uric acid as well as creatinine and excess water, hemodialysis helps restore or maintain acid-base and electrolyte balance and prevent the complications associated with uremia.

Hemodialysis can be performed in an emergency in acute renal failure or as regular long-term therapy in end-stage renal disease. In chronic renal failure, the frequency and duration of treatments depend on the patient's condition; up to several treatments a week, each lasting up to 6 hours, may be required.

Patient preparation. If the patient is undergoing hemodialysis for the first time, explain its purpose and what to expect during and after treatment. Explain that he first will undergo surgery to create vascular access. The site and type of hemodialysis access vary, depending on the expected duration of dialysis, the surgeon's preference, and the patient's condition. This includes arteriovenous fistula, arteriovenous shunt, arteriovenous vein graft, subclavian vein catheterization, and femoral vein catheterization.

After vascular access has been created and the patient is ready for dialysis, weigh him and take his vital signs. Be sure to take the patient's blood pressure in supine and standing positions. Place the patient in a supine position and make him as comfortable as possible. Keep the vascular access site well supported and resting on a sterile drape or sterile barrier shield.

As ordered, prepare the hemodialysis equipment, following the manufacturer's and your hospital's protocols and maintaining strict aseptic technique.

Monitoring and aftercare. Monitor the patient throughout dialysis. Once every 30 minutes, check and record vital signs to detect possible complications. Fever may point to infection from pathogens in the dialysate or equipment; notify the doctor, who may prescribe an antipyretic, an antibiotic, or both. Hypotension may indicate hypovolemia or a drop in hematocrit; give blood or fluid supplements I.V., as ordered. Rapid respirations may signal hypoxemia; give supplemental oxygen, as ordered.

About every hour, draw a blood sample for analysis of clotting time. Using the dialyzing unit's bed scale or a portable scale, check the patient's weight regularly to ensure adequate ultrafiltration during treatment. Also periodically check the dialyzer's blood lines to make sure all connections are secure, and monitor the lines for clotting.

Be especially alert for signs of air embolism—a potentially fatal complication characterized by sudden hypotension, dyspnea, chest pain, cyanosis, and a weak, rapid pulse. If these signs or symptoms develop, turn the patient onto his left side

and lower the head of the bed, and call the doctor immediately.

Assess for headache, muscle twitching, backache, nausea or vomiting, and seizures, which may indicate disequilibrium syndrome caused by rapid fluid removal and electrolyte changes. If this syndrome occurs, notify the doctor immediately; he may reduce the blood flow rate or stop dialysis. Muscle cramps also may result from rapid fluid and electrolyte shifts. As ordered, relieve cramps by injecting normal saline solution into the venous return line.

Observe the patient carefully for signs and symptoms of internal bleeding: apprehension; restlessness; pale, cold, clammy skin; excessive thirst; hypotension; rapid, weak, thready pulse; increased respirations; and decreased body temperature. Report any of these signs immediately and prepare to decrease heparinization; the doctor also may order blood transfusions.

After completion of hemodialysis, monitor the vascular access site for bleeding. If bleeding is excessive, maintain pressure on the site and notify the doctor. To prevent clotting or other problems with blood flow, make sure that the arm used for vascular access isn't used for any other procedure, including I.V. line insertion, blood pressure monitoring, or venipuncture. At least four times a day, assess circulation at the access site by auscultating for the presence of bruits and palpating for thrills. Lack of bruit at a venous access site for dialysis may indicate a blood clot, requiring immediate surgical attention.

Patient education. Teach the patient how to care for his vascular access site. Tell him to keep the incision clean and dry to prevent infection and to clean it with hydrogen peroxide solution daily until healing is complete and the sutures are removed (usually 10 to 14 days after surgery). Tell him to notify the doctor of pain, swelling, redness, or drainage in the accessed arm. Teach him how to use a stethoscope to auscultate for bruits.

Explain that once the access site has healed, he may use the arm freely. In fact, exercise is beneficial because it helps stimulate vein enlargement. Remind him not to allow any treatments or procedures on the accessed arm, including blood pressure monitoring or needle punctures. Also tell him to avoid putting excessive pressure on the arm; he shouldn't sleep on it, wear constricting clothing on it, or lift heavy objects or strain with it. He also should avoid showering, bathing, or swimming for several hours after dialysis.

Teach the patient exercises for the affected arm to promote vascular dilation and enhance blood flow. Explain the exercise routine as follows: 1 week after surgery, squeeze a small rubber ball or other soft object for 15 minutes, four times a day; 2 weeks after surgery, apply a tourniquet on the upper arm above the fistula site, making sure it's snug but not tight. With the tourniquet in place, squeeze the rubber ball for 5 minutes; repeat four times daily. After the incision has healed com-

pletely, perform the exercise with the arm submerged in warm water.

If the patient will be performing hemodialysis at home, make sure he thoroughly understands all aspects of the procedure. Give him the phone number of the dialysis center and encourage him to call if he has questions about the treatment. Also encourage him to arrange for another person to be present during dialysis in case problems develop.

Peritoneal dialysis

Like hemodialysis, peritoneal dialysis removes toxins from the blood of a patient with acute or chronic renal failure who doesn't respond to other treatments. But unlike hemodialysis, it uses the patient's peritoneal membrane as a semipermeable dialyzing membrane. In this technique, a hypertonic dialyzing solution (dialysate) is instilled through a catheter inserted into the peritoneal cavity. Then, by diffusion, excessive concentrations of electrolytes and uremic toxins in the blood move across the peritoneal membrane into the dialysis solution. Next, by osmosis, excessive water in the blood does the same. After an appropriate dwelling time, the dialysate is drained, taking toxins and wastes with it.

Peritoneal dialysis may be performed manually, by an automatic or semiautomatic cycler machine, or as continuous ambulatory peritoneal dialysis (CAPD). In manual dialysis, the nurse, the patient, or a family member instills dialysate through the catheter into the peritoneal cavity, allows it to dwell for a specified time, and then drains it from the peritoneal cavity.

The cycler machine requires sterile setup and connection technique, then it automatically completes dialysis. In contrast, CAPD is performed by the patient himself. Using careful aseptic technique, he instills dialysate from a special plastic bag through a catheter leading into his peritoneal cavity. With the solution in the peritoneal cavity, the patient can roll up the empty bag, place it under his clothing, and go about his normal activities. After 6 to 8 hours of dwell time, he drains the spent solution into the bag, removes and discards the filled bag, then attaches a new bag and instills a new batch of dialysate. He repeats the process to ensure continuous dialysis 24 hours a day.

Some patients use CAPD in combination with an automatic cycler, in a treatment called continuous cycling peritoneal dialysis (CCPD). In CCPD, the cycler performs dialysis at night while the patient sleeps, and the patient performs CAPD in the daytime.

Peritoneal dialysis can cause severe complications. The most serious one, peritonitis, results from bacteria entering the peritoneal cavity through the catheter or the insertion site. Besides causing infection, peritonitis can scar the peritoneum, causing thickening of the membrane and preventing its use as a dialyzing membrane.

Patient preparation. For the first-time peritoneal dialysis patient, explain the purpose of the treatment and what he can expect during and after the procedure. Explain the appropriate catheter insertion procedure.

Before catheter insertion, take and record the patient's baseline vital signs and weight. (Check blood pressure in both the supine and standing positions.) Ask him to urinate to reduce the risk of bladder perforation and increase comfort during catheter insertion. If he can't urinate, perform straight catheterization, as ordered, to drain the bladder.

While the patient undergoes peritoneal catheter insertion, warm the dialysate to body temperature in a warmer or heating pad. The dialysate may be a 1.5%, 2.5%, or 4.25% dextrose solution, usually with heparin added to prevent clotting in the catheter. It should be clear and colorless. Add any prescribed medication at this time.

Next, put on a surgical mask and prepare the dialysis administration set. Place the drainage bag below the patient to facilitate gravity drainage, and connect the outflow tubing to it. Then connect the dialysis infusion lines to the bags or bottles of dialysate, and hang the containers on an I.V. pole at the patient's bedside. Maintain sterile technique during solution and equipment preparation.

When the equipment and solution are ready, place the patient in a supine position, have him put on a surgical mask, and tell him to relax. Prime the tubing with solution, keeping the clamps closed, and connect one infusion line to the abdominal catheter.

To test the catheter's patency, open the clamp on the infusion line and rapidly instill 500 ml of dialysate into the patient's peritoneal cavity. Immediately unclamp the outflow line and let fluid drain into the collection bag; outflow should be brisk. Once you've established catheter patency, you're ready to start dialysis.

Monitoring and aftercare. During dialysis, monitor the patient's vital signs every 10 minutes until they stabilize, then every 2 to 4 hours or as ordered. Report any abrupt or significant changes. Also periodically check the patient's weight and report any gain. Using aseptic technique, change the catheter dressing every 24 hours or whenever it becomes wet or soiled.

Watch closely for developing complications. Peritonitis may be manifested by fever, persistent abdominal pain and cramping, slow or cloudy dialysis drainage, swelling and tenderness around the catheter, and an increased WBC count. If you detect these signs and symptoms, notify the doctor and send a dialysate specimen to the laboratory for smear and culture.

After the solution has dwelled in the peritoneal cavity for the prescribed length of time, allow the solution to drain from the peritoneal cavity into the collection bag. When emptying the collection bag and measuring the solution, wear protective eyewear and gloves.

Observe the outflow drainage for blood. Keep in mind that drainage is commonly blood-tinged after catheter placement but should clear after a few fluid exchanges. Notify the doctor of bright red or persistent bleeding. Watch for respiratory distress. If it's severe, drain the patient's peritoneal cavity and call the doctor.

Periodically check the outflow tubing for clots or kinks that may be obstructing drainage. If you can't clear an obstruction, notify the doctor. Have the patient change position frequently.

To help prevent fluid imbalance, calculate the patient's fluid balance at the end of each dialysis session or after every 8-hour period in a longer session. Record and report any significant imbalance, either positive or negative.

Patient education. If the patient will perform CAPD or CCPD at home, make sure he thoroughly understands and can do each step of the procedure. Usually, he'll go through a 2-week training program first. Tell him to keep the phone number of the dialysis center always at hand in case of an emergency.

Tell the patient to watch for and report signs of infection and fluid imbalance. Make sure he can take his vital signs to provide a record of response to treatment.

Calculi removal or destruction

This section covers treatment of calculi using basketing, extracorporeal shock waves, and percutaneous ultrasonic lithotripsy.

Calculi basketing

When ureteral calculi are too large for normal elimination, removal with a basketing instrument is the treatment of choice because it helps to relieve pain and prevent infection and renal dysfunction. In this technique, a basketing instrument is inserted through a cystoscope or ureteroscope into the ureter or a nephroscope into the renal pelvis to capture the calculus and then is withdrawn to remove it.

After calculus removal, the surgeon usually inserts a ureteral catheter or stent into the kidney to drain urine into the bladder. He also inserts an indwelling urinary catheter to aid bladder drainage. The calculus is examined and compared with the X-ray film to determine whether it has been totally removed.

Patient preparation. Review the procedure with the patient and explain why it's necessary. Prepare the patient for tests to determine calculi location and renal status. Such tests typically include abdominal X-rays and IVP.

Monitoring and aftercare. After the procedure, monitor the patient's vital signs and intake and output. Promote fluids to maintain a urine output of 3 to 4 qt (3 to 4 L) a day. Observe the color of urine drainage from the indwelling urinary catheter or voided urine; it should be slightly blood-tinged at first, gradually clearing within 24 to 48 hours. Notify the doctor if frank or persistent hematuria occurs. Irrigate the catheter, as ordered, using sterile technique.

Watch for and report any signs and symptoms of septicemia, which may result from ureteral perforation during basketing. If you suspect infection, obtain blood and urine samples, as ordered, and send them to the laboratory for analysis. Check drainage from the ureteral catheter, if one is implanted. Keep the catheter taped securely to the patient's thigh to prevent dislodgment or undue traction.

Patient education. Teach the patient and his family the importance of following prescribed dietary and medication regimens to prevent recurrence of calculi. For the same reason, encourage him to drink 3 to 4 qt (3 to 4 L) of fluid a day, unless contraindicated.

Tell him to immediately report signs and symptoms of recurrent calculi (flank pain, hematuria, nausea, fever, and chills) or acute ureteral obstruction (severe pain and inability to void). Explain that he should report urinary frequency or symptoms of irritation, which may indicate an ill-fitted stent or displacement.

Extracorporeal shock-wave lithotripsy

A revolutionary noninvasive technique for removing obstructive renal calculi, extracorporeal shock-wave lithotripsy (ESWL) uses high-energy shock waves to break up calculi and allow their normal passage. Repeat treatments may be necessary for large or multiple calculi.

Patient preparation. Review the doctor's explanation of ESWL. Tell the patient that he'll receive a general or epidural anesthetic. Also tell him that he'll have an I.V. line and an indwelling urinary catheter in place after ESWL.

Monitoring and aftercare. Check the patient's vital signs in 15 minutes, 30 minutes, and then hourly until discharge. Notify the doctor of any abnormal findings. Remove the indwelling urinary catheter once adequate urine output is established; the patient will be discharged after voiding. Strain all urine for calculi fragments and send these to the laboratory for analysis.

Assess for pain on the treated side, and give analgesics, as ordered. Promptly report severe pain, which may indicate ureteral obstruction.

Patient education. To help remove particles, instruct the patient to lie facedown with his head and shoulders over the edge of the bed for about 10 minutes. Have him perform this maneuver twice a day. Encourage fluids 30 to 45 minutes before starting.

Teach the patient how to strain his urine for fragments. Tell him to strain all urine for the first week after treatment, to save all fragments, and to bring the container with him on his first follow-up doctor's appointment.

Discuss expected adverse effects of ESWL, including pain in the treated side, slight redness or bruising on the treated side, blood-tinged urine for several days after treatment, and mild GI upset. Reassure the patient that these effects are normal. However, tell him to report severe, unremitting pain, persistent hematuria, inability to void, fever and chills, or recurrent nausea and vomiting.

Encourage him to resume normal activities when he feels able (unless the doctor instructs otherwise). Explain that physical activity will enhance the passage of calculi fragments.

Percutaneous ultrasonic lithotripsy

In percutaneous ultrasonic lithotripsy, an ultrasonic probe inserted through a nephrostomy tube into the renal pelvis generates ultrahigh-frequency sound waves to shatter calculi, while continuous suctioning removes the fragments. Percutaneous ultrasonic lithotripsy may be used in place of or following ESWL. It's particularly useful for radiolucent calculi lodged in the kidney, which aren't treatable by ESWL. (See *Using ultrasound to fracture calculi*, page 434.)

Patient preparation. Explain the procedure to the patient. Explain that the nephrostomy tube may cause discomfort; otherwise the treatment should be painless. Tell him he'll receive analgesics if needed.

The day before the scheduled treatment, as ordered, prepare the patient for IVP or lower abdominal X-rays to locate the calculi. Describe posttreatment care measures. Explain that if no complications develop, he may be discharged 2 to 4 days after treatment.

Using ultrasound to fracture calculi

In percutaneous ultrasonic lithotripsy, the lithotriptor's ultrasonic probe fractures calculi by vibration and continuously suctions the fragments from the kidney.

To perform the procedure, the surgeon establishes a nephrostomy tract with a needle puncture performed under fluoroscopic guidance. He then threads an angiographic wire through the needle and passes various-sized nephrostomy tubes over the wire to progressively dilate the tract. When the tract is sufficiently dilated, he removes the tube and inserts a nephroscope to visualize the calculus.

Next (or a day or two later if the procedure is being performed in two stages), the surgeon inserts a working tube resembling a small cystoscope through the nephrostomy tract and into the kidney's collecting system. He then passes an ultrasonic probe through the tube and positions it against the calculus. When the probe is in position, he turns on the device, producing ultrahigh-frequency sound waves that shatter the calculus into fragments. He then uses suction or, if necessary, irrigation or a basketing instrument to remove the fragments.

Once treatment is complete, the surgeon withdraws the probe and the working tube. Then he reinserts the nephrostomy tube.

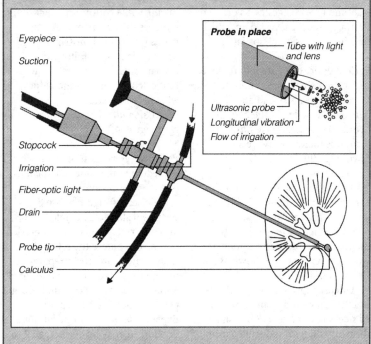

Eyepiece
Suction
Stopcock
Irrigation
Fiber-optic light
Drain
Probe tip
Calculus

Probe in place
Tube with light and lens
Ultrasonic probe
Longitudinal vibration
Flow of irrigation

Monitoring and aftercare. After treatment, check the volume of nephrostomy tube drainage hourly for the first 24 hours and then every 4 hours or so thereafter. Report absent or decreased drainage, which could indicate obstruction from retained calculi fragments. Also note urine color and test pH. Slight hematuria usually occurs for several days. However, if you detect frank or persistent bleeding, notify the doctor. Strain all urine for calculi and send any fragments to the laboratory for analysis.

Assess the patient for pain and give analgesics, as needed. Promptly report severe pain accompanied by decreased drainage, which may indicate obstruction from unremoved fragments. Also watch for and report signs of hemorrhage or infection. As ordered, gently irrigate the nephrostomy tube to ensure its patency. Maintain sterile technique and use no more than 10 ml of normal saline solution. Never clamp the tube; the resultant pressure increase could cause renal damage.

Encourage early ambulation. A day or two after treatment, prepare the patient for nephrotomography to check for retained fragments. If no fragments are revealed, the doctor usually will remove the nephrostomy tube. Occasionally, a patient will be discharged with the tube in place.

Patient education. Tell the patient to drink 3 to 4 qt (3 to 4 L) of fluid each day for about a month after treatment. Instruct him to promptly report persistent bloody or cloudy, foul-smelling urine; an inability to void; fever and chills; or severe, unremitting flank pain. He should also report redness, swelling, or purulent drainage from the nephrostomy tube insertion site.

Teach the patient how to strain his urine for calculi fragments. Tell him to strain all urine for the first week after treatment, to save all fragments, and to bring the container with him on his first follow-up doctor's appointment. If he's discharged with a nephrostomy tube in place, outline proper tube care.

Bladder management

This section covers catheterization—the insertion of a drainage device into the urinary bladder.

Catheterization

Intermittent catheterization drains urine remaining in the bladder after voiding. It may be used postoperatively and for patients with urinary incontinence, urethral strictures, cystitis, prostatic obstruction, neurogenic bladder, or other disorders that interfere with bladder emptying. Continuous catheterization can permit monitoring of urine output when normal voiding is impaired.

Patient preparation. Review the procedure and reassure the patient that although catheterization may produce slight discomfort, it shouldn't be painful. Explain that you'll stop the procedure if he experiences severe discomfort.

Assemble the necessary equipment, preferably a sterile catheterization package.

Monitoring and aftercare. During catheterization, note the difficulty or ease of insertion, any patient discomfort, and the amount and nature of urine drainage. Document this information, and notify the doctor if you observe hematuria or extremely foul-smelling or cloudy urine. Encourage fluids (up to 3 qt [3 L]/day if necessary) to maintain continuous urine flow and decrease the risk of complications.

Maintain good catheter care throughout treatment. Clean the urinary meatus and catheter junction at least daily, more often if you note a buildup of exudate. Expect a small amount of mucous drainage at the catheter insertion site from irritation of the urethral wall, but notify the doctor of excessive, bloody, or purulent drainage.

To prevent infection, avoid separating the catheter and tubing unless absolutely necessary. Remain alert for signs and symptoms of UTI and report them to the doctor. (See "Lower urinary tract disorders," page 404.) Monitor for signs of catheter obstruction. Watch for decreased or absent urine output (less than 30 ml/hour); severe, persistent bladder spasms; urine leakage around the catheter insertion site; and bladder distention.

Patient education. Instruct the patient to drink at least 2 qt (2 L) of water a day, unless the doctor orders otherwise. Teach him how to minimize the risk of infection by performing daily periurethral care. Stress the need for thorough hand washing before and after handling the catheter and collection system. Tell him that he may take showers but should avoid tub baths while the catheter is in place.

If the patient has an indwelling catheter, ensure that he knows how to secure the tubing and the leg bag. Tell him to alternate legs every other day. Instruct him to keep the leg bag or closed-system drainage bag lower than the level of the bladder to facilitate drainage. In male patients, tape the tubing upward onto the abdomen. Explain that he should empty the bag when it's about half-full. Teach him how to empty it. Demonstrate how he should apply a new bag.

Instruct the patient to notify the doctor if he notices urine leakage around the catheter. Also instruct him to report any signs and symptoms of UTI.

References and Readings

Guyton, A. *Textbook of Medical Physiology,* 8th ed. Philadelphia: W.B. Saunders Co., 1995.

Illustrated Guide to Diagnostic Tests, 2nd ed. Springhouse, Pa.: Springhouse Corp., 1997.

Nursing98 Drug Handbook. Springhouse, Pa.: Springhouse Corp., 1998.

Rakel, R.E., ed. *Conn's Current Therapy 1997.* Philadelphia: W.B. Saunders Co., 1997.

Sparks, S. M., et al. *Nursing Diagnosis Pocket Manual.* Springhouse, Pa.: Springhouse Corp., 1996.

Tanago, E., and McAninch, J. *Smith's General Urology,* 14th ed. East Norwalk, Conn.: Appleton & Lange, 1995.

9

GASTROINTESTINAL CARE

As the site of the body's digestive processes, the GI system has the critical task of supplying essential nutrients to fuel the brain, heart, and lungs. GI function also profoundly affects the quality of life by its impact on overall health.

ASSESSMENT

GI signs and symptoms can have many baffling causes. To help sort out significant symptoms, you'll need to take a thorough patient history. Using inspection, auscultation, palpation, and percussion, you'll probe further by conducting a thorough physical examination.

Physical assessment

Physical assessment of the GI system usually includes evaluation of the mouth, abdomen, liver, and rectum.

To perform a thorough abdominal and rectal assessment, gather the following equipment: gloves, stethoscope, flashlight, measuring tape, felt-tip pen, and a gown and drapes to cover the patient.

Assessing the oral cavity

Start by assessing the oral structures. Structural problems or disorders here may affect GI functioning. Here's what to look for when assessing oral structures:
• Mouth—asymmetry, motility, or malocclusion
• Lips—abnormal color, lesions, nodules, vesicles, or fissures
• Teeth—caries; missing, broken, or displaced teeth; dental appliances (such as dentures or braces)
• Gums—recession, redness, pallor, hypertrophy, ulcers, or bleeding
• Tongue—deviation to one side, tremors, redness, swelling, ulcers, lesions, or abnormal coatings
• Buccal mucosa—pallor, redness, swelling, ulcers, lesions, or leukoplakia
• Hard and soft palates—redness, lesions, patches, petechiae, or pallor
• Pharynx—uvular deviation, tonsil abnormalities, lesions, ulcers,

plaques, exudate, or unusual mouth odor (such as fruity or fetid).

Assessing the abdomen

Mentally divide the patient's abdomen into four regions, or quadrants. (See *Identifying abdominal landmarks.*) Then, when assessing the abdomen, perform the four basic steps in the following sequence: inspection, auscultation, percussion, and palpation. Unlike other body systems, in which auscultation is performed last, the GI system requires abdominal auscultation *before* percussion and palpation, because the latter can alter intestinal activity and bowel sounds.

When assessing a patient with abdominal pain, always auscultate, percuss, and palpate in the painful quadrant last. Otherwise, the patient may tense up, making further assessment difficult.

(See *Identifying areas of referred pain,* page 440.)

Inspection. Begin by inspecting the patient's entire abdomen, noting overall contour and skin integrity, appearance of the umbilicus, and any visible pulsations. Note any distention or irregular contours for further assessment.

Next, inspect the abdominal skin. Look for areas of discoloration, striae, rashes or other lesions, dilated veins, and scars. Document the location and character of these findings.

Observe the entire abdomen for movement from peristalsis or arterial pulsations. Normally, peristalsis isn't visible. In some patients, aortic pulsations may be seen in the epigastric area.

To detect any umbilical or incisional hernias, have the patient raise his head and shoulders while remaining in a supine position. Finally, inspect the umbilicus for position, contour, and color.

Auscultation. Auscultation provides information on bowel motility and the underlying vessels and organs. To auscultate for bowel sounds, lightly press the stethoscope diaphragm on the abdominal skin in all four quadrants. Normally, air and fluid moving through the bowel by peristalsis create soft, bubbling sounds with no regular pattern, often mixed with soft clicks and gurgles, every 5 to 15 seconds. Rapid, high-pitched, loud, and gurgling bowel sounds are *hyperactive* and may occur normally in a hungry patient. Sounds occurring at a rate of one every minute or longer are *hypoactive* and normally occur after bowel surgery or when the colon is feces filled.

Before reporting absent bowel sounds, be sure the patient has an empty bladder. Audible bowel sounds may be initiated by gently pressing on the abdominal surface or by having the patient eat or drink something.

Next, use the bell of the stethoscope to auscultate for vascular sounds. Normally, you should detect no vascular sounds. Note a bruit, venous hum, or friction rub.

Percussion. Abdominal percussion helps determine the size and location of abdominal organs and detects excessive accumulation of fluid and

Identifying abdominal landmarks

To aid accurate abdominal assessment and documentation of findings, you can mentally divide the patient's abdomen into regions. The quadrant method, the easiest and most commonly used, divides the abdomen into four equal regions by two imaginary lines crossing perpendicularly above the umbilicus.

Right upper quadrant (RUQ)
Liver and gallbladder
Pylorus
Duodenum
Head of pancreas
Hepatic flexure of colon
Portions of ascending and trans-
   verse colon

Left upper quadrant (LUQ)
Left liver lobe
Stomach
Body of pancreas
Splenic flexure of colon
Portions of transverse and descend-
   ing colon

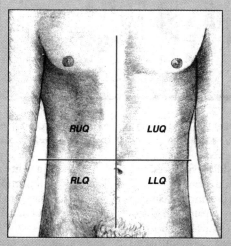

Right lower quadrant (RLQ)
Cecum and appendix
Portion of ascending colon
Lower portion of right kidney
Bladder (if distended)

Left lower quadrant (LLQ)
Sigmoid colon
Portion of descending colon
Lower portion of left kidney
Bladder (if distended)

air. Percuss in all four quadrants, keeping approximate organ locations in mind as you progress. Percuss the abdomen systematically, starting with the right upper quadrant and moving clockwise. If a patient complains of pain in a particular quadrant, percuss that quadrant last. Percussion sounds vary, depending on the density of underlying structures. The predominant abdominal percussion sound is tympany, created by

Identifying areas of referred pain

Pain may occur relatively near its source or distant from it. These illustrations will help you identify the areas and causes of referred pain.

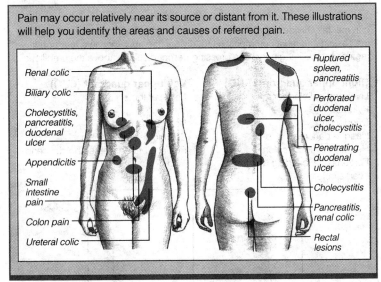

Renal colic

Biliary colic

Cholecystitis, pancreatitis, duodenal ulcer

Appendicitis

Small intestine pain

Colon pain

Ureteral colic

Ruptured spleen, pancreatitis

Perforated duodenal ulcer, cholecystitis

Penetrating duodenal ulcer

Cholecystitis

Pancreatitis, renal colic

Rectal lesions

percussing over an air-filled stomach or intestine. Dull sounds normally occur over the liver, the spleen, a lower intestine filled with feces, and a bladder filled with urine.

Note: Keep in mind that abdominal percussion or palpation is contraindicated in patients with suspected abdominal aortic aneurysm or those who have received abdominal organ transplants. It should be performed cautiously in patients with suspected appendicitis.

If the patient's abdomen is distended, assess its progression by taking serial measurements of abdominal girth.

Palpation. This maneuver elicits useful clues about the character of the abdominal wall, organs, any masses, and abdominal pain. Commonly used techniques include light palpation, deep palpation, and ballottement.

To perform light palpation, gently press your fingertips about ¹/₂″ to ³/₄″ (1.3 to 2 cm) into the abdominal wall. The light touch helps relax the patient.

To perform deep palpation, press the fingertips of both hands about 1¹/₂″ (4 cm) into the abdominal wall. Move your hands in a slightly circular fashion so that the abdominal wall moves over the underlying structures. If you detect a mass on light or deep palpation, note its location, size, shape, consistency, type of border, degree of tenderness, presence of pulsations, and degree of mobility.

Deep palpation may evoke rebound tenderness when you suddenly withdraw your fingertips, a possible sign of peritoneal inflammation.

Note: Don't palpate a pulsating midline mass; it may be a dissecting aneurysm, which can rupture under the pressure of palpation. Report such a mass to the doctor immediately. (See *Eliciting abdominal pain*, page 442.)

Ballottement involves lightly tapping or bouncing your fingertips against the abdominal wall. This technique helps elicit abdominal muscle resistance or guarding that can be missed with deep palpation or it may detect the movement or bounce of a freely movable mass. Your fingers should also bounce at the underlying dense liver tissue in the right upper quadrant. If the patient has ascites, use *deep ballottement* by pushing your fingertips deeply inward in a rapid motion; then quickly release the pressure, maintaining fingertip contact with the abdominal wall. You should feel the movement of an underlying organ or a movable mass toward your fingertips.

Assessing the liver

You can estimate the size and position of the liver through percussion and palpation.

Percussion. Use fist percussion (or blunt percussion) to detect tenderness, a common symptom of gallbladder or liver disease or inflammation. To perform this maneuver, place one hand flat over the patient's lower right rib cage along the midclavicular line, then strike the back of this hand with your other hand

clenched in a fist. Patient discomfort and muscle guarding indicate tenderness. **Note:** Use this maneuver only on a patient with unconfirmed but suspected inflammation or hepatomegaly, and defer it until the end of the abdominal assessment. If the patient complains of discomfort during the assessment, particularly over the spleen, do not perform this maneuver.

Palpation. Usually, it's impossible to palpate the liver in an adult. If palpable, the liver border usually feels smooth and firm, with a rounded, regular edge. A palpable liver may indicate hepatomegaly; it also may occur in an extremely thin patient or in the following variations.
• A low diaphragm, as occurs in emphysema, will displace a normal-sized liver downward.
• In a normal variation known as Riedel's lobe, the right lobe is elongated down toward the right lower quadrant and is palpable below the right costal margin.

Assessing the rectum

Usually, you'll perform a routine rectal examination only for patients over age 40. You may also perform it for a patient of any age with a history of bowel elimination changes or anal area discomfort and for an adult male of any age with a urinary problem. As a rule, you'll perform the rectal examination at the end of the physical assessment.

Inspection. To begin, ask an ambulatory patient to stand with his toes pointed inward and bend his body

Eliciting abdominal pain

Rebound tenderness and the iliopsoas and obturator signs can indicate such conditions as appendicitis or peritonitis. You can elicit these signs of abdominal pain.

Rebound tenderness
Position the patient supine with his knees flexed to relax the abdominal muscles. Place your hands gently on the right lower quadrant at McBurney's point—located about midway between the umbilicus and the anterior superior iliac spine.

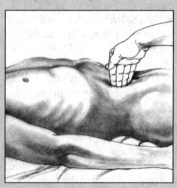

Slowly and deeply dip your fingers into the area, then release the pressure in a quick, smooth motion. Pain on release—rebound tenderness—is a positive sign. The pain may radiate to the umbilicus. *Caution:* Don't repeat this maneuver, to minimize the risk of rupturing an inflamed appendix.

Iliopsoas sign
Position the patient supine with his legs straight. Instruct him to raise his right leg upward as you exert slight pressure with your hand.

Repeat the maneuver with the left leg. When testing either leg, increased abdominal pain is a positive result, indicating irritation of the psoas muscle.

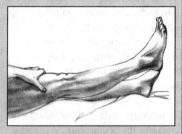

Obturator sign
Position the patient supine with his right leg flexed 90 degrees at the hip and knee. Hold the leg just above the knee and at the ankle, then rotate the leg laterally and medially. Pain in the hypogastric region is a positive sign, indicating irritation of the obturator muscle.

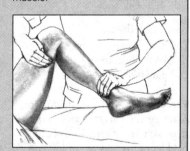

forward over the examination table. If the knee-chest position in bed isn't suitable for an ill, elderly, or pregnant patient, position such a patient in a left lateral Sims' position, with the knees drawn up and the buttocks near the edge of the bed or examination table.

Spread the patient's buttocks to expose the anus and surrounding area. Inspect for breaks in the skin, fissures, discharge, inflammation, lesions, scars, rectal prolapse, skin tags, and external hemorrhoids. Ask the patient to strain as though defecating to make internal hemorrhoids, polyps, rectal prolapse, and fissures visible.

Palpation. Next, palpate the external rectum. Put on a glove and apply lubricant to your index finger. As the patient strains again, palpate for any anal outpouchings or bulges, nodules, or tenderness. Then, palpate the internal rectum. Before beginning, explain to the patient what you'll be doing. Have the patient breathe through the mouth and relax. When the anal sphincter is relaxed, gently insert your finger approximately $2^1/2''$ to $4''$ (6.5 to 10 cm), angling it toward the umbilicus. (**Note:** Don't attempt to force entry through a constricted anal sphincter. Once you've inserted your finger, rotate it systematically to palpate all aspects of the rectal wall for nodules, tenderness, irregularities, and fecal impaction. The rectal wall should feel smooth and soft. In a female patient, try to feel the posterior side of the uterus through the anterior rectal wall. In a

male patient, assess the prostate gland when palpating the anterior rectal wall; the prostate should feel firm and smooth.

With your finger fully inserted, ask the patient to bear down again; this may cause any lesions higher in the rectum to move down to a palpable level. To assess anal sphincter competence, ask the patient to tighten the anal muscles around your finger. Finally, withdraw your finger and examine it for blood, mucus, or stool. If stool appears, note its color and test a sample for occult blood.

Ongoing assessment

Whenever a patient reports a GI complaint, he'll need reassessment. For example, the pain's nature and location may have changed, indicating more extensive involvement or perhaps a new disorder. Reassure him that ongoing assessment does not necessarily mean he has a significant health problem.

DIAGNOSTIC TESTS

Many tests provide information that will help direct your care of the patient with a GI problem. Even if you don't participate in testing, you'll need to know why the doctor ordered each test, what the results mean, and what responsibilities you'll need to carry out before, during, or after the test. Remember to take the patient's clinical status into account when interpreting results. (See *Diagnostic tests for gastrointestinal disorders*, pages 444 to 454.)

(Text continues on page 454.)

Diagnostic tests for gastrointestinal disorders

Test	Purpose	Nursing considerations
Blood tests		
Alkaline phosphatase (ALP)	To measure enzyme activity in bone, intestine, and liver and biliary systems	• Explain the procedure. • Instruct him to fast for at least 8 hours before the test. • Send sample to the laboratory immediately because ALP activity increases at room temperature. • After the test, observe venipuncture site for bleeding.
Bilirubin	To measure liver congutation and excretion of this pigmentary product of erythrocyte breakdown	• Explain the procedure. • Protect the sample from strong sunlight and ultraviolet light. • After the test, observe venipuncture site for bleeding.
Cholesterol	To measure liver metabolism and synthesis of bile acid precursor	• Explain the procedure. • Advise the patient to abstain from food and drink for 12 hours before the test. • After the test, observe venipuncture site for bleeding.
Serum aspartate aminotransferase (AST) Serum alanine aminotransferase (ALT)	To measure cytoplasmic enzymes that leak into plasma after cell damage	• Explain the procedure. • Withhold hepatotoxic and cholestatic medications as ordered. • For AST, draw specimens for 3 consecutive days at the same time. • For ALT a single sample is required. • After the test, observe venipuncture site for bleeding and resume withheld medications as ordered.
Plasma ammonia	To measure ability of the liver to detoxify ammonia	• Explain the procedure. • Instruct him to fast overnight. • Check the history for drugs that influence plasma ammonia levels. • Notify the laboratory before performing the venipuncture so that preparations can begin. Once collected, immediately send the sample, packed in ice, to the laboratory. • After the test, observe venipunc-

Diagnostic tests for gastrointestinal disorders *(continued)*

Test	Purpose	Nursing considerations
Blood tests *(continued)*		
Plasma ammonia *(continued)*		ture site for bleeding. • Tell patient to resume diet, if ordered.
Amylase	To measure pancreatic enzyme active in digestion and released with pancreatic damage	• Explain the procedure. • Instruct him to abstain from alcohol before the test. • For accurate results, obtain an early sample prior to diagnostic or therapeutic interventions. • After the test, observe venipuncture site for bleeding.
Lipase	To aid diagnosis of acute pancreatitis	• Explain the procedure. • Instruct the patient to fast overnight before the test. • Withhold cholinergics, codeine, meperidine, and morphine as ordered. If they're continued, note it on the slip. • After the test, he may resume diet and medications as ordered. Observe venipuncture site for bleeding.
Urine tests		
Urinary bilirubin	To measure liver function	• Explain the procedure. • Collect a random urine specimen in container. • If using Dipstrip, dip reagent strip into the specimen and remove immediately. After 20 seconds compare the strip color with the color standards. Record results on chart. • If using Ictotest, place five drops of urine on the asbestos-cellulose test mat. If bilirubin is present, it will be absorbed into the mat. Next, put a reagent tablet on the wet area of the mat and place two drops of water on the tablet. If bilirubin is present, a

(continued)

Diagnostic tests for gastrointestinal disorders *(continued)*

Test	Purpose	Nursing considerations
Urine tests *(continued)*		
Urinary bilirubin *(continued)*		blue to purple color will develop on the mat. Pink or red indicates a negative test. Record results on chart.
Urine urobilinogen	To aid in diagnosis of blockage of common bile duct and hepatic and hematologic disorders	• Explain the procedure. • Tell the patient to avoid bananas for 48 hours before the test. • Teach the patient how to collect the 2-hour urine sample. • Send sample to laboratory immediately.
Fecal contents		
Stool culture	To identify pathogenic organisms causing GI disease	• Explain that the procedure requires collection of a stool specimen on 3 consecutive days. • Collect specimen directly into container or transfer the specimen to container from a clean, dry bedpan. • Place specimen container in a leakproof bag before sending it to the laboratory.
Fecal occult blood	To detect GI bleeding and aid in early diagnosis of colorectal cancer	• Explain the procedure and that it requires three stool specimens or a random specimen. • Instruct him to maintain a high-fiber diet and to refrain from eating red meats, poultry, fish, turnips and horseradish for 48 to 72 hours before the test and throughout the collection period. • Withhold iron preparations, ascorbic acid, and anti-inflammatory agents for 48 to 72 hours before the specimens are collected.
Esophageal, gastric, and peritoneal contents		
Esophageal acidity test	To assess lower esophageal sphincter competence	• Explain the procedure. • Instruct him to fast and to avoid smoking after midnight before the test.

Diagnostic tests for gastrointestinal disorders *(continued)*

Test	Purpose	Nursing considerations
Esophageal, gastric, and peritoneal contents *(continued)*		
Esophageal acidity test *(continued)*		• Inform him that a tube will be passed through his mouth into his stomach and that he may experience coughing or gagging. • Monitor patient's vital signs before and during the test. • Withhold antacids, anticholinergics, cholinergics, corticosteroids, cimetidine, and reserpine for 24 hours before the test, as ordered. If they must be continued, note this on laboratory slip. • Clamp the catheter before removing it to prevent aspiration. • After the test, he may resume medications and diet as ordered.
Acid perfusion test	To distinguish chest pain caused by esophagitis from that caused by cardiac disorders	• Explain the procedure. • Instruct the patient that before the test he should not take antacids for 24 hours, eat for 12 hours, or drink fluids or smoke for 8 hours. • Inform him that the test requires passage of a tube through his nose into his esophagus and that he may experience discomfort, coughing, or gagging. • Monitor vital signs before and during the procedure and observe for cyanosis, coughing and arrhythmias. • After the test, if patient continues to experience burning, administer antacids as ordered. • He may resume diet and medications as ordered.
Basal gastric secretion test	To determine gastric output in the fasting state	• Explain the procedure. • Instruct the patient to restrict food for 12 hours and fluid and smoking for 8 hours before the test. • Withhold antacids, anticholinergics, cholinergics, alcohol, H_2 blockers, reserpine, adrenergic blockers, and *(continued)*

Diagnostic tests for gastrointestinal disorders *(continued)*

Test	Purpose	Nursing considerations
Esophageal, gastric, and peritoneal contents *(continued)*		
Basal gastric secretion test *(continued)*		adrenocorticosteroids for 24 hours before the test as ordered. If the medications must be continued, note on laboratory slip. • During insertion, be sure the nasogastric tube enters the esophagus and not the trachea; remove it immediately if the patient develops cyanosis or paroxysmal coughing. • Monitor vital signs and observe for arrhythmias. • After the test, if patient complains of sore throat, provide lozenges. He may resume diet and medications as ordered.
Gastric acid stimulation test	To aid diagnosis of duodenal ulcer, Zollinger-Ellison syndrome, pernicious anemia, and gastric carcinoma	• Explain the procedure. • Instruct the patient to refrain from eating, drinking, and smoking from midnight before the test. • Check the patient's history for hypersensitivity to pentagastrin. • As ordered, withhold antacids, anticholinergics, adrenergic blockers, H_2 blockers, and reserpine. If these drugs must be continued, note on laboratory slip. • Monitor vital signs before and during the test. • After the removal of the nasogastric tube, watch for nausea, vomiting, abdominal distention, and pain. • As ordered, he may resume his usual diet and medications.
Peritoneal fluid analysis	To help determine the cause of ascites and detect abdominal trauma	• Explain the procedure and that the patient will receive a local anesthetic. • Have him void before the test. • Monitor vital signs before and during the test. • Observe for dizziness, pallor, perspiration, increased anxiety, and increasing pain and tenderness.

Diagnostic tests for gastrointestinal disorders (continued)

Test	Purpose	Nursing considerations
Esophageal, gastric, and peritoneal contents (continued)		
Peritoneal fluid analysis (continued)		• After the test, apply a gauze dressing to puncture site. Check site frequently, and reinforce as needed. • Monitor vital signs as ordered and watch for hemorrhage and shock. • Monitor urine output for 24 hours and watch for hematuria.
Biopsy		
Percutaneous liver biopsy	To diagnose hepatic parenchymal disease, malignancies, and granulomatous infections	• Explain the procedure to the patient. • Instruct him to restrict food and fluid for at least 4 hours before the test. • Tell him he'll receive medication to help him relax and an anesthetic. • Inform him he will be asked to lie still and hold his breath as the doctor inserts the biopsy needle into the liver. • Monitor vital signs during and after the test. • After the test, he must remain in bed on his right side for 24 hours. • Watch for bleeding and symptoms of peritonitis, such as tenderness and rigidity at the biopsy site. • Watch for signs and symptoms of pneumothorax such as elevated respiratory rate, depressed breath sounds, and dyspnea. • Check dressing site frequently. Apply pressure as needed. • Monitor urine output for at least 24 hours and watch for hematuria.
Endoscopy		
Upper GI endoscopy (esophagogastroduodenoscopy)	To idenitfy abnormalities of the esophagus, stomach, and small intestine	• Explain the procedure to the patient and that he'll be awake. • Tell him to restrict food and fluid for at least 6 hours before the test. • Assure him he'll have no difficulty breathing once the tube is inserted.

(continued)

Diagnostic tests for gastrointestinal disorders *(continued)*

Test	Purpose	Nursing considerations
Endoscopy *(continued)*		
Upper GI endoscopy *(continued)*		• After the test, monitor his vital signs as ordered. • Withhold fluids until the gag reflex returns. • After the I.V. is discontinued, observe site for bleeding.
Lower GI endoscopy (colonoscopy)	To aid diagnosis of inflammatory and ulcerative bowel disease, pinpoint lower GI bleeding, and detect lower GI abnormalities	• Explain the procedure. • Inform the patient that he must maintain a clear liquid diet for up to 48 hours before the test and fast the morning of the test. • Tell him he will receive a laxative the afternoon before the test. • Explain that he'll be awake during the test and that he'll have an I.V. inserted and his vital signs monitored. • Inform him that he may feel the urge to defecate during the test. Tell him to take deep breaths. • After the test, monitor vital signs as ordered and venipuncture site. • Instruct him to report any blood in his stool.
Contrast radiography		
Barium swallow test	To detect hiatal hernia, esophageal disorders, ulcers, tumors, and strictures	• Explain the procedure and that the patient will be asked to swallow barium before and during the procedure. • Instruct him to fast after midnight before the test. • Withhold antacids as ordered. • Have him wear a hospital gown and remove metal objects and dentures. • After the test he may resume his usual diet as ordered. • Give a cathartic, as ordered. • Inform patient that stools will be chalky and light colored for 24 to 72 hours. Tell him to notify the doctor if he hasn't expelled the barium in 2 to 3 days.

Diagnostic tests for gastrointestinal disorders *(continued)*

Test	Purpose	Nursing considerations
Contrast radiography *(continued)*		
Upper GI and small bowel series	To detect hiatal hernia, diverticula, and varices; to aid diagnosis of stricture, ulcers, tumors, and malabsorption syndrome; to detect motility disorders	• Explain the procedure to the patient. Tell him he will swallow barium. • Instruct him to maintain a low-residue diet for 2 to 3 days before the test, then to fast and avoid smoking after midnight before the test. • As ordered, withhold oral medications before the test and anticholinergics and narcotics for 24 hours. • Have him wear a hospital gown and remove metal objects and dentures. • After the test, be sure additional radiographs haven't been ordered before allowing the patient food, fluid, or oral medications. • Administer a cathartic or enema, as ordered. Tell him that his stool will be light colored for 24 to 72 hours. • Tell him to notify the doctor if he doesn't pass barium within 2 to 3 days.
Barium enema	To evaluate suspected lower intestinal disorders	• Explain the procedure. • Instruct the patient to restrict dairy products and follow liquid diet for 24 hours before the test. Encourage fluids. • Administer bowel preparations supplied by the X-ray department and enemas, as ordered. • Withhold breakfast before the procedure. • Inform the patient that he may experience cramping pains or the urge to defecate as the barium or air is introduced into the intestines. Tell him to deep-breathe slowly through his mouth. Tell him to keep his anal sphincter tightly contracted around the rectal tube. • After the test, he should resume diet and drink fluids. • Administer a cathartic or enema as ordered. Tell him his stool will be light colored for 24 to 72 hours. *(continued)*

Diagnostic tests for gastrointestinal disorders *(continued)*

Test	Purpose	Nursing considerations
Contrast radiography *(continued)*		
Cholangiography (percutaneous and postoperative)	To determine the cause of upper abdominal pain; to detect calculi, strictures, neoplasms, and fistula in the biliary ducts	• Explain the procedure and check history for hypersensitivity to iodine, seafood, or contrast medium. *Percutaneous:* • Instruct the patient to fast for 8 hours before the test. • Warn him that injection of the local anesthetic may sting and produce transient pain when it punctures the liver capsule. • Advise him that injection of the contrast medium may produce a sensation of pressure, epigastric fullness, or right upper back pain. • If ordered, administer an antibiotic before the test. • After the test, monitor vital signs until stable. • Enforce bed rest for at least 6 hours after the test. • Check the injection site for bleeding, swelling, and tenderness. Watch for signs of peritonitis. Notify doctor immediately if such complications develop. • Clamp the T tube the day before the test, if ordered. • Withhold the meal just before the test and administer an enema 1 hour before the test, if ordered. • Warn him of adverse reactions to contrast medium. • After the test, if T tube was removed, observe dressing. • If the T tube is left in place, attach it to the drainage system, as ordered.
Endoscopic retrograde cholangiopancreatography	To help determine the cause of jaundice; evaluate tumors and inflammation of the pancreas, gallbladder, or liver; to locate	• Explain all procedures. • Instruct the patient to fast after midnight before the test. • Assure him that he will receive a sedative, but that he will remain conscious.

Diagnostic tests for gastrointestinal disorders *(continued)*

Test	Purpose	Nursing considerations
Contrast radiography *(continued)*		
Endoscopic retrograde cholangiopancreatography *(continued)*	obstruction in the pancreatic duct and hepatobiliary tree	• Have him void before the procedure and remove all metal objects. • Monitor vital signs during the procedure. • Tell him he'll receive an I.V. anticholinergic or glucagon and a contrast medium. Describe possible adverse reactions. • Watch for signs of respiratory depression. • After the test, observe for signs of cholangitis and pancreatitis. • Monitor vital signs as ordered. • Withhold food and fluid until the gag reflex returns. • Check for signs of urine retention. Notify doctor if patient hasn't voided within 8 hours.
Scanning tests		
Computed tomography scan	To help identify abscesses, cysts, hematomas, tumors and pseudocysts; to diagnose and evaluate pancreatitis	• Explain the procedure and that it will take 1½ hours. • Instruct the patient to restrict food and fluid after midnight before the test. • Tell him he must lie still, relax, and breathe normally. • If a contrast medium is being used, check for hypersensitivity. Warn him of possible adverse reactions. • After the test, have him resume his usual diet.
Liver-spleen scan	To detect tumors, cysts, and abscesses	• Explain the procedure. Tell the patient he will receive an injection of a radioactive substance. Assure him that the amount of radiation is minimal. Warn him of possible adverse reactions. • Instruct him to lie still and breathe normally. He may be asked to hold his breath briefly.

(continued)

Diagnostic tests for gastrointestinal disorders *(continued)*

Test	Purpose	Nursing considerations
Scanning tests *(continued)*		
Ultrasonography	To help differentiate between obstructive and nonobstructive jaundice and diagnose cholelithiasis or cholecystitis; to aid diagnosis of pancreatitis, pseudocysts, pancreatic cancer, and splenomegaly	• Explain the procedure. • Instruct him to drink three to four glasses of water beforehand and to avoid urinating until after the test. • For gallbladder evaluation, tell the patient not to eat solid food for 12 hours before the test. • For pancreas, liver, or spleen evaluation, have the patient fast for 8 hours. • After the test, the patient may resume his usual diet.

NURSING DIAGNOSES

When caring for patients with GI disorders, you'll find that several nursing diagnoses are commonly used. These diagnoses appear below, along with appropriate nursing interventions and rationales. (Rationales appear in italic type.)

Constipation

Related to inadequate intake of fluid and bulk, constipation may pertain to all patients undergoing periods of restricted food or fluid intake.

Expected outcomes

• Patient's fluid and fiber intake is documented.
• Patient uses bedside commode or walks to toilet facilities.
• Patient participates in development of a bowel program.
• Patient reports the urge to defecate, as appropriate.
• Patient reports easy and complete evacuation of stool.
• Patient describes measures that will help eliminate constipation.

Nursing interventions and rationales

• Record intake and output accurately *to ensure correct fluid replacement therapy.*
• Note color and consistency of stool and frequency of bowel movements *to form the basis of an effective plan of care.*
• Promote ample fluid intake *to increase intestinal fluid content.*
• Encourage patient to consume more fiber in diet *to promote comfortable elimination.*
• Discourage routine use of laxatives and enemas *to avoid eventual failure of defecation stimulus. (Bulk-adding laxatives are usually permitted.)*
• Teach patient to gently massage along the transverse and descending

colon *to stimulate the bowel's spastic reflex and aid stool passage.*
• Encourage patient to walk and exercise as much as possible *to stimulate intestinal activity.*

Diarrhea

Related to malabsorption, inflammation, or irritation of the bowel, diarrhea, may be associated with irritable bowel syndrome, colitis, and Crohn's disease.

Expected outcomes
• Patient regains and retains fluid and electrolyte balance.
• Diarrhea episodes decline or disappear.
• Patient's skin remains clean and free from irritation or ulcerations.
• Patient discusses the relationship of stress and anxiety to episodes of diarrhea.
• Patient demonstrates the ability to use at least one stress-reducing technique.

Nursing interventions and rationales
• Assess patient's level of dehydration and electrolyte imbalance. *Fluid loss secondary to diarrhea can be life-threatening.*
• Monitor patient's weight daily *to detect fluid loss or retention.*
• Note color and consistency of stools and frequency of bowel movements *to monitor treatment.*
• Test stool for occult blood, and obtain stool for culture *to help evaluate factors contributing to diarrhea.*
• Assess for fecal impaction. *Liquid stool may seep around an impaction.*

For acute diarrhea, provide dietary regimen as follows:
• Give clear fluids, including carbonated glucose and electrolyte-containing beverages or commercial rehydration preparations, orally. *Clear fluids provide rapidly absorbed calories and electrolytes.* After diarrhea has stopped for 24 to 48 hours, progress to a full fluid diet, then to a regular diet.
• Avoid milk, caffeine, and high-fiber foods for 1 week *to avoid irritating the intestinal mucosa.*
• In chronic diarrhea, encourage the patient to avoid foods and activities that may cause diarrhea. *Self-regulation of contributing factors helps manage chronic diarrhea.*

Altered tissue perfusion

Related to reduced blood flow, altered tissue perfusion may be associated with cirrhosis, hepatic failure, and other conditions.

Expected outcomes
• Patient's intake and output remain within normal limits.
• Laboratory values remain normal.
• Abdominal pain subsides.
• Normal bowel function returns.
• Patient understands role of regular exercise in maintaining bowel habits.
• Patient understands need to check stools for occult blood.

Nursing interventions and rationales
• Assess for bowel sounds, increasing abdominal girth, pain, nausea and vomiting, and electrolyte imbalance. *Acute changes may indicate surgical emergency.*

For chronic circulatory problems:
• Provide small, frequent feedings of bland foods *to promote digestion.*
• Encourage rest after feedings *to improve digestion.*

Bowel incontinence

Related to neuromuscular involvement, the diagnosis of bowel incontinence may be used in patients who've had a hemorrhoidectomy or other procedures.

Expected outcomes
• Patient or caregiver demonstrates increasing skill in performing bowel care routine independently.
• Patient or caregiver states understanding of the need to regulate food or fluids that cause constipation or diarrhea.
• Patient establishes and maintains a regular pattern of bowel care.

Nursing interventions and rationales
• Establish schedule for defecation; $1/2$ hour after meal is desirable for active peristalsis. *Regular pattern encourages routine physiologic function.*
• Instruct patient to use bathroom if possible *to allay anxiety.*
• If bedpan use is necessary, assist patient to most normal position possible for defecation *to increase comfort and reduce anxiety.*
• Instruct patient to bear down or help patient lean trunk forward *to increase intra-abdominal pressure.*
• Use gentle manual stimulation with lubricated finger in anal sphincter or glycerine suppository if

necessary. *This encourages regular physiologic function, stimulates peristalsis, and minimizes infection.*
• Provide meticulous skin care *to prevent infection.*
• Refrain from commenting about "accidents" *to avoid embarrassing patient.*

DISORDERS

This section discusses the most common disorders of the oropharyngeal area, stomach, intestines, anorectal area, and accessory organs (liver, gallbladder, pancreas, and bile ducts). For each disorder, you'll find information on causes, assessment findings, diagnostic tests, treatment, nursing interventions, patient education, and evaluation criteria.

Oral and esophageal disorders

The upper GI tract is susceptible to many serious disorders. Inflammation may cause ulcers and infections, which may lead to perforation and hemorrhage. Structural disorders such as hiatal hernia may interfere with esophageal valvular function and cause gastric reflux and possible strangulation of a portion of the stomach.

Stomatitis and other oral infections
An inflammatory disorder, stomatitis affects the oral mucosa and may also spread to the buccal mucosa, lips, and palate. The two main types are *acute herpetic stomatitis* and *aphthous stomatitis.* The acute form is usually

self-limiting; however, in neonates, it may be generalized and potentially fatal. Aphthous stomatitis usually heals spontaneously in 10 to 14 days. Other oral infections include gingivitis, periodontitis, Vincent's angina, and glossitis. (See *Understanding oral infections,* pages 458 and 459.)

Causes. Acute herpetic stomatitis may result from herpes simplex virus. Predisposing factors for aphthous stomatitis include stress, fatigue, anxiety, fever, trauma, immunosuppression, or overexposure to the sun.

Assessment findings. A patient with acute herpetic stomatitis may manifest these signs and symptoms: mouth pain, malaise, lethargy, anorexia, irritability, fever, swollen gums that bleed easily, tender mucous membranes, papulovesicular ulcers in mouth or throat, and possibly submaxillary lymphadenitis.

A patient with aphthous stomatitis may have burning, tingling, or slight swelling of the mucous membranes and single or multiple shallow ulcers (whitish centers and red borders) that heal at one site but then appear at another.

Diagnostic tests. A smear of ulcer exudate identifies the causative organism in Vincent's angina. Herpes culture also may be done.

Treatment. For acute herpetic stomatitis, treatment is conservative. For local symptoms, management includes warm-water mouth rinses and a topical anesthetic to relieve mouth ulcer pain. Supplementary treatment includes a bland or liquid diet and, in severe cases, I.V. fluids and bed rest.

For aphthous stomatitis, a topical anesthetic is the primary treatment.

Nursing interventions. Nursing care for these disorders primarily involves patient education.

Patient education. In acute herpetic stomatitis, teach the patient to use good oral hygiene to prevent the disorder's spread. In aphthous stomatitis, teach the patient to avoid precipitating factors. Instruct all patients with stomatitis to eat a bland, liquid diet high in vitamins and protein.

Evaluation. The patient should demonstrate good oral hygiene, good hydration and tolerance of diet, and an increased comfort level. He should also avoid transmitting herpes and should modify other contributing factors.

Hiatal hernia

Hiatal hernia is a structural defect in which a weakened diaphragm allows a portion of the stomach to pass through the esophageal diaphragmatic opening (hiatus) into the chest.

Three types of hiatal hernia can occur: sliding hernia (most common), paraesophageal (rolling) hernia, or mixed hernia, which includes features of the others. In a *sliding hernia,* both the stomach and the gastroesophageal junction slip up

Understanding oral infections

Disease and causes	Signs and symptoms	Treatment
Candidiasis (thrush) • *Candida albicans* • Predisposing factors: denture use, diabetes mellitus, and immuno-suppressant therapy	• Cream-colored or bluish white pseudomembranous patches on tongue, mouth, or pharynx • Pain, fever, and lymphadenopathy	• Peroxide and saline mouth rinses • Clotrimazole tablets dissolved in mouth five times/day • Nystatin troches (100,000 U) dissolved in mouth four times/day • Varied local or systemic antifungal therapies
Gingivitis (inflammation of the gingiva) • Early sign of hypovitaminosis, diabetes, or blood dyscrasias • Occasionally related to use of oral contraceptives	• Inflammation with painless swelling, redness, change of normal contours, bleeding, and periodontal pocket (gum detachment from teeth)	• Removal of irritating factors (calculus, faulty dentures) • Good oral hygiene, regular dental check-ups, and vigorous chewing • Oral or topical corticosteroids
Glossitis (inflammation of the tongue) • Streptococcal infection • Irritation or injury, jagged teeth, ill-fitting dentures, biting during convulsions, alcohol, spicy foods, smoking, and sensitivity to toothpaste or mouthwash • Vitamin B deficiency; anemia • Skin conditions: lichen planus, erythema multiforme, pemphigus vulgaris	• Reddened, ulcerated, or swollen tongue (may obstruct airway) • Painful chewing and swallowing • Speech difficulty • Painful tongue without inflammation	• Treatment of underlying cause • Topical anesthetic mouthwash or systemic analgesics (aspirin or acetaminophen) for painful lesions • Good oral hygiene, regular dental check-ups, and vigorous chewing • Avoidance of hot, cold, or spicy foods, and alcohol
Periodontitis (progression of gingivitis; inflammation of the oral mucosa)	• Acute onset of bright red gum inflammation, painless swelling of	• Scaling, root planing, and curettage for infection control

Understanding oral infections *(continued)*

Disease and causes	Signs and symptoms	Treatment
Periodontitis *(continued)* • Early sign of hypovitaminosis, diabetes, or blood dyscrasias • Occasionally related to use of oral contraceptives • Dental factors: calculus, poor oral hygiene, malocclusion; major cause of tooth loss after middle age	interdental papillae, easy bleeding • Loosening of teeth, typically without inflammatory symptoms, progressing to loss of teeth and alveolar bone • Acute systemic infection (fever, chills)	• Periodontal surgery to prevent recurrence • Good oral hygiene, regular dental check-ups, and vigorous chewing
Vincent's angina (trench mouth, necrotizing ulcerative gingivitis) • Fusiform bacillus or spirochete infection • Predisposing factors: stress, poor oral hygiene, insufficient rest, nutritional deficiency, smoking, and immunosuppressant therapy	• Sudden onset: painful, superficial, bleeding gingival ulcers (rarely, on buccal mucosa) covered with a gray-white membrane • Ulcers becoming punched out lesions after slight pressure or irritation • Malaise, mild fever, excessive salivation, bad breath, pain on swallowing or talking, and enlarged submaxillary lymph nodes	• Removal of devitalized tissue with ultrasonic cavitron • Antibiotics (penicillin or erythromycin P.O.) for infection • Analgesics, as needed • Hourly mouth rinses (with equal amounts of hydrogen peroxide and warm water) • Soft, nonirritating diet; rest; no smoking • With treatment, improvement common within 24 hours

into the chest so that the gastroesophageal junction is above the diaphragmatic hiatus. In a *paraesophageal hernia*, a part of the greater curvature of the stomach rolls through the diaphragmatic defect. (See *Understanding types of hiatal hernia,* page 460.)

Causes. This defect may be caused by muscle weakening associated with aging, esophageal carcinoma,

kyphoscoliosis, trauma, certain surgical procedures, and congenital diaphragmatic malformations.

Assessment findings. In a sliding hiatal hernia, symptoms occur in the presence of an incompetent gastroesophageal sphincter. Ask your patient about:
• pyrosis (heartburn). This occurs from 1 to 4 hours after eating and is aggravated by increased intra-ab-

Understanding types of hiatal hernia

The illustrations below show a normal stomach along with two types of hiatal hernia: sliding and paraesophageal.

Normal stomach

Diaphragm — Esophagus

Cardia —

— Duodenum

Sliding hernia

Peritoneum — — Esophagus

Pleura — — Hernia

Diaphragm —

Sac — — Cardia

— Duodenum

Paraesophageal hernia

Esophagus — Peritoneum

Pleura — — Hernia

Diaphragm —

— Duodenum

dominal pressure. It may be accompanied by regurgitation.
• retrosternal or substernal chest pain. This usually occurs after meals or at bedtime and is aggravated by reclining, belching, and increased intra-abdominal pressure.

In a paraesophageal hiatal hernia, the patient is typically asymptomatic. He may have a feeling of fullness in the chest or pain resembling angina pectoris.

Diagnostic tests. In chest X-ray, a large hernia may appear like an air shadow behind the heart. Infiltrates are seen in lower lobes if the patient has aspirated gastric contents.

In a barium study, the hernia may appear like an outpouching containing barium at the lower end of the esophagus. Diaphragmatic abnormalities are visible.

Endoscopy and biopsy differentiate among hiatal hernia, varices, and other small gastroesophageal lesions; identify the mucosal junction and the edge of the diaphragm indenting the esophagus; and can rule out malignancy.

Esophageal motility studies assess for esophageal motor abnormalities before surgical repair of the hernia. Measurement of pH assesses for reflux of gastric contents.

An acid perfusion test indicates that heartburn results from esophageal reflux when perfusion of hydrochloric acid through the nasogastric (NG) tube provokes this symptom.

Treatment. Therapy attempts to reduce reflux by changing the quantity or quality of gastric contents, by strengthening the gastroesophageal sphincter muscle pharmacologically, or by decreasing the amount of reflux through gravity.

Antacids are probably the best treatment for intermittent reflux. Intensive antacid therapy may call for hourly administration; however, the choice of antacid should take into consideration the patient's bowel function. Histamine$_2$-receptor antagonists (H$_2$ blockers) such as cimetidine are also used.

Drug therapy to strengthen gastroesophageal sphincter tone may include a cholinergic agent such as bethanechol. Metoclopramide has also been used to stimulate smooth muscle contraction, increase sphincter tone, and decrease reflux after eating.

Failure to control symptoms by medical means or onset of complications requires surgical repair. Also, a paraesophageal hiatal hernia,

even if asymptomatic, needs surgical treatment because of the high risk of strangulation. Techniques vary, but most create an artificial closing mechanism at the gastroesophageal junction. The surgeon may use an abdominal or a thoracic approach.

Laparoscopic surgery is an option for selected patients. The laparoscopic approach dramatically reduces recovery time.

Nursing interventions. If surgery is scheduled, reinforce the surgeon's explanation and any preoperative and postoperative considerations. Tell the patient that he probably won't be allowed to eat or drink and will have an NG tube in place, with low suction, for 2 to 3 days postoperatively.

While the NG tube is in place, provide meticulous mouth and nose care. Give ice chips to moisten oral mucous membranes.

If the surgeon uses a thoracic approach, the patient will have chest tubes in place. Carefully observe chest tube drainage and respiratory status, and perform chest physiotherapy.

Patient education. Before discharge, tell the patient what foods he can eat and recommend small, frequent meals. Warn against activities that cause increased intra-abdominal pressure, and advise a slow return to normal functions. Tell him he should be able to resume regular activity in 6 to 8 weeks.

For patients treated medically, advise losing weight, modifying the diet (for example, by eating small, frequent, bland meals; sitting up for 2 hours after eating; and avoiding smoking, coffee, alcohol, and heavy spices), elevating the head of the bed on 6″ blocks at home, and trying to avoid coughing or straining.

Evaluation. The patient should maintain optimal hydration and nutritional levels; make appropriate changes in diet, positioning, and activity; and report increased comfort.

Esophageal diverticula

In esophageal diverticula, hollow outpouchings develop in one or more layers of the esophageal wall. They occur in three main areas: just above the upper esophageal sphincter, near the midpoint of the esophagus, and just above the lower esophageal sphincter.

Esophageal diverticula usually occur in middle to late adulthood, Zenker's diverticula, the most common type, usually occur in men over age 60. Epiphrenic diverticula usually occur in middle-aged men.

Causes. Esophageal diverticula result from primary muscle abnormalities that may be congenital; they also may arise from inflammatory processes.

Assessment findings. The patient may be asymptomatic in mid- or lower-esophageal diverticulum with a motor disturbance, such as achalasia or spasm, or may experience dysphagia and heartburn.

Zenker's diverticulum may cause the following signs and symptoms:
• throat irritation initially (progressing to dysphagia and near-complete obstruction)
• regurgitation (may occur during sleep, leading to food aspiration and pulmonary infection)
• noise when liquids are swallowed
• chronic cough
• hoarseness
• bad taste in the mouth or foul breath
• bleeding (rare).

(For information about diagnostic tests, treatment, nursing interventions, patient education, and evaluation, see "Hiatal hernia," page 457.)

Gastroesophageal reflux

Gastroesophageal reflux is the backflow of gastric or duodenal contents, or both, into the esophagus and past the lower esophageal sphincter (LES), without associated belching or vomiting. Reflux may or may not cause symptoms or abnormal changes. The uncomfortable burning feeling associated with a transient relaxation of the LES is known commonly as "heartburn" or "acid indigestion." Persistent reflux may cause reflux esophagitis.

Causes. Reflux occurs when LES pressure is deficient or when pressure within the stomach exceeds LES pressure. Factors that lower esophageal sphincter pressure include fat, whole milk, orange juice, tomatoes, antiflatulents (simethicone), chocolate, high-dose ethanol, cigarette smoking, lying on the right or left side, and sitting. Factors that raise esophageal sphincter pressure include protein, nonfat milk, carbohydrates, and low-dose ethanol.

Predisposing factors include:
• pyloric surgery, which allows reflux of bile or pancreatic juice
• long-term NG intubation (more than 4 to 5 days)
• any agent that lowers esophageal sphincter pressure, such as food, alcohol, cigarettes, anticholinergics (atropine, belladonna, propantheline), or other drugs (morphine, diazepam, and meperidine)
• hiatal hernia
• any condition or position that increases intra-abdominal pressure.

Assessment findings. Gastroesophageal reflux doesn't always cause symptoms, and in patients showing clinical effects, physiologic reflux isn't always confirmable. The most common feature of gastroesophageal reflux is heartburn. Exercising vigorously, bending, or lying down may make the heartburn more severe; taking antacids or sitting upright may relieve it. The pain of esophageal spasm resulting from reflux esophagitis tends to be chronic and may mimic angina pectoris, radiating to the neck, jaws, and arms. Other signs and symptoms include odynophagia, which may be followed by a dull substernal ache from severe, long-term reflux; dysphagia from esophageal spasm, stricture, or esophagitis; and bleeding (bright red or dark brown).

Pulmonary symptoms, which result from reflux of gastric contents into the throat and subsequent aspiration, include chronic pulmonary disease or nocturnal wheezing, bronchitis, asthma, morning hoarseness, and cough.

Diagnostic tests. An acid perfusion (Bernstein) test can show that reflux is the cause of symptoms. Endoscopy and biopsy allow confirmation of any abnormal changes in the mucosa.

Treatment. Effective management relieves symptoms by reducing reflux through gravity, strengthening the LES with drug therapy, neutralizing gastric contents, and reducing intra-abdominal pressure. The patient should sleep with the head of the bed elevated and should avoid lying down after meals and late-night snacks. In uncomplicated cases, positional therapy is especially useful in infants and children.

Antacids given 1 hour and 3 hours after meals and at bedtime are effective for intermittent reflux. A nondiarrheal antacid containing aluminum carbonate or aluminum hydroxide (rather than magnesium) may be preferred, depending on the patient's bowel status. Bethanechol, a drug to increase esophageal sphincter pressure, stimulates smooth-muscle contraction and decreases esophageal acidity after meals (proven with pH probe). Metoclopramide and cisapride, which accelerates gastric emptying, and H_2 blockers have been used with beneficial results.

If possible, NG intubation should not be continued for more than 4 to 5 days because the tube interferes with sphincter integrity and itself allows reflux, especially when the patient lies flat.

Surgery may be necessary to control pulmonary aspiration, hemorrhage, obstruction, severe pain, perforation, incompetent LES, or associated hiatal hernia. Surgical procedures create an artificial closure at the gastroesophageal junction. Vagotomy or pyloroplasty may be combined with an antireflux regimen to modify gastric contents.

Nursing interventions. After surgery using a thoracic approach, carefully watch and record chest tube drainage and respiratory status. If needed, give chest physiotherapy and oxygen. Position the patient with an NG tube in semi-Fowler's position to help prevent reflux.

Patient education. Teach the patient what causes reflux, how to avoid reflux with an antireflux regimen (medication, diet, and positional therapy), and what symptoms to watch for and report.

Instruct the patient to avoid any circumstance that increases intra-abdominal pressure (such as bending, coughing, vigorous exercise, tight clothing, constipation, and obesity) and any substance that reduces sphincter control (such as cigarettes, alcohol, fatty foods, and certain drugs).

Advise the patient to sit upright, particularly after meals, and to eat small, frequent meals. Tell him to avoid highly seasoned food, acidic juices, alcoholic drinks, bedtime snacks, and foods high in fat or carbohydrates. He should eat meals at least 2 to 3 hours before lying down. Tell him to take antacids, as ordered (usually 1 hour and 3 hours after meals and at bedtime).

Evaluation. The patient should maintain optimal hydration and nutritional levels; modify his diet, positioning, and activity levels as needed; and report increased comfort.

Gastric, intestinal, and pancreatic disorders

This section covers various inflammations, infections, cancers and obstructions that affect the stomach, intestines, and pancreas.

Gastritis

An inflammatory disorder of the gastric mucosa, gastritis may be acute or chronic. Acute gastritis is the most common stomach disorder. In a person with epigastric discomfort or other GI symptoms (particularly bleeding), a history suggesting exposure to a GI irritant suggests gastritis. Gastritis commonly accompanies pernicious anemia (as chronic atrophic gastritis).

Causes. *Acute gastritis* may be caused by:
• chronic ingestion of irritating foods or an allergic reaction
• alcohol or drugs such as aspirin

• poisons, especially DDT, ammonia, mercury, and carbon tetrachloride
• hepatic disorders such as portal hypertension
• GI disorders such as sprue
• infectious disorders
• Curling's ulcer (after a burn)
• Cushing's ulcer
• GI injury (may be thermal [ingesting a hot fluid] or mechanical [swallowing a foreign object]).

Chronic gastritis may result from recurring ingestion of an irritating substance or from pernicious anemia. *Corrosive gastritis* may be caused by ingestion of strong acids or alkalies. *Acute phlegmonous gastritis* may be caused by a rare bacterial infection of the stomach wall.

Assessment findings. GI bleeding is the most common sign. However, the patient may experience only mild epigastric discomfort (postprandial distress).

Diagnostic tests. Gastroscopy (commonly with biopsy) confirms the diagnosis when done before lesions heal (within 24 hours). Gastroscopy is contraindicated after ingestion of a corrosive agent. X-rays rule out other diseases.

Treatment. Symptoms are usually relieved by eliminating the gastric irritant or other cause. The treatment for corrosive gastritis is neutralization with the appropriate antidote (emetics are contraindicated). Treatment for gastritis caused by other poisons includes emetics, anticholinergics such as methanthe-line, H_2 blockers such as cimetidine, and antacids to relieve GI distress.

When gastritis causes massive bleeding, treatment includes blood replacement; iced saline lavage, possibly with norepinephrine; angiography with vasopressin infused in normal saline solution; and surgery. Treatment for bacterial gastritis includes antibiotics, bland diet, and an antiemetic. For acute phlegmonous gastritis, antibiotic therapy is followed by surgical repair.

Nursing interventions. Give an antiemetic if the patient is vomiting, and, as ordered, replace I.V. fluids. Monitor fluid intake and output, and watch electrolyte balance.

Watch for signs and symptoms of GI bleeding (hematemesis, melena, drop in hematocrit, or bloody NG drainage) and hemorrhagic shock (hypotension, tachycardia, or restlessness). In corrosive gastritis, watch for nausea, vomiting, diarrhea, abdominal pain, or fever.

Patient education. Urge the patient to seek immediate attention for recurring signs and symptoms (hematemesis, nausea, vomiting, or unrelieved gastric distress). Advise the patient to prevent gastric irritation by taking medications with milk, food, or antacids; by taking antacids between meals and at bedtime; by avoiding aspirin-containing compounds and ibuprofen; and by avoiding spicy foods, hot fluids, alcohol, caffeine, and tobacco.

Evaluation. The patient should maintain optimal nutrition, follow his diet and medication regimens, and report increased comfort.

Gastroenteritis

Gastroenteritis is an inflammatory condition of the stomach and intestines that accompanies numerous GI disorders. It occurs in persons of all ages and is a major cause of morbidity and mortality in underdeveloped nations. In the United States, gastroenteritis ranks fifth as the cause of death among young children.

Causes. Gastroenteritis has many possible causes, such as:
• bacteria (responsible for acute food poisoning)—*Staphylococcus aureus, Salmonella, Shigella, Clostridium botulinum, Clostridium perfringens, Escherichia coli*
• amoebae, especially *Entamoeba histolytica*
• parasites—*Ascaris, Enterobius,* and *Trichinella spiralis*
• viruses—adenoviruses, echoviruses, or coxsackieviruses
• toxins—ingestion of plants or toadstools
• drug reactions—antibiotics
• enzyme deficiencies
• food allergens.

Assessment findings. Clinical manifestations vary. Assess your patient for diarrhea, abdominal discomfort (ranging from cramping to pain), nausea, vomiting, possible fever, malaise, and borborygmi.

Diagnostic tests. Stool culture (by direct swab) or blood culture identifies causative bacteria or parasites.

Treatment. Treatment is usually supportive and consists of bed rest, nutritional support, and increased fluid intake. When gastroenteritis is severe or affects a young child or an elderly or debilitated person, treatment may require hospitalization, specific antimicrobials, I.V. fluid and electrolyte replacement, bismuth-containing compounds such as Pepto-Bismol, and antiemetics (by mouth, I.M., or through rectal suppository), such as prochlorperazine or trimethobenzamide.

Nursing interventions. Give medications, as ordered. Correlate dosages, routes, and times appropriately with the patient's meals and activities. For example, give antiemetics 30 to 60 minutes before meals.

If the patient can eat, replace lost fluids and electrolytes with broth and ginger ale, as tolerated. Warn the patient to avoid milk products, which may provoke recurrence.

Record intake and output carefully. Watch for signs of dehydration, such as dry skin and mucous membranes, fever, and sunken eyes. To ease anal irritation, provide warm sitz baths.

If food poisoning is probable, contact public health authorities. Wash your hands thoroughly after providing care.

Patient education. Teach good hygiene to prevent recurrence. Instruct the patient to cook foods, especially pork, thoroughly and to refrigerate perishable foods, such as milk, mayonnaise, potato salad, and cream-filled pastry. Recommend that he always wash his hands with warm water and soap before handling food, especially after using the bathroom, and that he clean utensils thoroughly.

Evaluation. The patient should maintain an optimal hydration level, regain a regular pattern of bowel movements, maintain skin integrity of perianal area, and take steps to avoid infecting others.

Stomach cancer

Since 1960, stomach tumors have declined by 65% in the United States. Gastric cancer is difficult to detect early because its symptoms mimic other GI problems, such as ulcers, gastritis, and dyspepsia.

Causes. A specific cause of stomach cancer is not known; however, a number of genetic and environmental factors have been implicated. Pickled foods, salted foods, and nitrites have been associated with stomach cancer. Additional risk factors include low socioeconomic status, poor nutritional habits, vitamin A deficiency, family history, pernicious anemia, and benign peptic ulcer disease.

Assessment findings. Gastric cancer is usually locally advanced or metastatic at time of diagnosis. Patient may complain of bloating, a feeling of fullness in the abdomen, early satiety, or discomfort after eating. As the disease progresses he may experience weight loss, nausea, vomiting, abdominal pain, and hemate-

mesis. Assessment should include a thorough nutritional history. On physical examination, an abdominal mass, enlarged lymph nodes, or an enlarged spleen or liver may be palpated.

Diagnostic tests. If signs and symptoms suggest stomach cancer, then additional tests should be ordered. These include a double-contrast upper GI series to examine the mucosal pattern and characteristics of the walls of the stomach; a computed tomography (CT) scan to define tumor size, location, extension, and local metastases; and endoscopic gastroscopy to visualize the tumor and obtain biopsy specimens.

Treatment. Surgery is indicated in many cases to determine the resectability of the tumor. The specific surgical procedure depends on the location and extent of disease.

Gastric cancers are usually sensitive to radiation but difficult to radiate because of the depth and the proximity of the stomach to other organs affected by the radiation (liver, kidney, and spinal cord). However, radiation is administered as adjuvant therapy. Intraoperative radiation therapy has been used effectively in some centers.

Chemotherapy agents may be used in combination. Some of the most commonly used agents include 5-fluorouracil, doxorubicin, platinum analogues, and etoposide.

Nursing interventions. You'll initially focus on postoperative care of the patient undergoing gastric surgery. After the immediate recovery period, focus on maintaining nutritional status and restoring the patient's previous state of health.

Patient education. Preoperatively, you'll teach the patient and the family about the disease process and the effects of surgery on nutritional intake. Instruct the patient on necessary changes in dietary habits to decrease the incidence of dumping syndrome and therapy to reduce diarrhea. Explain that as a result of surgery vitamin B_{12} deficiency will occur but that replacement therapy can prevent pernicious anemia.

Peptic ulcers

Appearing as circumscribed lesions in the gastric mucosal membrane, peptic ulcers can develop in the lower esophagus, stomach, pylorus, duodenum, or jejunum from contact with gastric juice (especially hydrochloric acid and pepsin). About 80% of all peptic ulcers are duodenal ulcers.

Causes. *Helicobactor pylori* has been shown by research to be the primary cause of ulcers. An imbalance between the ability of the mucosal lining to defend itself and the presence of the powerful digestive fluids (hydrochloric acid and pepsin) was recognized as part of the pathophysiologic process. Lifestyle factors that play a role in ulcer development are smoking, caffeine, drugs (nonsteroidal anti-inflammatory drugs [NSAIDs], aspirin), alcohol, and stress.

Assessment findings. Patients with duodenal ulcers may experience attacks about 2 hours after meals, whenever the stomach is empty, or after consuming orange juice, coffee, aspirin, or alcohol. Exacerbations tend to recur several times a year, then fade into remission. Such patients may report heartburn and well-localized midepigastric pain, which is relieved by eating food. They may gain weight from eating.

Diagnostic tests. Upper GI tract X-rays show abnormalities in the mucosa. Gastric secretory studies show hyperchlorhydria. Upper GI endoscopy confirms the diagnosis.

Blood and breath tests should be performed to detect the presence of *H. pylori*. Biopsy rules out cancer and permits tissue testing for *H. pylori*. Stools may test positive for occult blood.

Treatment. Antibiotics to eradicate *H. pylori* include a 2-week triple therapy with metronidazole, tetracycline, and bismuth subsalicylate four times a day.

Nonbacterial ulcer disease may be treated with H_2 blockers—such as cimetidine and ranitidine—or an acid-pump inhibitor such as omeprazole. For short-term treatment and maintenance, mucosal protectors such as sucralfate coat the ulcer and shield it from stomach acid.

The incidence of severe bleeding has been reduced with the use of H_2 blockers. If GI bleeding does occur, gastroscopy to facilitate coagulation of the bleeding site by cautery or laser may be done.

Severe complications, such as hemorrhage or perforation, may require surgery. Surgical procedures include vagotomy, pyloroplasty, and gastrectomy. Laparoscopic procedures may be used more commonly in the future.

Nursing interventions. Give medications, as ordered, and watch for adverse effects such as stomach upset, loose stools and, in women, yeast infections (from antibiotic therapy).

Patient education. Instruct the patient to take antacids 1 to 2 hours after meals. Advise the patient who has a history of cardiac disease or who is on a sodium-restricted diet to take only low-sodium antacids. Warn that antacids may cause changes in bowel habits (diarrhea with magnesium-containing antacids or constipation with aluminum-containing antacids).

Stress the importance of quitting smoking. Advise the patient to avoid the use of aspirin and NSAIDs.

Explain that no evidence supports the notion of the need for a bland diet.

Tell the patient to avoid coffee, stress, and alcoholic beverages during exacerbations. Advise the patient to avoid milk products.

Evaluation. The patient should understand the disease process and comply with the treatment regimen. He should understand the need for follow-up care and know when to seek immediate attention.

Ulcerative colitis

An inflammatory—and in many cases—chronic disease, ulcerative colitis affects the mucosa and submucosa of the colon. It usually begins in the rectum and sigmoid colon and commonly extends upward into the entire colon. It rarely affects the small intestine, except for the terminal ileum. Severity ranges from a mild, localized disorder to a fulminant disease that may cause a perforated colon, progressing to potentially fatal peritonitis and toxemia. The disorder is more prevalent among whites, particularly those who are Jewish.

Causes. Unknown. Risk factors include a family history of the disease; bacterial infection; allergic reaction to food, milk, or other substances that release inflammatory histamine in the bowel; overproduction of enzymes that break down the mucous membranes; and emotional stress. Autoimmune disorders—such as rheumatoid arthritis, hemolytic anemia, erythema nodosum, and uveitis—may heighten the risk.

Assessment findings. Recurrent bloody diarrhea and asymptomatic remissions are the hallmark characteristics of ulcerative colitis. The stool typically contains pus and mucus. Assess for other signs and symptoms, such as spastic rectum and anus, abdominal pain, irritability, weight loss, weakness, anorexia, and nausea and vomiting.

Diagnostic tests. Sigmoidoscopy shows increased mucosal friability, decreased mucosal detail, and thick inflammatory exudate. Colonoscopy and barium enema may be done to determine the extent of the disease. Biopsy helps to confirm the diagnosis.

A stool specimen may be cultured and analyzed for leukocytes, ova, and parasites. The erythrocyte sedimentation rate (ESR) will be increased in relation to the severity of the attack. Other supportive laboratory values include decreased serum levels of potassium, magnesium, hemoglobin, and albumin as well as leukocytosis and increased prothrombin time (PT).

Treatment. The goals of treatment are to control inflammation, replace nutritional losses and blood volume, and prevent complications. For the most part, the patient will manage his own condition. For patients awaiting surgery or showing signs of dehydration and debilitation from excessive diarrhea, total parenteral nutrition (TPN) rests the intestinal tract, decreases stool volume, and restores positive nitrogen balance. Blood transfusions or iron supplements may be needed to correct anemia.

Drug therapy for mild and severe colitis usually includes sulfasalazine, which has anti-inflammatory and antimicrobial properties. Adrenal corticosteroids, such as prednisone, prednisolone, and hydrocortisone are also used. Antispasmodics such as tincture of belladonna and antidiarrheals such as diphenoxylate are used only for patients whose ulcerative colitis is under control but who have frequent, troublesome diarrheal stools. These drugs may precipitate massive dilation of the colon (toxic megacolon) and are usually contraindicated.

Surgery is the treatment of last resort if the patient has toxic megacolon, fails to respond to drugs and supportive measures, or finds symptoms unbearable. The most common surgical technique is proctocolectomy with ileostomy.

In pouch ileostomy, a pouch is created from a small loop of the terminal ileum and a nipple valve formed from the distal ileum. The resulting stoma opens just above the pubic hairline; the pouch empties through a catheter inserted in the stoma several times a day. (For more information, see "Bowel surgery with ostomy," page 509.)

Nursing interventions. Accurately record intake and output, particularly the frequency and volume of stools. Watch for signs of dehydration (poor skin turgor, furrowed tongue) and electrolyte imbalances, especially signs and symptoms of hypokalemia (muscle weakness, paresthesia) and hypernatremia (tachycardia, flushed skin, fever, dry tongue). Monitor hemoglobin levels and hematocrit, and give blood transfusions, as ordered. Provide good mouth care for the patient who is allowed nothing by mouth.

After each bowel movement, clean the skin around the rectum. Provide an air mattress or a sheepskin to help prevent skin break-down.

Watch for adverse effects of prolonged corticosteroid therapy (hyperglycemia, hypertension, hirsutism, edema, gastric irritation). Be aware that such therapy may mask infection.

Watch closely for signs and symptoms of complications, such as a perforated colon and peritonitis (fever, severe abdominal pain, abdominal rigidity and tenderness, cool, clammy skin), and toxic megacolon (abdominal distention, decreased bowel sounds).

Do a bowel preparation, as ordered. This usually involves keeping the patient on a clear-liquid diet, using cleansing enemas, and administering antimicrobials such as neomycin.

Patient education. Provide emotional support. Educate the patient about the disease and its association with stress, and teach stress-reducing activities. Explain the importance of follow-up medical care because of the high risk of colon cancer.

After a proctocolectomy and ileostomy, teach good stoma care. After a pouch ileostomy, teach the patient how to insert the catheter and take care of the stoma.

Evaluation. The patient should maintain optimal nutrition and hydration, report his feelings about his changed body image, and identify and avoid foods likely to cause distress. He should demonstrate proper ostomy care (if required),

use support groups, understand the need for follow-up care, and know when to seek immediate attention.

Crohn's disease

An inflammatory disorder that usually involves the small intestine, Crohn's disease can affect any part of the GI tract, extending through all layers of the intestinal wall. The terminal ileum is most commonly affected. The disease may also involve regional lymph nodes and the mesentery.

Causes. The cause is unknown. Possible causes include allergies, immune disorders, lymphatic obstruction, infection, and genetic factors. Studies find no causative link between this disease and emotional distress.

Assessment findings. Clinical effects vary according to the location and extent of inflammation and may be mild and nonspecific.

In *acute* disease, signs and symptoms include right lower abdominal quadrant pain, cramping, tenderness, flatulence, nausea, fever, diarrhea, and bleeding (usually mild but may be massive).

In *chronic* disease, look for diarrhea, four to six stools a day, right lower quadrant pain, steatorrhea, and marked weight loss.

Diagnostic tests. Laboratory findings typically indicate increased white blood cell (WBC) count and ESR, hypokalemia, hypocalcemia, hypomagnesemia, and decreased hemoglobin levels.

A barium enema showing the string sign (segments of stricture separated by normal bowel) supports this diagnosis. Sigmoidoscopy and colonoscopy may show patchy areas or inflammation, thus helping to rule out ulcerative colitis. Biopsy results confirm the diagnosis.

Treatment. Drug therapy is similar to ulcerative colitis with sulfasalazine and steroids as necessary. Immunosuppressant drugs may be used. In debilitated patients, therapy includes TPN to maintain nutrition while resting the bowel. Drug therapy may include anti-inflammatory corticosteroids, immunosuppressant agents such as azathioprine, and antibacterial agents such as sulfasalazine. Metronidazole has proved effective in some patients. Opium tincture and diphenoxylate may help combat diarrhea but are contraindicated in patients with significant intestinal obstruction.

Surgery may be necessary to correct bowel perforation, massive hemorrhage, fistulas, or acute intestinal obstruction. Patients with extensive disease of the large intestine and rectum may require colectomy with ileostomy. Surgery is not curative but may be necessary to relieve severe symptoms or to correct complications, such as perforation, bleeding, blockage, or fistula.

Some people follow an alternative therapy. (See *The "carbohydrate" diet and Crohn's disease.*)

Nursing interventions. Record fluid intake and output (including the amount of stool), and weigh the patient daily. Watch for dehydration and maintain fluid and electrolyte balance. Check stools daily for occult blood.

If the patient is receiving steroids, watch for adverse effects such as GI bleeding. Remember that steroids can mask signs of infection. Check hemoglobin level and hematocrit regularly. Give iron supplements, blood transfusions, and analgesics, as ordered.

Watch for fever and pain on urination, which may signal bladder fistula. Abdominal pain, fever, and a hard, distended abdomen may indicate intestinal obstruction. (See *Reducing social isolation via the Internet,* page 474.)

Before ileostomy, arrange for a visit by an enterostomal therapist. For postoperative care, see "Bowel surgery with ostomy," page 509.

Patient education. Teach the patient and family about the disease. Explain the medication regimen, including adverse effects. Educate the patient about dietary and stress management and the availability of support groups.

Evaluation. The patient should maintain optimal nutrition and hydration, maintain skin integrity, and use positive coping mechanisms. He should identify and avoid foods likely to cause distress, and demonstrate proper care of an ostomy, if required. He should use support groups, understand the need for follow-up care, and know when to seek immediate attention.

Pseudomembranous enterocolitis

Characterized by acute inflammation and necrosis involving the small and large intestines, pseudomembranous enterocolitis usually affects the mucosa but may extend into the submucosa. It has occurred postoperatively in debilitated patients who have undergone abdominal surgery or in patients who have been treated with broad-spectrum antibiotics. Marked by severe diarrhea, this rare condition is usually fatal in 1 to 7 days because of severe dehydration and toxicity, peritonitis, or perforation.

Causes. The most common cause is associated with antibiotic therapy. *Clostridium difficile* is thought to produce a toxin that may play a role in its development.

Assessment findings. The patient may experience a sudden onset of copious watery or bloody diarrhea as well as abdominal pain and fever.

Diagnostic tests. A rectal biopsy through sigmoidoscopy confirms pseudomembranous enterocolitis. Stool cultures can identify *C. difficile*.

Treatment. In most cases, antibiotic-associated pseudomembranous enterocolitis is treated with oral vancomycin. In some cases metronidazole or bacitracin may be used.

A patient with mild pseudomembranous enterocolitis may receive anion exchange resins such as cholestyramine to bind the toxin

ALTERNATIVE THERAPY

The "carbohydrate" diet and Crohn's disease

An alternative therapy that many people follow, the "carbohydrate" diet, calls for the avoidance of all disaccharides and polysaccharides. The theory is that people with Crohn's disease cannot break down these carbohydrate molecules. As a result, bacteria overgrow in the intestines because the bacteria eat these molecules.

By restricting the diet to monosaccharides, which the body can digest and absorb quickly, this bacterial overgrowth is prevented. Thus, the patient must avoid any food made with flour, rice, tofu, potatoes, or soy. Any product made with added starch sugar (canned or processed) and most dairy products are also forbidden.

produced by *C. difficile*. Supportive treatment must maintain fluid and electrolyte balance and combat hypotension and shock with pressors, such as dopamine and levarterenol.

Nursing interventions. Monitor vital signs, skin color, and level of consciousness (LOC). Immediately report signs of shock.

Record fluid intake and output, including fluid lost in stools. Watch for signs of dehydration (poor skin turgor, sunken eyes, and decreased urine output).

Check serum electrolyte levels daily, and watch for signs and symptoms of hypokalemia, especially malaise and weak, rapid, irregular pulse.

Evaluation. If treatment has been successful, the patient should maintain fluid and electrolyte balance, avoid shock and other complications, and regain a normal bowel elimination pattern.

Irritable bowel syndrome

Irritable bowel syndrome is a common syndrome, marked by chronic or periodic diarrhea alternating with constipation, and accompanied by straining and abdominal cramps. Diagnosis requires a careful history to determine contributing psychological factors such as a recent stressful life change. Diagnosis must also rule out other disorders, such as amebiasis, diverticulitis, colon cancer, and lactose intolerance. Supportive treatment or avoiding known irritants commonly relieves symptoms.

Causes. This disorder is usually associated with psychological stress but may also result from physical factors, such as diverticular disease, ingestion of irritants (coffee, raw fruits or vegetables), lactose intolerance, abuse of laxatives, food poisoning, or colon cancer.

Assessment findings. The following symptoms alternate with constipation or normal bowel function: lower abdominal pain (usually relieved by defecation or passage of gas), diarrhea, small stools that contain visible mucus, and possible dyspepsia and abdominal distention.

Diagnostic tests. Tests may include sigmoidoscopy, colonoscopy, barium enema, rectal biopsy, and stool examination for blood, parasites, and bacteria to rule out other disorders.

Treatment. Therapy aims to relieve symptoms and includes counseling to help the patient understand the relationship between stress and his illness. Strict dietary restrictions are not beneficial, but food irritants should be investigated and the patient should be instructed to avoid them. Rest and heat applied to the abdomen are helpful, as is judicious use of sedatives (phenobarbital) and antispasmodics (propantheline, diphenoxylate with atropine sulfate). With chronic use, however, the patient may become dependent on these drugs. If the cause of irritable bowel syndrome is chronic laxative abuse, bowel training may help correct the condition.

Nursing interventions. Focus your care on patient education.

Patient education. Tell the patient to avoid irritating foods, and how to develop regular bowel habits. Help him deal with stress, and warn against dependence on sedatives or antispasmodics. Encourage regular checkups because this syndrome is associated with a higher-than-normal incidence of diverticulitis and colon cancer. For patients over age 40, emphasize the need for an annual sigmoidoscopy and rectal examination.

Evaluation. The patient should modify his diet and lifestyle and demonstrate a regular bowel elimination pattern. He should understand the need for follow-up care and know when to seek immediate attention.

Diverticular disease
In diverticular disease, bulging pouchlike herniations (diverticula) in the GI wall push the mucosal lining through the surrounding muscle. Diverticula occur most commonly in the sigmoid colon, but they may develop anywhere, from the proximal end of the pharynx to the anus. Other typical sites are the duodenum, near the pancreatic border or the ampulla of Vater, and the jejunum.

Diverticular disease of the ileum (Meckel's diverticulum) is the most common congenital anomaly of the GI tract.

Diverticular disease has two clinical forms. In *diverticulosis*, diverticula are present but don't cause symptoms. In *diverticulitis*, diverticula are inflamed and may cause potentially fatal obstruction, infection, or hemorrhage.

Causes. Diverticula probably result from high intraluminal pressure on areas of weakness in the GI wall, where blood vessels enter. A diet low in fiber may be a contributing factor. Lack of fiber reduces fecal residue, narrows the bowel lumen, and leads to higher intra-abdominal pressure during defecation.

Assessment findings. This disorder is usually asymptomatic. However, in diverticulosis, recurrent left lower abdominal quadrant pain is relieved by defecation or passage of flatus.

Constipation and diarrhea alternate.

In diverticulitis, the patient may have moderate left lower abdominal quadrant pain, mild nausea, gas, irregular bowel habits, low-grade fever, leukocytosis, rupture of the diverticuli (in severe diverticulitis), and fibrosis and adhesions (in chronic diverticulitis).

Diagnostic tests. An upper GI series or barium enema confirms or rules out diverticulosis. Biopsy rules out cancer; however, a colonoscopic biopsy is not recommended during acute diverticular disease because of the strenuous bowel preparation it requires. Blood studies may show an elevated ESR in diverticulitis.

Treatment. Asymptomatic diverticulosis usually doesn't require treatment. Intestinal diverticulosis with pain, mild GI distress, constipation, or difficult defecation may respond to a liquid or bland diet, stool softeners, and occasional doses of mineral oil. These measures relieve symptoms, minimize irritation, and lessen the risk of progression to diverticulitis. After pain subsides, patients also benefit from a high-residue diet and bulk-forming laxatives such as psyllium.

Treatment for mild diverticulitis without signs of perforation must prevent constipation and combat infection. It may include bed rest, a liquid diet, stool softeners, a broad-spectrum antibiotic, meperidine, and an antispasmodic such as propantheline.

Diverticulitis unresponsive to medical treatment requires a colon resection to remove the involved segment. Complications that accompany diverticulitis may require a temporary colostomy to drain abscesses and rest the colon, followed by later anastomosis.

Patients who hemorrhage need blood replacement and careful monitoring of fluid and electrolyte balance. Angiography for catheter placement and infusion of vasopressin is used for severe bleeding.

Nursing interventions. If the patient with diverticulosis is hospitalized, observe his stools carefully for frequency, color, and consistency; keep accurate pulse and temperature charts because they may signal developing inflammation or complications.

Management of diverticulitis depends on the severity of symptoms, as follows:
• In mild disease, give medications, as ordered; explain diagnostic tests; observe stools carefully; and maintain accurate records of temperature, pulse rate, respiratory rate, and intake and output.
• Monitor carefully if the patient requires angiography and catheter placement for vasopressin infusion. Inspect the insertion site frequently for bleeding, check pedal pulses frequently, and keep the patient from flexing his legs at the groin.
• Watch for signs and symptoms of vasopressin-induced fluid retention (apprehension, abdominal cramps, convulsions, oliguria, or anuria) and severe hyponatremia (hypoten-

sion; rapid, thready pulse; cold, clammy skin; and cyanosis).

For postsurgical care, see "Bowel resection and anastomosis," page 513.

Patient education. Explain diverticula and how they form.

Make sure the patient understands the importance of dietary fiber and the harmful effects of constipation and straining at stool. Encourage increased intake of foods high in undigestible fiber. Caution the patient against intake of popcorn, nuts, and foods containing seeds. Advise the patient to relieve constipation with stool softeners or bulk-forming laxatives, but caution against taking bulk-forming laxatives without plenty of water.

Evaluation. The patient should observe and report character of stools and modify his diet as needed. He should understand the need for follow-up care and know when to seek immediate attention.

Appendicitis

Appendicitis is obstruction and inflammation of the vermiform appendix, which may lead to infection, thrombosis, necrosis, and perforation.

Causes. Appendicitis may result from an obstruction of the intestinal lumen caused by a fecal mass, stricture, barium ingestion, or a viral infection.

Assessment findings. Initially, your patient may experience abdominal pain, generalized or localized in the right upper abdomen, eventually localizing in the right lower abdomen (McBurney's point); anorexia; nausea; vomiting; boardlike abdominal rigidity; retractive respirations; and increasingly severe abdominal spasms and rebound spasms. (Rebound tenderness on the opposite side of the abdomen suggests peritoneal inflammation.)

Later symptoms include constipation (although diarrhea is also possible), temperature of 99° to 102° F (37.2° to 38.9° C), tachycardia, and sudden cessation of abdominal pain (indicates perforation or infarction of the appendix).

Diagnostic tests. The WBC count is moderately elevated, with increased immature cells. Enema using a diatrizoate meglumine and diatrizoate sodium solution combination may be used in diagnosis.

Treatment. Appendectomy is the only effective treatment. Laparoscopic appendectomy is an option in selected patients. If peritonitis develops, treatment involves GI intubation, parenteral replacement of fluids and electrolytes, and administration of antibiotics.

Nursing interventions. If appendicitis is suspected, or during preparation for appendectomy, follow these guidelines:
• Administer I.V. fluids to prevent dehydration. To prevent rupture, *never* administer cathartics or enemas.

- Give the patient nothing by mouth, and use analgesics judiciously because they may mask symptoms.
- Place the patient in Fowler's position to reduce pain. To prevent rupture, *never* apply heat to the right lower abdomen.

After appendectomy, follow these guidelines:
- Monitor vital signs and intake and output.
- Give analgesics, as ordered.
- Document bowel sounds, passing of flatus, or bowel movements— signs of peristalsis return. If these signs appear in a patient whose nausea and abdominal rigidity have subsided, he can resume oral fluids.
- Watch closely for possible surgical complications. Continuing pain and fever may signal an abscess. The complaint that "something gave way" may mean wound dehiscence. If an abscess or peritonitis develops, incision and drainage may be necessary. Frequently assess the dressing for wound drainage.
- If peritonitis complicated appendicitis, an NG tube may be needed to decompress the stomach and reduce nausea and vomiting. If so, record drainage, and provide good mouth and nose care.

Evaluation. The patient should demonstrate appropriate activity restrictions, resume a normal diet and bowel elimination pattern, and understand the importance of follow-up care.

Colorectal cancer

Colorectal cancer accounts for about 16% of all malignancies in the United States. Because this cancer spreads slowly, it's potentially curable with early diagnosis.

Malignant colorectal tumors are almost always adenocarcinomas. About one-half of these are sessile lesions of the rectosigmoid area; the rest are polypoid lesions.

Causes. The causes of colorectal cancer are unknown, but much research has linked dietary factors to the development of this cancer. A history of ulcerative colitis increases the risk of developing colorectal cancer. If left untreated, nearly all patients with familial adenomatous polyposis (an autosomal dominant inherited disease) will develop adenocarcinoma, many by the age of 40. Similarly, hereditary nonpolyposis colorectal cancer, formerly called the cancer family syndrome, significantly increases the risk of colorectal cancer.

Assessment findings. Signs and symptoms of colorectal cancer result from local obstruction and, in later stages, from direct extension to adjacent organs (bladder, prostate, ureters, vagina, sacrum) and distant metastasis (usually to the liver). Later, they generally include pallor, cachexia, ascites, hepatomegaly, or lymphangiectasis.

On the right side of the colon, early tumor growth causes no obstruction because this area of the bowel can accommodate a relatively large tumor without symptoms. It may, however, cause heme-positive stools, anemia, and abdominal aching, pressure, or dull cramps. As the disease progresses, the patient develops weakness, fatigue, exertional dyspnea, vertigo and, eventually, diarrhea, obstipation, anorexia, weight loss, vomiting, and other signs and symptoms of intestinal obstruction. A tumor on the right side may be palpable.

On the left side, where stools are denser, a tumor may be obstructive even in early stages and thus tends to be diagnosed. It commonly causes rectal bleeding (often ascribed to hemorrhoids), intermittent abdominal fullness or cramping, and rectal pressure. As the disease progresses, the patient develops obstipation, diarrhea, or "ribbon" or pencil-shaped stools. Typically, he notices that passage of a stool or flatus relieves the pain.

A rectal tumor is heralded by a change in bowel habits; for many it begins with an urgent need to defecate on arising (morning diarrhea) or obstipation alternating with diarrhea. Other signs and symptoms are blood or mucus in stool and a feeling of incomplete evacuation. Late in the disease, pain begins as a feeling of rectal fullness that later becomes a dull, and sometimes constant, ache in the rectum or sacral region that may radiate down the legs.

Diagnostic tests. Only tumor biopsy can verify colorectal cancer, but other tests help detect it.

Digital examination detects nearly 50% of rectal cancers. *Hemoccult test* (guaiac) detects blood in stools.

Flexible fiberoptic sigmoidoscopy detects up to 66% of colorectal cancers. *Colonoscopy* permits visual inspection of the colon up to the ileocecal valve and provides access for polypectomies and biopsies of suspected lesions.

The American Cancer Society recommends an annual digital examination after age 40, then annual Hemoccult after age 50. Proctosigmoidoscopy is recommended every 3 to 5 years for people age 50 and older after two initial normal tests 1 year apart. *Barium X-ray,* using a dual contrast with air, can locate lesions that are undetectable manually or visually. Barium examination should *follow* endoscopy because the barium sulfate interferes with this test. *Carcinoembryonic antigen* helps monitor a patient's response to treatment and detects metastasis or recurrence.

Treatment. Surgical treatment seeks to remove the malignant tumor and adjacent tissues as well as any lymph nodes that may contain cancer cells. The type of surgery performed depends on the location of the tumor: for *cecum and ascending colon,* right hemicolectomy for advanced disease; for *proximal and middle transverse colon,* transverse colectomy; for *tumors in the descending colon,* a left hemicolectomy. If possible, a more limited surgery—left partial colectomy—is performed to avoid the ligation of major arteries.

For *sigmoid colon* tumors, surgery is usually limited to the sigmoid colon and mesentery. Surgical procedures for cancers of the rectum depend on tumor size, location, and patient factors. Preserving continence is an important consideration. A low anterior resection is usually done for tumors in the upper rectum. For tumors in the lower rectum, an abdominal perineal resection is done, creating a permanent colostomy.

Chemotherapy may be used as adjuvant therapy or for patients with metastasis, residual disease, or a recurrent inoperable tumor. Drugs commonly used include 5-fluorouracil, with or without leucovorin; lomustine; mitomycin; methotrexate; vincristine; and levamisole.

Radiation therapy induces tumor regression and may be used before or after surgery. Biological response modifiers, particularly alpha-interferon, interleukin-2, and monoclonal antibodies, are being investigated.

Nursing interventions. Before surgery, monitor the patient's diet modifications, laxatives, enemas, and antibiotics; these clean the bowel and decrease abdominal and perineal cavity contamination during surgery.

For additional nursing care measures, see "Bowel surgery with ostomy" and "Bowel resection and anastomosis," pages 509 and 513.

Patient education. If the patient is to have a colostomy, teach him and his family about the procedure.

Patients who have had colorectal cancer are at increased risk for other primary cancers and should have yearly screening and follow-up testing as well as a high-fiber diet.

Evaluation. The patient should understand the treatment regimen, including ostomy care, and the need for long-term follow-up.

Peritonitis

An acute or chronic inflammation, peritonitis may extend throughout the peritoneum, the membrane that lines the abdominal cavity and covers the visceral organs, or be localized as an abscess. Peritonitis commonly reduces intestinal motility and causes intestinal distention with gas. Mortality is 10%, usually from bowel obstruction.

Causes. Peritonitis results from bacterial invasion of the peritoneum, which leads to infection, inflammation, and perforation of the GI tract. It usually arises as a complication of appendicitis, diverticulitis, peptic ulcer, ulcerative colitis, volvulus, a strangulated obstruction, an abdominal neoplasm, or a stab wound. Peritonitis may also result from chemical inflammation, as in ruptured fallopian tubes or bladder, perforated gastric ulcer, or released pancreatic enzymes.

Assessment findings. The main symptom is sudden, severe, diffuse abdominal pain that tends to intensify and localize in the area of the underlying disorder. Also assess your patient for weakness, pallor, excessive sweating, and cold skin; decreased intestinal motility and paralytic ileus; abdominal distention; an acutely tender abdomen associated with rebound tenderness; shallow breathing; diminished movement by the patient to minimize pain; hypotension, tachycardia, and signs of dehydration; temperature of 103° F (39.4° C) or higher; and possible shoulder pain and hiccups.

Diagnostic tests. Abdominal X-rays showing edematous and gaseous distention of the small and large bowel support the diagnosis. With perforation of a visceral organ, the X-ray shows air in the abdominal cavity. Chest X-ray may show an elevated diaphragm.

Blood studies show leukocytosis (WBC count above 20,000/mm³). Paracentesis reveals bacteria, exudate, blood, pus, or urine. Laparotomy may be done to identify the underlying cause.

Treatment. Emergency treatment aims to stop infection, restore intestinal motility, and replace fluids and electrolytes.

Massive antibiotic therapy usually includes administration of cefoxitin with an aminoglycoside, or penicillin G and clindamycin with an aminoglycoside, depending on the infecting organisms. To decrease peristalsis and prevent perforation, the patient should be given nothing by mouth and should receive supportive fluids and electrolytes parenterally.

Supplementary treatment measures include preoperative and postoperative analgesics such as meperidine, NG intubation to decompress the bowel, and possible use of a rectal tube to facilitate passage of flatus.

When peritonitis results from perforation, surgery is performed as soon as the patient can tolerate it. Surgery aims to eliminate the infection source by evacuating the spilled contents and inserting drains. Occasionally, paracentesis may be needed to remove accumulated fluid. Irrigation of the abdominal cavity with antibiotic solutions during surgery may be appropriate.

Nursing interventions. Regularly monitor vital signs, fluid intake and output, and the amount of NG drainage or vomitus. Place the patient in semi-Fowler's position to help him deep-breathe with less pain and thus prevent pulmonary complications.

After surgery to evacuate the peritoneum, watch for signs and symptoms of dehiscence and abscess formation. Frequently assess peristaltic activity by listening for bowel sounds and checking for gas, bowel movements, and soft abdomen. When peristalsis returns, and temperature and pulse rate are normal, gradually decrease parenteral fluids and increase oral fluids. If the patient has an NG tube in place, clamp it for short intervals. If neither nausea nor vomiting results, begin oral fluids, as ordered and tolerated.

Evaluation. The patient should have normal fluid and electrolyte balance, normal body temperature and WBC count, and lack of bowel obstruction or other complications.

He should resume normal oral intake and bowel elimination.

Inguinal hernia

In inguinal hernia, the large or small intestine, omentum, or bladder protrudes into the inguinal canal. This hernia may be *reducible* (if it can be moved back into place easily), *incarcerated* (if it can't be reduced because of adhesions in the hernial sac), or *strangulated* (if part of the herniated intestine becomes twisted or edematous, cutting off normal blood flow and peristalsis and possibly leading to intestinal obstruction and necrosis). Inguinal hernia can also be direct or indirect. When indirect, it causes the abdominal viscera to protrude through the inguinal ring and follow the spermatic cord (in males) or round ligament (in females). If direct, it results from a weakness in the fascial floor of the inguinal canal.

Causes. Inguinal hernia results from increased intra-abdominal pressure (due to heavy lifting, pregnancy, obesity, or straining) or from abdominal muscles weakened by congenital malformation, traumatic injury, or aging.

Assessment findings. Watch for a lump that appears over the herniated area when the patient stands or strains and disappears when the patient is supine. Note if tension on the herniated area causes sharp, steady groin pain that fades when the hernia is reduced. Severe pain, nausea, vomiting, and possibly diarrhea may indicate strangulation.

Palpate the inguinal area while the patient is performing Valsalva's maneuver to confirm the diagnosis.

To detect a hernia in a male patient, ask him to stand with the leg on the side being examined slightly flexed and to rest his weight on the other leg. Insert an index finger into the lower part of the scrotum and invaginate the scrotal skin so that the finger advances through the external inguinal ring to the internal ring (about $1^1/2''$ to $2''$ [4 to 5 cm] through the inguinal canal). Tell the patient to cough. If you feel pressure against your fingertip, an indirect hernia exists; if you feel pressure against the side of your finger, a direct hernia exists.

Diagnostic tests. X-rays and a WBC count are required for a suspected bowel obstruction.

Treatment. The pain of a reducible hernia may be relieved temporarily by moving the hernia back into place. A truss may keep the abdominal contents from protruding into the hernial sac, and is especially beneficial for an elderly or debilitated patient.

Herniorrhaphy is the preferred surgical treatment for infants, adults, and otherwise healthy elderly patients. Another effective procedure, hernioplasty, reinforces the weakened area with steel mesh, fascia, or wire. Laparoscopic herniorrhaphy is an option for selected patients but requires general anesthesia.

A strangulated or necrotic hernia requires bowel resection.

Nursing interventions. Apply a truss only after a hernia has been reduced. Apply it in the morning, before the patient gets out of bed.

Watch for and immediately report signs of incarceration and strangulation. Don't try to reduce an incarcerated hernia because this may perforate the bowel. If severe intestinal obstruction arises because of hernial strangulation, tell the doctor immediately. An NG tube may be inserted promptly to empty the stomach and relieve pressure on the hernial sac.

Before surgery, closely monitor vital signs. Administer I.V. fluids and analgesics for pain, as ordered. Control fever with acetaminophen or tepid sponge baths, as ordered. Place the patient in Trendelenburg's position.

For postoperative care, see "Hernia repair," page 507.

Patient education. To prevent skin irritation, tell the patient to bathe daily and apply liberal amounts of cornstarch or baby powder. Warn against applying the truss over clothing.

Before discharge, warn the patient against lifting or straining. Also, tell him to watch for signs and symptoms of infection (oozing, tenderness, warmth, redness) at the incision site and to keep the incision clean and covered until the sutures are removed.

Advise the patient not to resume normal activity nor return to work without the surgeon's permission.

Evaluation. The patient should have intact skin in the genital area, and no postsurgical complications. He should demonstrate proper use of a truss, restrict his activities appropriately, recognize symptoms of strangulation, and understand the need to obtain immediate care.

Intestinal obstruction

In intestinal obstruction, the lumen of the small or large bowel becomes partly or fully blocked. Small-bowel obstruction is far more common and usually more serious. Complete obstruction in any part of the bowel, if untreated, can cause death within hours from shock and vascular collapse. Intestinal obstruction is most likely to occur after abdominal surgery or in persons with congenital bowel deformities.

Causes. Mechanical obstruction can result from adhesions and strangulated hernias (these usually cause small-bowel obstruction), carcinomas (these usually cause large-bowel obstruction), foreign bodies (fruit pits, gallstones, worms), compression, stenosis, intussusception, volvulus of the sigmoid or cecum, tumors, and atresia.

Nonmechanical obstruction can result from paralytic ileus, electrolyte imbalances, toxicity, neurogenic abnormalities, and thrombosis or embolism of mesenteric vessels.

Assessment findings. To help detect *small-bowel obstruction,* assess for colicky pain, nausea, vomiting, and constipation. Auscultation may detect bowel sounds, borborygmi, and rushes. Palpation may reveal abdominal tenderness with moderate distention. Rebound tenderness may occur with strangulation and ischemia. In complete obstruction, the patient may vomit fecal contents.

In *large-bowel obstruction,* constipation may be the only clinical effect for days. Other symptoms include colicky abdominal pain, nausea (usually without vomiting at first), and abdominal distention. Eventually, pain is continuous and the patient may vomit fecal contents.

Diagnostic tests. X-rays confirm the diagnosis. Abdominal films show the presence and location of intestinal gas or fluid. In small-bowel obstruction, a typical "stepladder" pattern emerges, with alternating fluid and gas levels apparent in 3 to 4 hours. Free air beneath the diaphragm indicates perforation. In large-bowel obstruction, barium enema reveals a distended, air-filled colon or a closed loop of sigmoid with extreme distention (in sigmoid volvulus).

Laboratory results reveal decreased sodium, chloride, and potassium levels; slightly elevated WBC count; and increased serum amylase level. Endoscopy permits visualization, biopsy and sometimes treatment for lesions.

Treatment. Treatment aims to correct fluid and electrolyte imbalances, decompress the bowel to relieve vomiting and distention, and alleviate shock and peritonitis.

Strangulated obstruction usually requires blood replacement as well as I.V. fluid administration. Passage of a Levin tube, followed by use of the longer, weighted Miller-Abbott tube, usually accomplishes decompression, especially in small-bowel obstruction. If the patient fails to improve or his condition deteriorates, surgery is necessary. In large-bowel obstruction, surgical resection with anastomosis, colostomy, or ileostomy commonly follows decompression with a Levin tube.

TPN may be appropriate. Drug therapy includes analgesics or sedatives, such as meperidine or phenobarbital (but not opiates, which inhibit GI motility), and antibiotics for peritonitis. For intussusception, hydrostatic reduction may be attempted by infusing barium into the rectum. If this fails, manual reduction or bowel resection is performed in surgery.

Nursing interventions. Monitor vital signs frequently. Decreased blood pressure may indicate reduced circulating blood volume due to blood loss from a strangulated hernia. Remember, as many as 10.5 qt (10 L) of fluid can collect in the small bowel, drastically reducing plasma volume. Observe closely for signs of shock.

Stay alert for signs and symptoms of metabolic alkalosis (changes in sensorium; slow, shallow respirations; hypertonic muscles; tetany) or acidosis (shortness of breath on exertion, disorientation and, later, deep, rapid breathing, weakness, and malaise). Watch for signs and symptoms of secondary infection.

Monitor urine output carefully to assess renal function and possible urine retention. If you suspect bladder compression, catheterize the patient for residual urine immediately after he has voided. Also measure abdominal girth frequently to detect progressive distention.

Provide thorough mouth and nose care if the patient has undergone decompression by intubation or if he has vomited. Look for signs of dehydration (thick, swollen tongue; dry, cracked lips; dry oral mucous membranes). Record the amount and color of drainage from the decompression tube. Irrigate the tube, if necessary, with normal saline solution to maintain patency.

If a weighted tube has been inserted, check periodically to make sure it's advancing. Help the patient turn from side to side (or walk around, if he can) to facilitate passage of the tube.

Keep the patient in Fowler's position as much as possible to promote pulmonary ventilation and ease respiratory distress from abdominal distention. Listen for bowel sounds, and watch for signs of returning peristalsis.

Patient education. Provide emotional support after surgery. Arrange for an enterostomal therapist to visit the patient who has had a colostomy.

Evaluation. The patient should have normal fluid and electrolyte balance, normal oral intake, and regular bowel elimination patterns. You should detect bowel sounds and note the absence of abdominal distention and complications.

Pancreatitis

Inflammation of the pancreas occurs in acute and chronic forms and may result from edema, necrosis, or hemorrhage. In pancreatitis, the enzymes normally excreted by the pancreas attack and digest the surrounding pancreatic tissue. The prognosis is poor when pancreatitis follows alcoholism.

Causes. Most commonly caused by biliary tract disease and alcoholism, pancreatitis also results from pancreatic cancer; certain drugs, such as glucocorticoids, zidovudine (Retrovir), didanosine (ddI), sulfonamides, chlorothiazide, and azathioprine; and possibly peptic ulcer, mumps, or hypothermia. Less commonly, the disorder results from stenosis or obstruction of Oddi's sphincter, hyperlipidemia, metabolic and endocrine disorders, vascular disease, viral infections, mycoplasmal pneumonia, or pregnancy.

Assessment findings. Steady epigastric pain centered close to the umbilicus, radiating between the tenth thoracic and sixth lumbar vertebrae, and unrelieved by vomiting may be the first and only symptom of mild pancreatitis.

A severe attack may cause extreme pain (left upper quadrant) radiating to the back associated with oral food or fluid, persistent vomiting, abdominal rigidity, diminished bowel activity (suggesting peritonitis), crackles at lung bases, left pleural effusion, extreme malaise, restlessness, mottled skin, tachycardia, low-grade fever (100° to 102° F [37.8° to 38.9° C]), possible ileus, and cold, sweaty extremities.

Diagnostic tests. Dramatically elevated serum amylase levels—commonly more than 500 Somogyi U/dl—confirm pancreatitis. Similar elevations of amylase levels occur in urine, ascites, or pleural fluid. Characteristically, amylase levels return to normal 48 hours after onset of pancreatitis, despite continuing symptoms.

Serum lipase levels are increased. Serum calcium levels are low from fat necrosis and formation of calcium soaps. Glucose levels are elevated and may be as high as 900 mg/dl, indicating hyperglycemia. WBC counts range from 8,000 to 20,000/mm³, with increased polymorphonuclear leukocyte levels. Hematocrit occasionally exceeds 50% concentrations. Serum bilirubin and alkaline phosphatase are increased with liver impairment.

Abdominal X-rays may show dilation of the small or large bowel or calcification of the pancreas. GI series indicate extrinsic pressure on the duodenum or stomach caused by edema of the pancreas head. Abdominal ultrasound or CT scan differentiates acute cholecystitis from pancreatitis.

Treatment. Treatment must maintain circulation and fluid volume, relieve pain, and decrease pancreatic secretions. Emergency treatment for shock (the most common cause of death in early-stage pancreatitis) consists of vigorous I.V. replacement of electrolytes and proteins. Metabolic acidosis secondary to hypovolemia and impaired cellular perfusion requires vigorous fluid volume replacement.

Treatment may also include antibiotics and other medications. Hypocalcemia requires infusion of 10% calcium gluconate; serum glucose levels greater than 300 mg/dl require insulin therapy.

After the emergency phase, continue I.V. therapy for 5 to 7 days. Solutions should provide adequate electrolytes and protein without stimulating the pancreas (for example, glucose or free amino acids). If the patient isn't ready to resume oral feedings by then, TPN may be necessary. Nonstimulating elemental gavage feedings may be safer because of the decreased risk of infection and overinfusion. In extreme cases, laparotomy to drain the pancreatic bed, 95% pancreatectomy, or a combination of cholecystostomy-gastrostomy, feeding jejunostomy, and drainage may be necessary.

Nursing interventions. Monitor vital signs and pulmonary artery pressure closely. If the patient has a central venous pressure line, monitor it closely for volume expansion (it shouldn't exceed 10 cm H_2O). Give plasma or albumin, if ordered, to maintain blood pressure. Record fluid intake and output, check urine output hourly, and monitor electrolyte levels.

For bowel decompression, maintain constant NG suctioning, and give nothing by mouth. Perform good mouth and nose care.

Watch for signs and symptoms of calcium deficiency—tetany, cramps, carpopedal spasm, and convulsions. If you suspect hypocalcemia, keep airway and suction apparatus handy and pad side rails.

Give analgesics as needed. Watch for adverse reactions to antibiotics: nephrotoxicity with aminoglycosides, pseudomembranous enterocolitis with clindamycin, and blood dyscrasias with chloramphenicol.

Don't confuse thirst due to hyperglycemia (indicated by serum glucose levels of up to 350 mg/dl and glucose and acetone in urine) with dry mouth due to NG intubation and anticholinergics. Watch for complications due to TPN, such as sepsis, hypokalemia, overhydration, and metabolic acidosis.

Evaluation. The patient should have normal nutrition and hydration levels and balanced electrolyte levels. He should tolerate oral food and fluids without discomfort, and understand and modify lifestyle factors that aggravate his disease.

Pancreatic cancer

Pancreatic cancer is extremely difficult to diagnose early because its symptoms are insidious and often occur late. Most cases are locally advanced or metastatic at time of diagnosis. Hence, the percent of

patients alive after 5 years is only about 5%.

Causes. Few risk factors have been identified for pancreatic cancer. Some potential risk factors include tobacco use, diets high in fat or meat, history of peptic ulcer surgery, diabetes, and chronic pancreatitis.

Assessment findings. Clinical manifestations vary depending on whether the tumor is located in the head, body, or tail of the pancreas. Almost 70% of all pancreatic cancers are located in the head and present with jaundice, pain and weight loss. Other signs and symptoms include hemorrhage and bleeding disorders (with liver involvement), hepatomegaly, enlargement of the gallbladder, and portal hypertension as ducts are blocked. Physical examination of the pancreas is difficult; however, an enlarged gallbladder and a large smooth liver may be palpated. If the cancer is in the body or the tail of the pancreas, the mass may be palpable.

Diagnostic tests. Abdominal ultrasound (usually the first test ordered) can demonstrate a mass and dilated ducts. Endoscopic ultrasound may also be used. CT scans provide more detail about the location and extent of the tumor. Endoscopic retrograde cholangiopancreatography (ERCP) may be used to obtain biopsy samples. Several tumor markers have been identified in patients with pancreatic cancer, including CA 19-9, carcinoembryonic antigen, and pancreatic onco-fetal antigen. These markers help to measure response to therapy and may indicate recurrence.

Treatment. Surgery is the only treatment that offers a chance of cure to patients with pancreatic cancer. Surgery cures only a small percentage of patients with tumors in the head of the pancreas. Surgical approaches include total pancreatectomy, pancreatoduodenal resection (Whipple procedure), regional pancreatectomy, and distal pancreatectomy. Even when cure isn't possible, surgery may be palliative.

Radiation may be used as an adjunct to surgery but is most commonly used in unresectable tumors for local control and palliation of symptoms. Although no chemotherapy drugs are considered standard for pancreatic cancer, 5-fluorouracil appears to make radiation more effective, prolonging survival.

Nursing interventions. Nursing interventions involve intensive postoperative care as well as effective supportive care. Because most patients with pancreatic cancer die within a year of diagnosis, attention to all facets of caring for the dying patient are critical. Good palliative care with pain relief as a primary objective is crucial.

Patient education. Preoperatively answer patients questions and concerns. Explain postoperative expectations and procedures, including increased risk for disseminated intravascular coagulation (DIC), drains, fluid concerns, endocrine function and digestive function.

Hepatic disorders

This section reviews important hepatic disorders: viral and nonviral hepatitis, liver cancer, cirrhosis (and its critical complications—portal hypertension and esophageal varices), and hepatic coma.

Viral hepatitis

A fairly common systemic disease, viral hepatitis is marked by hepatic cell destruction, necrosis, and autolysis, leading to anorexia, jaundice, and hepatomegaly. In most patients, hepatic cells eventually regenerate with little or no residual damage, allowing ready recovery. However, old age and serious underlying disorders make complications more likely.

Today, five types of viral hepatitis are recognized:
• *type A* (infectious or short-incubation hepatitis)
• *type B* (serum or long-incubation hepatitis)
• *type C*
• *type D* (also called delta hepatitis), responsible for about 50% of all fulminant hepatitis, which has an extremely high mortality rate
• *type E* (formerly grouped with type C under the name of type non-A, non-B hepatitis), found primarily among patients who have recently returned from an endemic area (India, Africa, Asia, or Central America).

Causes. All forms of viral hepatitis are caused by hepatitis viruses:

HAV, HBV, HCV, HDV, and HEV. Type A is highly contagious and is usually transmitted by the fecal-oral route, commonly within institutions or families. However, it may also be transmitted parenterally. Hepatitis A usually results from ingestion of contaminated food, milk, or water. Many outbreaks of this type are traced to ingestion of seafood from polluted water.

Type B hepatitis is transmitted by contaminated blood as well as by contact with contaminated human secretions and feces. Transmission of this type also results from intimate sexual contact and through perinatal transmission.

Type C hepatitis is transmitted via blood, sexual contact, and perinatally.

Type D hepatitis is found only in patients with an acute or chronic episode of hepatitis B.

Type E hepatitis is a new form of hepatitis that is transmitted enterically, much like type A. Because this virus is inconsistently shed in feces, detection is difficult.

Assessment findings. In the *pre-icteric phase,* the patient may report fatigue, malaise, arthralgia, myalgia, photophobia, and headache. He may lose his appetite, become nauseous, and vomit. His sense of taste and smell may be altered. Fever may occur, possibly along with liver and lymph node enlargement.

The *icteric phase* lasts 1 to 2 weeks. Signs and symptoms include mild weight loss, dark urine, clay-colored stools, yellow sclera and skin, and continued hepatomegaly with tenderness.

The *convalescent phase* lasts 2 to 12 weeks or longer. Signs and symptoms include continued fatigue, flatulence, abdominal pain or tenderness, and indigestion.

Diagnostic tests. The following results help confirm the diagnosis:
• Antibody and seriologic tests confirm the diagnosis.
• Bilirubin (conjugated and unconjugated) may be elevated.
• Lactate dehydrogenase (LD) isoenzymes LD_4 and LD_5 are specific for liver damage.
• PT is prolonged (more than 3 seconds longer than normal indicates severe liver damage).
• Serum transaminase levels (alanine aminotransferase [ALT], and aspartate aminotransferase [AST]), are elevated.
• Serum alkaline phosphatase levels are slightly elevated.
• Serum and urine bilirubin levels are elevated (with jaundice).
• Serum albumin levels are low and serum globulin levels are high.
• Liver biopsy and scan show patchy necrosis.

Treatment. The patient should rest in the early stages of the illness and combat anorexia by eating small meals high in calories and protein. (Protein intake should be reduced if symptoms of precoma—lethargy, confusion, mental changes—develop.) Large meals are usually better tolerated in the morning.

Antiemetics (trimethobenzamide or benzquinamide) may be

given $1/2$ hour before meals to relieve nausea and prevent vomiting; phenothiazines have a cholestatic effect and should be avoided. If vomiting persists, the patient will require I.V. infusions.

In severe hepatitis, corticosteroids may stimulate appetite while decreasing itching and inflammation; however, their use is controversial.

Sexual contact should be avoided until the patient has normal serologic indicators.

Nursing interventions. Encourage fluids. Chipped ice and soft drinks promote adequate hydration without inducing vomiting.

Record weight daily, and keep accurate intake and output records. Observe feces for color, consistency, frequency, and amount. Watch for signs of hepatic coma, dehydration, pneumonia, vascular problems, and pressure sores.

Patient education. Warn the patient not to drink any alcohol during this time period, and teach him how to recognize signs of recurrence. Refer the patient for follow-up care, as needed.

Advise chronic carriers of hepatitis how to prevent exchange of body fluids during sex. Tell the patient to avoid contact sports while his liver is enlarged.

Evaluation. Optimal hydration and nutrition should be maintained. The patient should follow appropriate isolation precautions and modify diet and lifestyle as needed. He should obtain appropriate follow-up care and his close contacts should have sought evaluation and possible vaccination.

Nonviral hepatitis
Nonviral inflammation of the liver usually results from exposure to certain toxins or drugs. In toxic hepatitis, liver damage usually occurs within 24 to 48 hours after exposure to toxic agents. Alcohol, anoxia, and preexisting liver disease exacerbate the toxic effects of some of these agents. Drug-induced (idiosyncratic) hepatitis may stem from a hypersensitivity reaction, but toxic hepatitis appears indiscriminately with exposure.

Causes. Toxic hepatitis may result from exposure to various hepatotoxins, such as carbon tetrachloride, acetaminophen, trichloroethylene, poisonous mushrooms, or vinyl chloride. Drug-induced hepatitis may result from halothane, sulfonamides, isoniazid, methyldopa, and phenothiazines (cholestasis-induced hepatitis).

Assessment findings. Look for anorexia, nausea and vomiting, jaundice, dark urine, hepatomegaly, and possibly abdominal pain. With the cholestatic form, clay-colored stools and pruritus may occur.

Diagnostic tests. Test results may show elevated serum transaminase levels (AST and ALT), elevated total and direct serum bilirubin levels (with cholestasis), elevated alkaline

RESPIRATORY TRACT

The respiratory tract is divided into upper and lower tracts. The upper respiratory tract consists of the nose, mouth, nasopharynx, oropharynx, laryngopharynx, and larynx. The lower respiratory tract consists of the trachea, bronchi, bronchioles, and alveoli.

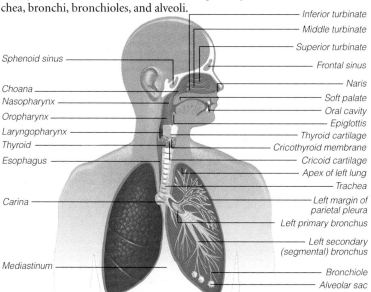

BRONCHIOLES AND ALVEOLI

The primary bronchi divide into bronchioles and then into increasingly smaller branches, such as the terminal and respiratory bronchioles. They terminate in alveolar sacs containing grapelike clusters of tiny air capsules called alveoli.

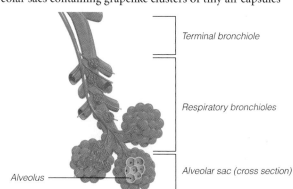

How the Brain Controls Breathing

Higher brain centers stimulate the respiratory centers in the pons and medulla to send impulses down the phrenic nerves to the diaphragm and then to the intercostal nerves and muscles. In the medullary respiratory center, neurons associated with inspiration interact with neurons associated with expiration to control respiratory rate and depth. In the pons, two additional centers interact with the medullary center to regulate rhythm. The apneustic center stimulates inspiratory neurons in the medulla to precipitate inspiration; these, in turn, stimulate the pneumotaxic center, allowing passive expiration.

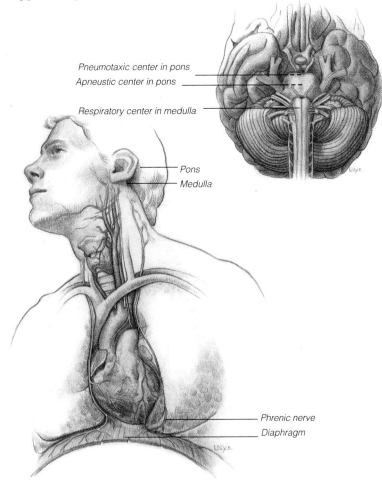

Pneumotaxic center in pons

Apneustic center in pons

Respiratory center in medulla

Pons

Medulla

Phrenic nerve

Diaphragm

HEART

The heart's internal structure consists of four chambers and valves, the pericardium, and three layers of heart wall.

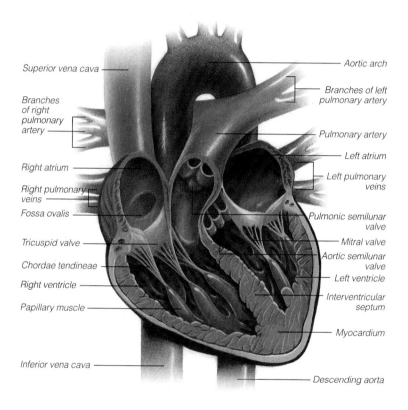

Superior vena cava

Aortic arch

Branches of right pulmonary artery

Branches of left pulmonary artery

Pulmonary artery

Right atrium

Left atrium

Left pulmonary veins

Right pulmonary veins

Fossa ovalis

Pulmonic semilunar valve

Tricuspid valve

Mitral valve

Aortic semilunar valve

Chordae tendineae

Left ventricle

Right ventricle

Interventricular septum

Papillary muscle

Myocardium

Inferior vena cava

Descending aorta

CIRCULATORY SYSTEM

Blood travels through the complex network of blood vessels formed by veins, arteries, and capillaries. This illustration shows the major veins and arteries.

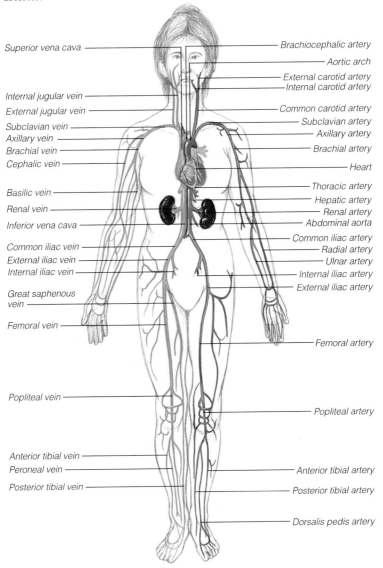

Superior vena cava

Internal jugular vein
External jugular vein
Subclavian vein
Axillary vein
Brachial vein
Cephalic vein

Basilic vein
Renal vein
Inferior vena cava

Common iliac vein
External iliac vein
Internal iliac vein

Great saphenous vein

Femoral vein

Popliteal vein

Anterior tibial vein
Peroneal vein
Posterior tibial vein

Brachiocephalic artery
Aortic arch
External carotid artery
Internal carotid artery
Common carotid artery
Subclavian artery
Axillary artery
Brachial artery

Heart

Thoracic artery
Hepatic artery
Renal artery
Abdominal aorta
Common iliac artery
Radial artery
Ulnar artery
Internal iliac artery
External iliac artery

Femoral artery

Popliteal artery

Anterior tibial artery

Posterior tibial artery

Dorsalis pedis artery

CRANIAL NERVES

The cranial nerves originate in the midbrain, pons, and medulla oblongata. They are assigned Roman numerals from I to XII to indicate the sequence in which they emerge, from the front to the back of the brain.

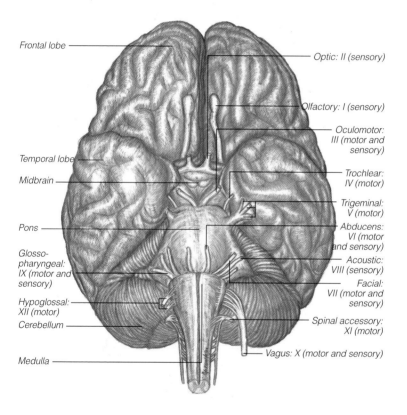

Frontal lobe

Temporal lobe

Midbrain

Pons

Glosso-pharyngeal: IX (motor and sensory)

Hypoglossal: XII (motor)

Cerebellum

Medulla

Optic: II (sensory)

Olfactory: I (sensory)

Oculomotor: III (motor and sensory)

Trochlear: IV (motor)

Trigeminal: V (motor)

Abducens: VI (motor and sensory)

Acoustic: VIII (sensory)

Facial: VII (motor and sensory)

Spinal accessory: XI (motor)

Vagus: X (motor and sensory)

CENTRAL NERVOUS SYSTEM

The central nervous system includes the brain and spinal cord. The brain has four major regions: the cerebrum, diencephalon, cerebellum, and brain stem. The nerves found in the spinal cord are identified by their origin: the cervical, thoracic, lumbar, sacral, and coccygeal nerves.

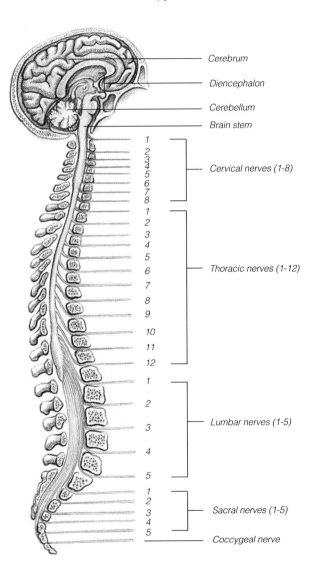

Cerebrum

Diencephalon

Cerebellum

Brain stem

Cervical nerves (1-8)

Thoracic nerves (1-12)

Lumbar nerves (1-5)

Sacral nerves (1-5)

Coccygeal nerve

SKELETAL MUSCLES

The human body contains more than 600 skeletal muscles (muscles that attach to and move bones).

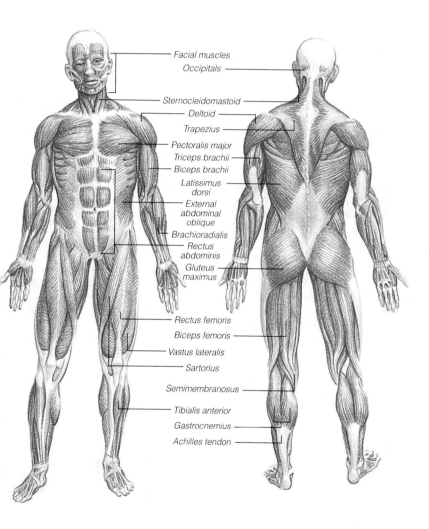

Facial muscles
Occipitals

Sternocleidomastoid
Deltoid
Trapezius

Pectoralis major
Triceps brachii
Biceps brachii
Latissimus dorsi
External abdominal oblique
Brachioradialis
Rectus abdominis
Gluteus maximus

Rectus femoris
Biceps femoris
Vastus lateralis
Sartorius
Semimembranosus
Tibialis anterior
Gastrocnemius
Achilles tendon

SKELETAL SYSTEM

The human skeleton consists of 206 bones and the joints between them.

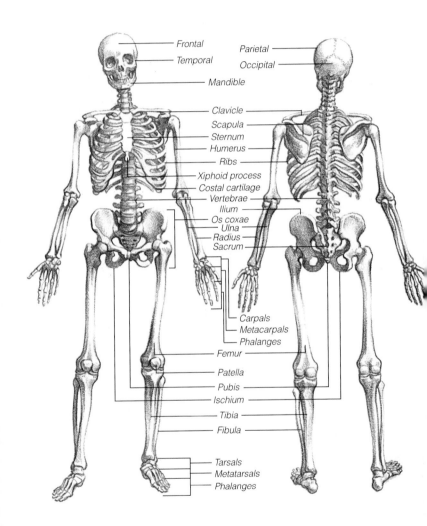

Frontal

Parietal

Temporal

Occipital

Mandible

Clavicle

Scapula

Sternum

Humerus

Ribs

Xiphoid process

Costal cartilage

Vertebrae

Ilium

Os coxae

Ulna

Radius

Sacrum

Carpals

Metacarpals

Phalanges

Femur

Patella

Pubis

Ischium

Tibia

Fibula

Tarsals

Metatarsals

Phalanges

KIDNEY

Shown below are a kidney, in cross section, and a nephron, the basic unit of the kidney.

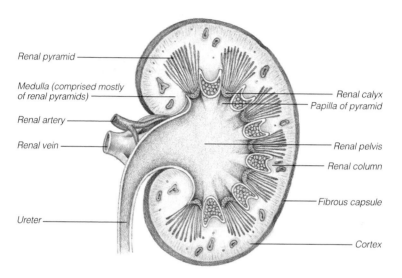

Renal pyramid

Medulla (comprised mostly of renal pyramids)

Renal artery

Renal vein

Ureter

Renal calyx

Papilla of pyramid

Renal pelvis

Renal column

Fibrous capsule

Cortex

Nephron

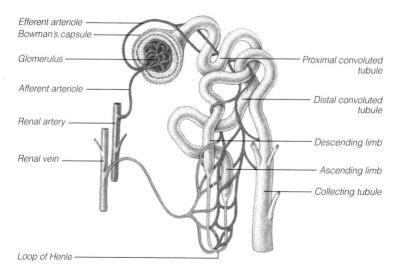

Efferent arteriole

Bowman's capsule

Glomerulus

Afferent arteriole

Renal artery

Renal vein

Loop of Henle

Proximal convoluted tubule

Distal convoluted tubule

Descending limb

Ascending limb

Collecting tubule

GASTROINTESTINAL TRACT

The GI tract is a hollow tube extending from the lips to the anal opening. Along its entire length are associated glands and accessory organs.

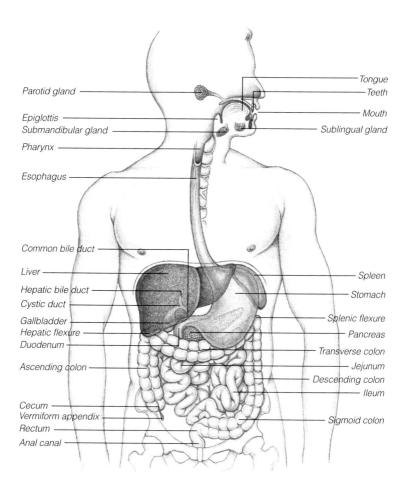

Parotid gland

Epiglottis
Submandibular gland
Pharynx

Esophagus

Common bile duct
Liver
Hepatic bile duct
Cystic duct
Gallbladder
Hepatic flexure
Duodenum
Ascending colon

Cecum
Vermiform appendix
Rectum
Anal canal

Tongue
Teeth
Mouth
Sublingual gland

Spleen
Stomach
Splenic flexure
Pancreas
Transverse colon
Jejunum
Descending colon
Ileum
Sigmoid colon

ENDOCRINE GLANDS

The endocrine glands secrete hormones directly into the blood stream to regulate body function. The illustration below shows their location.

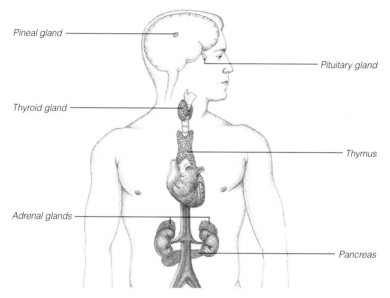

Pineal gland

Pituitary gland

Thyroid gland

Thymus

Adrenal glands

Pancreas

PARATHYROID GLANDS

Four parathyroid glands lie embedded on the posterior surface of the thyroid, one in each corner.

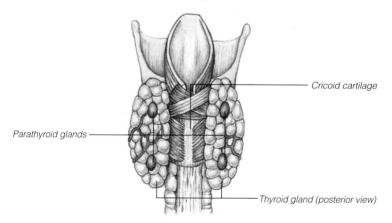

Cricoid cartilage

Parathyroid glands

Thyroid gland (posterior view)

IMMUNE RESPONSE TO BACTERIAL INVASION

Two types of immune responses reinforce the defense by white blood cells: antibody-mediated (humoral) and cell-mediated immunity. Both types involve lymphocytes, which develop into either B cells or T cells. B cells, aided by helper T cells, produce circulating antibody. Effector T cells kill antigen and produce lymphokines that induce inflammation and mediate the delayed hypersensitivity reaction. Suppressor T cells regulate T and B responses.

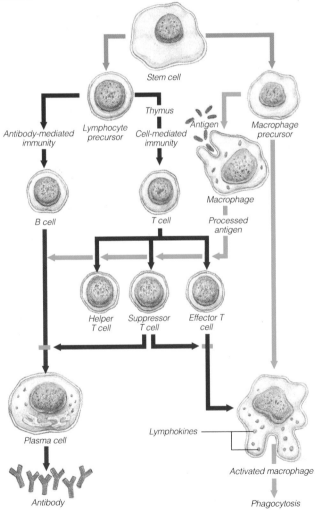

Stem cell

Thymus

Antibody-mediated immunity

Lymphocyte precursor

Cell-mediated immunity

Antigen

Macrophage precursor

Macrophage

B cell

T cell

Processed antigen

Helper T cell

Suppressor T cell

Effector T cell

Plasma cell

Lymphokines

Antibody

Activated macrophage

Phagocytosis

REPRODUCTIVE SYSTEM

The female reproductive system consists of the vagina, uterus, fallopian tubes, and ovaries. Associated structures include the external genitalia and the mammary glands.

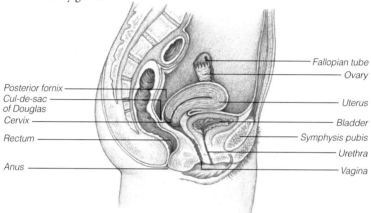

Posterior fornix
Cul-de-sac of Douglas
Cervix
Rectum
Anus

Fallopian tube
Ovary
Uterus
Bladder
Symphysis pubis
Urethra
Vagina

The male reproductive system consists of the testes and accessory organs, which include the epididymis, vas deferens, ejaculatory duct, and urethra. Supporting structures are the scrotum, penis, and spermatic cords.

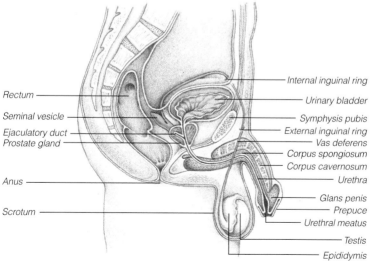

Rectum
Seminal vesicle
Ejaculatory duct
Prostate gland
Anus
Scrotum

Internal inguinal ring
Urinary bladder
Symphysis pubis
External inguinal ring
Vas deferens
Corpus spongiosum
Corpus cavernosum
Urethra
Glans penis
Prepuce
Urethral meatus
Testis
Epididymis

SKIN

Major components of the skin include the epidermis, dermis, and epidermal appendages.

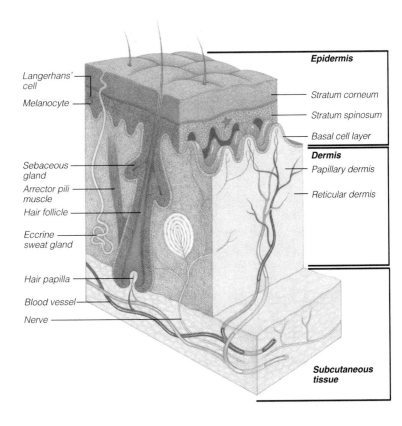

Langerhans' cell

Melanocyte

Sebaceous gland

Arrector pili muscle

Hair follicle

Eccrine sweat gland

Hair papilla

Blood vessel

Nerve

Epidermis

Stratum corneum

Stratum spinosum

Basal cell layer

Dermis

Papillary dermis

Reticular dermis

Subcutaneous tissue

EYE

Structures of the eye include the sclera, cornea, iris, pupil, anterior and posterior chambers, and the retina.

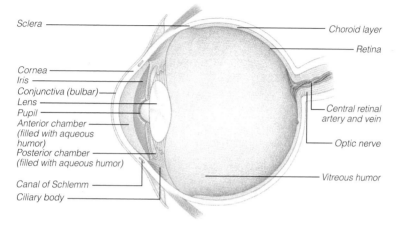

EAR

The ear is divided into three parts: the external, middle, and inner ear.

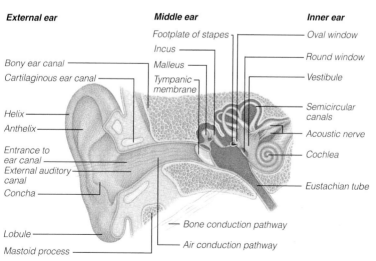

NOSE, MOUTH, AND NECK

The structures of the nose, mouth, and neck are illustrated below.

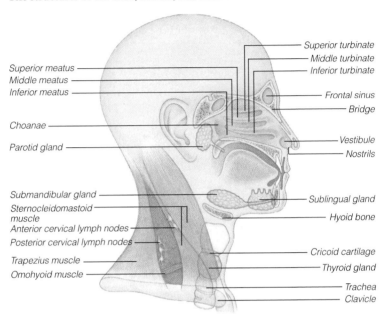

Superior meatus
Middle meatus
Inferior meatus
Choanae
Parotid gland
Submandibular gland
Sternocleidomastoid muscle
Anterior cervical lymph nodes
Posterior cervical lymph nodes
Trapezius muscle
Omohyoid muscle

Superior turbinate
Middle turbinate
Inferior turbinate
Frontal sinus
Bridge
Vestibule
Nostrils
Sublingual gland
Hyoid bone
Cricoid cartilage
Thyroid gland
Trachea
Clavicle

Anterior view of mouth structures

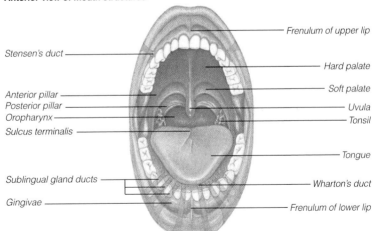

Stensen's duct
Anterior pillar
Posterior pillar
Oropharynx
Sulcus terminalis
Sublingual gland ducts
Gingivae

Frenulum of upper lip
Hard palate
Soft palate
Uvula
Tonsil
Tongue
Wharton's duct
Frenulum of lower lip

phosphatase levels, and elevated WBC count.

Eosinophil levels are increased in drug-induced nonviral hepatitis. Liver biopsy may help identify the underlying disorder, especially if it shows infiltration with WBCs and eosinophils.

Treatment. Effective treatment aims to remove the causative agent by lavage, catharsis, or hyperventilation, depending on the route of exposure. Dimercaprol may serve as an antidote for toxic hepatitis caused by gold or arsenic poisoning but does not prevent other drug-induced hepatitis. Corticosteroids may be ordered for patients with the drug-induced type. Transplant may be an option for selected patients.

Nursing interventions. Care of the patient with hepatitis involves close monitoring for complications of liver failure (bleeding, hepatic coma), maintaining hydration and nutrition, and relieving the patient of nausea, pruritus, and pain.

Patient education. Instruct the patient about the proper use of drugs and the proper handling of cleaning agents and solvents.

Evaluation. The patient should maintain normal nutrition and hydration. He should make lifestyle and dietary changes and seek follow-up care as needed.

Liver cancer

Primary liver tumors are relatively rare. However, the liver is one of the most common sites of metastasis from other primary cancers, particularly colon, rectum, stomach, pancreas, esophagus, lung, and breast cancers and melanoma.

Causes. The cause is unknown, though it may be congenital in children. Adult liver cancer is associated with alcohol-induced, nutritional, and posthepatitic cirrhosis. It may also result from environmental exposure to carcinogens, such as aflatoxins, thorium dioxide (a contrast dye medium formerly used), senecio alkaloids, and possibly androgens and oral estrogens. Exposure to hepatitis B and C viruses increases the risk of liver cancer.

Assessment findings. Clinical features of liver cancer include a mass in the right upper quadrant; tender, nodular liver on palpation; severe pain in the epigastrium or the right upper quadrant; bruit, hum, or rubbing sound if tumor involves a large part of the liver; jaundice; weight loss, weakness, anorexia, or fever; dependent edema; and ascites if portal vein is compressed.

Diagnostic tests. X-ray of the bladder confirms enlargement of the liver. CT scan, magnetic resonance imaging, and ultrasound help localize and delineate lesions. Hepatic arteriography is useful in evaluating tumor vascularity. Biopsy is required for definitive diagnosis. Many surgeons prefer to confirm diagnosis at the time of resection. If necessary, a CT-guided percutaneous needle biopsy is done. Patients with liver cancer may have abnormal liver function tests if no cirrhosis is present. Alpha-fetoprotein is elevated in many patients and is effectively used as a tumor marker.

Treatment. Because liver cancer is commonly in an advanced stage at diagnosis, few hepatic tumors are resectable. A resectable tumor must be solitary, in one lobe, and without cirrhosis, jaundice, or ascites. Resection is done by lobectomy or partial hepatectomy. Liver transplantation, a possibility for some patients, is still experimental. Surgical occlusion or embolization of the hepatic artery deprives the tumor of blood and nutrients, causing tumor regression and necrosis.

Radiation therapy for unresectable tumors is usually palliative. But because of the liver's low tolerance for radiation, this therapy has not increased survival.

Chemotherapy may include systemic administration of 5-fluorouracil, doxorubicin, cisplatin, streptozocin, etoposide, mitomycin C, mitoxantrone, epirubicin, methyl lomustine, or teniposide. For regional infusions, catheters are placed directly into the hepatic artery for continuous infusion of 5-fluorouracil, cisplatin, doxorubicin, mitomycin C, nitrogen mustard, and methotrexate. Permanent implantable pumps may be used for long-term infusion. Intraperitoneal administration of 5-fluorouracil is being investigated.

Appropriate treatment for metastatic cancer of the liver may include lobectomy or chemotherapy (with results similar to those in hepatoma).

Nursing interventions. Your plan of care should emphasize supportive care and emotional support.

To control edema and ascites, you'll need to monitor the patient's diet throughout. Most patients need a special diet that restricts sodium, fluids (no alcohol allowed), and protein. Weigh the patient daily, and record intake and output.

Signs of ascites include peripheral edema, orthopnea, or dyspnea on exertion. If ascites is present, measure and record abdominal girth daily. To increase venous return and prevent edema, elevate the patient's legs whenever possible.

Monitor respiratory function, and note any increase in respiratory rate or shortness of breath.

Watch for hepatic encephalopathy. Many patients develop symptoms of ammonia intoxication, including confusion, restlessness, irritability, agitation, delirium, asterixis, lethargy, and, finally, coma. Monitor the patient's serum ammonia level, vital signs, and neurologic status. Be prepared to control ammonia accumulation with sorbitol, neomycin, lactulose, and sodium polystyrene sulfonate.

Used to relieve obstructive jaundice, a transhepatic catheter requires frequent irrigation with prescribed solution (normal saline solution or sometimes 5,000 U of heparin in 500 ml of dextrose 5% in water). Monitor vital signs frequently for any indication of bleeding or infection.

Evaluation. The patient should receive adequate hydration and nutrition. He and his family should understand the treatment regimen and prognosis, know how to recognize signs of encephalopathy, and understand the need to notify the doctor immediately.

Cirrhosis

Cirrhosis is a chronic disorder marked by diffuse destruction and fibrotic regeneration of hepatic cells. As necrotic tissue yields to fibrosis, cirrhosis alters liver structure and normal vasculature, impairs blood and lymph flow, and ultimately causes hepatic insufficiency.

Causes. *Laënnec's cirrhosis* (also known as portal, nutritional, or alcoholic cirrhosis), the most common type, results from malnutrition, especially of dietary protein, and chronic alcohol ingestion. *Biliary cirrhosis* results from bile duct diseases, whereas *postnecrotic (posthepatitic) cirrhosis* stems from various types of hepatitis. *Pigment cirrhosis* may stem from disorders such as hemochromatosis. *Cardiac cirrhosis* may stem from prolonged elevation of venous pressure in the liver due to chronic right-sided heart failure.

Assessment findings. Palpation below the right costal margin may detect an enlarged liver. Similar examination on the left may detect splenomegaly. Cirrhosis has an insidious onset, causing few symptoms at first. As functioning liver cells diminish and scarring distorts the liver, symptoms occur. Cirrhosis affects many body systems. Assess your patient for these signs and symptoms:
• *GI (usually early and vague)*— anorexia, indigestion, nausea and vomiting, constipation or diarrhea, dull abdominal ache
• *Respiratory*—pleural effusion, limited thoracic expansion
• *Central nervous system*—progressive symptoms of hepatic encephalopathy, including lethargy, mental changes, slurred speech, asterixis (flapping tremor), peripheral neuritis, paranoia, hallucinations, extreme obtundation, and coma
• *Hematologic*—bleeding tendencies (nosebleeds, easy bruising, bleeding gums), anemia
• *Endocrine*—testicular atrophy, menstrual irregularities, gynecomastia, chest and axillary hair loss
• *Skin*—severe pruritus, extreme dryness, poor tissue turgor, abnormal pigmentation, spider angiomas, palmar erythema, possibly jaundice
• *Hepatic*—jaundice, hepatomegaly, ascites, edema of the legs
• *Miscellaneous*—musty breath, enlarged superficial abdominal veins, muscle atrophy, pain in the right upper abdominal quadrant that worsens when the patient sits up or leans forward, palpable liver or spleen, temperature of 101° to 103° F (38.3° to 39.4° C), bleeding from esophageal varices.

Diagnostic tests. Liver biopsy, the definitive test for cirrhosis, reveals destruction and fibrosis of hepatic tissue. Liver scan shows abnormal thickening and a liver mass. These tests also help confirm cirrhosis:

• Cholecystography and cholangiography visualize the gallbladder and the biliary duct system, respectively.

• Splenoportal venography visualizes the portal venous system.

• Percutaneous transhepatic cholangiography differentiates extrahepatic from intrahepatic obstructive jaundice and reveals hepatic disorders and gallstones.

• WBC count, hematocrit, and hemoglobin, albumin, serum electrolyte, and cholinesterase levels are decreased.

• Globulin, serum ammonia, total bilirubin, alkaline phosphatase, AST, ALT, and LD levels are increased.

• Anemia, neutropenia, and thrombocytopenia are present. PT and partial thromboplastin times are prolonged.

• Vitamins A, B_{12}, C, and K, folic acid, and iron levels are decreased.

• Glucose tolerance tests may be abnormal.

• Galactose tolerance and urine bilirubin tests are abnormal.

• Fecal and urine urobilinogen levels are elevated.

Treatment. Therapy aims to remove or alleviate the underlying cause of cirrhosis, to prevent further liver damage, and to prevent or treat complications. The patient may benefit from a high-protein diet, but this may be restricted by developing hepatic encephalopathy. Dietary protein will be adjusted through the course of the illness based on the patient's ability to handle nitrogenous by-products of protein metabolism. Sodium is usually restricted to 200 to 500 mg/day and fluids to 1,000 to 1,500 ml/day.

If the patient's condition continues to deteriorate, he may need tube feedings or TPN. Other supportive measures include supplemental vitamins—A, B complex, C, and K—to compensate for the liver's inability to store them, and vitamin B_{12}, folic acid, and thiamine for anemia. Rest, moderate exercise, and avoiding exposure to infections and toxic agents are essential. When absolutely necessary, antiemetics, such as trimethobenzamide or benzquinamide, may be given for nausea; vasopressin, for esophageal varices; and diuretics, such as furosemide or spironolactone, for edema. However, diuretics require careful monitoring because fluid and electrolyte imbalance may precipitate hepatic encephalopathy.

Paracentesis and infusions of salt-poor albumin may alleviate ascites. A LeVeen shunt may be used. Surgical procedures include sclerotherapy for varices and surgical shunts to relieve portal hypertension. Transplantation is an option for selected patients.

Cirrhosis prevention programs usually emphasize avoiding alcohol.

Nursing interventions. Check skin, gums, stools, and vomitus regularly for bleeding. Apply pressure to injection sites to prevent bleeding.

Observe closely for signs of behavioral or personality changes. Report increasing stupor, lethargy, hallucinations, or neuromuscular dysfunction. Watch for asterixis, a sign of hepatic encephalopathy.

Weigh the patient and measure abdominal girth daily, inspect ankles and sacrum for dependent edema, and accurately record intake and output.

Patient education. Warn the patient against taking aspirin, straining at stool, and blowing his nose or sneezing too vigorously. Suggest using an electric razor and a soft toothbrush.

Tell the patient that rest and good nutrition will conserve energy and decrease metabolic demands on the liver. Urge him to eat frequent, small meals. Stress the need to avoid infections and abstain from alcohol. Refer the patient to Alcoholics Anonymous if necessary.

Evaluation. The patient should maintain normal nutrition and skin integrity. He should adapt his lifestyle and diet to his disorder and understand the need for appropriate follow-up care.

Hepatic coma

Hepatic coma is a neurologic syndrome that develops as a complication of hepatic encephalopathy. This type of coma commonly occurs in patients with cirrhosis, resulting primarily from cerebral ammonia intoxication. It may be acute and self-limiting or chronic and progressive.

Causes. Rising blood ammonia levels may result from portal hypertension (which shunts portal blood past the liver), surgically created portal-systemic shunts, cirrhosis, excessive protein intake, sepsis, constipation or GI hemorrhage, and bacterial action on protein and urea.

Assessment findings. Clinical manifestations of hepatic encephalopathy vary and develop in four stages.
• *Prodromal stage:* Early signs and symptoms are so subtle they're commonly overlooked. They include slight personality changes and a slight tremor.
• *Impending stage:* Tremor progresses into asterixis (liver flap or flapping tremor), the hallmark of hepatic coma. Asterixis is characterized by quick, irregular extensions and flexions of the wrists and fingers when the wrists are held out straight and the hands flexed upward. Lethargy, aberrant behavior, and apraxia also occur.
• *Stuporous stage:* Hyperventilation occurs, and the patient is stuporous but noisy and abusive when aroused.
• *Comatose stage:* Signs include hyperactive reflexes, a positive Babinski's sign, fetor hepaticus (musty, sweet breath odor), and coma.

Diagnostic tests. Elevated venous and arterial ammonia levels, clinical features, and a positive history of liver disease confirm the diagnosis.

EEG shows slow waves as the disease progresses. Other suggestive test results include elevated serum bilirubin levels and prolonged PT.

Treatment. Effective treatment stops advancing encephalopathy by reducing blood ammonia levels. Ammonia-producing substances are removed from the GI tract by administering neomycin to suppress bacterial ammonia production, by using sorbitol to induce catharsis to produce osmotic diarrhea, by continuously aspirating blood from the stomach, by reducing dietary protein intake, and by giving lactulose to reduce blood ammonia levels.

Treatment may include potassium supplements (80 to 120 mEq/day, by mouth or I.V.) to correct alkalosis, especially if the patient is taking diuretics. Sometimes, hemodialysis can temporarily clear toxic blood. Exchange transfusions may provide dramatic but temporary improvement; however, these require a particularly large amount of blood. Salt-poor albumin may be used to maintain fluid and electrolyte balance, replace depleted albumin levels, and restore plasma.

Nursing interventions. Frequently assess and record the patient's LOC. Continually orient him to place and time. Remember to keep a daily record of the patient's handwriting to monitor neurologic deterioration.

Monitor intake, output, and fluid and electrolyte balance. Check daily weight and measure abdominal girth. Watch for, and immedi-

ately report, signs of anemia, infection, alkalosis, and GI bleeding.

Ask the dietary department to provide the specified low-protein diet, with carbohydrates supplying most of the calories. Provide good mouth care.

Promote rest, comfort, and a quiet atmosphere. Discourage stressful exercise. Use restraints, if necessary, but avoid sedatives. Protect the comatose patient's eyes from corneal injury by using artificial tears or eye patches.

Provide emotional support for the patient's family in the terminal stage of hepatic coma.

Evaluation. The patient should have normal hydration and skin integrity. His relatives should express anticipatory grieving and seek appropriate support services.

Gallbladder and biliary tract disorders

This section includes cholecystitis, cholelithiasis, choledocholithiasis, cholangitis, and gallstone ileus.

Cholecystitis, cholelithiasis, and related disorders

Gallbladder and biliary tract disorders are common and frequently painful conditions that usually require surgery and may be life-threatening. They often accompany calculus deposition and inflammation. (See *Understanding gallbladder and biliary tract disorders.*)

Causes. The cause of gallstone formation is unknown, but abnormal

Understanding gallbladder and biliary tract disorders

Cholecystitis, acute or chronic inflammation of the gallbladder, is usually associated with a gallstone impacted in the cystic duct, causing painful distention of the gallbladder. The acute form is most common during middle age; the chronic form, among the elderly. Prognosis is good with treatment.

Cholangitis, infection of the bile duct, is commonly associated with choledocholithiasis and may follow percutaneous transhepatic cholangiography. Widespread inflammation may cause fibrosis and stenosis of the common bile duct and biliary radicles. Prognosis for this rare condition is poor—stenosing or primary sclerosing cholangitis is almost always fatal.

Cholelithiasis, stones or calculi in the gallbladder (gallstones), results from changes in bile components. The leading biliary tract disease, it

affects over 20 million Americans and accounts for the third most common surgical procedure performed in the United States—cholecystectomy. Prognosis is usually good with treatment unless infection occurs, in which case prognosis depends on the infection's severity and response to antibiotics.

Choledocholithiasis occurs when gallstones passed out of the gallbladder lodge in the common bile duct, causing partial or complete biliary obstruction. Prognosis is good unless infection develops.

Gallstone ileus involves small-bowel obstruction by a gallstone. Typically, the gallstone travels through a fistula between the gallbladder and small bowel and lodges at the ileocecal valve. This condition is most common in the elderly. Prognosis is good with surgery.

metabolism of cholesterol and bile salts is a likely cause. Risk factors include:

• a high-calorie, high-cholesterol diet, associated with obesity
• elevated estrogen levels from oral contraceptives, postmenopausal therapy, pregnancy, or multiparity
• use of the antilipemic clofibrate
• diabetes mellitus, ileal disease, hemolytic disorders, liver disease, or pancreatitis.

Assessment findings. In *acute cholecystitis, acute cholelithiasis,* and *choledocholithiasis,* look for a classic

attack with severe midepigastric or right upper quadrant pain radiating to the back or referred to the right scapula, frequently after meals rich in fats. Also note recurring fat intolerance, belching that leaves a sour taste in the mouth, flatulence, indigestion, diaphoresis, nausea, chills and low-grade fever, and possible jaundice and clay-colored stools with common duct obstruction.

In *cholangitis,* look for abdominal pain, high fever and chills, possible jaundice and related itching, weakness, and fatigue.

Where calculi collect

Besides the kidneys and ureters, calculi also may collect at the following sites and may move from one site to another.

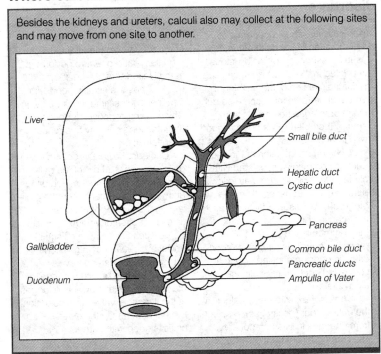

In *gallstone ileus,* look for nausea and vomiting, abdominal distention, absent bowel sounds (in complete bowel obstruction), and intermittent colicky pain over several days.

Diagnostic tests. Ultrasonography reveals calculi in the gallbladder with up to 96% accuracy. Percutaneous transhepatic cholangiography distinguishes between gallbladder disease and cancer of the pancreatic head in patients with jaundice.

ERCP visualizes the biliary tree after endoscopic examination of the duodenum, cannulation of the common bile and pancreatic ducts, and injection of a contrast medium. Technetium-labeled iminodiacetic acid (HIDA) scan of the gallbladder detects obstruction of the cystic duct.

Abdominal X-ray identifies calcified calculi with 15% accuracy. Oral cholecystography shows calculi in the gallbladder and biliary duct obstruction.

Laboratory tests showing an elevated icteric index and elevated total bilirubin, urine bilirubin, and alkaline phosphatase levels support the diagnosis. WBC count is slightly elevated during a cholecystitis attack. Serum amylase levels distinguish gallbladder disease from pancreatitis.

Serial enzyme tests and electrocardiogram should precede other diagnostic tests if heart disease is suspected. (See *Where calculi collect.*)

Treatment. Surgery, usually elective, is the treatment of choice for gallbladder and duct disease. Procedures may include cholecystectomy, cholecystectomy with operative cholangiography, and possibly exploration of the common bile duct. Cholescyctectomy by laparoscopic procedure is the preferred surgical method. Other treatments include a low-fat diet to prevent attacks and vitamin K for itching, jaundice, and bleeding tendencies caused by vitamin K deficiency. Treatment during an acute attack may include insertion of an NG tube and an I.V. line, and antibiotic administration.

A nonsurgical treatment for choledocholithiasis involves insertion of a flexible catheter through the sinus tract into the common bile duct. Guided by fluoroscopy, the doctor directs the catheter toward the stone. A Dormia basket is threaded through the catheter to entrap the calculi.

The relative ease, short length of stay, and cost effectiveness of laparoscopic cholecystectomy have made dissolution (by ursodiol) and lithotripsy less viable options.

Nursing interventions. For information on preoperative and postoperative care of surgical patients, see "Gallbladder surgery," page 516.

Evaluation. The patient should receive adequate hydration and nutrition and have no complications.

Anorectal disorders

This section covers disorders of the anus and rectum, including hemorrhoids, polyps, anorectal abscess, fistulas, strictures, stenoses and contractures, proctitis, and anal fissure.

Hemorrhoids

Hemorrhoids are varicosities in the superior or inferior hemorrhoidal venous plexus. Dilation and enlargement of the superior plexus produces internal hemorrhoids; dilation and enlargement of the inferior plexus produces external hemorrhoids.

Causes. Hemorrhoids result from increased intravenous pressure in the hemorrhoidal venous plexus. Risk factors include occupations that require prolonged standing or sitting; straining due to constipation, diarrhea, coughing, sneezing, or vomiting; heart failure, hepatic disease, alcoholism, and anorectal infections; loss of muscle tone due to old age, rectal surgery, or episiotomy; anal intercourse; and pregnancy.

Assessment findings. Patients may be asymptomatic, but painless, intermittent bleeding during defecation is the characteristic symptom. Other symptoms include pruritus, discomfort and prolapse in response to an increase in intra-abdominal pressure, sudden rectal pain, and a large, firm, subcutaneous lump with thrombosed external hemorrhoids.

Diagnostic tests. Physical examination confirms external hemorrhoids. Proctoscopy confirms internal hemorrhoids and rules out rectal polyps.

Treatment. Typically, treatment aims to ease pain, combat swelling and congestion, and regulate bowel habits. Local swelling and pain can be decreased with local anesthetic agents, astringents, or cold compresses, followed by warm sitz baths or thermal packs. Rarely, the patient with chronic, profuse bleeding may require a blood transfusion.

Other nonsurgical treatments include injection of a sclerosing solution to produce scar tissue that decreases prolapse, manual reduction, and freezing. Techniques used to burn hemorrhoids include laser coagulation and infrared photo coagulation, both of which can be performed in a doctor's office. Hemorrhoidectomy is performed as an ambulatory procedure.

Hemorrhoidectomy, the most effective treatment, is required for most patients with severe bleeding, intolerable pain and pruritus, and large prolapse.

Nursing interventions. Prepare the patient for hemorrhoidectomy. For information, see "Hemorrhoidectomy," page 514.

Patient education. Stress the importance of regular bowel habits and good anal hygiene. Warn against too-vigorous wiping with washcloths and using harsh soaps. Encourage the use of medicated astringent pads and white toilet paper (the fixative in colored paper can irritate the skin).

Advise the patient to relieve constipation by increasing the amount of raw vegetables, fruit, and whole grain cereal in the diet or by using stool softeners. Also tell him to avoid venous congestion by not sitting on the toilet longer than necessary. Teach the patient how to use local medications and to take sitz baths to relieve pain. Instruct the patient to report significant bleeding, increased pain, or fever.

Evaluation. The patient should report a regular bowel elimination pattern, improved diet, and return to normal activity levels.

Polyps

Polyps are masses of tissue that rise above the mucosal membrane and protrude into the large intestine and rectum. Types of polyps include common polypoid adenomas, villous adenomas, familial polyposis, focal polypoid hyperplasia, and juvenile polyps (hamartomas). Most rectal polyps are benign. However, villous and hereditary polyps show a marked inclination to become malignant. Familial polyposis is frequently associated with rectosigmoid adenocarcinoma.

Causes. Polyps are caused by unrestrained cell growth in the upper epithelium. Risk factors include heredity, age (incidence rises after age 70), infection, and diet.

Assessment findings. Patients with polyps are usually asymptomatic, but look for rectal bleeding (most common sign) and diarrhea.

Diagnostic tests. Lower GI endoscopy with rectal biopsy confirms the diagnosis. Stool may be positive for occult blood. Hemoglobin level and hematocrit are low because of bleeding.

Treatment. This varies with the type and size of polyps and their location within the colon. Common polypoid adenomas less than $^3/_8''$ (1 cm) require polypectomy, commonly by fulguration (destruction by high-frequency electricity) during endoscopy. Common polypoid adenomas over $1^1/_2''$ (4 cm) and all invasive villous adenomas are typically treated by abdominoperineal resection. Focal polypoid hyperplasia necessitates local fulguration. Depending upon GI involvement, familial polyposis requires total abdominoperineal resection with a permanent ileostomy, subtotal colectomy with ileoproctostomy, or ileoanal anastomosis.

Nursing interventions. During evaluation, check sodium, potassium, and chloride levels daily as appropriate. Adjust fluid and electrolyte levels, as necessary. Administer normal saline solution with potassium I.V., as ordered. Weigh the patient daily, and record the amount of diarrhea. Watch for signs of dehydration (decreased urine, increased blood urea nitrogen [BUN] levels).

After biopsy and fulguration, check for signs and symptoms of perforation and hemorrhage, such as sudden hypotension, decrease in hemoglobin level or hematocrit, shock, abdominal pain, and passage of red blood through the rectum.

Watch for and record the first bowel movement, which may not occur for 2 to 3 days. Provide sitz baths for 3 days.

For care after ileostomy or subtotal colectomy with ileoproctostomy, see "Bowel surgery with ostomy," page 509.

Patient education. Prepare the patient with precancerous or familial lesions for abdominoperineal resection.

Tell the patient to watch for and report evidence of rectal bleeding. If he has benign polyps, stress the need for routine follow-up studies to check their growth rate.

Evaluation. The patient should have a regular bowel elimination pattern. He should understand the potential for hemorrhage and the need for immediate follow-up care.

Anorectal abscess and fistula

Anorectal abscess appears as a localized collection of pus resulting from inflammation of the soft tissue near the rectum or anus. As the abscess produces more pus, a fistula may form in the soft tissue beneath the muscle fibers of the sphincters, usually extending into the perianal skin. The internal (primary) opening of the abscess or fistula is usually near the anal glands and crypts; the external (secondary) opening, in the perianal skin.

Causes. Typically, the lining of the anal canal, rectum, or perianal skin is abraded or torn by such objects as enema tips or ingested eggshells or fish bones. The injury becomes infected by *Escherichia coli*, staphylococci, or streptococci. The disorder may also be caused by systemic illness such as ulcerative colitis.

Assessment findings. A patient with anorectal abscess characteristically manifests throbbing pain and tenderness at the abscess site; a hard, painful lump that prevents comfortable sitting may also be present.

A patient with anorectal fistula may have pruritic drainage and perianal irritation; a pink, red, elevated, discharging sinus or ulcer on the skin near the anus; possible chills, fever, nausea, vomiting, and malaise, depending on the severity of infection; or a palpable indurated tract, a drop or two of pus, and a depression or ulcer in the midline anteriorly or at the dentate line posteriorly (found on digital examination).

Diagnostic tests. Sigmoidoscopy, barium studies, and colonoscopy may be done to rule out other conditions.

Treatment. Anorectal abscesses require surgical incision to promote drainage. Fistulas require fistulotomy. If the fistula tract is epithelialized, treatment requires fistulectomy—removal of the fistulous tract—followed by insertion of drains, which remain in place for 48 hours.

Nursing interventions. Provide adequate medication for pain relief, as ordered. Examine the wound frequently to assess proper healing.

Instruct the patient to be alert for the first postoperative bowel movement.

Patient education. Stress the importance of perianal cleanliness. Instruct the patient to report significant bleeding, increasing pain, or fever. If a drain is in place, explain about dressing changes and have the patient observe drainage amount and color.

Evaluation. The patient should understand prescribed medications and know how to perform dressing changes and observe drainage.

Rectal prolapse

In rectal prolapse, one or more layers of the rectal mucous membrane protrude through the anus. Prolapse may be complete or partial.

Causes. Rectal prolapse may be caused by weakened sphincters or weakened longitudinal, rectal, or levator ani muscles. Risk factors include conditions affecting the pelvic floor or rectum, including neurologic disorders, injury, tumor, aging, chronic wasting diseases, and nutritional disorders.

Assessment findings. Assess for protrusion of tissue from the rectum, which may occur during defecation or walking. Also check for a persistent sensation of rectal fullness, bloody diarrhea, and pain in the lower abdomen.

In complete prolapse, look for protrusion of the full thickness of the bowel wall and, possibly, the sphincter muscle and for mucosa falling into bulky, concentric folds. In partial prolapse, you may find only partially protruding mucosa and a smaller mass of radial mucosal folds. Asking the patient to strain during the examination may disclose the full extent of prolapse.

Diagnostic tests. Typical clinical features and visual examination confirm the diagnosis.

Treatment. Treatment varies according to the underlying cause. Eliminating the cause (straining, coughing, or nutritional disorders) may be the only treatment necessary. In a child, prolapsed tissue usually diminishes with age. In an older patient, a sclerosing agent may be injected to cause a fibrotic reaction that fixes the rectum in place. Severe or chronic prolapse requires surgical repair.

Nursing interventions. Before surgery, explain possible complications, including permanent rectal incontinence. After surgery, watch for hemorrhage, then for pelvic abscess, fever, pus drainage, pain, rectal stenosis, constipation, or pain on defecation.

Patient education. Teach correct diet and stool-softening regimen. Advise the patient with severe prolapse and incontinence to wear a perineal pad.

Teach perineum-strengthening exercises: Have the patient lie down, with his back flat on the mattress; then ask him to take a deep breath and pull in his abdomen and squeeze. Or have the patient repeatedly squeeze and relax his buttocks while sitting on a chair.

Evaluation. The patient should have adequate rectal mucosal integrity and maintain a regular bowel elimination pattern. He should report that he performs perineum-strengthening exercises and has modified his diet as needed.

Proctitis

An acute or chronic inflammation of the rectal mucosa, proctitis has a good prognosis unless hemorrhage occurs.

Causes. Many factors contribute to proctitis, including chronic constipation, habitual laxative use, emotional upset, radiation (especially for cancer of the cervix and of the uterus), endocrine dysfunction, rectal injury, rectal medications, bacterial infections, allergies (especially to milk), vasomotor disturbance that interferes with normal muscle control, and food poisoning.

Assessment findings. Assess your patient for tenesmus, constipation, a feeling of rectal fullness, or cramps in the left abdomen. He may have an intense urge to defecate, which produces a small stool that may contain blood and mucus.

Diagnostic tests. Sigmoidoscopy confirms the diagnosis. In chronic proctitis, sigmoidoscopy shows thickened mucosa, loss of vascular pattern, and stricture of the rectal lumen. A biopsy to rule out carcinoma may be performed, and bacteriologic examination may be necessary.

Treatment. Primary treatment aims to remove the underlying cause (fecal impaction or laxatives or other medications). Soothing enemas or steroid (hydrocortisone) suppositories or enemas may be helpful in radiation-induced proctitis. Tranquilizers may be appropriate.

Nursing interventions. Offer reassurance during rectal examinations and treatment.

Patient education. Tell the patient to watch for and report bleeding and other persistent symptoms. Fully explain proctitis and its treatment to help him understand the disorder and prevent its recurrence.

Evaluation. The patient should be free from exacerbating factors. He should report an increased comfort level, understand the potential for hemorrhage, and know when to seek immediate care.

Anal fissure

In anal fissure, the lining of the anus develops a laceration or crack that extends to the circular muscle. An anal fissure may be an acute or chronic condition.

Causes. Anal fissure may be caused by the passage of large, hard stools that severely stretch the anal lining and by strain on the perineum during childbirth (anterior fissure). Occasionally, it may result from proctitis, anal tuberculosis, or carcinoma; rarely, from scar stenosis (anterior fissure).

Assessment findings. A patient with acute anal fissure may show tearing, cutting, or burning pain during or immediately after a bowel movement; drops of blood seen on toilet paper or underclothes; painful anal sphincter spasms, and pain and bleeding on digital examination.

A patient with chronic anal fissure may show scar tissue that hampers normal bowel evacuation and pain and bleeding on digital examination.

In both cases, the fistula may be seen upon eversion by gentle traction on perianal skin.

Diagnostic tests. Anoscopy revealing a longitudinal tear helps establish the diagnosis.

Treatment. This varies with the severity of the tear. For superficial fissures without hemorrhoids, forcible digital dilation of anal sphincters under local anesthesia stretches the lower portion of the ana' sphincter. For complicated fissures, treatment includes surgical excision of tissue, adjacent skin, and mucosal tags, and division of internal sphincter muscle from external.

Nursing interventions. Prepare the patient for rectal examination, and explain the necessity of the procedure. Provide hot sitz baths, warm soaks, and local anesthetic ointment to relieve pain.

Patient education. Teach the patient to eat a high-fiber diet and drink plenty of fluids.

Evaluation. The patient should report a regular bowel elimination pattern and an increased comfort level, and modification of his diet to prevent constipation.

TREATMENTS

GI dysfunction presents many treatment challenges. These include tumors, hyperactivity and hypoactivity, malabsorption, infection and inflammation, vascular disorders, intestinal obstruction, and degenerative disease. Treatments for these disorders include drug therapy, surgery, and related measures.

Drug therapy

Among the commonly used GI drugs are antacids, such as calcium carbonate and aluminum hydroxide; digestants such as pancrelipase; antiflatulents such as simethicone; H_2 blockers such as cimetidine; anticholinergics, such as dicyclomine and anisotropine; antidiarrheal

agents such as bismuth subgallate; laxatives such as bisacodyl; emetics such as ipecac; and antiemetics such as metoclopramide. Some of these drugs, such as antacids and antiemetics, provide relief immediately. Other drugs, such as laxatives and H_2 blockers, may take several days or longer to ameliorate the problem.

Surgery

Laparoscopic techniques for GI surgery have resulted in reduced lengths of stay. However, not all GI problems can be corrected with minimally invasive surgery. Following major GI surgery, a patient may need special support to make permanent and difficult changes in his lifestyle. For example, besides teaching a colostomy patient about stoma care, you'll also have to help him adjust to body-image changes. Or, you'll have to draw on your own emotional strengths to help a patient through a lengthy bowel training program.

Esophageal surgeries

Surgery may be necessary to manage a constriction or provide palliative care for an incurable disease such as advanced esophageal cancer. In one common laparoscopic procedure, Nissen fundoplication, the lower esophageal sphincter is repaired through several small puncture wounds made in the abdomen. The upper part of the stomach fundus is used to wrap around the lower esophageal sphincter. The Belsey Mark IV procedure involves going through the chest and bringing the stomach up into the chest cavity where the fundoplication is performed. Other esophageal surgeries include cardiomyotomy, cricopharyngeal myotomy, esophagectomy, esophagogastrostomy, and esophagomyotomy. The surgical approach is through the neck, chest, or abdomen, depending on the location of the problem.

Serious complications may follow esophageal surgeries. For example, mediastinitis may result from leakage of esophageal contents into the thorax. Severe inflammation can produce obstruction of the mediastinal structures, such as the superior vena cava, the tracheobronchial tree, and the esophagus. The patient is also at risk for aspiration pneumonia.

Patient preparation. Explain the procedure to the patient. Inform him that when he awakens from the anesthetic he'll probably have an NG tube inserted to aid feeding and relieve abdominal distention. Discuss possible postoperative complications and measures to prevent or minimize them. Warn him of the risk of aspiration pneumonia. Demonstrate coughing and deep-breathing exercises, and show the patient how to splint his incision.

Monitoring and aftercare. After surgery, place the patient in semi-Fowler's position to help minimize esophageal reflux. Provide antacids as needed for symptomatic relief.

If surgery involving the upper esophagus produces hypersalivation, the patient may be unable to swallow the excess saliva. Control drooling with gauze wicks or suctioning. Place an emesis basin within reach.

To reduce the risk of aspiration pneumonia, elevate the head of the patient's bed and encourage him to turn frequently. Carefully monitor his vital signs and auscultate his lungs. Encourage coughing and deep-breathing exercises.

Watch for developing mediastinitis, especially if surgery involved extensive thoracic invasion (as in esophagogastrostomy). Note and report fever, dyspnea, and complaints of substernal pain. If ordered, give antibiotics.

Watch for signs of leakage at the anastomosis site. Check drainage tubes for blood, test for occult blood in stool and drainage, and monitor hemoglobin levels for evidence of slow blood loss. If the patient has an NG tube in place, avoid handling the tube because this may damage the internal sutures or anastomoses. (See *Documenting NG tube drainage.*) Avoid deep suctioning in a patient who has undergone extensive esophageal repair.

Patient education. Advise the patient to sleep with his head elevated to prevent reflux. Suggest that he use three pillows or raise the head of his bed on blocks.

If the patient smokes, encourage him to stop. Explain that nicotine adversely affects the lower esophageal sphincter. Advise the patient to avoid alcohol, aspirin, and effervescent over-the-counter products (such as Alka-Seltzer) because they may damage the tender esophageal mucosa.

Also advise him to avoid heavy lifting, straining, and coughing.

Instruct him to report any respiratory symptoms, such as wheezing, coughing, and nocturnal dyspnea.

Hernia repair

Hernia surgery includes herniorrhaphy or hernioplasty. Herniorrhaphy, for inguinal and other abdominal hernias, returns the protruding intestine to the abdominal cavity, repairing the abdominal wall defect. Laparoscopic hernia repair is done on an ambulatory or one-night stay basis. Hernioplasty corrects larger hernias by reinforcing the weakened area around the repair with plastic, steel, or wire.

If the patient is having elective surgery, recovery is usually rapid; without complications, he may return home the day of surgery and usually resume normal activities within 4 to 6 weeks. Emergency herniorrhaphy may be required to reduce a strangulated hernia and prevent ischemia and gangrene. In this case, he may be hospitalized from 7 to 10 days.

Patient preparation. Explain to the patient that this procedure will relieve the discomfort caused by his hernia. If he's having elective surgery, tell him he may return home the day of surgery and resume normal activities in 4 to 6 weeks. If he's having emergency surgery for a strangulated or incarcerated hernia, explain that he may be hospitalized for a longer period and may have an NG tube in place

CHARTING TIPS

Documenting NG tube drainage

When documenting intake and output, don't forget to include the drainage from the patient's nasogastric (NG) tube. If the tube is clamped and the patient develops nausea and vomits before the tube is unclamped, don't forget to include the amount of vomitus on the intake and output record as well.

Equally important, remember to document any irrigating solutions that you instilled through the NG tube on the input record.

for several days before he's allowed to eat or get out of bed.

Before surgery, shave the surgical site and administer a cleansing enema and a sedative.

Monitoring and aftercare. Teach the patient how to reduce pressure on the incision site (for example, how to get up from a lying or sitting position). Teach him how to splint his incision when he coughs or sneezes.

Encourage early ambulation, but warn against bending, lifting, or other strenuous activities. Make sure the patient voids within 12 hours after surgery.

Provide comfort measures. Administer analgesics, as ordered.

Regularly check the dressing for drainage and the incision site for inflammation or swelling. Assess the patient for other symptoms of infection. Report possible infection to the doctor, and expect to administer antibiotics, as ordered.

Patient education. Instruct the patient to avoid lifting, bending, and pushing or pulling movements for 8 weeks after surgery or until his doctor allows them. Tell him to watch for and report signs and symptoms of infection, including fever, chills, diaphoresis, malaise, and lethargy as well as pain, inflammation, swelling, and drainage at the incision site. Instruct him to keep the incision clean and covered until the sutures are removed.

Stress the importance of regular follow-up examinations. If the patient's job involves heavy lifting or other strenuous activity, encourage him to think about changing jobs.

Gastric surgeries

Gastric surgery is used to remove diseased or malignant tissue or to relieve an obstruction or perforation. In an emergency, it may be performed to control severe GI hemorrhage or perforation. Surgery may also be necessary when laser endoscopic coagulation for control of severe GI bleeding isn't possible.

Gastric surgeries are varied. For example, a partial gastrectomy reduces the amount of acid-secreting mucosa. A bilateral vagotomy relieves ulcer symptoms and eliminates vagal nerve stimulation of gastric secretions. A pyloroplasty improves drainage and prevents obstruction. Most commonly, two gastric surgeries are combined, such

as vagotomy with gastroenterostomy or vagotomy with antrectomy.

Gastric surgery carries the risk of serious complications, including hemorrhage, obstruction, dumping syndrome, paralytic ileus, vitamin B_{12} deficiency, and atelectasis.

Patient preparation. Before surgery, evaluate and begin stabilizing the patient's fluid and electrolyte balance and nutritional status—which may be severely compromised. Monitor intake and output, and draw serum samples for hematologic studies. As ordered, begin I.V. fluid replacement and parenteral nutrition. Also as ordered, prepare the patient for abdominal X-rays. On the night before surgery, administer cleansing laxatives and enemas, as necessary. On the morning of surgery, insert an NG tube.

Monitoring and aftercare. Follow these directions:
• When the patient awakens from surgery, place him in low or semi-Fowler's position.
• Check the patient's vital signs every 2 hours until his condition stabilizes. Periodically check the wound site, NG tube, and abdominal drainage tubes for bleeding.
• Maintain tube feedings or TPN, and I.V. fluid and electrolyte replacement therapy, as ordered. Monitor blood studies daily. Monitor and record intake and output, including NG tube drainage.
• Auscultate the abdomen daily for bowel sounds. When they return, notify the doctor, who'll order

clamping or removal of the NG tube and gradual resumption of oral feeding. During NG tube clamping, watch for nausea and vomiting; if they occur, unclamp the tube immediately and reattach it to suction.

• Throughout recovery, have the patient cough, deep-breathe, and change position frequently.

• Assess for other complications, including vitamin B_{12} deficiency, anemia (especially common following total gastrectomy), and dumping syndrome, a potentially serious digestive complication marked by weakness, nausea, flatulence, and palpitations within 30 minutes after a meal.

Patient education. Tell the patient to notify the doctor immediately if he has any signs of life-threatening complications, such as hemorrhage, obstruction, or perforation.

Explain dumping syndrome and how to avoid it. Advise the patient to eat small, frequent meals evenly spaced throughout the day and to drink fluids between meals rather than with them. In his diet, he should decrease intake of carbohydrates and salt while increasing fat and protein. After a meal, he should lie down for 20 to 30 minutes. As needed, teach the patient and his family how to give tube feedings.

Advise the patient to avoid or limit foods high in fiber.

Encourage the patient and his family to identify and eliminate stress at home and in the workplace. Advise the patient to avoid smoking.

Bowel surgery with ostomy

In bowel surgery with ostomy, the surgeon removes diseased colonic and rectal segments and creates a stoma on the outer abdominal wall to allow fecal elimination. This surgery is performed for such intestinal maladies as inflammatory bowel disease, familial polyposis, diverticulitis, and advanced colorectal cancer if conservative surgery and other treatments aren't successful.

The surgeon can choose from several types of surgery. For instance, intractable obstruction of the colon requires permanent colostomy and removal of the affected bowel segments. Cancer of the rectum and lower sigmoid colon commonly calls for abdominoperineal resection, which involves creation of a permanent colostomy and removal of the remaining colon, rectum, and anus. (See *Reviewing types of ostomies*, page 510.)

Perforated sigmoid diverticulitis, rectovaginal fistula, and penetrating trauma commonly require temporary colostomy. After healing occurs (usually within 6 to 8 weeks), the divided segments are anastomosed to restore bowel integrity and function. In a double-barrel colostomy, the transverse colon is divided and both ends are brought out through the abdominal wall to create a proximal stoma for fecal drainage and a distal stoma leading to the nonfunctioning bowel. Loop colostomy, done to relieve acute obstruction in an emergency, involves creating proximal and distal stomas from a loop of intestine that has been

Reviewing types of ostomies

The type of ostomy depends on the patient's condition. Temporary ones, such as a double-barrel or loop colostomy, help treat perforated sigmoid diverticulitis, penetrating trauma, and other conditions in which intestinal healing is expected.

Permanent colostomy or ileostomy typically accompanies extensive abdominal surgery such as for removal of a malignant tumor.

Ileostomy

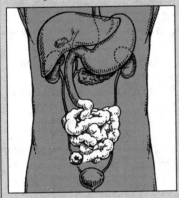

Permanent colostomy

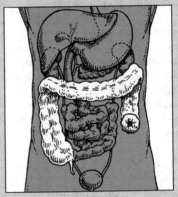

Loop colostomy

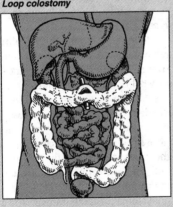

Double-barrel colostomy

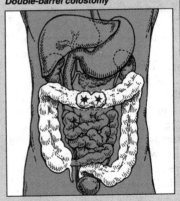

pulled through an abdominal incision and supported with a plastic or glass rod.

Severe, widespread colonic obstruction may require total or near-total removal of the colon and rectum and creation of an ileostomy from the proximal ileum. A permanent ileostomy requires that the patient wear a drainage pouch or bag over the stoma to receive the constant fecal drainage. In contrast, a continent, or Kock, ileostomy doesn't require an external pouch.

Common complications of ostomies include hemorrhage, sepsis, ileus, and fluid and electrolyte imbalance from excessive drainage through the stoma. The skin around the stoma may be excoriated from contact with acidic digestive enzymes in the drainage, and irritation may result from pressure of the ostomy pouch. Excoriation occurs more commonly with an ileostomy than with a colostomy because of the greater acidity of fecal drainage.

Ostomates commonly exhibit depression and anxiety related to altered body image and worries about lifestyle changes associated with the stoma and ostomy pouch.

Patient preparation. Before surgery, arrange for the patient to visit with an enterostomal therapist. The therapist can also help him select the best location for the stoma.

Evaluate the patient's nutritional and fluid status before surgery (if time permits). Typically, the patient will be receiving TPN to prepare him for the physiologic stress of surgery. Record the patient's fluid intake and output and weight daily, and watch for early signs of dehydration. Expect to draw periodic blood samples for hematocrit and hemoglobin determinations. Be prepared to transfuse blood if ordered.

Monitoring and aftercare. After surgery, carefully monitor intake and output and weigh the patient daily. Maintain fluid and electrolyte balance, and watch for signs of dehydration (decreased urine output, poor skin turgor) and electrolyte imbalance. Provide analgesics, as ordered. Be especially alert for pain in the patient with an abdominoperineal resection.

Note and record the color, consistency, and odor of fecal drainage from the stoma. If the patient has a double-barrel colostomy, check for mucus drainage from the inactive (distal) stoma. The nature of fecal drainage is determined by the type of ostomy surgery; generally, the less colon tissue is removed, the more closely drainage will resemble normal stool. For the first few days after surgery, fecal drainage probably will be mucoid (and possibly slightly blood-tinged) and mostly odorless. Report excessive blood or mucus content, which could indicate hemorrhage or infection.

Observe the patient for signs of peritonitis or sepsis, caused by bowel contents leaking into the abdominal cavity. Patients receiving antibiotics or TPN are at an increased risk for sepsis.

Provide meticulous wound care, changing dressings often. Check dressings and drainage sites frequently for signs of infection (purulent drainage, foul odor) or fecal drainage. If the patient has had an abdominoperineal resection, irrigate the perineal area, as ordered.

Regularly check the stoma and surrounding skin for irritation and excoriation, and take corrective measures. Also observe the stoma's appearance. The stoma should look smooth, cherry red, and slightly edematous; immediately report any discoloration or excessive swelling, which may indicate circulatory problems that could lead to ischemia.

Don't neglect the patient's emotional needs. Encourage him to express his feelings and concerns; reassure an anxious or depressed patient that these common postoperative reactions should subside. Continue to arrange for visits by an enterostomal therapist if possible.

Patient education. If the patient has a colostomy, teach him or a caregiver how to apply, remove, and empty the pouch. When appropriate, teach him how to irrigate the colostomy with warm tap water to gain some control over elimination. Reassure him that he can regain continence with dietary control and bowel retraining.

Instruct the colostomy patient to change the stoma appliance as needed, to wash the stoma site with warm water and mild soap every 3 days, and to change the adhesive layer. These measures help prevent skin irritation and excoriation.

If the patient has an ileostomy, instruct him to change the drainage pouch only when leakage occurs. Also emphasize meticulous skin care and use of a protective skin barrier around the stoma site.

Discuss dietary restrictions and suggestions to prevent stoma blockage, diarrhea, flatus, and odor. Tell the patient to stay on a low-fiber diet for 6 to 8 weeks and to add new foods to his diet gradually.

Identify foods that cause odor, such as corn, dried beans, onions, cabbage, fish, and spicy dishes. Some vitamin and mineral supplements and antibiotics may also cause odor. Suggest that the patient use an ostomy deodorant or an odorproof pouch if he includes odor-producing foods in his diet.

Trial and error will help the patient determine which foods cause gas. Gas-producing fruits and vegetables include apples, melons, avocados, beans, corn, and cabbage.

The patient is susceptible to fluid and electrolyte losses. He must drink plenty of fluids, especially in hot weather or when he has diarrhea. Suggest fruit juice and bouillon, which contain potassium. Warn the patient to avoid alcohol, laxatives, and diuretics.

Tell the patient to report persistent diarrhea through the stoma.

If the patient had an abdominoperineal resection, suggest sitz baths to help relieve perineal discomfort. Recommend refraining from intercourse until the perineum heals.

Encourage the patient to discuss his feelings about resuming sexual relations. Mention that the drainage pouch won't dislodge if the device is empty and fitted properly. Suggest avoiding food and fluids for several hours before intercourse.

Remind the patient and his family that depression commonly occurs after ostomy surgery. Recommend counseling if depression persists.

Bowel resection and anastomosis

Resection of diseased intestinal tissue (colectomy) and anastomosis of the remaining segments help treat localized obstructive disorders, including diverticulosis, intestinal polyps, bowel adhesions, and malignant or benign intestinal lesions. This procedure is the preferred surgical technique for localized bowel cancer, but not for widespread carcinoma, which usually requires massive resection with creation of a temporary or permanent colostomy or an ileostomy.

The patient who undergoes simple resection and anastomosis usually retains normal bowel function. Still, he's at risk for postoperative complications, including bleeding from the anastomosis site, peritonitis and resultant sepsis, wound infection, and atelectasis.

Patient preparation. Before surgery, as ordered, administer antibiotics and laxatives or enemas.

Monitoring and aftercare. Follow these guidelines:
• For the first few days after surgery, carefully monitor the patient's intake, output, and weight daily. Maintain fluid and electrolyte balance through I.V. replacement therapy, and check regularly for signs of dehydration, such as decreased urine output and poor skin turgor.
• Keep the NG tube patent. Warn the patient that, if the tube becomes dislodged, he should never attempt to reposition it himself; doing so could damage the anastomosis.
• Carefully monitor the patient's vital signs and closely assess his overall condition. Because anastomotic leakage may produce only vague symptoms initially, watch for low-grade fever, malaise, slight leukocytosis, and abdominal distention and tenderness. Also be alert for more extensive hemorrhage from acute leakage; watch for signs and symptoms of hypovolemic shock (precipitous drop in blood pressure and pulse rate, respiratory difficulty, decreased LOC) and bloody stool or wound drainage.
• Observe the patient for signs of peritonitis or sepsis, caused by leakage of bowel contents into the abdominal cavity. He's at increased risk for sepsis if he's receiving antibiotics or TPN. To prevent sepsis, provide frequent mouth and tube care.
• Provide meticulous wound care, changing dressings often. Frequently check dressings and drainage sites for signs of infection (purulent drainage, foul odor) and fecal drainage. Watch for sudden fever, especially when accompanied by abdominal pain and tenderness.
• Regularly assess the patient for signs of postresection obstruction. Examine the abdomen for distention and rigidity, auscultate for bowel sounds, and note the passage of any flatus or feces.
• Once the patient regains peristalsis and bowel function, help him avoid constipation and straining during defecation. Encourage him to drink plenty of fluids, and administer a stool softener or other laxatives, as ordered. Note and record the fre-

quency, character, and amount of all bowel movements.

• Encourage regular coughing and deep breathing to prevent atelectasis; remind the patient to splint the incision site as necessary.

Patient education. Instruct the patient to record the frequency and character of bowel movements and to tell the doctor if he notices any changes in his normal pattern. Warn against using laxatives without consulting his doctor.

Caution the patient to avoid abdominal straining and heavy lifting until the sutures are completely healed and the doctor allows him. Instruct him to maintain the prescribed semibland diet until his bowel has healed completely (usually 4 to 8 weeks after surgery). Stress the need to avoid carbonated beverages and gas-producing foods.

Emphasize the importance of taking prescribed vitamin supplements.

Hemorrhoidectomy

Hemorrhoidectomy involves removing hemorrhoidal varicosities through various methods including cauterization (infrared coagulation or electric current) and laser. Excision, the most effective treatment for intolerable hemorrhoidal pain, excessive bleeding, or large prolapse, is used when conservative measures fail.

Though uncomplicated, hemorrhoidectomy risks one potentially serious complication—hemorrhage. This risk is greatest during the first 24 hours after surgery and then

again after 7 to 10 days when the tissue sloughs off. Hemorrhoidectomy is contraindicated in patients with blood dyscrasias or certain GI cancers, or during the first trimester of pregnancy.

Postoperative healing of delicate rectoanal tissues can be slow and painful.

Patient preparation. The patient receives instructions prior to surgery, which includes following a full liquid diet prior to surgery and self-administration of an enema on the morning of the procedure. He is also instructed to clean the perineal area.

Monitoring and aftercare. After surgery, position the patient comfortably in bed, and support his buttocks with pillows if necessary. Encourage him to shift position regularly and to lie prone for 15 minutes every few hours to reduce edema at the surgical site.

• Keep alert for hemorrhage and hypovolemic shock. Monitor vital signs every 2 to 4 hours, check and record intake and output, and assess for signs of fluid volume deficit.

• Check the dressing regularly, and immediately report any excessive bleeding or drainage.

• Make sure the patient voids within 24 hours after surgery.

• Clean the perianal area with warm water and a mild soap to prevent infection and irritation, and gently pat the area dry. After spreading petroleum jelly on the wound site to prevent skin irritation, apply a wet dressing (a 1:1 solution of cold water and witch hazel) to the perianal area.

• As needed, give analgesics and sitz baths or hot compresses to reduce local pain, swelling, and inflammation and to prevent rectoanal spasms.

• Explain that he needs to pass stools shortly after surgery to dilate the anus and prevent the formation of strictures during wound healing.

Patient education. Before discharge, teach the patient proper perianal hygiene: wiping gently with soft, white toilet paper (dyes in colored paper may cause irritation), cleaning with mild soap and warm water, and applying a sanitary pad. Encourage him to take sitz baths three to four times daily and after each bowel movement to reduce swelling and discomfort. Instruct him to report increased rectal bleeding, purulent drainage, fever, constipation, or rectal spasm. Use of a stool softener is recommended.

Stress the importance of regular bowel habits. Provide tips on avoiding constipation, including regular exercise and adequate intake of dietary fiber and fluids. Warn against overusing stool-softening laxatives; however, fiber supplements may be necessary.

Appendectomy

With rare exceptions, the only effective treatment for acute appendicitis is to remove the inflamed vermiform appendix. A common emergency surgery, appendectomy aims to prevent imminent rupture or perforation of the appendix. When

completed before these complications can occur, this procedure is usually effective and uneventful. Laparoscopy is successfully used to perform uncomplicated appendectomies. If the appendix ruptures or perforates before surgery, life-threatening peritonitis may result.

Patient preparation. Before surgery, reduce the patient's pain by placing him in Fowler's position. Avoid giving analgesics, which can mask the pain that heralds rupture. *Never* apply heat to the abdomen or give cathartics or enemas; these measures could trigger rupture.

Monitoring and aftercare. As soon as possible, depending on the type of anesthetic used, the patient should be placed in a Fowler's position to decrease the risk of any contaminated peritoneal fluid infecting the upper abdomen. Carefully monitor his vital signs and record intake and output for 2 days after surgery. Auscultate the abdomen for bowel sounds, which signal the return of peristalsis.

Regularly check the wound dressing for drainage, and change it as necessary. If abdominal drains are in place, check and record the amount and nature of drainage, and maintain drain patency.

Encourage ambulation within 8 hours after surgery if possible. Assist the patient as needed. Encourage coughing, deep breathing, and frequent position changes. After bowel sounds return, gradually resume oral foods and fluids.

Assess the patient closely for signs of peritonitis. Watch for and report continuing pain and fever, excessive wound drainage, hypotension, tachycardia, pallor, weakness, and other signs and symptoms of infection and fluid and electrolyte loss. If peritonitis develops, expect to assist with emergency treatment, including GI intubation, parenteral fluid and electrolyte replacement, and antibiotic therapy.

Patient education. The patient with an uncomplicated laparoscopic appendectomy will be discharged on the evening of surgery or the next day. Abdominal appendectomies (uncomplicated) are discharged within 48 to 72 hours. Instruct the patient to watch for and immediately report fever, chills, diaphoresis, nausea, vomiting, or abdominal pain and tenderness. Encourage him to keep his scheduled follow-up appointments to monitor healing and detect any developing complications. Most patients can resume normal activities within 2 to 3 weeks.

Gallbladder surgery

Gallbladder removal, or *cholecystectomy*, restores biliary flow in gallstone disease (cholecystitis or cholelithiasis). Cholecystectomy is one of the most commonly performed surgeries. Conventional cholecystectomy requires a large incision and produces considerable discomfort, and patients require weeks of recovery time.

Following *laparoscopic laser cholecystectomy*, patients are usually discharged from the hospital and are able to resume a normal diet after 24 to 36 hours. Typically, patients can return to the workplace after 2 to 3 days. Laparoscopic laser cholecystectomy is contraindicated in pregnancy as well as in acute cholangitis, septic peritonitis, and severe bleeding disorders.

Alternatives to cholecystectomy include *cholecystostomy* (incision into the fundus of the gallbladder to remove and drain any retained gallstones or inflammatory debris) and *choledochotomy* (incision into the common bile duct to remove any gallstones or other obstructions).

Complications of gallbladder surgery, though unusual, can be life-threatening. Peritonitis may arise from obstructed biliary drainage and resultant bile leakage into the peritoneum. Postcholecystectomy syndrome, marked by fever, jaundice, and pain, may occur. Postoperative atelectasis may result from impaired respiratory excursion.

Patient preparation. Monitor and, if necessary, help stabilize the patient's nutritional status and fluid balance. Administer vitamin K, blood transfusions, or glucose and protein supplements, as ordered. For 24 hours before surgery, give the patient clear liquids only.

Monitoring and aftercare. After laparoscopic laser cholecystectomy, follow these guidelines:
• Watch for anesthesia-related nausea and vomiting.

• Be aware that the small stab wounds closed with staples may have small dressings.

• To alleviate right shoulder pain caused by phrenic irritation from carbon dioxide under the diaphragm, apply heat to the shoulder. To decrease discomfort, place the patient in semi-Fowler's position. Early ambulation also helps.

• The patient may usually eat a light meal the same evening.

• The day after discharge, the ambulatory surgery nurse should phone the patient's home to follow-up on his progress.

After conventional surgery, follow these guidelines:

• Place the patient in low Fowler's position. If an NG tube is being used, attach it to low intermittent suction. Monitor the amount and character of drainage from the NG tube as well as from any abdominal drains. Check the dressing frequently and change it as necessary.

• If the patient has a T tube in place, frequently assess the position and patency of the tube and drainage bag. Make sure the bag is level with the abdomen to prevent excessive drainage. Also note the amount and character of drainage; bloody or blood-tinged bile usually occurs for only the first few hours after surgery. Provide meticulous skin care around the tube insertion site to prevent irritation.

• After a few days, expect to remove the NG tube and begin introducing foods: first liquids, then gradually soft solids. As ordered, clamp the T tube for an hour before and after each meal to allow bile to travel to the intestine to aid digestion.

• Watch for signs of postcholecystectomy syndrome (such as fever, abdominal pain, and jaundice) and other complications involving obstructed bile drainage. For several days after surgery, monitor vital signs and record intake and output every 8 hours. Report unusual signs to the doctor, and collect urine and stool samples for laboratory analysis of bile content.

• Help the patient to ambulate on the first postoperative day, unless contraindicated. Have him cough, deep-breathe, and perform incentive spirometry every 4 hours; as ordered, provide analgesics to ease discomfort. Assess respiratory status every 3 hours to detect hypoventilation and signs of atelectasis.

Patient education. After laparoscopic laser cholecystectomy, give written instructions to the patient on the use of analgesics, how to clean the surgical stab sites, and when to call the doctor. Recommend activity as tolerated, but tell the patient to avoid heavy lifting for about 2 weeks. Many patients return to a normal schedule within 8 to 10 days. The patient will be given a follow-up appointment within 7 days for removal of the staples. Scarring is usually minimal.

After conventional surgery, if the patient is being discharged with a T tube in place, stress the need for meticulous tube care. Tell him to immediately report any signs or symptoms of biliary obstruction:

fever, jaundice, pruritus, pain, dark urine, and clay-colored stools.

Instruct the patient to maintain a diet low in fats and high in carbohydrates and protein. Tell him that his ability to digest fats will improve. As this occurs, usually within 6 weeks, he may gradually add fats to his diet.

Liver transplantation

For the patient with a life-threatening liver disorder that doesn't respond to any other treatment, a liver transplant is the last resort. Transplant surgery is reserved for those terminally ill patients with a realistic chance of surviving the surgery and postoperative complications. Candidates include patients with congenital biliary abnormalities, inborn errors of metabolism, or end-stage liver disease.

Many qualified transplant candidates are awaiting suitable donor organs, but few survive the wait. If a compatible healthy liver is located and transplantation performed, the patient faces many obstacles to recovery, including a risk of tissue rejection.

The outcome for liver transplantation has improved considerably. The survival rate has increased, largely as a result of improved immunosuppressants that inhibit rejection response.

Patient preparation. Transplant candidates become active participants with the nurse coordinator who helps arrange the specialty teams. These teams include medical, surgical and hepatology, anesthesia, nephrology, cardiology, social workers, and mental health care professionals.

Before transplant surgery, address the patient's (and the family's) emotional needs. Discuss the stages of emotional adjustment to a liver transplant: overwhelming relief and elation at surviving the operation, followed by—as complications set in—anxiety, frustration, and depression. The transplant coordinators should provide teaching packets that include patient education material.

Monitoring and aftercare. Focus your aftercare on maintaining immunosuppressant therapy to combat tissue rejection; monitoring for early signs of rejection and other complications; preventing opportunistic infections, which can lead to rejection; and providing emotional support throughout the prolonged recovery period.

Patient education. Teach the patient and his family to recognize and immediately report early indicators of tissue rejection. These include pain and tenderness in the right upper quadrant, right flank, or center of the back; fever; tachycardia; jaundice; and changes in the color of urine or stool.

Instruct them to watch for and report any signs or symptoms of liver failure, such as abdominal distention, bloody stool or vomitus, decreased urine output, abdominal pain and tenderness, anorexia, or altered LOC.

Advise the patient to avoid contact with any person who has or may have a contagious illness. Emphasize the importance of reporting any early signs or symptoms of infection, including fever, weakness, lethargy, and tachycardia.

Urge the patient to strictly comply with the prescribed immunosuppressive drug regimen. Explain that noncompliance can trigger rejection, even of a liver that has been functioning well for years. Also warn about adverse effects of immunosuppressive therapy, such as infection, fluid retention, acne, glaucoma, diabetes, and cancer.

Emphasize the importance of regular follow-up examinations. These will be continued until the transplant team discharges the patient into the care of the primary care doctor. If appropriate, suggest that the patient and the family seek psychological counseling.

Liver resection or repair

Resection or repair of diseased or damaged liver tissue may be indicated for various hepatic disorders, including cysts, abscesses, tumors, and lacerations or crush injuries from blunt or penetrating trauma. Usually surgery is performed only after conservative measures prove ineffective.

Liver resection procedures include a partial or subtotal hepatectomy (excision of a portion of the liver) and lobectomy (excision of an entire lobe). Lobectomy is the surgery of choice for primary liver tumors, but partial hepatectomy may be effective for small tumors.

However, because liver cancer is usually advanced at diagnosis, few tumors are resectable. Only single tumors confined to one lobe are considered resectable, and then only if the patient is free from complicating cirrhosis, jaundice, or ascites.

Surgery usually is performed through a thoracoabdominal incision. As a result, it carries many of the risks associated with both thoracic and abdominal surgery, such as atelectasis, ascites, and renal failure. What's more, impaired liver function due to surgery can result in such diverse complications as hypoglycemia, hypovolemia, and hepatic encephalopathy. And acute hemorrhage remains a threat during and after surgery.

Patient preparation. Explain the procedure and the purpose of coagulation studies, blood chemistry tests, arterial blood gas analysis, and blood typing and crossmatching. Depending on the results of these tests, give fluid and electrolyte replacements, transfuse blood or blood components, or provide protein supplements, as ordered. Encourage rest and good nutrition and provide vitamin supplements, as ordered.

Prepare the patient for additional diagnostic tests, which may include liver scan, CT scan, ultrasonography, percutaneous needle biopsy, hepatic angiography, and cholangiography.

Explain postoperative care measures. Tell the patient he'll awaken from surgery with an NG tube, a chest tube, and hemodynamic lines in place. If possible, allow the patient to visit the intensive care unit.

To reduce the risk of postoperative atelectasis, encourage the patient to practice coughing and deep-breathing exercises.

Monitoring and aftercare. Follow these guidelines:
• After surgery, frequently assess for complications, such as hemorrhage and infection. Monitor the patient's vital signs and evaluate fluid status every 1 to 2 hours. Report any signs of volume deficit, which could indicate intraperitoneal bleeding. Keep an I.V. line patent for possible emergency fluid replacement or blood transfusion. Provide analgesics, as ordered.
• At least daily, check laboratory test results for hypoglycemia, increased PT, increased ammonia levels, azotemia (increased BUN and creatinine levels), and electrolyte imbalances (especially potassium, sodium, and calcium imbalances). Promptly report adverse findings and take corrective steps, as ordered. For example, give vitamin K I.M. to decrease PT, or infuse hypertonic glucose solution to correct hypoglycemia.
• Check wound dressings often and change them as needed. Note and report excessive bloody drainage on the dressings or in the drainage tube. Also note the amount and character of NG tube drainage; excessive drainage could trigger metabolic alkalosis. If the patient has a chest tube in place, maintain tube patency by milking it as necessary, and make sure the suction equipment is operating properly.
• Encourage the patient to cough, deep-breathe, and change position frequently. Regularly auscultate his lungs and report any adventitious breath sounds.
• Watch for symptoms of hepatic encephalopathy: confusion, forgetfulness, lethargy or stupor, and hallucinations. Observe for asterixis, apraxia, and hyperactive reflexes.
• Throughout the recovery period, promote rest and relaxation, and provide a quiet atmosphere. Help the patient to ambulate, as ordered.

Patient education. Advise the patient that adequate rest and good nutrition conserve energy and speed healing. For the first 6 to 8 months after surgery, he should gradually resume normal activities, balance periods of activity and rest, and avoid overexertion.

As ordered, instruct the patient to maintain a high-calorie, high-carbohydrate, and high-protein diet during this period to help restore the liver mass. However, if the patient had hepatic encephalopathy, advise him to follow a low-protein diet, with carbohydrates making up the balance of caloric intake.

Emphasize the importance of follow-up examinations.

LeVeen shunt insertion

Intractable ascites resulting from chronic liver disease can be controlled by draining ascitic fluid from the abdominal cavity into the superior vena cava, using the LeVeen peritoneovenous shunt.

Commonly used with diuretic therapy, the LeVeen shunt provides an effective alternative to traditional treatments for ascites such as paracentesis. However, it can cause potentially serious complications, such as ascitic fluid leakage from incisions, wound infection, subcutaneous bleeding, disseminated intravascular coagulation (DIC), and heart failure. These complications, serious in any patient, are even more threatening to a patient with chronic liver disease.

Patient preparation. Show the shunt to the patient and describe how it works. Tell him that he'll receive a local anesthetic to prevent discomfort during shunt insertion. Before surgery, measure and record the patient's weight and abdominal girth to serve as a baseline.

Monitoring and aftercare. Follow these guidelines:
• After the patient returns from surgery, place him in low- or semi-Fowler's position, whichever he prefers, and give analgesics, as ordered.
• Monitor vital signs frequently, and watch for hypervolemia or hypovolemia. As ordered, administer an I.V. or I.M. diuretic such as furosemide to reduce fluid retention. Check and record intake and output hourly for the first 24 hours after surgery, then daily until discharge. Measure abdominal girth and weight daily; compare the findings with baseline data to assess fluid drainage.

• As ordered, draw serum samples for a complete blood count; serum electrolyte, creatinine, albumin, and BUN levels; and other studies. Monitor the results of these tests and notify the doctor of any abnormalities.
• Teach the patient to use the blow bottle four times daily, for at least 15 minutes at a time. As ordered, apply an abdominal binder for the first 24 hours after surgery. Tell the patient that these measures raise intra-abdominal pressure and enhance ascitic fluid drainage.
• Regularly check the incision site for bleeding, swelling, inflammation, drainage, and hematoma, and change dressings as needed. Also be alert for signs of heart failure, DIC, and GI bleeding.

Patient education. Instruct the patient to continue using the blow bottle for as long as the shunt is in place. Tell him to avoid putting pressure on the shunt to prevent clot formation and shunt occlusion.

Advise the patient to watch for and immediately report bleeding or drainage from the incision site as well as fever, chills, diaphoresis, or other signs of infection. Stress the importance of regular follow-up examinations.

Portal-systemic shunting

A portal-systemic shunt reduces portal pressure and prevents or controls bleeding from esophageal varices in patients with intractable portal hypertension. Typically, portal-systemic shunting is performed if more conservative measures fail.

If possible, it's done after esophageal bleeding is controlled and the patient's condition stabilized. However, emergency surgery may be necessary if esophagogastric tamponade or vasopressor drugs can't control hemorrhage.

Three types of portal-systemic shunting are performed. *Portacaval shunting,* the most common, diverts blood from the portal vein to the inferior vena cava, thereby reducing portal pressure. *Splenorenal shunting,* used in portal vein obstruction and when hypersplenism accompanies portal hypertension, diverts blood from the splenic vein to the left renal vein. *Mesocaval shunting,* indicated in portal vein thrombosis, previous splenectomy, or uncontrollable ascites, routes blood from the superior mesenteric vein to the inferior vena cava.

Portal-systemic shunting is complicated and risky. For example, diverting large amounts of blood into the inferior vena cava may cause pulmonary edema and ventricular overload. And shunting of blood away from the liver inhibits the conversion of ammonia to urea, possibly causing hepatic encephalopathy, which can progress rapidly to hepatic coma and death. Other possible complications include hemorrhage leading to peritonitis, and respiratory complications.

Portal-systemic shunting has a mortality of 25% to 50%. In fact, research suggests that the surgery does little to prolong survival; patients are more likely to succumb to hepatic complications than to uncontrolled esophageal bleeding.

Patient preparation. In emergencies, you'll need to focus on stabilizing the patient's condition and helping to control bleeding. If surgery is planned, however, explain the procedure to him and discuss what he can expect after surgery and during the recovery period. Inform him that he'll return from surgery with an NG tube and chest tube in place. He'll also be connected to a cardiac monitor and have pulmonary artery, arterial, and central venous pressure catheters in place to monitor hemodynamic status. Tell him to expect frequent vital sign checks and neurologic assessments.

If the patient's esophageal varices and portal hypertension are related to alcoholism, explain the need to stop drinking. As appropriate, refer the patient to a local chapter of Alcoholics Anonymous.

Monitoring and aftercare. Careful postoperative assessment can help you detect complications and perhaps even prevent death. For 48 to 72 hours after surgery, closely monitor the patient's fluid balance. At least hourly, check his vital signs and record intake and output. Monitor cardiac output and other hemodynamic measurements. Auscultate the patient's lungs at least every 4 hours to detect signs of pulmonary edema such as crackles.

Observe for neurologic changes, such as lethargy, disorientation, apraxia, or hyperreflexia, which may indicate hepatic encephalopathy and developing hepatic coma. As ordered, draw a serum sample to determine ammonia levels. Also as ordered, draw blood for liver function and electrolyte studies.

Encourage the patient to cough, deep-breathe, and change position at least once every hour. Teach him how to use an incentive spirometer.

Patient education. Explain to the patient that although surgery has stopped the bleeding and reduced the risk of future rupture, it has not corrected the underlying liver disease. Urge the patient to comply with his prescribed dietary and drug regimens, including strict abstention from alcohol. Also stress the need for adequate rest to reduce the risk of bleeding and infection.

Tell the patient and his family to watch for and immediately report disorientation, lethargy, amnesia, slurred speech, asterixis, apraxia, and hyperreflexia. Explain that these signs and symptoms may herald hepatic encephalopathy, a potentially fatal complication.

Stress the importance of regular follow-up examinations.

Endoscopic retrograde sphincterotomy

First used to remove retained gallstones from the common bile duct after cholecystectomy, endoscopic retrograde sphincterotomy (ERS) is now also used to treat high-risk patients with biliary dyskinesia and to insert biliary stents for draining malignant or benign strictures in the common bile duct.

In this procedure, a fiber-optic endoscope is advanced through the stomach and duodenum to the ampulla of Vater. A papillotome is passed through the endoscope to make a small incision to widen the biliary sphincter. If the stone does not drop out into the duodenum on its own, the doctor may introduce a Dormia basket, a balloon, or a lithotriptor through the endoscope to remove or crush the stone.

ERS allows treatment without general anesthesia or a surgical incision, ensuring a quicker and safer recovery. Complications of ERS include hemorrhage, transient pancreatitis, cholangitis, and sepsis.

Patient preparation. Explain the treatment to the patient, and answer any questions he may have. Tell him his throat will be sprayed with an anesthetic to avoid discomfort during the insertion and that he may also receive a sedative to help him relax. Reassure him that the sphincterotomy should cause little or no discomfort.

Position him on the fluoroscopy table in a left side-lying position, with his left arm behind him. Encourage him to relax and, if ordered, administer a sedative.

Monitoring and aftercare. After treatment, take steps to help the patient maintain good pulmonary hygiene. Instruct him to cough, deep-breathe, and expectorate regularly to avoid aspirating secretions. Keep in mind that the anesthetic's effects may hinder expectoration and swallowing. Withhold food and fluids until the anesthetic wears off and the patient's gag reflex returns.

Check the patient's vital signs frequently and monitor carefully for signs of hemorrhage: hematemesis, melena, tachycardia, and hypotension. If any of these signs develops, notify the doctor immediately.

Observe for other complications. Cholangitis, for instance, produces hyperbilirubinemia, high fever and chills, abdominal pain, jaundice, and hypotension. Pancreatitis may be marked by abdominal pain and rigidity, vomiting, low-grade fever, tachycardia, diaphoresis, and elevated serum amylase levels. If you note any complications, call the doctor and prepare to draw serum samples for culture and sensitivity studies and to administer antibiotics, as ordered.

Patient education. Instruct the patient to immediately report any signs of hemorrhage, sepsis, cholangitis, or pancreatitis. Advise him to report any recurrence of jaundice and pain from biliary obstruction. He may need repeat ERS to remove new stones or replace a malfunctioning biliary stent.

Intubation

Nasoenteric, esophageal, and other specialized tubes may be used to treat acute intestinal obstruction, bleeding esophageal varices, and other GI dysfunctions.

Nasoenteric decompression

In nasoenteric decompression, a doctor or a specially trained nurse inserts a long, weighted nasoenteric tube through the patient's stomach and into the intestinal tract. Peristalsis propels the tube through the intestine down to, and possibly through, the obstruction, thereby relieving it.

Nasoenteric decompression is used along with fluid and electrolyte replacement as the initial treatment for acute intestinal obstruction resulting from polyps, adhesions, fecal impaction, volvulus, or localized carcinoma. It usually relieves the obstruction, especially in the small intestine.

Use of nasoenteric tubes for decompression is less common than formerly. Many doctors believe decompression can be achieved with an NG tube.

If paralytic ileus occurs as a post-surgical complication, the nasoenteric tube may remain in place for several weeks. However, if the patient fails to improve, or if his condition deteriorates, bowel resection may be necessary.

This procedure can also be performed to aspirate gastric contents or to prevent GI upset after abdominal surgery, but possible complications include reflex esophagitis, nasal or oral inflammation, and nasal or laryngeal ulcers. Rarely, atelectasis and pneumonia may result. And excessive intestinal drainage can produce acid-base imbalance or malposition of the tube within the intestine. Fortunately, these complications can be prevented by scrupulous postoperative care.

Patient preparation. Explain the procedure to the patient. Tell him he'll feel mild discomfort as the doctor advances the tube, but he'll be given a mild sedative if intubation proves difficult or painful.

Gather and prepare the equipment. If you're using a Cantor tube, inject the proper amount of mercury into the balloon. If you're using a Miller-Abbott tube, inflate the balloon and check for leaks. Be sure to deflate the balloon completely before insertion; it will be filled with mercury only after it passes through the pylorus and into the duodenum.

After preparing the equipment, place the patient in semi-Fowler's position and help him to relax.

Before intubation, remove the patient's dentures or bridgework.

Monitoring and aftercare. Once the tube is inserted the premeasured distance (or until it meets an obstruction), its location is confirmed with abdominal X-rays. If these confirm proper tube placement, secure the tube to prevent it from advancing further or being pulled out. (Don't tape the tube directly to the patient's skin; wrap it with gauze, then tape the gauze to the cheek.) As ordered, connect the tube to intermittent suction.

The patient with a nasoenteric tube in place requires special care and continuous monitoring. Frequently check the tube's patency and the effectiveness of intestinal suction and decompression. Note and record the amount and nature of drainage.

Mucus tends to plug the openings of these tubes. You'll need to irrigate the tubes as ordered to maintain patency.

Regularly check the patient's vital signs and assess his fluid and electrolyte status. Record his intake and output and watch for signs of fluid imbalance, such as decreased urine output, poor skin turgor, skin and mucous membrane dryness, lethargy, and fever.

Monitor for acid-base imbalance. Watch for signs and symptoms of metabolic alkalosis (altered LOC, slow and shallow respirations, hypertonic muscles, and tetany) or metabolic acidosis (dyspnea, disorientation and, later, weakness, malaise, and deep, rapid respirations). Also watch for signs and symptoms of secondary infection, such as fever and chills.

Provide mouth care and moisten the nostril openings with petroleum jelly at least every 4 hours. Check for the presence of bowel sounds, decreased abdominal distention, flatus, or a spontaneous bowel movement, which indicate the return of peristalsis. If these signs occur, notify the doctor and assist with tube removal.

Esophagogastric tamponade

Esophagogastric tamponade is an emergency treatment in which insertion of a multilumen esophageal tube helps to control esophageal or gastric hemorrhage resulting from ruptured varices. The most commonly used esophageal tubes include the Minnesota, the Linton, and the Sengstaken-Blakemore tubes.

The tube is inserted through a nostril, or sometimes through the mouth, and then passed through the esophagus into the stomach. The tube's esophageal and gastric balloons are inflated to exert pressure on the varices and stop bleeding, while a suction lumen allows esophageal and gastric contents to be aspirated.

An NG tube may also be used to aspirate oral secretions and to check for bleeding above the esophageal balloon. Balloon inflation pressures are monitored by a pressure gauge.

Typically, the balloons are deflated within 48 hours, after measures have been taken to identify and control the source of the bleeding. Balloon inflation for more than 48 hours may produce further hemorrhage.

Other potential complications include airway obstruction from tube migration or balloon rupture and tissue necrosis at the insertion site.

Patient preparation. Place the patient in semi-Fowler's position to aid gastric emptying and prevent aspiration of vomitus. However, if the patient is unconscious, position him on his left side with the head of the bed raised about 15 degrees.

Next, gather and prepare the equipment: an esophageal tube (as ordered), an NG tube, an irrigation set, a piston syringe, a bulb syringe, a large basin with ice, a water-soluble lubricant, four hemostats, a small sponge block or a football helmet with face mask, a Hoffman clamp, and adhesive tape.

Make sure a suction machine is on hand and in good working order. Keep emergency resuscitation equipment readily available. Tape a pair of scissors to the head of the bed to cut the tube in case of acute respiratory distress.

Check the balloons for air leaks and the tubes for patency. Before intubation, remove the patient's dentures or bridgework.

Monitoring and aftercare. Follow these care guidelines:
• Never leave the patient unattended during esophagogastric tamponade. Closely monitor his condition and the tube's lumen pressure. If pressure changes or drops, notify the doctor immediately before attempting reinflation or pressure readjustment. Check vital signs every 30 to 60 minutes; changes may indicate new bleeding or other complications.
• As ordered, maintain drainage and suction on the esophageal and gastric aspiration ports to prevent fluid accumulation. Irrigate the gastric aspiration port with normal saline solution to prevent clogging.
• Watch for signs of respiratory distress while the esophageal tube is in place. If it develops, have someone else notify the doctor. Then quickly pinch the tube at the patient's nose

and cut it with scissors. Next, remove the tube.

• Be alert for esophageal rupture, heralded by signs of shock, increased respiratory difficulty, and increased bleeding. Rupture can occur at any time but is most common during intubation or esophageal balloon inflation. Be prepared to transfuse blood if needed.

• Keep the patient warm and comfortable. Instruct him to remain as still and quiet as possible; if ordered, administer a sedative to help him relax. Provide frequent mouth and nose care, applying a water-soluble ointment to the nostrils to prevent tissue irritation and pressure sores.

• When bleeding has been controlled, assist the doctor with tube removal.

REFERENCES AND READINGS

Centers for Disease Control and Prevention. *Prevention of Hepatitis A Through Active or Passive Immunization: Advisory Committee on Immunization Practices (ACIP).* MMWR Recommendations and Reports, CDC publication, December 27, 1996.

Forkner, D. "Clinical Pathways: Benefits and Liabilities," *Nurse Management* (11):35-38, November 1996.

Granisetron Approved for Chemotherapy-induced Vomiting. Electronic Publication. Reprinted from Medical Sciences Bulletin, Pharmaceutical Information Associates, Ltd., March 1994. URL: http://pharminfo.com/pubs/msb.

Greenberg, P. *Fecal Occult Blood Testing in Patients Taking Low-Dose Aspirin for Cardiovascular Disease.* Proceedings of the Annual Scientific Meeting of the American College of Gastroenterology, October 21, 1996.

H. pylori Breath Test Receives FDA Clearance. Electronic Publication. Reprinted from Medical Sciences Bulletin, Pharmaceutical Information Associates, Ltd., December 1996. URL: http://aaac.org/cln/profiles/96profiles/12/indpro9602.html.

Ignativicius, D., and Hausman, K. *Clinical Pathways for Collaborative Practice.* Philadelphia: W.B. Saunders Co., 1995.

Ignativicius, et al. *Medical-Surgical Nursing: A Nursing Process Approach.* Philadelphia: W.B. Saunders Co., 1995.

Kosche, K. *C. difficile in the Elderly.* Proceedings of the Annual Scientific Meeting of the American College of Gastroenterology, October 21, 1996.

Letters from the Specific Carbohydrate Diet Support Group. Electronic Publication. URL: http://www.inform.dk/djembe.

Lilley, L., et al. *Pharmacology and the Nursing Process.* St. Louis: Mosby–Year Book, Inc., 1996.

Malarkey, L., and McMorrow, M. *Nurse's Manual of Laboratory Tests and Diagnostic Procedures.* Philadelphia: W.B. Saunders Co., 1996.

National Digestive Disease Information Clearinghouse. *Gastroesophageal Reflux Disease.* NIH Publication No. 94-882, September 1994.

National Digestive Disease Information Clearinghouse. *Stomach and Duodenal Ulcers.* NIH Publication No. 95-38, January 1995.

Nedrud, J., and Czinn, S. "Update on *Helicobacter pylori*," *Current Opinion in Gastroenterology* 12(1):62-67, January 1996.

Nursing98 Drug Handbook. Springhouse, Pa.: Springhouse Corp., 1998.

Oral Granisetron Antiemetic for High Dose Chemotherapy. Electronic Publication. Reprinted from Medical Sciences Bulletin, Pharmaceutical Information Associates, Ltd., May 1995. URL: http://pharminfo.com/pubs/msb.

Polanski, A., and Tatro, S. *Core Principles and Practice of Medical-Surgical Nursing.* Philadelphia: W.B. Saunders Co., 1996.

Sackier, J. "New Applications of Laparoscopy in Gastrointestinal Surgery," *American Family Physician* 53(1):237-42, January 1996.

Table, F., et al. *Laparoscopic Cholecystomy in the Elderly.* Electronic publication: URL: http://pharminfo.com/cgi~bin.

10

ENDOCRINE CARE

Endocrine disorders may affect the patient's growth and development, reproductive system, energy level, metabolic rate, or ability to adapt to stress. Many of these disorders, such as Cushing's syndrome or goiter, can cause disfigurement. Others such as diabetes mellitus may require extensive lifestyle changes.

ASSESSMENT

To thoroughly assess the endocrine system, you must take an accurate health history—including family history—and conduct a physical examination.

Physical examination

A physical examination should include a total body evaluation and a complete neurologic assessment. Begin by measuring the patient's vital signs, height and weight. Then, to obtain the most objective findings, inspect, palpate, and auscultate the patient.

Inspection

Continue your physical assessment by systematically inspecting the patient's overall appearance and examining all areas of his body.

General appearance. Assess the patient's physical appearance and mental and emotional status. Note such factors as overall affect, speech, level of consciousness (LOC) and orientation, appropriateness and neatness of dress and grooming, and activity level. Evaluate general body development, including posture, body build, body proportion, and distribution of body fat.

Skin, hair, and nails. Assess the patient's overall skin color, and inspect the skin and mucous membranes for any lesions or areas of increased, decreased, or absent pigmentation. Consider racial and ethnic variations. In a dark-skinned patient, color variations are best assessed in the sclera, conjunctiva, mouth, nail beds, and palms. Next, assess skin texture and hydration.

Inspect the patient's hair for amount, distribution, condition, and texture. Assess scalp and body hair, looking for abnormal patterns of growth or loss. Again, consider normal racial, ethnic, and sexual differences in hair growth and texture. Then, check the patient's fingernails for cracking, peeling, separation from the nail bed (onycholysis), and clubbing, and the toenails for fungal infection, ingrown nails, discoloration, length, and thickness.

Head and neck. Assess the patient's face for overall color and presence of erythematous areas, especially in the cheeks. Note facial expression. Note the shape and symmetry of the eyes and look for eyeball protrusion, incomplete eyelid closure, or periorbital edema. Have the patient extend his tongue, and inspect it for color, size, lesions, positioning, and any tremors or unusual movements.

Standing in front of the patient, examine the neck—first with it held straight, then slightly extended, and finally while the patient swallows water. Check for neck symmetry and midline positioning and for symmetry of the trachea.

Chest. Evaluate the overall size, shape, and symmetry of the chest, noting any deformities. In females, assess the breasts for size, shape, symmetry, pigmentation (especially on the nipples and in skin creases), and nipple discharge (galactorrhea). In males, observe for bilateral or unilateral breast enlargement

(gynecomastia) and nipple discharge.

Genitalia. Inspect the patient's external genitalia—particularly the testes and clitoris—for normal development.

Extremities. Inspect the patient's arms and hands for tremors. To do so, have him hold both arms outstretched in front with the palms down and fingers separated. Then place a sheet of paper on the outstretched fingers and watch for any trembling. Note any muscle wasting, especially in the upper arms, and have him grasp your hands to assess his grip.

Next, inspect the legs for muscle development, symmetry, color, and hair distribution. Then, assess muscle strength by having the patient sit on the edge of the examination table and extend the legs horizontally. A patient who can maintain this position for 2 minutes usually exhibits normal strength. Examine the feet for size, and note any lesions, corns, calluses, or marks made from socks or shoes. Inspect the toes and the spaces between them for maceration and fissures.

Palpation

Use the following guidelines to palpate the thyroid gland and testes.

In many patients, you may not be able to palpate the thyroid gland. But if you can, it should be smooth, finely lobulated, nontender, and either soft or firm. If palpable, you should be able to feel the gland's sections.

Palpating the thyroid

To palpate the thyroid *from the front,* stand in front of the patient and place your index and middle fingers below the cricoid cartilage on both sides of the trachea. Palpate for the thyroid isthmus as he swallows. Then ask the patient to flex his neck to the side being examined as you gently palpate each lobe. In most cases, you'll feel only the isthmus connecting the two lobes. However, if the patient has a thin neck, you may feel the whole gland. If he has a short, stocky neck, you may have trouble palpating even an enlarged thyroid.

To locate the right lobe, use your right hand to displace the thyroid cartilage slightly to your left. Hook your left index and middle fingers around the sternocleidomastoid muscle to palpate for thyroid enlargement. Then examine the left lobe, using your left hand to displace the thyroid cartilage and your right hand to palpate the lobe.

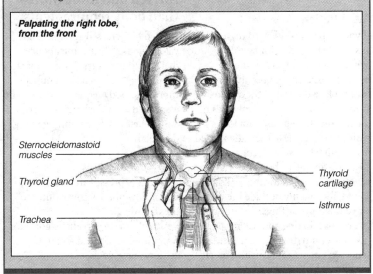

Palpating the right lobe, from the front

Sternocleidomastoid muscles

Thyroid gland

Trachea

Thyroid cartilage

Isthmus

Use tangential lighting to aid visualization. An enlarged thyroid may be diffuse and asymmetrical. Thyroid nodules feel like a knot, a protuberance, or a swelling; a firm, fixed nodule may be a tumor. Be careful not to confuse thick neck musculature with an enlarged thyroid or a goiter. (See *Palpating the thyroid.*)

If you suspect that a patient has hypocalcemia (low serum calcium levels) related to deficient or ineffective parathyroid hormone (PTH) secretion from hypoparathyroidism or surgical removal of the parathyroid glands, attempt to elicit Chvostek's sign and Trousseau's sign. To elicit Chvostek's sign, tap the facial nerve in front of the ear with a finger;

if the facial muscles contract toward the ear, the test is positive for hypocalcemia. To elicit Trousseau's sign, place a blood pressure cuff on the arm and inflate it above the patient's systolic pressure. If the patient has a positive reaction, he will exhibit carpal spasm (ventral contraction of the thumb and digits) within 3 minutes.

Milk the testes to the bottom of the scrotal sac for palpation. The testes should feel firm and smooth. The normal testis is about 2″ (5 cm) in length.

Auscultation

If you palpate an enlarged thyroid, auscultate the gland for systolic bruits. Such bruits may indicate hyperthyroidism. To auscultate for bruits, place the bell of the stethoscope over one of the lateral lobes of the thyroid, then listen for a low, soft, rushing sound. Have the patient hold his breath while you auscultate.

To distinguish a bruit from a venous hum, listen for the rushing sound, then gently occlude the jugular vein with your fingers on the side you're auscultating and listen again. A venous hum disappears during venous compression; a bruit doesn't.

DIAGNOSTIC TESTS

Various tests can suggest, confirm, or rule out an endocrine disorder. Some of these tests also can identify a dysfunction as hyperfunction or hypofunction or as primary, secondary, or functional. Endocrine function can be tested by direct, indirect, provocative, and radiographic studies. (See *Diagnostic tests for endocrine disorders.*)

NURSING DIAGNOSES

When caring for patients with endocrine disorders, you'll find that several nursing diagnoses are commonly used. These diagnoses appear below, along with appropriate nursing interventions and rationales. (Rationales appear in italic type.)

Altered nutrition: More than body requirements

Related to increased appetite, high calorie intake, slowed metabolic rate, inability to use nutrients, and inactivity, the diagnosis of altered nutrition, more than body requirements, can be associated with Cushing's syndrome and diabetes mellitus, among many disorders.

Expected outcomes

• Patient expresses an understanding of how obesity contributes to the disorder.
• Patient develops realistic goals for weight reduction and a plan to achieve these goals.
• Patient loses the specified number of pounds each week.
• Patient carries out an exercise and activity plan.

Nursing interventions and rationales

• Obtain the patient's dietary history. *Permanent weight change starts with examination of contributing factors.* Teach the patient about a

(Text continues on page 536.)

Diagnostic tests for endocrine disorders

Test	Purpose	Nursing considerations
Cortisol	Evaluates the status of adrenocortical function	• Explain the procedure and that the specimens will be drawn between 6 to 8 am and 4 to 6 pm. • Instruct the patient to maintain a 2 to 3 g/day salt diet for 3 days before the test and to fast and limit physical activity for 10 to 12 hours before the test. • Withhold all medications that may interfere with plasma cortisol levels such as estrogens, androgens, and phenytoin for 48 hours before the test. • Make sure the patient is relaxed and recumbent for at least 30 minutes before the test. • After the test, observe the venipuncture site for bleeding. • The patient should resume diet and medications.
Catecholamines	Assesses adrenal medulla function	• Explain the procedure and that the sample will be drawn between 6 to 8 am. • Instruct the patient to refrain from cold or allergy medication for 2 weeks before the test. • Tell him to exclude amine-rich foods and beverages from his diet for 48 hours before the test, to maintain Vitamin C intake, and to fast 10 to 12 hours before the test. • Instruct him to abstain from smoking 24 hours before the test. • Make sure the patient is relaxed and recumbent for 45 to 60 minutes before the test. • After the test, pack the blood sample in crushed ice and send to laboratory immediately. • Observe the venipuncture site for bleeding. • Instruct the patient to resume normal diet and medications.
Parathyroid hormone	Evaluates parathyroid function	• Explain the procedure including venipuncture. • Instruct the patient to fast overnight. • After the test, observe the venipuncture site for bleeding. • The patient should resume normal diet.

(continued)

Diagnostic tests for endocrine disorders *(continued)*

Test	Purpose	Nursing considerations
Serum calcium	Helps detect bone and parathyroid disorders	• Explain the procedure including venipuncture. • When drawing the sample, avoid using a tourniquet as it may cause venous stasis, which may alter calcium results. • After the test, observe the venipuncture site for bleeding.
Serum phosphorous	Helps detect parathyroid disorders and renal failure	• Explain the procedure including venipuncture. • When drawing the sample avoid using a tourniquet as this causes venous stasis, which may alter results. • After the test, observe the venipuncture site for bleeding.
Oral glucose tolerance	Detects diabetes mellitus and hypoglycemia	• Explain the procedure and that it requires 5 blood samples and possible urine samples. • Advise the patient to maintain a high-carbohydrate diet for 3 days and then to fast 10 to 16 hours before the test. • Withhold drugs that may affect test results, as ordered. If these drugs must be continued, note on laboratory slip. • Teach the patient to recognize the symptoms of hypoglycemia, such as weakness, restlessness, nervousness, hunger and sweating and to report them immediately. • Tell him to lie down if he feels faint. • Encourage him to drink water throughout the test. • After the test, observe venipuncture sites for bleeding. • Resume medications withheld before the test. • Provide a balanced meal or snack, but observe for hypoglycemic reaction.
Glycosylated hemoglobin	Monitors the degree of glucose control in diabetes mellitus over 3 months	• Explain the procedure and that the patient should maintain his prescribed medication and diet regimen. • After the test, observe venipuncture site for bleeding.

Diagnostic tests for endocrine disorders *(continued)*

Test	Purpose	Nursing considerations
Growth hormone radioimmunoassay	Helps evaluate growth hormone oversecretion	• Explain the procedure. • Instruct the patient to fast and limit physical activity for 10 to 12 hours before the test. • Make sure he is relaxed and recumbent for 30 minutes before the test. • After the test, resume diet and observe the venipuncture site for bleeding.
Insulin-induced hypoglycemia	Helps detect hypopituitarism	• Explain that the procedure involves I.V. infusion of insulin and obtaining multiple blood samples. • Instruct the patient to fast and restrict physical activity for 10 to 12 hours before the test. • Make sure he is relaxed and recumbent for 90 minutes before the test. • Have concentrated glucose solutions available in the event that the patient has a severe hypoglycemic reaction to insulin. • After the test, observe the venipuncture site for bleeding. • Instruct him to resume diet, activity and medications.
T_4 RIA	Evaluates thyroid function and monitors iodine or antithyroid therapy	• Explain the procedure. • Withhold any medications that may interfere with the test. If these must be continued, note this on the laboratory slip. • After the test, observe the venipuncture site for bleeding. • Resume any medications discontinued before the test.
T_3 RIA	Detects hyperthyroidism if T_4 levels are normal	• Explain the procedure. • Withhold medications that may interfere with the test results such as estrogens, androgens, phenytoin, and salicylates, as ordered. If these must be continued, note this on the laboratory slip. • After the test, observe the venipuncture site for bleeding. • Resume medications discontinued before the test.

(continued)

Diagnostic tests for endocrine disorders *(continued)*

Test	Purpose	Nursing considerations
17-Ketosteroids, urine	Evaluates adrenocortical and gonadal function	• Explain the procedure and that he should avoid excessive exercise and stressful situations during collecting period. • Tell him the test requires a 24-hour urine collection and instruct him in the proper collection technique. • Collect in a container with a preservative to keep specimen pH at 4 to 4.5. • Refrigerate the specimen or place it on ice during the collection period. • After the test the patient may resume activity restricted during the test.
17-Hydroxycorticosteroids, urine	Evaluates adrenal function	• Explain the procedure. • Tell him the test requires a 24-hour urine collection and instruct him in proper collection technique. • Collect in a bottle containing a preservative to keep specimen pH at 4 to 4.5. • Refrigerate the specimen or place it on ice during the collection period.
Urine free cortisol	Aids in diagnosis of Cushing's syndrome	• Explain the procedure. • Tell him the test requires a 24-hour collection and instruct him in proper collection technique. • Collect in a bottle containing a preservative to keep specimen pH at 4 to 4.5. • Refrigerate the specimen or place it on ice during the collection period.

calorie-based meal plan and provide a written copy of it. Obtain dietary consultation as necessary and available. Evaluate the patient's eating habits, include preferred foods in his meal plan, and help him set realistic weight-loss goals.
• Encourage activity and exercise based on the patient's physical abilities. *Activities offer a positive alternative to eating to alleviate stress.*

• Refer to community resources as needed and available.

Risk for injury

Related to incoordination, fatigue, inattentiveness, and small muscle tremors, risk for injury is associated with hyperthyroidism.

Expected outcomes
• Patient identifies factors that increase potential for injury.
• Patient and family develop strategies to maintain safety.
• Patient is as active and independent as possible.

Nursing interventions and rationales
• Assist the patient with tasks needing fine motor skills such as shaving. Reduce environmental obstacles. *This helps the patient provide self-care.*
• Assist the patient with ambulation. Provide support as indicated; for example, supply a cane or walker. *This allows independence and promotes bone metabolism.*
• Instruct the patient and his family in safety measures, such as removing throw rugs or using nonskid surfaces in the bathroom. *Preventive measures decrease injuries from falls.*

Sleep pattern disturbance
Related to anxiety or hormone imbalance, sleep pattern disturbance can be associated with hyperthyroidism, diabetes insipidus, and diabetes mellitus, among many disorders.

Expected outcomes
• Patient identifies measures that aid sleep.
• Patient stays out of bed during normal waking hours and participates in activities during the day.
• Patient reports getting adequate sleep.
• Patient sleeps 6 hours each night.

Nursing interventions and rationales
• Promote usual sleep and rest practices. Decrease environmental stimuli. Provide a quiet, darkened room that's private, if possible.
• Encourage frequent, short periods of ambulation.
• Give antihormone medications as ordered and sedatives as needed.
• Instruct the patient and his family to eliminate caffeine-containing foods from his diet.
• Provide and encourage quiet diversionary activities.
  All of these measures promote rest and sleep.

Disorders

Endocrine dysfunction takes one of two forms: hyperfunction, which results in excessive hormone production or response, or hypofunction, which results from a relative or absolute hormone deficiency. Hormonal imbalance resulting from disease within an endocrine gland is known as *primary* dysfunction. Dysfunction outside a particular endocrine gland that affects the gland or its hormone(s) is termed *secondary* dysfunction. (See *Assessing endocrine dysfunction: Some common signs and symptoms*, page 538.)

Pituitary disorders
The most common pituitary disorders include hypopituitarism, hyperpituitarism, and diabetes insipidus.

Assessing endocrine dysfunction: Some common signs and symptoms

Sign or symptom	Possible cause
Abdominal pain	Diabetic ketoacidosis (DKA), myxedema, addisonian crisis, thyroid storm
Anemia	Hypothyroidism, panhypopituitarism, adrenal insufficiency, Cushing's disease, hyperparathyroidism
Anorexia	Hyperparathyroidism, Addison's disease, DKA, hypothyroidism
Body temperature changes	*Increase:* Thyrotoxicosis, thyroid storm, primary hypothalamic disease (after pituitary surgery) *Decrease:* Addison's disease, hypoglycemia, myxedema coma, DKA
Hypertension	Primary aldosteronism, pheochromocytoma, Cushing's syndrome
Libido changes, sexual dysfunction	Thyroid or adrenocortical hypofunction or hyperfunction, diabetes mellitus, hypopituitarism, gonadal failure
Skin changes	*Hyperpigmentation:* Addison's disease (after bilateral adrenalectomy for Cushing's disease), corticotropin-secreting pituitary tumor *Hirsutism:* Cushing's syndrome, adrenal hyperplasia, adrenal tumor, acromegaly *Coarse, dry skin:* Myxedema, hypoparathyroidism, acromegaly *Excessive sweating:* Thyrotoxicosis, acromegaly, pheochromocytoma, hypoglycemia
Tachycardia	Hyperthyroidism, pheochromocytoma, hypoglycemia, DKA
Weakness, fatigue	Addison's disease, Cushing's syndrome, hypothyroidism, hyperparathyroidism, hyperglycemia or hypoglycemia, pheochromocytoma
Weight gain	Cushing's syndrome, hypothyroidism, pituitary tumor
Weight loss	Hyperthyroidism, pheochromocytoma, Addison's disease, hyperparathyroidism, hyperglycemia, diabetes mellitus and insipidus

Hypopituitarism

Also called dwarfism when occurring in childhood, hypopituitarism is a complex syndrome marked by metabolic dysfunction, sexual immaturity, and growth retardation resulting from a deficiency of the hormones secreted by the anterior pituitary gland. Panhypopituitarism refers to a generalized condition caused by partial or total failure to secrete all six of this gland's vital hormones: corticotropin, thyroid-stimulating hormone (TSH), luteinizing hormone (LH), follicle-stimulating hormone (FSH), growth hormone (GH), and prolactin.

Causes. Primary hypopituitarism may result from a tumor (most common), congenital defects (hypoplasia or aplasia of the pituitary gland), pituitary ischemia (in most cases from postpartum hemorrhage), or partial or total hypophysectomy by surgery, radiation therapy or chemical agents, or head injury.

Secondary hypopituitarism results in a deficiency of hypothalamic releasing hormones produced by the hypothalamus or of vascular or neural connections to the pituitary from the pituitary stalk and hypothalamus or other central nervous system (CNS) disease. It can be idiopathic or result from infection or a tumor.

Assessment findings. Clinical features of hypopituitarism usually develop slowly and vary greatly with the severity of the disorder.

In adults, signs and symptoms can include decreased libido, impotence, infertility, tiredness, weakness, lethargy, sensitivity to cold, and menstrual disturbances. Other indications are pale skin, hypoglycemia, anorexia, nausea, abdominal pain, hypotension, and failure of lactation, menstruation, and growth of pubic and axillary hair.

In children, signs include growth retardation and absence of secondary sexual characteristics during puberty.

Diagnostic tests. The following tests are used to detect hypopituitarism.
• Assays showing decreased plasma levels of pituitary hormones, accompanied by end-organ hypofunction, suggests pituitary failure rather than target gland disease.
• Failure of thyrotropin-releasing hormone administration to increase TSH concentrations rules out hypothalamic dysfunction as the cause of hormonal deficiency.
• Provocative tests: To pinpoint the source of low cortisol levels, a corticotropin stimulation test can be used; a cortisol response that fails to increase indicates primary adrenal failure. Insulin-induced hypoglycemia stimulates corticotropin secretion. Persistently low levels of corticotropin indicate pituitary or hypothalamic failure. (These tests require careful medical supervision because they may precipitate an adrenal crisis.)
• Magnetic resonance imaging (MRI) and computed tomography (CT) scans confirm intrasellar or extrasellar tumors.
• Exercise tests evaluate GH levels.

Treatment. Removal of the tumor and replacement of hormones secreted by the target glands is the treatment for hypopituitarism and panhypopituitarism. Hormonal replacement includes cortisol, thyroxine (T_4), and testosterone or estrogen (but not prolactin). Patients of reproductive age may benefit from administration of FSH, LH, and human chorionic gonadotropin to boost fertility.

GH is effective for treating dwarfism and stimulates growth increases as great as 4″ to 6″ (10 to 15 cm) in the first year of treatment. The growth rate tapers off in later years. After pubertal changes have occurred, the effects of GH therapy are limited.

Nursing interventions. Keep track of the results of all laboratory tests for hormonal deficiencies. Until replacement therapy is complete, check for signs and symptoms of thyroid deficiency (increasing lethargy) and adrenal deficiency (weakness, orthostatic hypotension, hypoglycemia, fatigue, and weight loss).

During insulin testing, monitor closely for signs of hypoglycemia (initially tachycardia, nervousness and slow cerebration progressing to convulsions). Keep dextrose 50% in water available for I.V. administration to correct hypoglycemia.

Record temperature, blood pressure, and heart rate every 4 to 8 hours. Check for pallor, which indicates anemia, a complication of panhypopituitarism.

Prevent infection by providing meticulous skin care; use oil or lotion instead of soap. If body temperature is low, keep the patient warm. To prevent falls related to postural hypotension, encourage the patient to rise slowly and hold onto a secure object.

Darken the room if the patient has a tumor that is causing headaches and visual disturbances. Help with any activity that requires good vision.

Patient education. Stress the need to take replacement medicines as directed and to obtain follow-up care. Instruct the patient to wear a medical identification bracelet. Teach him to administer steroids parenterally in case of an emergency.

Evaluation. The patient should take prescribed medication, return for appropriate follow-up care, identify when to take extra steroids, demonstrate correct I.M. injection technique and, if needed, receive psychological counseling.

GH excess: A type of hyperpituitarism

A chronic, progressive disease marked by excess GH secretion and tissue overgrowth, hyperpituitarism appears in two forms: gigantism and acromegaly. *Gigantism* begins before epiphyseal closure and causes proportional overgrowth of all body tissues. *Acromegaly* occurs after epiphyseal closure, causing bone thickening and transverse growth and visceromegaly.

Cause. GH oversecretion is usually caused by a tumor of the anterior pituitary gland.

Assessment findings. The clinical features of acromegaly are a gradual, marked enlargement of the bones of the face, jaw, and extremities; diaphoresis; oily skin; weakness and hirsutism. Gigantism is marked by a proportional overgrowth of all body tissues with remarkable height increases.

Diagnostic tests. This type of hyperpituitarism can be confirmed from a set of tests. Plasma GH levels are increased, although a random sampling may be misleading. Somatomedin C (insulin-like growth factor I) levels are increased, and because these vary less than GH, this test is a good indicator of GH excess. A glucose tolerance test also offers reliable information. CT scans and MRI identify pituitary lesions.

Treatment. Treatment aims to curb overproduction of GH through removal of the underlying tumor by transsphenoidal hypophysectomy, pituitary radiation therapy, bromocriptine or octreotide administration (which inhibits GH synthesis), or a combination of these. Postoperative therapy requires replacement of thyroid, cortisone, and (if the entire pituitary must be removed) gonadal hormones.

Nursing interventions. Provide support to help the patient cope with severe psychological stress and an altered body image.

To promote maximum joint mobility and prevent injury, perform or assist with range-of-motion (ROM) exercises. Evaluate muscle weakness, especially in the patient with late-stage acromegaly.

Keep the skin dry. Avoid oily lotions.

Be aware that a pituitary tumor may cause visual problems. If the patient has hemianopia, stand where he can see you. Reassure the family that inexplicable mood changes are hormonal and can be modified with treatment.

Before surgery, reinforce the surgeon's explanation and reassure the patient. After surgery, diligently monitor vital signs and neurologic status.

Patient education. Before discharge, emphasize the importance of continuing hormone replacement therapy, if ordered.

Advise the patient to wear a medical identification bracelet at all times and to bring his hormone replacement schedule with him whenever he returns for follow-up care. Instruct him to have follow-up examinations at least once a year for the rest of his life because there's a slight chance the tumor may recur.

Evaluation. The patient should comply with prescribed follow-up care, such as hormone replacement therapy, periodic medical visits, and other measures.

Diabetes insipidus

Resulting from a deficiency of circulating antidiuretic hormone (ADH) (vasopressin), this uncommon condition occurs equally in both sexes. In uncomplicated diabetes insipidus, the prognosis is good. With adequate water replacement, patients usually lead normal lives.

Causes. Diabetes insipidus may be familial, acquired, or idiopathic. It can be acquired as the result of intracranial neoplastic or metastatic lesions. Other causes may include hypophysectomy or other neurosurgery; head trauma, which damages the neurohypophyseal structures; infection; granulomatous disease; vascular lesions; and autoimmune disorders.

Assessment findings. Signs and symptoms of diabetes insipidus include extreme polyuria (usually 4 to 17 qt [4 to 16 L]/day of dilute urine but sometimes as much as 32 qt [30 L]/day) with a low specific gravity (less than 1.005); polydipsia, particularly for cold, iced drinks; nocturia; fatigue (in severe cases); and dehydration, characterized by weight loss, poor tissue turgor, dry mucous membranes, constipation, muscle weakness, dizziness, tachycardia, and hypotension.

Diagnostic tests. Urinalysis reveals almost colorless urine of low osmolality (less than 200 mOsm/kg and less than that of plasma) and low specific gravity (less than 1.005). Patients also exhibit hypernatremia and increased blood urea nitrogen (BUN). A water deprivation test confirms the diagnosis by showing renal inability to concentrate urine (evidence of ADH deficiency). Subcutaneous injection of 5 U of vasopressin produces decreased urine output with increased specific gravity if the patient has central diabetes insipidus.

Treatment. Until the cause of diabetes insipidus can be identified and eliminated, administration of vasopressin can control fluid balance and prevent dehydration.

Nursing interventions. Record fluid intake and output carefully. Maintain fluid intake to prevent severe dehydration. Watch for signs of hypovolemic shock, and monitor blood pressure and heart and respiratory rates regularly, especially during the water deprivation test. Check weight daily. If the patient is dizzy or has muscle weakness, remember to keep the side rails up and assist with walking.

Monitor urine specific gravity between vasopressin doses. Watch for a decrease in specific gravity, with increasing urine output, indicating the return of the inability to concentrate urine and necessitating administration of the next dose or a dosage increase. Check laboratory values for hypernatremia or hyponatremia.

If constipation develops, add more bulk foods and fruit juices to the diet. If necessary, obtain an order for a mild laxative. Provide meticulous skin and mouth care.

Patient education. Before discharge, teach the patient how to monitor fluid intake and output. Instruct him to administer desmopressin by nasal insufflation or by mouth. Advise the patient about possible drug adverse effects, for example headache. Tell him to report any weight gain; it may mean the dosage is too high. Recurrence of polyuria, as reflected on the intake and output sheet, indicates that the dosage is too low.

Advise the patient to wear a medical identification bracelet and to carry his medication with him at all times. Give him written instructions on his medication and the signs and symptoms he should report to his doctor. Remind him to schedule regular follow-up appointments.

Evaluation. The patient should maintain an adequate fluid volume and electrolyte balance and should resume his normal elimination pattern.

If diabetes insipidus hasn't been eliminated, the patient should also know how to administer his medication correctly and how to record his intake and output. If using a nasal preparation, he should self-medicate while still an inpatient.

Thyroid disorders

Common thyroid disorders include hyperthyroidism and hypothyroidism.

Hyperthyroidism

This metabolic imbalance results from excessive thyroid hormone. The most common form of hyperthyroidism is Graves' disease, which increases T_4 and triiodothyronine (T_3) production, enlarges the thyroid gland (goiter), and causes multisystemic changes. With treatment, most patients can lead normal lives. However, thyroid storm—an acute exacerbation of hyperthyroidism—is a medical emergency that may lead to cardiac failure. (See *Under-*

standing forms of hyperthyroidism, page 544.)

Cause. Graves' disease is an autoimmune disease and is usually familial. Thyroid receptor antibodies are present in most patients with this disorder.

Assessment findings. Classic signs and symptoms of Graves' disease include a diffusely enlarged thyroid, nervousness, heat intolerance, weight loss despite increased appetite, sweating, diarrhea or hyperdefecation, tremor, palpitations, and possibly exophthalmos. (In thyroid storm [thyrotoxicosis], these signs and symptoms can be accompanied by extreme restlessness, systolic hypertension, tachycardia, vomiting, temperature up to 106° F [41.1° C], delirium, and coma.) Other signs and symptoms include:
• *CNS*—difficulty concentrating, excitability or nervousness, fine tremor, clumsiness, and mood swings, ranging from occasional outbursts to overt psychosis
• *Skin, hair, and nails*—smooth, warm, paper thin, flushed skin; pretibial myxedema (dermopathy), producing thickened skin, accentuated hair follicles, raised red patches of skin that are itchy and sometimes painful, with occasional nodule formation; fine, soft hair; premature graying and increased hair loss in both sexes; friable nails and onycholysis
• *Cardiovascular system*—tachycardia; full, bounding pulse; wide pulse pressure; cardiomegaly; increased cardiac output and blood volume; a

Understanding forms of hyperthyroidism

In addition to Graves' disease, hyperthyroidism occurs in several other forms, including the following.

Toxic adenoma
This small, benign nodule in the thyroid gland that secretes thyroid hormone is the second most common cause of hyperthyroidism. The cause of toxic adenoma is unknown; incidence is highest in the elderly. Clinical effects are essentially similar to those of Graves' disease, except that toxic adenoma does not induce ophthalmopathy, pretibial myxedema, or acropachy. Toxic adenoma is confirmed by radioactive iodine 131 (^{131}I) uptake and thyroid scan, which show a single hyperfunctioning nodule suppressing the rest of the gland. Treatment includes ^{131}I therapy or surgery to remove the adenoma after antithyroid drugs achieve a euthyroid state.

Thyrotoxicosis factitia
This form results from chronic ingestion of thyroid hormone for thyrotropin suppression in patients with thyroid carcinoma or from thyroid hormone abuse by persons who are trying to lose weight.

Functioning metastatic thyroid carcinoma
This form is a rare disease that causes excess production of thyroid hormone.

Thyroid-stimulating-hormone-secreting pituitary tumor
This form causes overproduction of thyroid hormone.

Subacute thyroiditis
This form is a virus-induced granulomatous inflammation of the thyroid, producing transient hyperthyroidism associated with fever, pain, pharyngitis, and tenderness in the thyroid gland.

Silent thyroiditis
This is a self-limiting, transient form of hyperthyroidism with histologic thyroiditis but no inflammatory symptoms.

visible point of maximal impulse; paroxysmal supraventricular tachycardia and atrial fibrillation (found especially in elderly patients); occasionally, a systolic murmur at the left sternal border
• *Musculoskeletal system*—weakness, fatigue, and proximal muscle atrophy; periodic paralysis; occasional acropachy—soft-tissue swelling, accompanied by underlying bone changes where new bone formation occurs

• *Reproductive system*—in females, oligomenorrhea or amenorrhea, decreased fertility, and higher incidence of spontaneous abortions; in males, gynecomastia; in both sexes, diminished libido
• *Eyes*—exophthalmos; occasional inflammation of conjunctivae, corneas, or eye muscles; diplopia; increased tearing; lid lag; lid retraction
• *Respiratory system*—dyspnea on exertion and possibly at rest

• *GI system*—increased appetite, but occasional anorexia; increased defecation; soft stools or, with severe disease, diarrhea; liver enlargement.

Diagnostic tests. Radioimmunoassay (RIA) tests shows elevated T_4 levels. Free T_4 is also elevated as is T_3, although T_3 may not be elevated in the elderly. Thyroid scan reveals increased radioactive iodine 131 (^{131}I) uptake. Immunometric assay shows suppressed sensitive TSH levels. Orbital sonography and CT scan confirm subclinical ophthalmopathy.

Treatment. The primary forms of treatment for hyperthyroidism are antithyroid drugs, ^{131}I, beta-adrenergic blockers, sedation, and surgery. Appropriate treatment depends on the size of the goiter, the causes, the patient's age and parity, and how long surgery (if planned) will be delayed.

Antithyroid drug therapy with propylthiouracil (PTU) and methimazole blocks thyroid hormone synthesis. It is used for pregnant women, children, and patients who refuse surgery or ^{131}I treatment.

During pregnancy, PTU and subtotal (partial) thyroidectomy are the preferred therapies. Antithyroid medication should be kept at the minimum dosage required to keep maternal thyroid function testing at high-normal or slightly elevated levels. A few (1%) of the infants born to mothers receiving antithyroid medication will be hypothyroid.

Another major form of therapy for hyperthyroidism is a single oral dose of ^{131}I. This is the treatment of choice in the United States, except for pregnant patients.

Subtotal thyroidectomy is indicated for the patient younger than age 40 who has a large goiter and whose hyperthyroidism has repeatedly relapsed after drug therapy. Subtotal thyroidectomy removes part of the thyroid gland, thus decreasing its size and capacity for hormone production.

Before surgery, the patient may receive iodides (Lugol's solution or saturated solution of potassium iodide), antithyroid drugs, or high doses of propranolol, a beta blocker, to help prevent thyroid storm. If euthyroidism is not achieved, surgery should be delayed and propranolol administered to decrease the systemic effects (such as cardiac arrhythmias) caused by hyperthyroidism.

After ablative treatment with ^{131}I or surgery, patients require lifelong, regular, frequent medical supervision. They usually develop hypothyroidism.

Therapy for hyperthyroid ophthalmopathy includes local applications of topical medications but may require high doses of corticosteroids, given systemically or, in severe cases, injected into the retrobulbar area. A patient with severe exophthalmos that causes pressure on the optic nerve may require surgical decompression.

Treatment of thyroid storm includes administration of an antithyroid drug such as PTU, propranolol I.V. to block sympathetic effects, a corticosteroid to replace depleted cortisol levels, and an iodide to block release of thyroid hormone. Supportive measures include nutrients, vitamins, fluid administration, and sedation, as necessary.

If iodine is part of the treatment, mix it with water or juice and administer it through a straw.

Nursing interventions. Provide vigilant care to prevent acute exacerbations and complications. Record vital signs and weight. Monitor serum electrolyte levels, and check periodically for hyperglycemia and glycosuria. Carefully monitor cardiac function. Check LOC and urine output.

Additionally, if the patient is in her first trimester of pregnancy, report any signs of spontaneous abortion (spotting, occasional mild cramps) to the doctor immediately.

Remember, patient may exhibit bizarre behavior. Reassure the patient and family that such behavior subsides with treatment. Provide sedatives, as necessary.

To promote weight gain, provide a balanced diet, with six meals a day. If the patient has edema, suggest a low-sodium diet.

Watch for signs of thyroid storm. Check intake and output carefully to ensure adequate hydration and fluid balance. Closely monitor blood pressure, cardiac rate and rhythm, and temperature. Take steps to reduce high fever (sponging, hypothermia blankets, and acetaminophen); avoid aspirin, which raises T_4 levels. Maintain an I.V. line and give drugs, as ordered.

Thyroidectomy necessitates meticulous postoperative care to prevent complications.

Patient education. If the patient has exophthalmos or another ophthalmopathy, suggest sunglasses or eye patches to protect his eyes from light. Moisten the conjunctivae often with artificial tears. Warn the patient with severe lid retraction to avoid sudden physical movements that might cause the lid to slip behind the eyeball. Elevate the head of the bed to reduce periorbital edema. (See *Caring for the patient with Graves' disease.*)

Stress the importance of regular medical follow-up care after discharge because hypothyroidism may develop from 2 to 4 weeks postoperatively. Antithyroid, beta blockers and iodine therapy require careful monitoring and comprehensive patient education. If the patient is taking antithyroid drugs, instruct him to report any adverse reactions to the drugs.

If the patient is pregnant, tell her to watch closely during the first trimester for signs and of spontaneous abortion and to report them to the doctor immediately.

Evaluation. The patient should maintain an adequate fluid volume and electrolyte balance, normal cardiac function, and normal body temperature. He should gain weight. He should have no complications.

The patient should schedule return appointments. If he's taking an antithyroid drug or is on ^{131}I therapy, he should have a handout listing the signs and symptoms to report to his doctor.

Hypothyroidism

A state of low serum thyroid hormone levels or cellular resistance to thyroid hormone, hypothyroidism results from hypothalamic, pituitary, or thyroid insufficiency. Most prevalent in women, hypothyroidism can progress to life-threatening myxedema coma—usually precipitated by infection, exposure to cold, or sedatives.

Causes. Hypothyroidism in adults may result from thyroidectomy; radiation therapy; chronic autoimmune thyroiditis (Hashimoto's disease); inflammatory conditions, such as amyloidosis and sarcoidosis; pituitary failure to produce TSH; or hypothalamic failure to produce thyrotropin-releasing hormone (TRH). Other causes include inborn errors of thyroid hormone synthesis, an inability to synthesize thyroid hormone because of iodine deficiency, and the use of antithyroid medications such as PTU.

Assessment findings. Signs and symptoms include fatigue; forgetfulness; cold intolerance; unexplained weight gain; constipation; goiter; decreasing mental stability; cool, dry, flaky, yellowish, inelastic skin; puffy face, hands, and feet; periorbital edema; dry, sparse hair; and thick, brittle nails. Other indications include a slow pulse rate, anorexia, abdominal distention, menorrhagia, decreased libido, infertility, ataxia, intention tremor,

> ### FOCUS ON CARING
> ### Caring for the patient with Graves' disease
>
> Your patient has ophthalmopathy from Graves' disease and complains of eye discomfort. Keep the room darkened as much as possible. Arrange for sunglasses to be brought in or supplied for the patient. Moist compresses may also relieve the discomfort.
>
> If your patient has been hyperactive from the hyperthyroidism, help her to decrease her pace. Counsel her that it will take time for her behaviors to return to normal, and assist her with problem solving. With her permission, discuss behaviors that might have caused problems with her family. Then, relate the behaviors to the hyperthyroidism, and prepare the family for the pending behavior changes.

nystagmus, delayed reflex relaxation time (especially in the Achilles tendon), muscle cramps, and carpal tunnel syndrome.

If hypothyroidism progresses to clinical effects of myxedema coma, signs include progressive stupor, hypoventilation, hypoglycemia, hyponatremia, hypotension, and hypothermia.

Diagnostic tests. Low free T_4 levels indicate hypothyroidism. TSH level is increased in primary hypothyroidism and decreased in secondary hypothyroidism. TRH level is decreased in hypothalamic insufficiency. Serum cholesterol, carotene, alkaline phosphatase, and triglyceride levels are increased.

In myxedema coma, laboratory tests may also show low serum sodium levels, and decreased pH and increased partial pressure of carbon dioxide in arterial blood, indicating respiratory acidosis.

Treatment. Therapy for hypothyroidism consists of gradual thyroid replacement with levothyroxine. During myxedema coma, effective treatment supports vital functions while restoring euthyroidism. To support blood pressure and pulse rate, treatment includes I.V. administration of levothyroxine and hydrocortisone in cases of pituitary or adrenal insufficiency. Hypoventilation necessitates oxygenation and vigorous respiratory support. Other supportive measures include careful fluid replacement and antimicrobials for infection.

Nursing interventions. To manage the hypothyroid patient, provide a high-bulk, low-calorie diet and encourage activity. Administer cathartics and stool softeners, as needed. After thyroid replacement therapy begins, watch for signs or symptoms of hyperthyroidism, such as restlessness, sweating, and excessive weight loss. (See *Managing myxedema coma.*)

Patient education. Tell the patient to report any signs of aggravated cardiovascular disease, such as chest pain and tachycardia. To prevent myxedema coma, tell him to continue his course of antithyroid medication even if his symptoms subside. Instruct him to report infection immediately and to make sure any doctor who prescribes drugs for him knows about his hypothyroidism. Advise the patient how to obtain a medical identification bracelet and a wallet identification card.

Evaluation. If therapy succeeds, the patient has a normal bowel elimination pattern and adequate cardiac function. He knows which cardiac symptoms to report and understands the need for lifelong thyroid replacement and regular medical follow-up care to monitor replacement therapy.

A patient with myxedema should show signs of adequate cardiac output and function, including blood pressure and pulse rate; adequate urine output; intact skin; adequate fluid volume and electrolyte balance; and adequate gas exchange.

Parathyroid disorders

Common parathyroid disorders include hypoparathyroidism and hyperparathyroidism.

Hypoparathyroidism

Hypoparathyroidism stems from a deficiency of PTH. Because PTH primarily regulates calcium balance, hypoparathyroidism causes hypocalcemia, producing neuromuscular symptoms ranging from paresthesia to tetany. The clinical effects are usually correctable with replacement therapy. However, some complications of this disorder, such as cataracts and basal ganglion calcifications, are irreversible.

Managing myxedema coma

A medical emergency, myxedema coma commonly has a fatal outcome. Progression is usually gradual, but when stress aggravates severe or prolonged hypothyroidism, coma may develop abruptly. Examples of severe stress are infection, exposure to cold, and trauma. Other precipitating factors include thyroid medication withdrawal and the use of sedatives, narcotics, or anesthetics.

Patients in myxedema coma have significantly depressed respirations, so their partial pressure of carbon dioxide in arterial blood may rise. Decreased cardiac output and worsening cerebral hypoxia may also occur. The patient is stuporous and hypothermic, and her vital signs reflect bradycardia and hypotension.

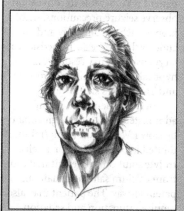

Lifesaving interventions

If your patient becomes comatose, begin these interventions as soon as possible:

• Maintain airway patency with ventilatory support if needed.
• Maintain circulation through I.V. fluid replacement.
• Provide continuous electrocardiogram monitoring.
• Monitor arterial blood gas measurements to detect hypoxia and metabolic acidosis.
• Warm the patient by wrapping her in blankets. Don't use a warming blanket because it might increase peripheral vasodilation, causing shock.
• Monitor body temperature until stable with a low-reading thermometer.
• Replace thyroid hormone by giving large I.V. levothyroxine doses, as ordered. Monitor vital signs because rapid correction of hypothyroidism can cause adverse cardiac effects.
• Monitor intake and output and daily weight. With treatment, urine output should increase and body weight decrease; if not, report this to the doctor.
• Replace fluids and other substances such as glucose. Monitor serum electrolyte levels.
• Administer corticosteroids, as ordered.
• Check for possible sources of infection, such as blood, sputum, or urine, which may have precipitated coma. Treat infections or any other underlying illness.

Causes. Hypoparathyroidism may result from a congenital absence or malfunction of the parathyroid glands, autoimmune destruction, removal of or injury to one or more parathyroid glands during neck surgery or, rarely, from massive thyroid radiation therapy. Other causes include ischemic infarction of the parathyroids during surgery or from disease, such as amyloidosis or neoplasms, suppression of normal gland function caused by hypercalcemia (reversible), and hypomagnesemia-induced impairment of hormone secretion (reversible).

Assessment findings.
Hypoparathyroidism may be asymptomatic in mild cases. Otherwise, signs and symptoms relate to hypocalcemia, and include neuromuscular irritability, increased deep tendon reflexes, positive Chvostek's and Trousseau's signs, circumoral numbness, dysphagia, paresthesia, psychosis, and mental deficiency in children. (See *Eliciting signs of hypocalcemia.*) Other indications are tetany; seizures; arrhythmias; cataracts; abdominal pain; dry, lusterless hair; spontaneous hair loss; and brittle fingernails that develop ridges or fall out. The patient's skin may be dry and scaly. Teeth may be stained, cracked, and decayed.

Diagnostic tests. Test results that confirm hypoparathyroidism include decreased, or "normal," PTH and decreased serum calcium levels and elevated serum phosphorus levels. X-rays reveal increased bone density, and an electrocardiogram (ECG) shows prolonged QT and ST intervals caused by hypocalcemia.

Treatment. Therapy includes vitamin D, with high doses of supplemental calcium. Such therapy is usually lifelong, except in the rever-

sible form of the disease. Types of vitamin D given include dihydrotachysterol if renal function is adequate and calcitriol if renal function is severely compromised.

Acute life-threatening tetany calls for immediate I.V. administration of calcium to raise serum calcium levels. Sedatives and anticonvulsants may control spasms until calcium levels rise. Chronic tetany calls for maintenance of serum calcium levels with vitamin D and possibly oral calcium supplements.

Nursing interventions. While awaiting diagnosis of hypoparathyroidism in a patient with a history of tetany, maintain a patent I.V. line and keep 10% calcium gluconate solution available. Because the patient is vulnerable to convulsions, observe seizure precautions. Also, keep a tracheostomy tray and an endotracheal tube at the bedside, as laryngospasm may result from hypocalcemia. Monitor Chvostek's and Trousseau's signs.

For the patient with tetany, administer 10% calcium gluconate by slow I.V. infusion (1 mg/minute) diluted in 50 to 100 ml of an electrolyte solution to prevent irritation from calcium salts, and maintain a patent airway. The patient may also require intubation and sedation with I.V. diazepam. Monitor vital signs often after I.V. administration of diazepam to make certain blood pressure and heart rate return to normal.

When caring for the patient with hypoparathyroidism, particularly a child, stay alert for minor muscle

Eliciting signs of hypocalcemia

When your patient complains of muscle spasms and paresthesia in his limbs, try eliciting Chvostek's and Trousseau's—indications of tetany associated with calcium deficiency.

Follow the procedures described below, keeping in mind the discomfort they typically cause. If you detect these signs, notify the doctor immediately. During these tests, watch the patient for laryngospasm, monitor his cardiac status, and have resuscitation equipment nearby.

Chvostek's sign

To elicit this sign, tap the patient's facial nerve just in front of the ear-lobe and below the zygomatic arch or between the zygomatic arch and the corner of the mouth, as shown below.

A positive response (indicating latent tetany) ranges from simple mouth-corner twitching to twitching of all facial muscles on the side tested. Simple twitching may be normal in some patients. However, a more pronounced response usually confirms Chvostek's sign.

Trousseau's sign

To elicit this sign, occlude the brachial artery by inflating a blood pressure cuff on the patient's upper arm to a level between diastolic and systolic blood pressure. Maintain this inflation for 3 minutes while observing the patient for carpal spasm (shown below), which is Trousseau's sign.

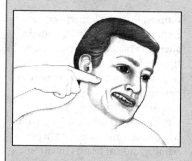

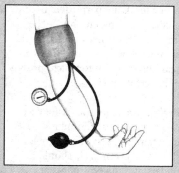

twitching (especially in the hands) and for signs of laryngospasm (respiratory stridor or dysphagia) because these effects may signal the onset of tetany.

Because the patient with chronic disease has prolonged QT intervals on an ECG, watch for heart block and signs of decreasing cardiac output. Closely monitor the patient receiving both digitalis glycosides and calcium because calcium potentiates the effect of these drugs. Stay alert for signs and symptoms of digitalis toxicity (arrhythmias, nausea, fatigue, and changes in vision).

Patient education. Advise the patient to follow a high-calcium, low-phosphorus diet, and tell him

Bone resorption in primary hyperparathyroidism

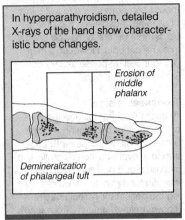

In hyperparathyroidism, detailed X-rays of the hand show characteristic bone changes.

Erosion of middle phalanx

Demineralization of phalangeal tuft

which foods are permitted. If he's on drug therapy, emphasize the importance of checking serum calcium levels at least three times a year. Instruct him to watch for signs of hypercalcemia.

Evaluation. After successful treatment, the patient should not develop tetany. His serum calcium levels should be normal. He should understand the symptoms of hypocalcemia and hypercalcemia and state reportable ones. He should also be able to identify high-calcium, low-phosphorus foods.

Hyperparathyroidism

Overactivity of one or more of the four parathyroid glands, resulting in excessive secretion of PTH, characterizes hyperparathyroidism. Hypersecretion of PTH promotes bone resorption and leads to hyper-

calcemia and hypophosphatemia. Increased renal and GI absorption of calcium also occurs. (See *Bone resorption in primary hyperparathyroidism.*)

In primary hyperparathyroidism, one or more of the parathyroid glands enlarge, increasing PTH secretion and causing elevated serum calcium levels.

In secondary hyperparathyroidism, excessive compensatory production of PTH stems from a hypocalcemia-producing abnormality outside the parathyroid gland, which is not responsive to the metabolic action of PTH. Complications associated with hyperparathyroidism include renal calculi, which may lead to renal failure, osteoporosis, pancreatitis, and peptic ulcer.

Causes. Primary hyperparathyroidism may result from a single adenoma (a genetic disorder), multiple endocrine neoplasia, or prior neck irradiation, or it may be idiopathic. Secondary hyperparathyroidism may be caused by rickets, vitamin D deficiency, or phenytoin or laxative abuse. Tertiary hyperparathyroidism occurs in chronic renal failure.

Assessment findings. Hyperparathyroidism is usually asymptomatic but may be indicated by these symptoms:
• *Renal*—symptoms of recurring nephrolithiasis, which may lead to renal insufficiency, polyuria, nocturia
• *Skeletal and articular*—chronic low back pain, easy fracturing from

bone degeneration, and bone tenderness

• *GI*—anorexia, nausea, vomiting, dyspepsia, and constipation

• *Neuromuscular*—fatigue and marked muscle weakness and atrophy, particularly in the legs

• *CNS*—psychomotor and personality disturbances, loss of memory for recent events, depression, overt psychosis, stupor, and possibly coma

• *Other*—skin pruritus, vision impairment from cataracts, anemia, subcutaneous calcification, hypertension.

Secondary hyperparathyroidism may produce the same clinical features as primary hyperparathyroidism, with possible skeletal deformities of the long bones (rickets, for example) as well as symptoms of the underlying disease.

Diagnostic tests. RIA tests reveal elevated serum PTH levels. Along with increased serum calcium and possibly decreased phosphorus levels, this confirms the diagnosis of hyperparathyroidism. X-rays may show diffuse demineralization of bones, bone cysts, outer cortical bone resorption, and subperiosteal erosion of the radial aspect of the middle fingers.

Laboratory tests reveal elevated urine and serum calcium, chloride, and alkaline phosphatase levels, and decreased serum phosphorus levels. Alkaline phosphatase (bone specific) gives an indication of bone formation, as does measurement of urinary pyrinoline and deoxypyridoline. Serum 1, 25 di-hyaroxyvitamin D (1,25[OH]$_2$D) may also be

elevated. Bone biopsies and quantitative histomorphometry may also be done.

Secondary hyperparathyroidism can be confirmed if serum calcium levels are normal or slightly decreased, with variable serum phosphorus levels. Other laboratory values may identify the cause of secondary hyperparathyroidism.

Treatment. For primary hyperparathyroidism, treatment may include surgery to remove the adenoma or, depending on the extent of hyperplasia, all but one-half of one gland (the remaining part of the gland is necessary to maintain normal PTH levels). Such surgery may relieve bone pain within 3 days. Renal damage may be irreversible.

Other treatments can decrease calcium levels preoperatively or if surgery isn't feasible or necessary. Such treatments include forcing fluids; limiting dietary calcium and vitamin D intake; promoting sodium and calcium excretion through forced diuresis, using normal saline solution (up to 6.5 qt [6 L] in life-threatening circumstances). After the patient is adequately hydrated, furosemide or ethacrynic acid may be given as well as oral sodium or potassium phosphate, calcitonin, or mithramycin. Ambulation will also help maintain calcium levels and bone mineralization.

Postoperative therapy includes I.V. administration of magnesium and phosphate, or sodium phosphate solution given by mouth or by retention enema. During the first 4 or 5 days after surgery, when serum calcium falls to low-normal levels, supplemental calcium also may be necessary. Vitamin D or calcitriol may also be used.

Treatment of secondary hyperparathyroidism must correct the underlying cause of parathyroid hypertrophy and includes vitamin D therapy or, in the patient with renal disease, aluminum hydroxide for hyperphosphatemia. In the patient with chronic secondary hyperparathyroidism, if the enlarged glands don't revert to normal size and function, they should be surgically removed.

Nursing interventions. Care emphasizes prevention of complications from the underlying disease and its treatment. During hydration to reduce serum calcium levels, record intake and output accurately. Strain urine to check for stones. Monitor sodium, potassium, and magnesium levels frequently. Auscultate for lung sounds often. Listen for signs of pulmonary edema in the patient receiving large amounts of saline solution I.V., especially if he has pulmonary or cardiac disease. Take measures to avoid trauma to prevent pathologic fractures.

Patient education. Before discharge, advise the patient of the possible adverse effects of drug therapy. Emphasize the need for periodic follow-up through laboratory blood tests. Instruct the patient in calcium content of foods. If hyperparathyroidism was not corrected surgically, warn the patient to avoid thiazide diuretics.

Evaluation. The patient should understand the need for regular determinations of serum calcium levels. He should understand the signs and symptoms of hypercalcemia and hypocalcemia and be able to identify reportable ones. He should also understand drug therapy and possible adverse drug effects.

Pancreatic disorders
Diabetes mellitus and hypoglycemia are the most common pancreatic disorders.

Diabetes mellitus
A chronic insulin deficiency or resistance, diabetes mellitus is characterized by disturbances in carbohydrate, protein, and fat metabolism. Diabetes is a major risk factor for myocardial infarction, cerebrovascular accident (CVA), renal failure, and peripheral vascular disease. It's also the leading cause of new blindness and end-stage renal disease in adults.

Two forms exist: type I (insulin-dependent diabetes mellitus, or juvenile-onset diabetes) and the more prevalent type II (non-insulin-dependent diabetes mellitus, or maturity-onset diabetes). Secondary diabetes may be caused by several medications in genetically susceptible people. (See *How types I and II diabetes mellitus develop*.)

Type I diabetes usually occurs before age 30; the patient is usually thin and will require exogenous insulin and dietary management to achieve control. Conversely, type II generally occurs in obese adults after age 30 and is usually treated

How types I and II diabetes mellitus develop

Both types I and II diabetes mellitus are strongly influenced by hereditary factors. However, type I is an autoimmune disorder, whereas type II is associated with insulin resistance and obesity.

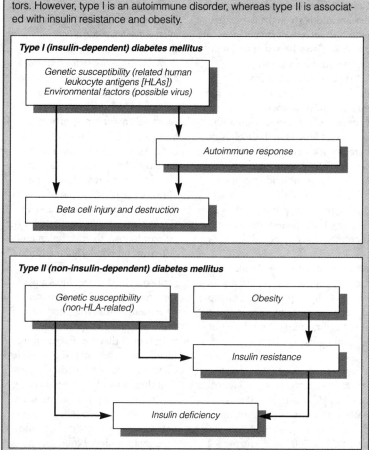

Type I (insulin-dependent) diabetes mellitus

Genetic susceptibility (related human leukocyte antigens [HLAs]) Environmental factors (possible virus)

Autoimmune response

Beta cell injury and destruction

Type II (non-insulin-dependent) diabetes mellitus

Genetic susceptibility (non-HLA-related)

Obesity

Insulin resistance

Insulin deficiency

with medical nutrition therapy and exercise (often in combination with drugs). Treatment may include insulin therapy.

In diabetic ketoacidosis (DKA) or hyperosmolar hyperglycemic nonketotic syndrome (HHNS), dehydration may cause hypovolemia and shock. Long-term effects of diabetes may include retinopathy, nephropathy, atherosclerosis, and autonomic neuropathy. Sensory peripheral neuropathy usually affects the legs and may cause numbness and loss of sensation.

Causes. Type I is an autoimmune disease and is strongly associated with human leukocyte antigens DR 3 and 4. It may be associated with certain viral infections.

Type II may result from impaired insulin secretion, peripheral insulin resistance, and increased hepatic glucose production. Other associated factors include obesity, heredity, a sedentary lifestyle, oral contraceptives, and excess corticosteroids, nicotinic acid and phenytoin. Gestational diabetes occurs during pregnancy and resolves after delivery, but affected women are at increased risk for type II diabetes.

Assessment findings. Look for fatigue, polyuria especially nocturia related to hyperglycemia, polydipsia, dry mucous membranes, poor skin turgor, unintentional weight loss, and polyphagia.

Diagnostic tests. Two fasting plasma glucose tests above 140 mg/dl, a random glucose over 200 mg/dl with symptoms or, with normal fasting glucose, two blood glucose levels above 200 mg/dl during a 2-hour glucose tolerance test confirm the diagnosis. Ophthalmologic examination may show diabetic retinopathy. Other tests include plasma insulin level determination, urine testing for glucose and acetone, and glycosylated hemoglobin (hemoglobin A$_{1c}$) determination.

Treatment. Medical nutrition therapy, exercise, and perhaps insulin or glucose-lowering agents are prescribed to normalize carbohydrate, fat, and protein metabolism and avert long-term complications while avoiding hypoglycemia.

All types of diabetes require adherence to individualized meal plans to meet nutritional needs, control blood glucose levels, and reach and maintain appropriate body weight. The American Diabetes Association (ADA) recommends a plan, based on an individualized assessment to determine appropriate distribution of carbohydrate, protein, and fat calories. Glycemic control is facilitated if the patient follows the meal plan consistently and regularly. In addition, aerobic exercise is generally prescribed at least three times a week for a minimum of 45 to 60 minutes.

Patients with type I diabetes must take insulin daily. Patients with type II diabetes may require insulin to control blood glucose levels unresponsive to medical nutrition therapy and glucose lowering agents, or during periods of acute stress. Patients with sedentary diabetes usually require daily insulin therapy to achieve blood glucose control. Patients with gestational diabetes are treated with meal planning, exercise and, if indicated, insulin.

Type II patients unresponsive to meal planning and exercise may require glucose-lowering agents. Sulfonylureas initially regulate blood glucose levels by increasing beta cell insulin secretion. This effect diminishes after several months, but the drugs also decrease cellular insulin resistance, enhancing blood glucose regulation.

Biguanides (metformin) increase insulin sensitivity and decrease inappropriate hepatic glucose production. Alpha-glucosidase inhibitors (Precose) decrease intestinal absorption of carbohydrate. Thiazolidinedione (triglitazone) is a new type of glucose-lowering agent currently being investigated for type II diabetes. Pancreatic and islet cell transplants are performed occasionally but remain experimental.

Exercise. Exercise provides many benefits, such as improved glucose control, increased insulin sensitivity, and decreased risk of atherosclerosis. It can also promote weight loss in conjunction with dietary measures.

Help the patient choose an aerobic exercise. Aerobic exercises decrease blood glucose levels and improve cardiovascular fitness. Have the patient avoid anaerobic exercises, such as weight-lifting or push-ups, because they can increase blood pressure and cause rapid heart rate. The patient should test his blood glucose level before and after each exercise session and know the safety guidelines.

Insulin therapy. Administer insulin as prescribed, most likely by subcutaneous injection using a standard insulin syringe. Insulin may also be injected subcutaneously using an insulin injector (a penlike device), which uses a disposable needle and replaceable insulin cartridges, eliminating the need to draw insulin up into a syringe. Jet-injection devices may disperse insulin more rapidly, speeding absorption. These devices draw up insulin from standard bottles (which allows the patient to mix insulins, if necessary, but requires a special procedure for drawing up) and deliver it into the subcutaneous tissue with a pressure jet.

The multiple-dose regimens may use an insulin pump to deliver rapid or fast-acting insulin continuously into subcutaneous tissue. The infusion rate selector automatically releases about one-half the total daily insulin requirement over 24 hours. The patient releases the remainder in bolus amounts before eating.

When giving insulin injections subcutaneously, rotate the injection sites. Diabetes specialists recommend rotating the injection site within a specific area, preferably the abdomen. (See *Preventing an insulin overdose,* page 558.)

Rapid and fast-acting insulin may also be administered I.M. or I.V. during severe episodes of hyperglycemia. *Never* administer any other type of insulin by these routes.

Two experimental methods of insulin administration are the intranasal delivery method and the programmable implantable medication system (PIMS). Intranasal administration uses aerosolized insulin in a nasal spray. Because nasal solutions are less potent than subcutaneous insulin, dosages are much higher.

CRITICAL THINKING

Preventing an insulin overdose

When giving medication at bedtime, you notice that Mrs. Benton's blood glucose is 283 mg/dl, which calls for sliding scale insulin coverage. However, on review of her medication and capillary blood glucose monitoring records, you note that her blood glucose was 320 mg/dl before her evening meal. At that time she received an extra 10 U of fast-acting insulin in addition to her usual dose of 10 U of fast-acting insulin and 45 U of intermediate-acting insulin. Should you give her more insulin based on her high blood glucose reading?

Suggested response
You realize that even though she ate all her dinner, her blood glucose is now on the way down, and her intermediate insulin will start to peak during the night. Therefore, you don't give the ordered sliding scale, fast-acting insulin. You reason that this insulin will most likely cause hypoglycemia during the night because your patient won't be eating until the next morning. Document your reason for not giving the sliding scale coverage. Discuss the appropriateness of administration of fast-acting insulin at bedtime with the patient's doctor the next day. Because this insulin peaks 3 to 4 hours after administration, bedtime administration commonly causes severe nocturnal hypoglycemia.

The PIMS has an implantable infusion pump unit that holds and delivers the insulin and a delivery catheter that feeds insulin directly into the peritoneal cavity. The patient uses a handheld external radio transmitter to control insulin release. As the PIMS lacks a blood glucose sensor, the patient must monitor glucose levels several times a day.

Nursing interventions. Develop a teaching plan that considers the patient's desires, capabilities, motivation, and barriers. It's crucial to bring the patient's blood glucose level within an acceptable range (less than 180 mg/dl) and alleviate or avert DKA or HHNS.

For the patient with unstable diabetes who isn't experiencing DKA or HHNS, monitor blood glucose levels several times a day as prescribed until they stabilize. Also monitor the type I diabetic patient's urine for ketones. Administer regular insulin as prescribed until blood glucose levels are under control and keep the doctor informed. Then expect to begin the patient on an insulin regimen. If the patient has type II diabetes, he may need an oral hypoglycemic agent or a trial period with only diet therapy. Check all meals and snacks to ensure patient is getting the prescribed meal plan on time.

Monitor the patient closely for signs and symptoms of DKA or HHNS as well as for hypoglycemia (caused by too-rapid reduction in blood glucose level). If you suspect DKA (if your patient begins to exhibit Kussmaul's respirations, develops a fruity odor to his breath and signs and symptoms of severe dehydration) or HHNS, test his blood sugar and urine for ketones, and notify the doctor immediately.

Treatment may include fluid and electrolyte replacement, increased insulin therapy, and possibly antiacidosis therapy. Administer doses of insulin I.V. or I.M., as prescribed. Monitor the patient's blood glucose levels frequently during insulin infusion. Alert the doctor when it reaches 250 to 300 mg/dl, as he may wish to change the saline infusion to glucose to prevent hypoglycemia. Typically, insulin decreases blood glucose levels by about 75 to 100 mg/dl each hour. After the crisis, expect to resume the patient's usual insulin regimen.

Administer I.V. fluids rapidly at the prescribed rate. Expect to give 1,000 to 2,000 ml over the first 2 hours. The solution prescribed may be either hypotonic or isotonic saline solution. When the glucose level is slightly above normal, the doctor may switch to a glucose solution. Monitor your elderly patient closely for evidence of fluid overload. Monitor electrolyte levels closely. Administer potassium replacement therapy as ordered.

Your patient must control his food intake to prevent widely fluctuating blood glucose levels. If he's taking insulin or glucose-lowering agents, he'll have to adhere to his meal plan even more carefully.

Monitor the patient for complications related to insulin therapy, which include hypoglycemia, the dawn phenomenon (early morning rise in blood glucose), insulin allergy, and insulin resistance.

Administer oral glucose-lowering agents as prescribed. Check the patient's history for contraindications, such as pregnancy, lactation, stressful concurrent conditions or illnesses that have increased insulin requirements, and known allergies to sulfa-agents if sulfonylureas are prescribed. Monitor the patient for adverse reactions.

Blood glucose monitoring. The patient with diabetes must measure his glucose level often. Although urine testing may be used to monitor blood glucose control, it's rapidly being replaced with blood glucose monitoring. However, urine testing is the only way to detect ketone bodies—particularly important for the ketosis-prone diabetic patient.

Blood glucose self-monitoring allows the patient (and the nurse) to determine metabolic status quickly and as needed. With this feedback, the patient can make immediate adjustments to his nutrition therapy or drug regimen. It's especially useful for those on a tight-control regimen. The landmark Diabetes Control and Complications Trial showed that tight control can delay and prevent the long-term complications of diabetes.

Blood glucose monitoring equipment varies greatly, so it's important to follow the manufacturer's instructions precisely. Monitor the patient's hemoglobin A_{1c} level as ordered to assess long-term diabetes control. The amount of glycosylation directly correlates with blood glucose levels. Ideally, the patient's hemoglobin A_{1c} level should measure no more than 1.5 times the normal level (which ranges from 3% to 6%). A high hemoglobin A_{1c} level over several weeks suggests hyperglycemia.

Keep accurate records of vital signs, weight, fluid intake, urine output, and caloric intake besides monitoring serum glucose and urine acetone levels.

Monitor the patient closely for signs and symptoms of hyperglycemia and hypoglycemia. Should a hypoglycemic reaction occur, immediately give carbohydrates in the form of fruit juice, hard candy, honey or, if the patient is unconscious, glucagon or I.V. dextrose. Notify the doctor of any significant change in the patient's blood glucose levels.

Provide meticulous skin care, especially to the feet and legs, to avert problems associated with peripheral vascular disease and neuropathy because even a tiny skin break can eventually lead to complications necessitating amputation. Avoid constricting hose, slippers, or bed linens. Refer the patient to a podiatrist, if indicated.

Patient education. Explain the type of diabetes the patient has.

Review the prescribed meal plan, and teach the patient how to adjust his meal plan when engaged in extra activity. Encourage the type II patient to control his weight, and suggest Weight Watchers or Overeaters Anonymous if necessary.

Advise the patient about aerobic exercise programs. Explain how exercise affects blood glucose levels, and provide safety guidelines.

Instruct the patient on insulin administration, if prescribed, including type, peak times, dosage, drawing up the insulin, mixing (if applicable), administration technique, site rotation, and storage.

Instruct the patient on oral hypoglycemic therapy, if prescribed, including dosage, frequency and time of administration, and potential adverse reactions. Stress that the drug doesn't replace dietary measures. Advise the patient to take the drug only as ordered and never to discontinue the drug without consulting his doctor. Review guidelines for alcohol use.

Demonstrate urine testing for ketones and blood glucose monitoring. Instruct him to test himself when prescribed and if he feels his blood glucose level needs checking. Have the patient demonstrate all procedures. Encourage the patient to use the data from self-monitoring of his blood glucose to make changes, as indicated, in his diabetes regimen. Help him obtain both a medical identification bracelet and wallet identification card.

Evaluation. The patient should have optimal blood glucose levels, maintain an adequate nutritional intake, understand his drug regimen, and monitor himself for any complications. (See *Management of new onset of hyperglycemia [new onset diabetes]*, pages 562 to 564.)

Hypoglycemia

Characterized by an abnormally low glucose level, hypoglycemia occurs when glucose is used too rapidly, when the glucose release rate falls behind tissue demands, or when excessive insulin enters the bloodstream. True hypoglycemia in persons not taking glucose lowering agents must meet the following criteria: symptoms of confusion, aberrant behavior, light-headedness, loss of consciousness, seizures, serum glucose level less than 40 mg/dl, and relief with glucose administration. Classified as reactive postprandial or fasting, hypoglycemia is a specific endocrine imbalance, yet its symptoms may be vague and depend on how quickly the patient's glucose levels drop. If not corrected, severe hypoglycemia may result in coma and irreversible brain damage. (See *Comparing hypoglycemia, DKA, and HHNS*, pages 566 to 568.)

Causes. Reactive hypoglycemia can result from rapid movement of food into the small intestine caused by gastrectomy or other GI procedures or from congenital abnormalities (idiopathic). It can be caused by exogenous factors, such as alcohol or drug ingestion (particularly too much insulin and sulfonylureas by patients with diabetes), or endogenous factors, such as insulin-secreting tumors or hepatic or renal disease. Fasting hypoglycemia causes discomfort during long periods without food.

Assessment findings. Any of the following signs and symptoms can indicate hypoglycemia: hunger, weakness, cold sweats, shakiness, trembling, headache, irritability, tachycardia, pallor, blurred vision, confusion, motor weakness, hemiplegia, convulsions, or coma.

Diagnostic tests. A 5-hour glucose tolerance test may be administered to provoke reactive hypoglycemia. Laboratory testing to detect serum insulin and glucose levels may identify fasting hypoglycemia after a 48-hour fast.

A self-monitoring blood glucose test is a quick way to screen blood glucose levels. A color change or value that corresponds to less than 45 mg/dl indicates the need for a venous blood sample. Laboratory testing confirms the diagnosis.

Treatment. For acute hypoglycemia, the first priority is to restore the patient's glucose level. For an unconscious patient, I.M. or subcutaneous glucagon or an I.V. bolus of 50 ml of dextrose 5% in water is usually administered first. For a conscious patient, administer 15 to 20 g of a fast-acting carbohydrate such as sweetened orange juice.

When the patient's condition improves, in about 15 to 20 minutes, a snack should be given to prevent another hypoglycemic episode. Effective long-term treatment of reactive hypoglycemia may require dietary modification to help delay glucose absorption and gastric emptying. Usually, this includes small, frequent meals; ingestion of complex carbohydrates, fiber, and fat;

(*Text continues on page 564.*)

Management of new onset of hyperglycemia (new onset diabetes)

DRG#: 250
Length of Stay (LOS): 6 days (Goal: 4 days)
Actual LOS:

	Day 1

Medical interventions	• History and physical
	• Order the following:
	  –Fingersticks (before meals and bedtime)
	  –American Dietetic Association (ADA) diet
	  –Intake and output (I & O)
	  –No dextrose in routine I.V. fluids unless patient is having nothing by mouth
	  –Hypoglycemic therapy.
	• Initiate assessment for precipitating factors.

Nursing interventions	• Complete database—assessment. • Document patient's self-care ability. • Obtain fingersticks as ordered and as needed (p.r.n.). • Administer glycemic medications as ordered. • Assess learning ability. • Obtain I & O as ordered.
Social work	• Respond to assessed need if patient has inadequate support systems or needs assistance with discharge.
Nutrition	• Dietary screening • ADA diet
Tests	• Urinalysis • Chemistries: sodium, potassium, carbon dioxide, glucose, creatinine
Consults	• Dietitian • Endocrinologist
Activity	• Screen ability to perform activities of daily living (ADLs).
Patient/significant other education	• Screen ability to learn. • Initiate teaching protocol.
Discharge planning	• Identify support system: family and significant other involvement. • Identify lifestyle, health habits prior to admission.

Days 2–3	Day 4 (Discharge)
• Assessment for precipitating factors complete. • Reassess need for ongoing glycemic control. • Assess need for home glucose monitoring. • Day prior to discharge: "Tentative DC in AM" order on chart; DC medications, supplies ordered.	• Address need for home health referral • Complete discharge instructions, discuss with patient. • Dictate discharge summary. • Discharge order on order sheet
• Fingersticks, I & O as ordered • Glycemic medications as ordered • Initiate educational activities.	• Document on teaching protocol form: –Reinforcement of self-care activities –Reinforcement of medication information.
• Assess support systems.	
• Individualized caloric assessment • Instruction in diet	• Complete caloric assessment. • Reinforce diet.
• Continue to document glucose monitoring.	
• Dietitian and endocrine consults in progress	• Arrange follow-up with ophthalmology, podiatry, and diabetic management class. • Ensure that endocrine consult is completed by day 4 or endocrine clinic appointment is scheduled.
• Assess ability to perform ADLs.	• Document ability to perform ADLs.
• Distribute educational literature. • Discuss disease process, self-care (and home glucose monitoring). • Demonstrate/observe return demonstration of medication administration.	• Address use of home glucose monitor. • Reinforce medication administration.
• Order glucometer if applicable. • Initiate referral for home care (if applicable).	• Stress importance of maintaining medical regimen, clinic appointments, diet. *(continued)*

Management of new onset of hyperglycemia (new onset diabetes) *(continued)*

	Day 1
Discharge planning *(continued)*	
Key patient outcomes	Therapy initiated. Assessment for the presence or absence of precipitating factors initiated.
	Signature _____ Initials _____ _____ _____

Adapted with permission from Veterans Affairs Maryland Health Care System, Baltimore.

and avoidance of simple sugars, alcohol, and fruit drinks. The patient may also receive anticholinergic drugs.

For fasting hypoglycemia, drug therapy—including adjustment of insulin or sulfonylureas—is usually required. In patients with insulinoma, removal of the tumor is the treatment of choice. Drug therapy may include nondiuretic thiazides such as diazoxide to inhibit insulin secretion, streptozocin, and hormones such as glucocorticoids and long-acting glycogen.

Nursing interventions. Explain the purpose and procedure for any diagnostic tests. Collect blood samples at the appropriate times, as ordered. Monitor the effects of drug therapy, especially development of adverse effects.

Patient education. Teach the patient which foods to include in his diet and which foods to avoid. Refer the patient and family for dietary counseling, as appropriate.

Evaluation. The patient should know the disorder's signs and how to maintain an appropriate diet. Blood glucose levels should be normal.

Adrenal disorders

Adrenal disorders include pheochromocytoma, hyperaldosteronism, adrenal hypofunction (Addison's disease, adrenal insufficiency), and adrenal hyperfunction (Cushing's syndrome).

Pheochromocytoma

In pheochromocytoma, a chromaffin-cell tumor of the sympathetic nervous system, usually in the

Days 2–3	Day 4 (Discharge)
	• Review discharge and procedure for mail-in renewal for supplies. • Provide telephone numbers for clinic, doctor, support groups.
Random blood sugar (BS) > 60 and <300 Fasting BS > 60 and < 240 Therapy for precipitating factors indicated (if applicable)	• Fasting blood sugar >60, <180; or random blood sugar >60, <280 • Home glucose monitoring initiated (if applicable). • Patient or significant other verbalizes understanding of self-care, knowledge of follow-up, medications renewal.

adrenal medulla, secretes an excess of the catecholamines epinephrine and norepinephrine. A history of acute episodes of hypertension strongly suggests the presence of this tumor. The tumor is usually benign but may be malignant in as many as 10% of patients.

Occasionally, pheochromocytoma is diagnosed during pregnancy, when uterine pressure on the tumor induces more frequent attacks. This can be fatal for mother and fetus as a result of CVA, acute pulmonary edema, cardiac arrhythmias, or hypoxia.

Cause. Pheochromocytoma may result from an inherited autosomal dominant trait.

Assessment findings. Symptomatic episodes may recur as seldom as every 2 months or as often as 25 times a day. They may occur spontaneously or may follow certain precipitating events, such as postural change, exercise, laughter, smoking, anesthesia, urination, or temperature change (body or environment).

The cardinal signs and symptoms are persistent or paroxysmal hypertension accompanied by headache, diaphoresis, and palpitations. Other signs and symptoms include tachycardia, visual disturbances, pallor, warmth or flushing, paresthesia, tremor, and excitation. Other indications can include fright, nervousness, feelings of impending doom, abdominal or chest pain, tachypnea, nausea and vomiting, fatigue, weight loss, constipation, postural hypotension, paradoxical response to antihypertensive drugs (common), glycosuria,

(*Text continues on page 568.*)

Comparing hypoglycemia, DKA, and HHNS

Hypoglycemia	Diabetic ketoacidosis (DKA)	Hyperosmolar hyperglycemic nonketotic syndrome (HHNS)
Precipitating factors		
Delayed or omitted meal, insulin overdose, excessive exercise without food or insulin adjustments	Undiagnosed diabetes, neglected treatment, infection, cardiovascular disorders, physical stress, emotional distress Exercise in uncontrolled diabetes	Undiagnosed diabetes, infection or other stress, acute or chronic illnesses, certain drugs and medical procedures, severe burns treated with high glucose concentrations
Symptom onset		
Rapid (minutes to hours)	Slow (hours to days)	Slow (hours to days), but more gradual than DKA
Signs and symptoms		
Skin and mucous membranes Cold, clammy skin; pallor; profuse sweating; normal mucous membranes	Warm, flushed, dry, loose skin; dry, crusty mucous membranes; soft eyeballs	Warm, flushed, dry, extremely loose skin; dry, crusty mucous membranes; soft eyeballs
Neurologic status *Initial*—irritability, nervousness, giddiness; hand tremors; difficulty speaking, concentrating, focusing, and coordinating; paresthesias *Late*—hyperreflexia, dilated pupils, coma	*Initial*—dullness, confusion, lethargy; diminished reflexes *Late*—coma	*Initial*—dullness, confusion, lethargy, diminished reflexes *Late*—coma
Muscle strength Normal or reduced	Extremely weak	Extremely weak
GI None	Anorexia, nausea, vomiting, diarrhea, abdominal tenderness and pain	None

Comparing hypoglycemia, DKA, and HHNS *(continued)*

Hypoglycemia	Diabetic ketoacidosis (DKA)	Hyperosmolar hyperglycemic nonketotic syndrome (HHNS)
Signs and symptoms *(continued)*		
Temperature Normal (subnormal if in deep coma)	Hypothermia Possible fever (from dehydration or infection)	Possible fever (from dehydration or infection)
Pulse Tachycardic (bradycardic in deep coma)	Mildly tachycardic, weak	Usually rapid
Blood pressure Normal or above normal	Subnormal	Subnormal
Respirations *Initial*—normal to rapid *Late*—slow	*Initial*—deep, fast *Late*—Kussmaul's	Rapid (but no Kussmaul's)
Breath odor Normal	Fruity, acetone	Normal
Weight Stable	Decreased	Decreased
Other Hunger	Thirst	*Initial*—thirst *Late*—thirst may be absent
Laboratory findings		
Blood glucose level Below normal (<50 mg/dl)	Above normal	Markedly above normal
Serum sodium level Normal	Normal or subnormal	Above normal, normal, or subnormal
Serum potassium level Normal	Normal or above normal	Normal or above normal *(continued)*

Comparing hypoglycemia, DKA, and HHNS *(continued)*

Hypoglycemia	Diabetic ketoaci-dosis (DKA)	Hyperosmolar hyper-glycemic nonketotic syndrome (HHNS)
Laboratory findings *(continued)*		
Serum ketones Negative	Positive, large	Negative, small
Serum osmolarity Normal (290 to 310 mOsm/L)	Above normal but usually less than 330 mOsm/L	Markedly above normal—350 to 450 mOsm/L
Hematocrit Normal	Above normal	Above normal
Arterial blood gas levels Normal or slight respiratory acidosis	Metabolic acidosis with compensatory respiratory alkalosis	Normal or slight metabolic acidosis
Urine glucose level Normal	Above normal	Markedly above normal
Urine output Normal	*Initial*—polyuria *Late*—oliguria	*Initial*—marked polyuria *Late*—oliguria
Treatment		
Glucose, glucagon, epinephrine	Insulin, fluid replacement, electrolyte replacement, antiacidosis therapy (if needed)	Fluid replacement, insulin, electrolyte replacement

hyperglycemia, and hypermetabolism.

Diagnostic tests. Increased urinary excretion of total free epinephrine and norepinephrine and their metabolites, vanillylmandelic acid (VMA), and metanephrine, as measured by analysis of a single voided urine specimen or a 24-hour urine collection, confirms pheochromocytoma. Labile blood pressure necessitates urine collection after a hypertensive episode to be compared with a baseline specimen. Total plasma catecholamines levels 14 to 50 times higher than normal indicate a pheochromocytoma.

A clonidine suppression test may help confirm the diagnosis. After obtaining baseline catecholamine levels, administer 0.3 mg clonidine by mouth, then measure plasma or urine catecholamine levels 3 hours afterwards. Clonidine should suppress catecholamines. A CT or MRI scan helps locate the tumor. Palpation of the area surrounding the tumor may induce a typical acute attack and help confirm the diagnosis if the tumor is palpable.

Treatment. Surgical removal of the tumor is the treatment of choice. To decrease blood pressure, an alpha-adrenergic blocking agent (phentolamine, prazosin, or phenoxybenzamine) or metyrosine (which blocks catecholamine synthesis) is administered from 1 day to 2 weeks before surgery. A beta-adrenergic blocking agent (propranolol) may also be used after achieving alpha blockade if the patient develops serious tachycardia or arrhythmias. Calcium channel blockers, such as nifedipine or nicardipine, may also be used to prevent the release of catecholamines from the tumor. Postoperatively, I.V. fluids, plasma volume expanders, vasopressors, and transfusions may be required if marked hypotension occurs.

The first 24 to 48 hours immediately after surgery are the most critical, as blood pressure can drop drastically. If hypotension develops, the patient needs volume replacement.

Usually large volumes of fluid are required—$1/2$ to $1 1/2$ times calculated blood volume during the first 24 to 48 hours. When renal output increases and blood pressure and heart rate stabilize, decrease the I.V. volume replacement to 125 ml per hour.

If the patient is receiving vasopressors I.V., check blood pressure every 3 to 5 minutes and regulate the drip to maintain a safe pressure. Arterial pressure lines facilitate constant monitoring.

Postoperative hypertension may occur because the stress of surgery and manipulation of the adrenal gland stimulate secretion of catecholamines or because some pheochromocytoma tissue remains. Because this excess secretion causes profuse sweating, keep the room cool and change the patient's clothing and bedding often. If the patient is receiving phentolamine, monitor blood pressure closely. Observe and record adverse reactions, such as dizziness, hypotension, and tachycardia.

Watch for abdominal distention and return of bowel sounds. Check dressings and vital signs for indications of hemorrhage (increased pulse rate, decreased blood pressure, cold and clammy skin, pallor, unresponsiveness). Give analgesics for pain, as ordered, but monitor blood pressure carefully because many analgesics, especially meperidine, can cause hypotension.

If surgery isn't feasible, alpha- and beta-adrenergic blocking agents are beneficial in controlling catecholamine effects and preventing attacks. An acute attack or a hypertensive crisis requires I.V. administration of phentolamine (push or drip) or nitroprusside to normalize blood pressure.

Nursing interventions. Be aware of foods high in vanillin and drugs that may interfere with the accurate determination of VMA levels (such as guaifenesin and salicylates). Collect the urine in a special container, with hydrochloric acid, that has been prepared by the laboratory.

Obtain blood pressure readings often because transient hypertensive attacks are possible. Tell the patient to report headaches, palpitations, nervousness, or other acute attack symptoms. If hypertensive crisis develops, monitor blood pressure and heart rate every 2 to 5 minutes until blood pressure stabilizes acceptably.

Check blood for glucose, and watch for weight loss from hypermetabolism. If autosomal dominant transmission of pheochromocytoma is suspected, the patient's family should also be evaluated for this condition.

Patient education. To ensure the reliability of urine catecholamine measurements, make sure the patient avoids foods high in vanillin (such as coffee, nuts, chocolate, and bananas) for 2 days before urine collection for VMA measurements.

Evaluation. The patient should have normal blood pressure and plasma catecholamine levels and should understand the need for follow-up care.

Hyperaldosteronism

Hyperaldosteronism is characterized by the adrenal cortex's hypersecretion of aldosterone with resultant hypokalemia. It occurs as a primary disease of the adrenal cortex or, more commonly, as a secondary disorder in response to extra-adrenal disorders commonly associated with increased plasma renin activity. Aldosterone hypersecretion causes excessive reabsorption of sodium and water and excessive renal excretion of potassium.

Causes. Primary hyperaldosteronism can result from a benign adrenal adenoma, primary adrenocortical hyperplasia (in children), adenocortical cancer, or unknown causes.

Secondary hyperaldosteronism can result from renal artery stenosis, renin-secreting tumors, malignant hypertension, Wilms' tumor, pregnancy, oral contraceptive use, nephrotic syndrome, cirrhosis with ascites, idiopathic edema, heart failure (HF), Bartter's syndrome, and extrarenal sodium loss.

Assessment findings. Any of these signs and symptoms may be apparent: hypertension, hypokalemia, hypernatremia (140 to 150 mEq/L), decreased hematocrit, muscle weakness, tetany, paresthesia, arrhythmias, fatigue, headache, polyuria, polydipsia, or visual disturbances.

Diagnostic tests. To assess hypokalemia, the patient follows a normal sodium diet, with 1 g sodium (as tablets or an extra $\frac{1}{2}$ teaspoon of table salt) for 4 days; on the fifth day, electrolytes are measured. To assess plasma renin levels, the patient must be off diuretic and angiotensin-converting enzyme inhibitor therapy for 3 weeks, with the first sample drawn while the patient is recumbent, early in the morning or after 30 minutes of bedrest, and the second drawn 2 to 4 hours after the patient has been upright. Normally, the value should increase at least twofold. Serum bicarbonate levels are often elevated, with ensuing alkalosis from hydrogen and potassium ion loss in the distal renal tubules.

Other tests show markedly increased 24-hour urinary aldosterone levels after infusion of 2 qt [2 L] of normal saline over 4 hours; increased plasma aldosterone levels; and, in secondary hyperaldosteronism, increased plasma renin levels. Aldosterone levels greater than 10 ng/dl indicated failure to suppress. CT scan and MRI may be used for tumor localization as may bilateral catheterization of the adrenal veins for corticosteroids.

Treatment. Use of a potassium-sparing diuretic (such as spironolactone or amiloride) and sodium restriction may control the disease without unilateral adrenalectomy. Treatment may also include calcium channel blockers.

After adrenalectomy, watch for weakness, hyponatremia, rising serum potassium levels, and signs of adrenal insufficiency, especially hypotension. Treatment of secondary hyperaldosteronism requires correction of the underlying cause.

Nursing interventions. Monitor and record urine output, blood pressure, weight, and serum potassium levels. Watch for signs of tetany and for hypokalemia-induced cardiac arrhythmias, paresthesia, or weakness. Give potassium replacements, as ordered, and keep I.V. calcium gluconate available. Ask the dietitian to provide a low-sodium, high-potassium diet.

Patient education. If the patient is taking spironolactone, advise him to watch for signs and symptoms of hyperkalemia. Tell him that loss of libido, impotence, and gynecomastia may follow long-term use. Instruct females that menstrual irregularities and breast discomfort may occur.

Evaluation. The patient should maintain an adequate fluid and electrolyte balance, have normal blood pressure and plasma aldosterone levels, and have follow-up examinations.

Adrenal hypofunction

Addison's disease, the most common form of adrenal insufficiency, occurs when more than 90% of the adrenal gland is destroyed. In this autoimmune process, circulating antibodies react specifically against the adrenal tissue.

Adrenal hypofunction can also occur secondary to a disorder outside the gland, but aldosterone secretion commonly continues intact.

Acute adrenal insufficiency, or adrenal crisis (addisonian crisis), is a medical emergency requiring immediate, vigorous treatment.

Causes. Autoimmune causes, the most common cause, are associated with polyendocrine deficiency syndrome. Addison's disease can result from tuberculosis, bilateral adrenalectomy, hemorrhage into the adrenal gland, neoplasms, acquired immune deficiency syndrome, or fungal infections.

Secondary adrenal hypofunction can be caused by hypopituitarism, the abrupt withdrawal of long-term corticosteroid therapy, or removal of a nonendocrine, corticotropin-secreting tumor.

Adrenal crisis occurs when the body's stores of glucocorticoids are exhausted in a person with adrenal hypofunction caused by trauma or surgery.

Assessment findings. The signs and symptoms of Addison's disease are weakness, fatigue, weight loss, nausea and vomiting, anorexia, chronic diarrhea, and conspicuous bronze skin coloration, especially in creases. Other indications include darkening of scars and areas of vitiligo (absence of pigmentation); increased pigmentation of the mucous membranes, especially the buccal mucosa; cardiovascular abnormalities, such as postural hypotension, decreased heart size and cardiac output, and a weak, irregular pulse; decreased tolerance for even minor stress; poor coordination; fasting hypoglycemia; and craving for salt. In female patients, amenorrhea may occur.

Secondary adrenal hypofunction has similar clinical effects, but without hyperpigmentation, hypotension, and electrolyte abnormalities.

Adrenal crisis is characterized by profound weakness and fatigue, severe nausea and vomiting, hypotension, dehydration, clouded sensorium, occasionally high fever, and muscle, joint and abdominal pain.

Diagnostic tests. Adrenal hypofunction can be confirmed if plasma cortisol and serum sodium levels are decreased and corticotropin, serum potassium, and BUN levels are increased. In secondary hypoadrenalism, potassium is usually normal and corticotropin is normal or low.

Provocative tests that determine if adrenal hypofunction is primary or secondary include metyrapone and corticotropin stimulation tests. CT scans showing large adrenals indicate primary adrenal disease.

Treatment. For all patients with primary or secondary adrenal hypofunction, lifelong corticosteroid replacement, usually with cortisone or hydrocortisone, is the primary treatment. The usual replacement dose is increased during stress. Drug therapy may also include fludrocortisone.

Adrenal crisis requires prompt I.V. administration of 400 mg hydrocortisone per day. Up to 300 mg/day of hydrocortisone and 3 to 5.5 qt (3 to 5 L) of I.V. dextrose 5% in saline solution may be required during the acute stage. With proper treatment, the crisis usually subsides quickly; blood pressure stabilizes, and fluid and sodium levels return

to normal. Subsequent oral maintenance doses of hydrocortisone preserve stability.

Nursing interventions. In an
adrenal crisis, monitor vital signs
carefully, especially for hypotension,
volume depletion, and other signs
of shock (decreased LOC and urine
output). Watch for hyperkalemia
before treatment and for hypokalemia after treatment (from
excessive mineralocorticoid effect).

If the patient also has diabetes,
check blood glucose levels periodically because steroid replacement
may require adjustment of glucose-
lowering agent dosage. Record
weight and intake and output carefully because the patient may have
volume depletion. Until onset of
mineralocorticoid effects, force fluids to replace excessive fluid loss.

Ask the dietitian to provide a
diet high in protein and carbohydrates that maintains sodium and
potassium balance. If the patient is
anorexic, suggest six small meals a
day to increase calorie intake.

Observe the patient receiving
steroids for cushingoid signs such as
fluid retention around the eyes and
face. Watch for fluid and electrolyte
imbalance.

Patient education. Explain that lifelong cortisone replacement therapy
is necessary. Advise the patient of
symptoms of overdose and underdose and concerning his need to
increase the dosage during times of
stress (when he has a cold, for
example). Warn that infection,

injury, or profuse sweating in hot
weather may precipitate crisis.

Instruct the patient to always
carry a medical identification card
and to wear a bracelet giving the
name of the steroid and the dosage.
Teach the patient how to give himself an injection of hydrocortisone.
Tell him to keep available an emergency kit containing hydrocortisone
in a prepared syringe for use in
times of stress. Warn that any stress
may necessitate additional cortisone
to prevent a crisis.

Evaluation. The patient should
maintain a proper diet; maintain
normal serum sodium, potassium,
and plasma cortisol levels; understand the need to take his medication routinely; and make necessary
adjustments in times of stress.

Adrenal hyperfunction (Cushing's syndrome)

Cushing's syndrome results from
excessive levels of adrenocortical
hormones (particularly cortisol) or
related corticosteroids and, to a lesser extent, androgens and aldosterone. Its unmistakable signs include
rapidly developing adiposity of the
face (moon face), neck, and trunk,
and purple striae on the skin.

Steroid-induced diabetes, pathologic fractures, and osteoporosis are
associated complications.

Causes. Adrenal hyperfunction can
be caused by pituitary hypersecretion of corticotropin or corticotro-
pin-releasing hormone (CRH)
(Cushing's disease), a corticotropin-
secreting tumor in another organ

(particularly bronchogenic or carcinoma in the pancreas), or the administration of synthetic glucocorticoids. Adrenal tumor, which is usually benign in adults, is a less common cause of the syndrome. The most common cause in infants is adrenal carcinoma.

Assessment findings. As with other endocrine disorders, Cushing's syndrome induces multiple body system changes, depending on the adrenocortical hormone involved. (See *Signs of Cushing's syndrome.*) In addition to obesity, clinical effects may include:
- *Musculoskeletal system*— muscle weakness, back pain, skeletal growth retardation in children
- *Skin*—purplish striae; fat pads above the clavicles, over the upper back (buffalo hump), on the face (moon face), and throughout the trunk, with slender arms and legs; little or no scar formation; facial plethora; poor wound healing; acne and hirsutism in women
- *CNS*—irritability and emotional lability, ranging from euphoric behavior to depression or psychosis; insomnia; headache
- *Cardiovascular system*—hypertension; bleeding, petechiae, HF, and ecchymosis
- *Immune system*—increased susceptibility to infection, decreased resistance
- *Renal and urinary systems*—sodium and secondary fluid retention, renal calculi
- *Reproductive system*—increased androgen production, causing gynecomastia in males and clitoral hypertrophy, mild virilism, and amenorrhea or oligomenorrhea in females.

Diagnostic tests. An inability to suppress cortisol with a low-dose (overnight) dexamethasone suppression test and elevated 24-hour urinary free cortisol levels confirms the diagnosis of Cushing's syndrome. A plasma corticotropin test and high-dose dexamethasone suppression test can determine the cause of Cushing's syndrome. With an adrenal tumor, corticotropin levels are undetectable and cortisol levels are not suppressed. Ectopic corticotropin syndrome is indicated by elevated corticotropin or unsuppressed cortisol levels. Cushing's disease is indicated by normal to elevated corticotropin with steroid suppressed to less than 50% of baseline. The pituitary response to multiple dose metyrapone and dexamethasone may also be elevated as well as the corticotropin response to CRH. Ultrasonography, CT scan, or MRI localizes tumors.

Treatment. Radiation, drug therapy, or surgery may be necessary to restore hormone balance and reverse Cushing's syndrome.

For example, transsphenoidal resection of the corticotropin-secreting pituitary microadenoma is the therapy of choice for Cushing's disease, although pituitary radiation may be used in children and young adults. Adrenal tumors are treated by unilateral adrenalectomy, but patients require glucocorticoid therapy perioperatively and postoperatively. Nonendocrine corticotropin-

Signs of Cushing's syndrome

Long-term treatment with corticosteroids may produce Cushing's syndrome—a condition marked by obvious fat deposits between the shoulders and around the waist and by widespread systemic abnormalities. In addition to the signs shown below, observe for renal disorders, hyperglycemia, tissue wasting, muscular weakness, and labile emotional state.

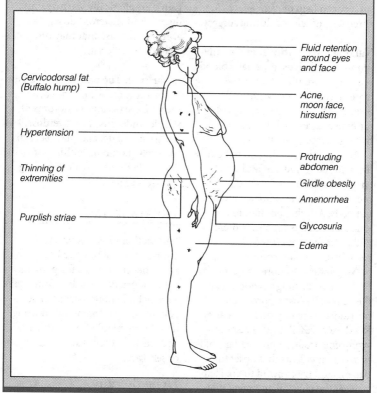

Cervicodorsal fat (Buffalo hump)

Hypertension

Thinning of extremities

Purplish striae

Fluid retention around eyes and face

Acne, moon face, hirsutism

Protruding abdomen

Girdle obesity

Amenorrhea

Glycosuria

Edema

secreting tumors require excision. Drug therapy (ketoconazole, mitotane, metyrapone, or aminoglutethimide) is also used to decrease cortisol levels if symptoms persist or the tumor is inoperable. Mitotane may be used in combination with irradiation.

Aminoglutethimide and cyproheptadine decrease cortisol levels. Cyproheptadine and valproate can suppress corticotropin secretion and lead to remission. Aminoglutethimide alone or in combination with metyrapone may be useful in metastatic adrenal carcinoma.

Before surgery, the patient with cushingoid signs and symptoms needs management to control hypertension, edema, diabetes, and cardiovascular manifestations and to prevent infection. Glucocorticoid administration on the morning of surgery can help prevent acute adrenal insufficiency during surgery.

Nursing interventions. Frequently monitor vital signs, especially blood pressure. Carefully observe the hypertensive patient with cardiac disease. Check laboratory reports for hypernatremia, hypokalemia, hyperglycemia, and glycosuria.

Because the cushingoid patient is likely to retain sodium and water, check for edema, and carefully monitor weight and intake and output daily. Ask the dietitian to provide a diet that is high in protein and potassium but low in calories, carbohydrates, and sodium.

Watch for infection—a particular problem in Cushing's syndrome. If the patient has osteoporosis and is bedridden, carefully perform passive ROM exercises. Because Cushing's syndrome produces emotional lability, record incidents that upset the patient, and try to avoid them. Help him get the physical and mental rest he needs—by sedation if necessary. Offer emotional support throughout the difficult testing period.

Patient education. Advise the patient to take replacement steroids with antacids or meals, to minimize gastric irritation.

Have the patient carry a medical identification card and report immediately any physiologically stressful situations such as infections, which require increased dosage.

Instruct him to recognize signs and symptoms of steroid underdose (fatigue, weakness, dizziness) and overdose (severe edema, weight gain). Emphatically warn against discontinuing steroid dosage abruptly because that may produce a fatal adrenal crisis.

Evaluation. The patient should take his medication as prescribed, and recognize signs and symptoms of steroid underdose and overdose. His fluid, electrolyte, and plasma cortisol levels should be within normal limits. He should seek counseling for stress as needed.

TREATMENTS

This section provides practical information about drugs, surgery, and other treatments for patients with endocrine disorders. You'll play a crucial role in preparing these patients for treatment, monitoring them during and after treatment, and teaching them various aspects of self-care.

Drug therapy

Many different drugs are used to treat patient with endocrine disorders. Corticosteroids—such as cortisone acetate and hydrocortisone—are used to treat adrenal insufficiency. Glucose-lowering agents—such as insulins, tolazamide, and chlorpropamide and glucagon—are used to treat types I and II diabetes.

Drugs that affect calcium levels include calcitonin and calcitriol. Calcitonin is used to treat Paget's disease; calcitriol, to manage hypocalcemia in patients undergoing renal dialysis.

Pituitary hormones—such as desmopressin and lypressin—are used to treat pituitary diabetes insipidus. Thyroid hormone antagonists—such as methimazole and PTU—are used to treat hyperthyroidism. Liotrix is used to treat hypothyroidism.

Surgery

Surgical treatment for endocrine disorders includes hypophysectomy, thyroidectomy, parathyroidectomy, pancreatectomy, and adrenalectomy.

Hypophysectomy

Transsphenoidal hypophysectomy is the treatment of choice for pituitary tumors, which can cause gigantism, acromegaly, and Cushing's disease. It can also be used as a palliative measure for patients with metastatic breast or prostate cancer to relieve pain and reduce hormonal secretions.

Hypophysectomy is usually performed transsphenoidally (entering from the inner aspect of the upper lip through the sphenoid sinus). (See *Transsphenoidal hypophysectomy,* page 578.)

The transsphenoidal approach may preserve pituitary gland function and reduce the risk of postoperative illness and death. New techniques can remove microadenomas.

After surgery, transient diabetes insipidus may occur, requiring careful patient monitoring for 24 to 48 hours. Other potential complications include infection, cerebrospinal fluid (CSF) leakage, hemorrhage, and visual defects. Total removal of the pituitary gland causes a hormonal deficiency that requires close monitoring and replacement therapy; usually, the anterior pituitary is preserved.

Patient preparation. Explain to the patient that this surgery will remove a tumor from his pituitary gland. Tell him that he will receive a general anesthetic and, after surgery, may go to the intensive care unit (ICU) to permit careful monitoring. Mention that he will have a nasal catheter and packing in place for at least 1 day after surgery as well as an indwelling urinary catheter.

Arrange for appropriate tests and examinations, as ordered. For example, if the patient has acromegaly, he will need a thorough cardiac evaluation because he may have incipient myocardial ischemia. If the patient has Cushing's disease, he will need blood pressure checks and serum potassium determinations. For all patients, arrange visual field tests to serve as a baseline.

Review the preoperative medication regimen if appropriate. If the patient is hypothyroid, he may need hormone replacement therapy. If he has a prolactin-secreting tumor, find out if he has been taking bromocriptine for 6 weeks before surgery to help shrink and soften the tumor. Many patients receive I.V. hydrocortisone preoperatively and postoperatively.

Transsphenoidal hypophysectomy

When a pituitary tumor is confined to the sella turcica, the doctor will perform transsphenoidal hypophysectomy. For this procedure, the patient is placed in a semirecumbent position and given a general anesthetic. The doctor incises the upper lip's inner aspect so that he can enter the sella turcica through the sphenoid sinus to remove the tumor.

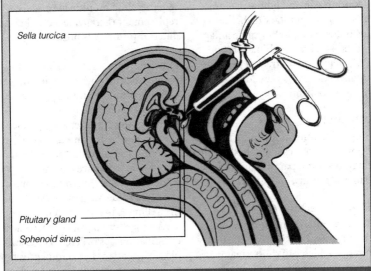

Sella turcica

Pituitary gland

Sphenoid sinus

Monitoring and aftercare. Keep the patient on bed rest for 24 hours after surgery and then encourage ambulation. Keep the head of his bed elevated to avoid placing tension or pressure on the suture line. Tell him not to sneeze, cough, blow his nose, or bend over for several days to avoid disturbing the muscle graft. (See *Documenting surgical incision care.*)

Give mild analgesics, as ordered, for headache caused by CSF loss during surgery or for paranasal pain. Paranasal pain typically subsides when the catheters and pack-ing are removed—usually 24 to 72 hours after surgery.

The patient may develop transient diabetes insipidus, usually 24 to 48 hours after surgery. Be alert for increased thirst and increased urine volume with a low specific gravity. If diabetes insipidus occurs, replace fluids and administer aqueous vasopressin, or give sublingual desmopressin, as ordered. With these measures, diabetes insipidus quickly resolves.

Arrange for visual field testing as soon as possible because visual defects can indicate hemorrhage. Collect a serum sample to measure pituitary hormone levels and evaluate the need for hormone replacement. As ordered, give prophylactic antimicrobials.

Patient education. Instruct the patient to report signs of diabetes insipidus immediately. Explain that he may need to limit fluid intake or take prescribed medications. Tell the patient with hyperprolactinemia that he will need follow-up visits for several years because relapse is possible. Explain that he may be placed on bromocriptine if relapse occurs.

If ordered, tell the patient not to brush his upper teeth for 2 weeks to avoid suture line disruption. Mention that he can use a mouthwash. He may need hormone replacement therapy as a result of decreased pituitary secretion of tropic hormones. If he needs cortisol or thyroid hormone replacement, teach him to recognize the signs of excessive or insufficient dosage. Advise him to wear a medical identification bracelet. Stress the importance of regular follow-up appointments.

Thyroidectomy

Surgery to remove all or part of the thyroid gland is performed to treat hyperthyroidism, respiratory obstruction from goiter, and thyroid cancer. Subtotal thyroidectomy, which reduces secretion of thyroid hormone, is used to correct hyperthyroidism when drug therapy fails or radiation therapy is contraindicated. It may also effectively treat diffuse goiter. After surgery, the remaining thyroid tissue usually supplies enough thyroid hormone

CHARTING TIPS

Documenting surgical incision care

When a patient returns from surgery, pay particular attention to maintaining records on the surgical incision, the drains, and the care you provide—in addition to documenting vital signs and level of consciousness. Make certain that you read the records from the postanesthesia care unit.

Also document these important points:
• the date, time, and type of wound care provided
• the wound's appearance (size, condition of margins, necrotic tissue, if any), odor (if any), location of any drains, and drainage characteristics (type, color, consistency, and amount)
• dressing information such as type and amount of new dressing or pouch applied
• additional wound care procedures provided, such as drain management, irrigation, packing, or application of a topical medication
• the patient's tolerance of the procedure
• the amount and color of measurable drainage. Record this on the intake and output record.

for normal function, although hypothyroidism may occur later.

Total thyroidectomy is usually performed for extensive cancer. After this surgery, the patient requires lifelong thyroid hormone replacement therapy.

Thyroidectomy is usually performed under general anesthesia. Potential complications include thyrotoxicosis; hemorrhage; parathyroid damage, resulting in postoperative hypocalcemia or tetany; and laryngeal nerve damage.

Patient preparation. Explain to the patient that thyroidectomy will remove diseased thyroid tissue or, if necessary, the entire gland. Tell him that he'll have an incision in his neck; that he'll have a drain and dressing in place after surgery; and that he may experience some hoarseness and a sore throat from intubation and anesthesia. Reassure him that he'll receive analgesics.

Ensure that the patient has followed his preoperative drug regimen, which will prevent thyrotoxicosis during surgery. He probably will have received either PTU or methimazole, usually starting 4 to 6 weeks before surgery. Expect him to be receiving iodine as well for 10 to 14 days before surgery to reduce the gland's vascularity and thus prevent excess bleeding. He may also be receiving propranolol to reduce excess sympathetic effects. Notify the doctor immediately if the patient has failed to follow his medication regimen. (See *Caring for the patient undergoing thyroidectomy.*)

Collect samples for serum thyroid hormone determinations to check for euthyroidism. If necessary, arrange for an ECG to evaluate cardiac status.

Monitoring and aftercare. Keep the patient in high semi-Fowler's position to promote venous return from the head and neck and to decrease oozing into the incision. Check for laryngeal nerve damage by asking the patient to speak as soon as he awakens from anesthesia.

Watch for signs of respiratory distress. Tracheal collapse, mucus accumulation in the trachea, laryngeal edema, and vocal cord paralysis can all cause respiratory obstruction, with sudden stridor and restlessness. Keep a tracheostomy tray at the patient's bedside for 24 hours after surgery, and be prepared to assist with emergency tracheotomy if necessary.

Assess for signs of hemorrhage, which may cause shock, tracheal compression, and respiratory distress. Check the patient's dressing and palpate the *back* of his neck, where drainage tends to flow. Expect about 50 ml of drainage in the first 24 hours; if you find none, check for drain kinking or the need to reestablish suction. Expect only scant drainage after 24 hours.

As ordered, give a mild analgesic. Reassure the patient that the discomfort should resolve quickly.

Assess for hypocalcemia, which may occur when bones depleted of calcium from hyperthyroidism begin to heal, rapidly taking up calcium from the blood, or if the parathyroid glands are injured or destroyed. Test for positive Chvostek's and Trousseau's signs, indicators of neuromuscular irritability from hypocalcemia. Keep calcium gluconate available for emergency I.V. administration.

Be alert for signs of thyroid storm, a rare but serious complication.

Patient education. If the patient has had a subtotal or total thyroidectomy, explain the importance of regularly taking the prescribed thyroid hormone replacement. Teach him to recognize and report signs of hypothyroidism and hyperthyroidism.

If parathyroid damage occurred during surgery, tell the patient he may need to take calcium supplements. Teach him to recognize the warning signs of hypocalcemia.

Tell the patient to keep the incision site clean and dry. Help him cope with concerns about its appearance. Suggest clothing to hide the incision until it has healed.

Arrange follow-up appointments as necessary, and explain to the patient that the doctor needs to check the incision and serum thyroid hormone levels.

Parathyroidectomy

The surgical removal of one or more of the four parathyroid glands treats primary hyperparathyroidism. In this disorder, the parathyroids secrete excessive PTH, causing high serum calcium and low serum phosphorus levels, which affect the kidneys or bones or cause peptic ulcer or pancreatitis.

The number of glands removed depends on the underlying cause of excessive PTH secretion. For example, if the patient has a single adenoma, excision of the affected gland corrects the problem. In subtotal parathyroidectomy, all but part of the fourth gland is removed. This

FOCUS ON CARING

Caring for the patient undergoing thyroidectomy

Your patient is having her thyroid removed. Because she's concerned about the appearance of the scar, reassure her that it will fade with time.

Suggest that, in the meantime, she might want to hide the scar with high-necked clothing or a scarf. It might be helpful to ask a family member to bring in some scarves.

remaining glandular segment decreases the risk of postoperative hypoparathyroidism.

Total parathyroidectomy is necessary when glandular hyperplasia results from a malignant tumor. In this case, the patient will require lifelong treatment for hypoparathyroidism.(See *What happens in parathyroidectomy?* page 582.)

Serum calcium levels typically decrease within 24 to 48 hours after surgery and become normal within 4 to 5 days. Complications seldom occur but may include hemorrhage, damage to the recurrent laryngeal nerve, and hypoparathyroidism.

Patient preparation. Explain to the patient that this surgery will remove diseased parathyroid tissue. Tell him that he will be intubated and receive a general anesthetic. Then, the doctor will make a neck incision and remove parathyroid tissue as necessary. Explain that the doctor may

What happens in parathyroidectomy?

The surgeon makes a transverse cervical incision and explores the exposed area to identify the parathyroid gland (or glands). The superior glands prove easier to locate than the inferior glands.

In this illustration, the surgeon has located the left inferior parathyroid gland. Before removing the gland, he will take a tissue sample for biopsy to ensure correct gland identification.

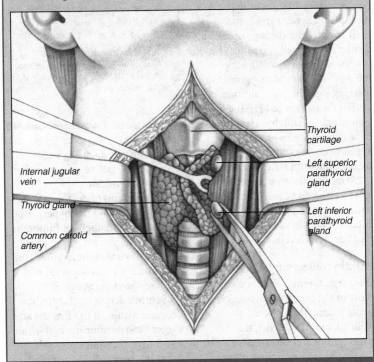

need to perform a subtotal thyroidectomy.

Maintain calcium restrictions, as ordered, before surgery. If the patient's hypercalcemia causes renal calculi, provide plenty of fluids to dilute the excess calcium. If hypercalcemia is severe, give saline solution with potassium I.V., as ordered, and expect to give a diuretic such as furosemide. If his calcium level remains elevated once diuresis has begun, you may give mithramycin I.V. (an antihypercalcemic agent), as ordered. As an adjunct, the doctor may also order inorganic phosphates.

Monitoring and aftercare. Keep the patient in high semi-Fowler's position after surgery to promote venous return from the head and neck and to decrease oozing into the incision. As soon as he begins to awaken from anesthesia, check for laryngeal nerve damage by asking him to speak.

Check the patient's dressing and palpate the *back* of his neck, where drainage tends to flow. Expect about 50 ml of drainage in the first 24 hours; if you find no drainage, check for drain kinking or the need to reestablish suction. Expect only scant drainage after 24 hours.

Check the patient for hemorrhage. Keep a tracheostomy tray at the bedside for the first 24 hours after surgery, and assess the patient frequently for signs of respiratory distress, such as dyspnea and cyanosis. Upper airway obstruction may result from tracheal collapse, mucus accumulation in the trachea, laryngeal edema, or vocal cord paralysis.

Give mild analgesics, as ordered, for postoperative pain.

Because transient hypoparathyroidism with resulting hypocalcemia can occur 1 to 4 days after surgery, watch closely for signs of increased neuromuscular excitability. Check for positive Chvostek's and Trousseau's signs, and tell the patient to report numbness and tingling of his fingers and toes or around his mouth (early symptoms of hypocalcemia) as well as muscle cramps. Keep I.V. calcium on hand in case tetany occurs.

Patient education. Tell the patient to keep the incision site clean and dry, and explain that it will be checked in follow-up appointments. Also tell him that he will need periodic serum calcium determinations.

Advise him not to take any over-the-counter drugs without consulting his doctor. In particular, tell him to avoid magnesium-containing laxatives and antacids, mineral oil, and vitamins A and D.

If the patient has had a total parathyroidectomy, instruct him to follow a high-calcium, low-phosphorus diet, as ordered, and to take his calcium medications. If he'll be receiving dihydrotachysterol or calciferol, tell him not to take vitamins without consulting his doctor. Tell him to call his doctor if he develops symptoms of hypercalcemia, such as excessive thirst, headache, vertigo, tinnitus, and anorexia.

Pancreatectomy

Pancreatectomy may be used to treat pancreatic diseases after more conservative techniques have failed. It includes various resections, drainage procedures, and anastomoses. This procedure is indicated for palliative treatment of pancreatic cancer and chronic pancreatitis, which often stems from prolonged alcohol abuse. Pancreatectomy is also used to treat islet cell tumors (insulinomas).

The type of procedure used depends on the patient's condition, the extent of the disease and its metastases, and the amount of endocrine and exocrine function the pancreas retains. Often, the procedure is determined only after surgical exploration of the abdomen.

Major complications of pancreatectomy include hemorrhage (during and after surgery), fistulas, abscesses (common with distal pancreatectomy), common bile duct obstruction, and pseudocysts. Subtotal resection sometimes causes insulin dependence, whereas total pancreatectomy always causes permanent insulin dependence.

Patient preparation. Explain that the surgeon selects the specific procedure during abdominal exploration. Provide emotional support. Give analgesics, as ordered.

Arrange for necessary diagnostic studies, as ordered, to help the surgeon determine the existing endocrine and exocrine structure of the pancreas and any anatomic anomalies.

For the patient with chronic pancreatitis or cancer, provide enteral or parenteral nutrition before surgery. As ordered, give low-fat, high-calorie feedings to combat the malnutrition and steatorrhea that result from malabsorption. Provide meticulous skin care. If the patient is hyperglycemic, give oral hypoglycemic agents or insulin, as ordered, and monitor blood glucose and urine ketone levels.

Monitor the patient with a recent history of alcohol abuse for withdrawal signs: agitation, tachycardia, tremors, anorexia, and hypertension. Alcohol withdrawal syndrome may occur 72 to 96 hours after the patient's last drink; surgery should be delayed until then.

If the patient smokes, advise him to stop smoking before surgery.

Evaluate his pulmonary status to provide baseline information, and instruct him in deep-breathing and coughing techniques. Explain to the patient that he should turn in bed, perform deep-breathing exercises, and cough every 2 hours for 24 to 72 hours after surgery. If incentive spirometry is indicated, instruct him as appropriate.

Assess the patient for jaundice and increased hematoma formation—signs of liver dysfunction, which commonly accompanies pancreatic disease. As ordered, arrange for liver function and coagulation studies before surgery. If the patient has a prolonged prothrombin time, expect to give vitamin K to prevent postoperative hemorrhage.

Because resection of the transverse colon may be necessary, the doctor may order mechanical and antimicrobial bowel preparation as well as prophylactic systemic antimicrobials (begun 6 hours before surgery and continuing for 72 hours after surgery). Carry out these measures as directed, and expect to assist with nasogastric (NG) tube and indwelling urinary catheter insertion.

Monitoring and aftercare. After surgery, the patient usually spends 48 hours in the ICU. Monitor his vital signs closely and administer plasma expanders, as ordered. Use central, arterial, or pulmonary catheter readings to evaluate hemodynamic status; correlate these readings with urine output and wound drainage. If central venous pressure and urine output drop, give fluids to avoid hypovolemic shock.

Evaluate NG tube drainage, which should be green-tinged as bile drains from the stomach. A T tube may be placed in the common bile duct; normal bile drainage is 600 to 800 ml daily, decreasing as more bile goes to the intestine. Notify the doctor if bile drainage doesn't decrease because this may indicate a biliary obstruction leading to possibly fatal peritonitis. Assess Penrose drainage from the abdomen, and inspect the dressing and drainage sites for frank bleeding, which may signal hemorrhage. If a pancreatic drain is in place, prevent skin breakdown from highly excoriating pancreatic enzymes by changing dressings frequently or by using a wound pouching system to contain the drainage.

Monitor the patient's fluid and electrolyte balance closely, evaluate arterial blood gas levels, and provide I.V. fluid replacements, as ordered. Be alert for metabolic alkalosis, signaled by apathy, irritability, dehydration, and slow, shallow breathing. Report these signs to the doctor, and expect to administer isotonic fluids. Also watch for metabolic acidosis, signaled by elevated blood pressure, rapid pulse and respiratory rates, and arrhythmias. Report these signs to the doctor and give I.V. bicarbonate, as ordered.

Have I.V. calcium ready because serum amylase levels commonly rise after pancreatic surgery, and amylase can bind to calcium. Evaluate serum calcium levels periodically. Also check urine or blood glucose levels periodically to assess for pos-

sible fluctuations. If ordered, give insulin.

Monitor the patient's respiratory status. Watch for shallow breathing, decreased respiratory rate, and respiratory distress. Administer oxygen, if ordered. Reinforce deep-breathing techniques and encourage the patient to cough.

Be alert for absent bowel sounds, severe abdominal pain, vomiting, or fever—evidence of such complications as fistula and paralytic ileus. Also, check the patient's wound for redness, pain, edema, unusual odor, or suture line separation. Report any of these findings to the doctor.

If no complications develop, expect the patient's GI function to return in 24 to 48 hours. Remove his NG tube, as ordered, and start him on fluids.

Patient education. Teach the patient wound care, including careful cleaning and dressing each day. Tell him to report signs of wound infection promptly.

As needed, teach the patient how to test his urine for ketones or how to monitor his blood glucose levels. If he had a total pancreatectomy, teach him about diabetes, and show him how to administer insulin.

Because pancreatic exocrine insufficiency leads to malabsorption, provide dietary instructions and inform the patient that he may eventually need pancreatic enzyme replacements.

Adrenalectomy

Adrenalectomy—the resection or removal of one or both adrenal glands—is the treatment of choice for adrenal hyperfunction and hyperaldosteronism. It's also used to treat adrenal tumors such as adenomas and has been used to aid treatment of breast and prostate cancer.

Total bilateral adrenalectomy eliminates the body's reserve of corticosteroids, which the adrenal cortex synthesizes. As these hormones disappear from the circulation, the symptoms produced by their excess also disappear. However, excessive levels of adrenal hormones can also stem from pituitary oversecretion of corticotropin. In this case, treatment first focuses on removal of a pituitary adenoma by radiation therapy or surgery. Only if this is impossible will unilateral or bilateral adrenalectomy be considered.

Careful postoperative monitoring reduces the risk of life-threatening conditions.

Patient preparation. Explain the procedure to the patient. If he has hyperaldosteronism, draw blood, as ordered, for laboratory evaluation. Expect to give oral or I.V. potassium supplements to correct low serum potassium levels. Monitor for muscle twitching and a positive Chvostek's sign (indications of tetany). Keep the patient on a low-sodium, high-potassium diet, as ordered, to help correct hypernatremia. Give aldosterone antagonists, as ordered, and beta blockers for blood pressure control. Explain to the patient that surgery will probably cure his hypertension if it results from an adenoma. Observe for signs and symptoms of HF and arrhythmias.

The patient with adrenal hyperfunction needs a controlled environment to offset emotional lability. If ordered, give a sedative. Expect to give medications to control his hypertension, edema, diabetes, and cardiovascular symptoms as well as his susceptibility to infections. As ordered, give glucocorticoids the morning of surgery.

Monitoring and aftercare. Monitor vital signs carefully, observing for indications of shock from hemorrhage. Observe the patient's dressing for bleeding, and correlate this with your reading of his vital signs. Report wound drainage or fever immediately. Keep in mind that postoperative hypertension is common.

Watch for weakness, nausea, vomiting, and abdominal pain. If preoperative steroids were used, observe the patient closely for wound infections and abscess as steroids may mask infection.

Use aseptic technique when changing dressings. Administer analgesics for pain, and give replacement steroids, as ordered. Glucocorticoids from the adrenal cortex are essential to life and must be replaced to prevent adrenal crisis until the hypothalamic–pituitary–adrenal axis resumes functioning.

If the patient had primary hyperaldosteronism, he will have had preoperative renin suppression with resulting postoperative hypoaldosteronism. Monitor his serum potassium levels carefully.

Patient education. Stress the importance of taking his prescribed medications as directed. If the patient had a unilateral adrenalectomy, explain that he may be able to taper his medications in a few months, when his remaining gland resumes function.

Emphasize that sudden withdrawal of steroids can precipitate adrenal crisis and that he needs continued medical follow-up to adjust his steroid dosage during stress or illness.

Describe the signs of adrenal insufficiency, and make sure the patient knows this can progress to adrenal crisis if not treated. Explain that he should consult his doctor if he has weight gain, acne, headaches, fatigue, and increased urinary frequency, which can indicate steroid overdosage. Advise him to take his steroids with meals or antacids.

If the patient had adrenal hyperfunction, explain that he will see a reversal of the physical characteristics of his disease over the next few months. However, caution him not to stop his medications when his physical appearance improves.

Provide wound care instructions. Advise him to keep the incision clean and to follow his doctor's instructions regarding application of ointments or dressings. Tell him to report fever or any increased drainage, inflammation, or pain at the incision site.

Advise the patient to wear a medical identification bracelet. Stress the importance of a follow-up visit 1 to 2 weeks after surgery. Instruct patient that full corticotropin recovery may take up to 2 years.

Radiation

Radiation and ^{131}I treatments may be performed for certain pituitary and thyroid disorders.

Pituitary radiation

Pituitary radiation therapy helps control the growth of a pituitary adenoma or relieves its signs and symptoms. Accelerated proton beam therapy focuses narrowly on the pituitary, reducing damage to surrounding tissue. Treatment may also involve the implantation of radioactive substances, such as yttrium and other radionuclides.

The most common method, conventional radiation therapy, has a slow onset of action and may not take full effect for up to 10 years. Therefore, it may best be used to treat a slow-growing tumor.

[131]I administration

A form of radiation therapy, the administration of ^{131}I treats hyperthyroidism and is used adjunctly for thyroid cancer. After oral ingestion, ^{131}I is rapidly absorbed and concentrated in the thyroid. It gradually shrinks functioning thyroid tissue and destroys malignant cells.

[131]I causes symptoms to subside after about 3 weeks and exerts its full effect only after 3 months. A patient with acute hyperthyroidism may require ongoing antithyroid drug therapy during this period. A patient with cardiac disease must be made euthyroid before the start of ^{131}I therapy, to withstand the initial hypermetabolism.

Although one ^{131}I treatment usually suffices, a second or third treatment may be needed several months later. Complications include transient or permanent hypothyroidism, requiring thyroid hormone replacements. Rarely, acute exacerbation occurs, resulting in thyroid storm.

Patient preparation. Before ^{131}I administration, explain the procedure and check the patient's history for allergies to iodine. Unless contraindicated, instruct the patient to stop thyroid hormone antagonists 4 to 7 days before ^{131}I administration. Also tell the patient to fast overnight. Make sure the patient isn't taking lithium carbonate. Inform the patient that ^{131}I won't be given if he develops severe vomiting or diarrhea.

Monitoring and aftercare. After ^{131}I administration, the patient usually is discharged with appropriate instructions. However, he may stay in the hospital if he received an unusually large dose or if treatment was for cancer. In such cases, observe radiation precautions for 3 days.

Patient education. Advise the patient to drink plenty of fluids for 48 hours to speed excretion of ^{131}I. Tell him to urinate into a lead-lined container for 48 hours. Give him disposable eating utensils, and tell him to avoid close contact with young children and pregnant women for 7 days after therapy. (If you're pregnant, arrange for another nurse to care for this patient.)

Explain that his urine and saliva will be slightly radioactive for 24 hours and that any vomitus will be highly radioactive for 6 to 8 hours after therapy. Teach him to dispose of these properly. Tell him he'll start to see improvement in several weeks, but the maximum effects won't occur for up to 3 months. Instruct him to take his prescribed thyroid hormone antagonist as ordered. He will need follow-up laboratory tests.

The patient should report pain, swelling, fever, and other signs and symptoms. Reassure him that they can be treated. Advise patients of childbearing age to avoid conception for several months.

REFERENCES AND READINGS

American Diabetes Association. "Position Statement: Nutrition Recommendations and Principles for People with Diabetes Mellitus," *Diabetes Care* 19(Suppl 1): S16-S19, 1996.

American Diabetes Association. "Position Statement: Insulin Administration," *Diabetes Care* 19(Suppl 1):S31-S34, 1996.

Felig, P., et al., eds. *Endocrinology and Metabolism*, 3rd ed. New York: McGraw-Hill Book Co., 1995.

Haas, L.B. "Nursing Assessment: Endocrine System" and "Nursing Role in Management: Endocrine Problems," in *Medical-Surgical Nursing: Assessment and Management of Clinical Problems*, 3rd ed. Edited by Lewis, S.M., et al. St. Louis: Mosby–Year Book, 1996.

Jankowski, C.B. "Irradiating the Thyroid: How to Protect Yourself and Others," *AJN* 96(10):51-54, October 1996.

Tietgens, S.T., et al. "Thyroid Storm," *Medical Clinics of North America* 79:169-84, 1995.

11

IMMUNOLOGIC AND HEMATOLOGIC CARE

When caring for a patient with an immunologic or hematologic disorder, you face a range of complex tasks. One reason is the immune system's diverse nature. This system consists of billions of circulating cells and specialized structures such as the lymph nodes located throughout the body. And immunologic and hematologic disorders can result from—or cause—problems in other systems. This interaction makes accurate assessment and intervention challenging.

ASSESSMENT

Besides examining the patient's spleen and lymph nodes, you need to evaluate his general appearance, vital signs, and related body structures. Because an immunologic or hematologic disorder can involve almost every body system, be sure to perform a complete physical examination.

Assessing appearance and vital signs

Begin by observing the patient's physical appearance. Look for signs of acute illness, such as grimacing or profuse perspiration, and of chronic illness, such as emaciation and listlessness. Determine whether the patient's stated age and appearance agree. Chronic disease and nutritional deficiencies related to immune dysfunction may make a patient look older than he is.

Next, measure the patient's height and weight. Compare the findings with normal values for the patient's bone structure. Weight loss may result from GI problems related to immune disorders.

Observe the patient's posture, movements, and gait for abnormalities that may indicate joint, spinal, or neurologic changes caused by an immune disorder.

Assess his vital signs, noting especially whether they vary from his normal baseline measurements. Fever, with or without a chill, suggests infection, whereas a subnormal temperature usually occurs with gram-negative infections. Other signs and symptoms of inflammation, such as redness, swelling, or tenderness, may accompany a fever. These effects may be absent if the patient has a white blood cell (WBC) deficiency.

Assess the patient's pulse rate and respiratory rate and character. Note the heart rate. The heart may pump harder or faster to compensate for a decreased oxygen supply resulting from anemia or decreased blood volume from bleeding. This problem can cause tachycardia, palpitations, or arrhythmias. Check respirations for tachypnea. Measure blood pressure with the patient lying, sitting, and standing. Check for orthostatic hypotension as well as hypotension possibly caused by septicemia or hypovolemia.

Finally, assess your patient's level of consciousness (LOC), which may be impaired by hypoxia, fever, or even an active intracranial hemorrhage. Be alert for critical changes that require the doctor's immediate attention. Look for the impairment's cause only after you've begun interventions and have stabilized the patient hemodynamically.

Inspecting related body structures

Immunologic and hematologic disorders affect many body systems, but special attention should be given to the skin, mucous membranes, fingernails, eyes, lymph nodes, liver, and spleen.

Skin and mucuous membranes. Your patient's skin color directly reflects body fluid composition. Observe for pallor, cyanosis, or jaundice. Because normal skin color can vary widely, ask the patient if his present skin tone is normal. Decreased hemoglobin content can cause pallor. Cyanosis, in turn, can result from excessive deoxygenated hemoglobin in cutaneous blood vessels, a condition caused by hypoxia, which appears in some anemias. Check for erythema (redness), indicating a local inflammation, and plethora (red, florid complexion), which appears in polycythemia.

Focus on the skin over your patient's lymph nodes and note any color abnormalities. Nodes covered by red-streaked skin suggest a lymphatic disorder, including acute lymphadenitis. With lymphadenitis, also look for an obvious infection site. Also note other infection signs, such as poor wound healing, wound drainage, induration (tissue hardening), or lesions. Pay close attention to sites of recent invasive procedures for evidence of wound healing.

When assessing the patient's mucous membranes and skin for jaundice, observe him in natural light if possible. With dark-skinned patients, inspect the buccal mucosa, palms, and soles for a yellowish tinge. For an edematous patient, examine the inner forearm for jaundice. An elevated bilirubin level may appear secondary to increased erythrocyte hemolysis—either acquired or hereditary. *Note:* Excessive carrot or yellow-vegetable intake may cause yellow skin but doesn't change sclerae or mucous membrane color.

Also check for rashes and note their distribution. For example, a butterfly-shaped rash over the nose and cheeks may indicate systemic lupus erythematosus (SLE). Palpable, nonpainful, purplish lesions may indicate Kaposi's sarcoma, which occurs with acquired immunodeficiency syndrome (AIDS).

If you suspect a blood clotting abnormality, check the patient's skin for purpuric lesions. These are variable-sized and usually result from thrombocytopenia. With dark-skinned patients, check the oral mucosa or conjunctivae for petechiae or ecchymoses.

Check your patient's skin for dryness and coarseness, which may indicate iron deficiency anemia. Ask him whether his skin itches. Itching (pruritus) can signal Hodgkin's disease, chronic lymphocytic leukemia, or polycythemia vera.

Inspect the mucous membranes, especially the gingivae. Bleeding, redness, swelling, or ulceration may indicate leukemia. A smooth tongue can signify vitamin B_{12} deficiency or iron deficiency anemia. An ulcerated tongue may mean leukemia or neutropenia or SLE. Fluffy white patches scattered throughout the oral cavity indicate candidiasis, a fungal infection. Hairy leukoplakia, a lacy white plaque found typically on the buccal mucosa, appears with AIDS.

Fingernails. Note any abnormalities in the patient's nails. Longitudinal striation can indicate anemia. Koilonychia (spoon nail) characterizes iron deficiency anemia. The fingers may become clubbed; in this abnormality, the nail angle may change from 160 degrees to 180 degrees or more. Finger clubbing indicates chronic hypoxia.

Eyes. Inspect the color of the patient's conjunctivae (normally pink) and sclerae (normally white). Conjunctival pallor may accompany anemia. Yellowish sclerae may indicate an accumulation of bile pigment from excessive hemolysis. Retinal hemorrhages and exudates, seen with an ophthalmoscope, suggest severe anemia and thrombocytopenia. Also observe the eyelids for signs of infection or inflammation, such as swelling, redness, or lesions.

Respiratory system. Observe the patient's respiratory rate, rhythm, and energy expenditure related to respiratory effort. Note the position he assumes to ease breathing. During an asthma attack, the patient may sit up to use every accessory muscle of respiration. Exertional dyspnea, tachypnea, and orthopnea (difficulty breathing except in an upright position) commonly accompany hypoxia.

Percuss the anterior, lateral, and posterior thorax, comparing one side with the other. A dull sound indicates consolidation, which may occur with pneumonia. Hyperresonance may result from trapped air, as in bronchial asthma.

Auscultate over the lungs to assess for adventitious (abnormal) sounds. Wheezing suggests asthma or an allergic response. Crackles may denote a respiratory infection such as pneumonia.

Cardiovascular system. Assess the pulse rate and rhythm for anemia-related tachycardia or other arrhythmias. Then palpate and auscultate the heart and vessels for other signs of immune or blood disorders. First, palpate the point of maximal impulse (PMI), normally located in the fifth intercostal space at the mid-clavicular line. The PMI may be broadened, displaced, or less distinct because of ventricular enlargement, the body's compensatory mechanism for severe anemia. Auscultate for heart sounds over the precordium. Normally, auscultation reveals only the first and second heart sounds (*lub-dub*). Any auscultated apical systolic murmurs may signify severe anemia; mitral, aortic, or pulmonary murmurs; sickle cell anemia; pericardial friction rub; endocarditis; or pericardial effusion, which occurs in about 50% of SLE patients.

Assess the patient's peripheral circulation. Begin by inspecting for Raynaud's phenomenon (intermittent arteriolar vasospasm of the fingers or toes and sometimes of the ears and nose). This phenomenon, which may be caused by SLE or scleroderma, produces blanching in the affected area, followed by cyanosis, pallor, and then reddening. Next, palpate the peripheral pulses, which should be symmetrical and regular. Weak, irregular pulses may indicate anemia.

GI system. With the patient lying down, auscultate the abdomen *before* palpation and percussion to avoid altering bowel sounds. In autoimmune disorders that cause diarrhea, bowel sounds increase. In scleroderma and in autoimmune disorders that cause constipation, bowel sounds decrease. Listen for loud, high-pitched tinkling sounds, which herald the early stages of intestinal obstruction. Next, auscultate the liver and spleen. Listen carefully over both organs for friction rubs—grating sounds that fluctuate with respiration. These sounds usually indicate inflammation of the organ's peritoneal covering. Splenic friction rubs also suggest infarction and inflammation. Next, percuss the liver. Normally, the liver produces a dull sound over a span of $2^1/2''$ to $4^3/4''$ (6.5 to 12 cm). Hepatomegaly (liver enlargement) may accompany many immune disorders.

Palpate the abdomen to detect enlarged organs and tenderness. An enlarged liver that feels smooth and tender suggests hepatitis; one that feels hard and nodular suggests a neoplasm. Abdominal tenderness may result from infections.

Finally, inspect the anus, which should be pink and puckered without inflammation or breaks in the mucosal surface. Defer internal examination of the anus and rectal vault if you suspect or know that the patient has a low platelet count or granulocyte level.

Urinary system. Because the urinary system also may be affected by immune dysfunctions, obtain a urine specimen and evaluate its color, clarity, and odor. Cloudy, malodorous urine may result from a urinary tract infection.

Inspect the urinary meatus. In a patient with a WBC deficiency or an immunodeficiency, the external genitalia may be focal points for inflammation.

Nervous system. Evaluate the patient's LOC and mental status. Impaired neurologic function may occur secondary to hypoxia or fever. An anemic patient may not be able to concentrate or may become confused, especially if he's elderly. Hemorrhage also compromises oxygen supply to nerve tissues, resulting in similar symptoms. If bleeding occurs within the cranial vault, disorientation, progressive loss of consciousness, changes in motor and sensory capabilities, changes in pupillary responses, and seizures may result.

Other neurologic effects may provide clues to an underlying disorder. For example, a patient with SLE may experience altered mentation, depression, or psychosis.

Musculoskeletal system. Ask the patient to perform simple maneuvers, such as standing up, walking, and bending over. He should be able to do so effortlessly. Then test joint range of motion (ROM), particularly in the hand, wrist, and knee. Palpate the joints to assess for swelling, tenderness, and pain. Autoimmune disorders such as SLE can limit ROM and cause joint enlargement. If palpation reveals bone tenderness, the

cause may be bone marrow hyperactivity, a compensatory mechanism for oxygen-carrying deficits prevalent in anemias. Bone tenderness may also result from a leukemic or immunoproliferative disorder such as plasma cell myeloma.

Lymph nodes, liver, and spleen. Inspect the abdominal area for enlargement, distention, and asymmetry, possibly indicating a tumor. Hepatomegaly and splenomegaly may result from polycythemia, leukemia, or hemolytic anemia.

When assessing the patient's immune system, percuss and palpate the spleen. First, percuss the spleen to estimate its size. On percussion, the spleen normally produces dullness in the left upper quadrant between the sixth and tenth ribs. Spleen enlargement (splenomegaly) may indicate an immune disorder.

Next, palpate the spleen to detect tenderness and confirm splenomegaly. The spleen must be enlarged approximately three times normal size to be palpable. Splenic tenderness may result from infections, commonly seen in a patient with an immunodeficiency disorder.

The first step in regional lymph node assessment is to inspect areas where the patient reports "swollen glands" or "lumps" for color abnormalities and visible lymph node enlargement. Then inspect all other nodal regions. Proceed from head to toe to avoid missing any region. Normally, lymph nodes can't be seen. (See *Documenting lymph node findings,* page 594.)

Documenting lymph node findings

If palpation reveals nodal enlargement or other abnormalities, document the location of the node. Use reference points, such as body axis and lines, to pinpoint the site, or sketch the location, if appropriate. Then indicate the nodal length, width, and depth in centimeters, and describe or sketch the shape. Accurately describe its surface as smooth, nodular, or irregular. Identify the consistency of the node as hard, soft, firm, resilient, spongy, or cystic. Evaluate its symmetry, comparing the node with similar structures on the other side of the body.

Document the node's degree of mobility. If it's immobile, indicate whether it's fixed to overlying tissues, underlying tissues, or both. During palpation, note whether any tenderness is elicited by palpation, movement, or rebound phenomenon (tenderness that occurs after the pressure of the palpating fingerpads is released).

Describe any color change, such as pallor, erythema, or cyanosis, in overlying skin. Note whether the site feels warm. If the node exhibits increased vascularity, describe any changes in the overlying blood vessels.

Palpating lymph nodes. Use the pads of your index and middle fingers to palpate the patient's superficial lymph nodes in the head and neck, and in the axillary, epitrochlear, inguinal, and popliteal areas.

Apply gentle pressure and rotary motion to feel the underlying nodes without obscuring them by pressing them into deeper soft tissues. (See *Palpating the lymph nodes.*) Lymph nodes usually can't be felt in a healthy patient.

DIAGNOSTIC TESTS

The doctor may order various tests to evaluate the patient's immune and hematologic response. Commonly ordered studies include general cellular tests, such as T- and B-lymphocyte assays, to aid diagnosis of primary and secondary immunodeficiency diseases and general humoral tests such as complement assays to help detect immunomediated disease. Diagnostic tests allow direct analysis of the blood, its formed elements (cells), and the bone marrow, where blood cells originate. These tests include red blood cell (RBC) and platelet studies, coagulation and agglutination tests, bone marrow aspiration, and needle biopsy. (For more information, see *Diagnostic tests for immunologic and hematologic disorders,* pages 598 to 604.)

NURSING DIAGNOSES

In this section, nursing diagnoses commonly used in patients with immunologic and hematologic problems are discussed. For each diagnosis, you'll find nursing interventions along with rationales (which appear in italic type).

Palpating the lymph nodes

When assessing a patient for signs of an immune disorder, you'll need to palpate the superficial lymph nodes of the head and neck, and of the axillary, epitrochlear, inguinal, and popliteal areas, using the pads of the index and middle fingers. Always palpate gently; begin with light pressure and gradually increase the pressure.

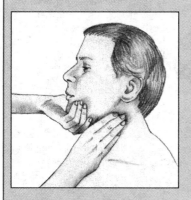

To palpate the submandibular, submental, anterior cervical, and occipital nodes, position your fingers as shown. Palpate over the mandibular surface and continue moving up and down the entire neck. Flex the head forward or to the side being examined. This relaxes the tissues and makes enlarged nodes more palpable. Reverse your hand position to palpate the opposite side.

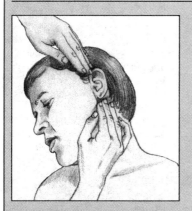

To palpate the preauricular, parotid, and mastoid nodes, position your fingers as shown.

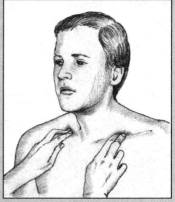

To palpate the posterior cervical nodes, place your fingertip pads along the anterior surface of the trapezius muscle. Then move your fingertips toward the posterior surface of the sternocleidomastoid muscle.

(continued)

Palpating the lymph nodes *(continued)*

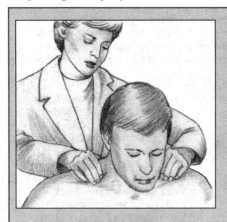

To palpate the supraclavicular nodes, encourage the patient to relax so that the clavicles drop. To relax the soft tissues of the anterior neck, flex the patient's head slightly forward with your free hand. Then hook your left index finger over the clavicle lateral to the sternocleidomastoid muscle. Rotate your fingers deeply into this area to feel these nodes.

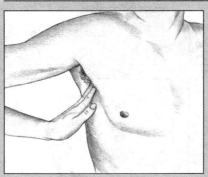

To palpate the axillary nodes, use your nondominant hand to support the patient's relaxed right arm, and put your other hand as high in his right axilla as possible. Then palpate the axillary nodes, gently pressing the soft tissues against the chest wall and the muscles surrounding the axilla (the pectorals, latissimus dorsi, subscapular, and anterior serratus). Repeat this procedure for the left axilla.

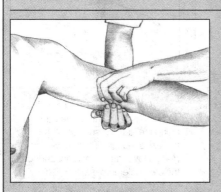

To palpate the epitrochlear lymph nodes, place your fingertips in the depression above and posterior to the medial area of the elbow and palpate gently.

Palpating the lymph nodes *(continued)*

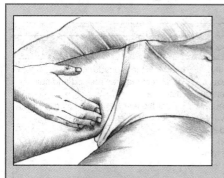

To palpate the inferior superficial inguinal (femoral) lymph nodes, gently press below the junction of the saphenous and femoral veins.

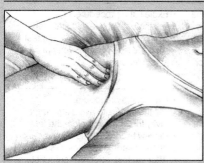

To palpate the superior superficial inguinal lymph nodes, press along the course of the saphenous veins from the inguinal area to the abdomen.

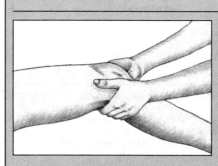

To palpate the popliteal nodes, press gently along the posterior muscles at the back of the knee.

Risk for infection

This diagnosis may be associated with AIDS, severe combined immunodeficiency disease, pernicious anemia, and other immune disorders.

Expected outcomes

• Patient maintains good personal and oral hygiene.
• Patient shows no evidence of diarrhea or skin breakdown.

(Text continues on page 604.)

Diagnostic tests for immunologic and hematologic disorders

Test	Purpose	Nursing considerations
T and B lympho-cytes	To help identify immunoregula-tions associated with autoimmune disorders, evalu-ate immunodefi-ciencies, and characterize lym-phoid cancers	• Explain the procedure. • This test requires no food and fluid restrictions. • After the test, observe venipuncture site for bleeding.
White blood cell (WBC) count	To help determine infection or inflam-mation and moni-tor response to chemotherapy or radiation therapy	• Explain the procedure. • Tell the patient to avoid strenuous exercise for 24 hours before the test. • After the test, observe venipuncture site for bleeding.
WBC differential	To evaluate the body's capacity to resist and over-come infection, detect and identi-fy various types of leukemia, determine the stage and severi-ty of infection, and detect aller-gic reactions	• Explain the procedure. • Tell the patient to avoid strenuous activity for 24 hours before the test. • Review history for use of medications that may interfere with test results. • After the test, observe venipuncture site for bleeding.
Erythrocyte sedi-mentation rate	To monitor inflam-matory or malig-nant disease and aid detection and diagnosis of occult disease	• Explain the procedure. • After collecting the sample, send it to the laboratory immediately. It must be tested within 2 hours. • After the test, observe venipuncture site for bleeding.
Patch and scratch allergy test	To evaluate the immune system's ability to respond to known aller-gens	• Explain the procedure. To perform a patch test: • Thoroughly clean the area with alco-hol. Then wipe with acetone and allow to dry. • After removing protective cover, apply

Diagnostic tests for immunologic and hematologic disorders *(continued)*

Test	Purpose	Nursing considerations
Patch and scratch allergy test *(continued)*		allergen disk to skin and secure with tape. • Leave in place for the prescribed period. Then remove the patch and wait 30 minutes. • Examine the site for erythema, papules, vesicles, or edema. If such signs are absent, reexamine the site 96 hours after application of the allergen. Record test results. To perform a scratch test: • Thoroughly clean the skin with alcohol. Then wipe with acetone and allow to dry. • Stretch the skin taut at scratch site; then make a scratch 1 to 4 mm long and about 2 mm deep with a sterile lancet or tine. If you draw blood, apply an adhesive bandage and scratch another site. • With an eyedropper, apply a drop of the allergen to the scratch site. • Examine the test site after waiting 30 to 40 minutes. Measure the diameter of any reaction and record the results in millimeters.
Intradermal skin tests	To evaluate immune response by injecting recall antigens into the superficial skin layer	• Explain the procedure. • Clean the volar surface of the arm with alcohol and allow to dry. To perform the tine test or Aplitest: • Remove the protective cap from the unit. • Hold the forearm with one hand and stretch the skin taut. Grasp the unit with the other hand and firmly depress the tines completely into the patient's skin, without twisting the unit. • Hold the device in place for 1 second. Recap device and discard. • Read results 48 to 72 hours after injection. Record test results. To perform recall antigen and Mantoux tests: • With your free hand, hold the needle at a 15-degree angle to the patient's arm, with its bevel up. *(continued)*

Diagnostic tests for immunologic and hematologic disorders *(continued)*

Test	Purpose	Nursing considerations
Intradermal skin tests *(continued)*		• Insert the needle about 3 mm below the epidermis site. Stop when the needle bevel is under the skin, and inject the antigen slowly and gently. A wheal should form as you inject the antigen. • Withdraw the needle and apply gentle pressure. Don't rub the site. Circle the test site with a marking pen. • After waiting 48 to 72 hours, inspect the injection site. Record induration in millimeters.
Red blood cell (RBC) count	To help diagnose anemia and polycythemia	• Explain the procedure. • This test requires no food or fluid restrictions. • After the test, observe venipuncture site for bleeding.
Total hemoglobin concentration	To help indicate the severity of anemia or polycythemia	• Explain the procedure. • This test requires no food or fluid restrictions. • After the test, observe venipuncture site for bleeding.
Hematocrit	To help diagnose anemia, polycythemia, and abnormal hydration states	• Explain the procedure. • This test requires no food or fluid restrictions. • After the test, observe venipuncture site for bleeding.
Platelet count	To evaluate platelet production, assess effects of chemotherapy or radiation therapy on platelet production, and aid diagnosis of thrombocytopenia and thrombocytosis	• Explain the procedure. • This test requires no food or fluid restriction. • Check patient history for drugs that may affect test results. • After the test, observe venipuncture site for bleeding.

Diagnostic tests for immunologic and hematologic disorders (continued)

Test	Purpose	Nursing considerations
Bleeding time	To help assess overall hemostatic function and detect congenital and acquired platelet function disorders	• Explain the procedure. • This test requires no food or fluid restrictions. • Reassure the patient that, although he may feel some discomfort from the incisions, the antiseptics and the tightness of the blood pressure cuff, the test takes only 10 to 20 minutes to perform. • Advise him that the incisions will leave two small hairline scars that should be barely visible when healed. • Check his history for recent ingestion of drugs that prolong bleeding time. • Maintain a pressure of 40 mm Hg throughout the test. • If the bleeding doesn't diminish after 15 minutes, discontinue the test. • After the test, in a patient with a bleeding tendency, maintain a pressure bandage over the incision for 24 to 48 hours to prevent further bleeding. Check the test area frequently.
Activated partial thromboplastin time	To screen for deficiencies of the clotting factors in the intrinsic pathways and monitor heparin therapy	• Explain the procedure. • This test requires no food or fluid restrictions. • For a patient on anticoagulant therapy, additional pressure may be needed at venipuncture site to control bleeding.
Prothrombin time	To evaluate the extrinsic coagulation system and monitor response to oral anticoagulant therapy	• Explain the procedure. • This test requires no food or fluid restrictions. • Check patient history for use of medications that may interfere with accurate determination of test results. • When appropriate, explain that the test will be performed daily to monitor therapy and will be repeated at longer intervals when medication levels stabilize. • After the test, observe venipuncture site for bleeding.

(continued)

Diagnostic tests for immunologic and hematologic disorders *(continued)*

Test	Purpose	Nursing considerations
Plasma thrombin time	To detect fibrinogen deficiency or defect, aid diagnosis of disseminated intravascular coagulation and hepatic disease, and monitor the effectiveness of treatment with heparin or thrombolytic agents	• Explain the procedure. • If possible, withhold heparin therapy before the test, as ordered. If it must be continued, note this on the laboratory slip. • After the test, observe venipuncture site for bleeding.
ABO blood typing	To establish blood group according to the ABO system and check compatibility of donor and recipient blood before transmission	• Explain the procedure. • Check patient history for recent administration of blood, dextran, or I.V. contrast medium, which causes cells to aggregate. • Before the transmission, compare current and past ABO typing and crossmatching to detect mistaken identification and prevent transfusion reaction. • After the test, observe venipuncture site for bleeding.
Rh typing	To establish blood type according to the Rh system, help determine the compatibility of donor before transmission, and determine if the patient will require an Rh immune globulin (Rh-IG) injection	• Explain the procedure. • Check patient history for recent administration of dextran, I.V. contrast medium, or drugs that may alter results. • After the test, observe venipuncture site for bleeding.
Crossmatching	To establish compatibility or incompatibility of the donor and the recipient's blood	• Explain the procedure. • Check patient's history for recent administration of blood, dextran, or I.V. contrast medium, which can cause aggregation resembling agglutination.

Diagnostic tests for immunologic and hematologic disorders *(continued)*

Test	Purpose	Nursing considerations
Crossmatch-ing *(continued)*		• If more than 72 hours have elapsed since previous transfusion, previously crossmatched blood must be recross-matched with a new blood sample from the recipient. • After the test, observe venipuncture site for bleeding.
Direct antiglobulin test (Direct Coombs' test)	To diagnose hemolytic disease of the newborn, investigate hemolytic transfu-sion reactions, and aid differential diagnosis of hemolytic anemias	• Explain the procedure. • As ordered, withhold medications that can induce autoimmune hemolytic ane-mia. • Send sample to the laboratory imme-diately. The test must be performed within 24 hours. • After the test, observe venipuncture site for bleeding. • As ordered, resume administration of medications withheld before the test.
Antibody screening test (Indirect Coombs' test)	To determine un-expected circulat-ing antibodies to RBC antigens in the recipient's or donor's serum be-fore transfusion, determine the pre-sence of anti-$Rh_o(D)$ (Rh-posi-tive) antibody in maternal blood, evaluate the need for Rh-IG adminis-tration, and aid diagnosis of acquired hemolyt-ic anemia	• Explain the procedure. • Check patient history for recent administration of blood, dextran, or I.V. contrast medium. • After the test, observe venipuncture site for bleeding.
Bone marrow aspiration and needle biopsy	To help diagnose thrombocytopenia, leukemias, granu-lomas and aplas-	• Explain the procedure. • This test requires no food or fluid restrictions. *(continued)*

Diagnostic tests for immunologic and hematologic disorders *(continued)*

Test	Purpose	Nursing considerations
Bone marrow aspiration and needle biopsy *(continued)*	tic, hypoplastic and pernicious anemia; to aid in staging of disease; and to evaluate the effectiveness of chemotherapy	• Inform the patient that he'll receive a local anesthetic but that he'll feel pressure on biopsy needle insertion and a brief pulling pain on marrow removal. • As ordered, administer a mild sedative 1 hour before the test. • After the procedure, check biopsy site for bleeding and inflammation. • Change the dressing over the site every 24 hours.

• Patient takes the prescribed amount of fluid and protein daily.
• Respiratory secretions are clear and odorless.
• Urine remains clear, yellow, odorless, and free from sediment.
• Wounds and incisions are clean, pink, and free from drainage.
• Patient states infection risk factors.
• Patient identifies signs and symptoms of infection.
• Patient remains free from all signs and symptoms of infection.

Nursing interventions and rationales

• Practice strict hand washing before and after all patient contact. *Hand washing is the best way to avoid spreading pathogens.*
• Monitor closely for signs and symptoms of infection. Check vital signs every 4 hours. *Close monitoring permits timely intervention.*
• Maintain skin integrity. Encourage ambulation; assist patient in turning every 2 hours. Don't administer enemas or suppositories, or take rectal temperatures. Encourage mouth care with sodium bicarbonate and saline rinse (1 tsp/8 oz) to inhibit microbial growth. Perform daily hygiene and oral assessment. *Healthy skin is the best barrier against infection.*
• Assist patient in performing coughing and deep-breathing exercises. *Removal of secretions helps prevent pulmonary infections.*
• Require visitors and staff members with upper respiratory infections to wear masks when with patient. *Masks protect patient.*
• Teach patient measures to minimize infection risk. *Participation in care encourages patient's compliance.*

Fatigue

Related to the disease process, fatigue may be associated with hematologic and immunologic problems, such as rheumatoid arthritis, chronic graft-versus-host (GVH) disease, AIDS, SLE, anemias, and leukemia.

Expected outcomes

• Patient explains the relationship of fatigue to disease process and activity level.
• Patient expresses feeling of increased energy.
• Patient identifies and employs measures to prevent fatigue.

Nursing interventions and rationales

• Help patient prioritize activities of daily living to allow for maximum independence. Provide assistance as needed. *Planning and pacing activities prevent fatigue.*
• Provide for uninterrupted periods of rest and sleep. *Scheduled rest periods help decrease fatigue.*
• Teach patient relaxation techniques. *Relaxation restores energy.*

Altered protection

Related to bleeding disorders, altered protection can be associated with hemophilia, thrombocytopenia, various purpuras, and disseminated intravascular coagulation (DIC).

Expected outcomes

• Patient has no chills, fever, or other signs and symptoms of illness.
• Patient demonstrates personal cleanliness and maintains a clean, safe environment.
• Patient uses protective measures, including conservation of energy, balanced diet, and adequate rest.
• Patient demonstrates increased strength and resistance.
• Patient shows improved immunity and no evidence of bleeding.

Nursing interventions and rationales

• Monitor the patient's vital signs every 4 hours. Assess for signs of minor bleeding. Also assess for serious bleeding (headache or changed mental status, hypotension, tachycardia, orthostatic changes, hemoptysis, hematemesis, melena). *Detecting bleeding early helps control complications.*
• Take steps to prevent bleeding. Avoid invasive measures, such as injections, rectal suppositories or enemas, or urinary catheterization. Avoid giving aspirin or aspirin-containing products, if possible. Shave patient with electric razor only. Give oral care with soft toothbrush. *These measures prevent complications by maintaining skin integrity.*
• Use stool softener and daily cathartic *to maintain regular defecation and avoid straining.*
• Help the unsteady patient ambulate. Avoid use of restrictive or tight clothing. Inflate blood pressure cuff as little as possible. *These measures help prevent injury.*

Ineffective individual coping

Related to perceived or impending personal loss, ineffective individual coping may be associated with life-threatening immunodeficiencies.

Expected outcomes

• Patient communicates feelings about the present crisis.
• Patient develops therapeutic relationship with member of the staff.

- Patient gradually increases participation in self-care activities.
- Patient identifies at least two new coping techniques.
- Patient describes efforts to implement coping techniques.

Nursing interventions and rationales

- Encourage patient and family to discuss past coping mechanisms and their effectiveness. *This reinforces successful coping behaviors.*
- Encourage patient and family to participate in care and decision making. *Participation in care allows progress at patient's own pace.*
- Refer patient and family to appropriate community resources, as needed. *Community resources help restore psychological equilibrium.*

DISORDERS

This section discusses immune disorders that may result from hyperreactivity, as in allergic rhinitis; autoimmunity, as in SLE; or immunodeficiency, as in AIDS. They range from mild ailments such as hypersensitivity vasculitis to life-threatening ones such as GVH disease. Some are congenital, whereas others are acquired. Also discussed are common hematologic disorders, from anemias—such as sickle cell anemia and pernicious anemia—to hemorrhagic disorders—such as thrombocytopenia and hemophilia. For each disorder, you'll find information on causes, assessment findings, diagnostic tests, treatment, nursing interventions, patient education, and evaluation criteria.

Hyperreactivity disorders

Besides asthma, disorders of hyperreactivity include allergic rhinitis, urticaria, and angioedema.

Asthma

A chronic reactive airway disorder, asthma produces episodic, reversible airway obstruction by way of bronchospasms, increased mucus secretion, and mucosal edema. Children under age 10 account for one-half of all cases. A predisposition to asthma is inherited.

Causes. *Extrinsic asthma* follows exposure to pollen, animal dander, house dust or mold, kapok or feather pillows, food additives containing sulfites, or other sensitizing substances. *Intrinsic asthma* can result from irritants, emotional stress, fatigue, endocrine changes, temperature and humidity changes, or exposure to noxious fumes.

Other asthma causes can include aspirin, various nonsteroidal anti-inflammatory drugs (such as indomethacin and mefenamic acid), tartrazine (a yellow food dye), exercise, or occupational exposure to various allergenic factors such as platinum.

Assessment findings *Extrinsic asthma* is usually accompanied by manifestations of atopy (type I immunoglobulin [Ig] E–mediated allergy), such as eczema and allergic rhinitis. It commonly follows a severe respiratory infection, especially in adults.

An *acute asthma attack* may begin dramatically or insidiously. Asthma that occurs with cyanosis, confusion, and lethargy indicates the onset of life-threatening status asthmaticus and respiratory failure.

Signs and symptoms of asthma include sudden dyspnea, wheezing, and tightness in the chest. Coughing produces thick, clear or yellow sputum. Tachypnea may occur along with use of accessory respiratory muscles. Other findings include rapid pulse, profuse perspiration, hyperresonant lung fields, and diminished breath sounds.

Diagnostic tests. Pulmonary function studies reveal signs of airway obstructive disease (decreased flow rates and forced expiratory volume in 1 second [FEV_1]), low-normal or diminished vital capacity, and increased total lung and residual capacity. Typically, the patient has lowered partial pressure of oxygen and partial pressure of carbon dioxide ($PaCO_2$) in arterial blood. In severe asthma, $PaCO_2$ may be normal or elevated, indicating severe bronchial obstruction. In fact, FEV_1 will probably be less than 25% of the predicted value. Complete blood count (CBC) with differential shows an increased eosinophil count.

Chest X-ray shows possible hyperinflation, with areas of local atelectasis (mucus plugging). Skin testing for specific allergens may be necessary if no allergic history exists. Inhalation bronchial challenge testing evaluates the significance of allergens identified by skin testing.

Treatment. Treatment aims to identify and avoid precipitating factors, such as allergens or irritants. Usually, such stimuli cannot be removed entirely. Desensitization to specific antigens may be helpful but is rarely totally effective or persistent.

Drug therapy usually includes some form of bronchodilator and proves more effective when begun soon after the onset of symptoms. Drugs used include rapid-acting epinephrine; epinephrine in oil, which isn't recommended for infants; terbutaline; aminophylline; theophylline and oral preparations containing theophylline; oral sympathomimetics; corticosteroids; and aerosolized sympathomimetics, such as isoproterenol or albuterol.

Nursing interventions. During an acute attack, maintain respiratory function and relieve bronchoconstriction, while allowing mucus plug expulsion. If the attack is induced by exertion, you may be able to control it by having the patient sit down, rest, and sip warm water. These measures help slow breathing, promote bronchodilation, and loosen secretions.

Loss of breath is terrifying, so reassure the patient that you'll help him. Then, place him in semi-Fowler's position, encourage diaphragmatic breathing, and urge him to relax as much as possible.

Consider status asthmaticus unrelieved by epinephrine a medical emergency. Give humidified oxygen by nasal cannula at 2 L/minute to ease breathing and to increase arterial oxygen saturation. Later, adjust oxygen according to the patient's vital functions and arterial blood gas measurements. Administer drugs and I.V. fluids as ordered.

Patient education. Identify and explain asthma triggers. Explain the importance of diet and adequate hydration in treating asthma. Teach the patient how to recognize and prevent respiratory infection. Inform him and his family about the availability of support groups such as the American Lung Association.

Tell the patient how to control an asthma attack. Discuss ordered drugs and their use. Teach him how to use an oral inhaler. Explain that he should have his nebulizer readily available at all times, but not overuse it. Explain that nebulizer overuse can weaken his response and diminish the therapeutic effect. Extended overuse can even lead to cardiac arrest and death.

Evaluation. The patient's respirations should be regular and unlabored. He should exhibit signs of adequate gas exchange, such as absence of cyanosis and confusion. The patient and family should be able to identify predisposing factors and state how to eliminate them.

Allergic rhinitis

Allergic rhinitis is a reaction to airborne (inhaled) allergens. Depending on the allergen, the resulting rhinitis and conjunctivitis may be seasonal (hay fever) or occur year-round (perennial allergic rhinitis). Pollen allergy may exacerbate symptoms of perennial rhinitis.

Causes. Hay fever results from wind-borne pollens, such as tree pollens in spring, grass pollens in summer, and weed pollens in fall as well as from mold (fungal spores) in summer and fall. Perennial allergic rhinitis results from dust, feather pillows, mold, cigarette smoke, upholstery, and animal dander.

Assessment findings. Signs and symptoms of hay fever include paroxysmal sneezing, profuse watery rhinorrhea, and nasal obstruction or congestion. The patient's nose and eyes may itch, and his nasal mucosa may appear pale, cyanotic, and edematous. His eyelids and conjunctivae may appear red and edematous. He may also have excessive lacrimation, headache or sinus pain, dark circles under the eyes, occasional itching in the throat, malaise, and fever.

Signs and symptoms of perennial allergic rhinitis include chronic nasal obstruction commonly extending to eustachian tube obstruction, particularly in children, and dark circles under the eyes.

Diagnostic tests. Microscopic examination of sputum and nasal secretions reveals large numbers of eosinophils. Blood chemistry shows normal or elevated IgE levels. Skin testing can pinpoint the responsible allergens when paired with tested responses to environmental stimuli and interpreted in light of the patient's history.

Treatment. Treatment aims to control symptoms by eliminating the environmental antigen, if possible, and by drug therapy and immunotherapy. Antihistamines effectively block histamine effects. Topical intranasal steroids produce local anti-inflammatory effects with minimal systemic effects.

The most commonly used drugs are flunisolide and beclomethasone. These drugs usually aren't effective for acute exacerbations; nasal decongestants and oral antihistamines may be needed instead. Cromolyn sodium may be helpful in preventing allergic rhinitis. However, this drug may take up to 4 weeks to produce a satisfactory effect and must be taken regularly during allergy season.

Nursing interventions. Long-term management includes immunotherapy, or desensitization with injections of extracted allergens. Seasonal allergies require close dosage regulation.

Before drug injections, assess the patient's symptoms. Afterward, watch for adverse reactions, including anaphylaxis and severe localized erythema. Keep epinephrine and emergency resuscitative equipment available. Observe the patient for 30 minutes after the injection. Tell him to call the doctor if a delayed reaction occurs.

Patient education. To reduce exposure to airborne allergens, advise the patient to sleep with the windows closed and to avoid the countryside during pollination seasons. Suggest that he use air-conditioning to filter allergens and keep down moisture and dust. Advise him to eliminate dust-collecting items, such as wool blankets, deep-pile carpets, and heavy drapes from the home. If allergic rhinitis is severe, suggest that he consider relocation to a pollen-free area.

Evaluation. The patient should be free from nasal congestion or obstruction and from excessive nasal and lacrimal discharge.

Urticaria and angioedema

Urticaria is an episodic, usually self-limited skin reaction characterized by local dermal wheals surrounded by an erythematous flare. Angioedema is a subcutaneous and dermal eruption that produces deeper, larger wheals and a more diffuse swelling of loose subcutaneous tissue.

Causes. Urticaria and angioedema are common allergic reactions. Their causes include allergy to drugs, foods, insect stings and, occasionally, inhalant allergens (animal danders, cosmetics) that provoke an IgE-mediated response to protein allergens.

Nonallergic urticaria and angioedema are probably also related to histamine release by some still-unknown mechanism. External physical stimuli, such as cold (usually in young adults), heat, water, or sunlight, may also provoke urticaria and angioedema. *Dermographism urticaria* appears after stroking or scratching the skin. Such urticaria develops with varying pressure, most commonly under tight clothing, and worsens with scratching.

Several different mechanisms and underlying disorders may provoke urticaria and angioedema. These include IgE-induced release of mediators from cutaneous mast cells; binding of IgG or IgM to an antigen, resulting in complement activation; and such disorders as localized or secondary infection (respiratory infection), neoplastic disease (Hodgkin's lymphoma), connective tissue disease (SLE), collagen vascular disease, and psychogenic disease.

Assessment findings. Urticaria produces distinct, raised, evanescent dermal wheals surrounded by an erythematous flare. These lesions may vary in size.

Angioedema characteristically produces nonpitted swelling of deep subcutaneous tissue, usually on the eyelids, lips, genitalia, and mucous membranes. These swellings don't itch but may burn and tingle.

Diagnostic tests. An accurate patient history can help determine the cause of urticaria. It should include drug history, including over-the-counter preparations (vitamins, aspirin, antacids), diet (strawberries, milk products, fish), and environmental influences (pets, carpet, clothing, soap, inhalants, cosmetics, hair dye, insect bites and stings).

Diagnosis also requires physical assessment to rule out similar conditions, and CBC, urinalysis, erythrocyte sedimentation rate (ESR), and chest X-ray to rule out inflammatory infections.

Skin testing, an elimination diet, and a food diary (recording time and amount of food eaten) can pinpoint allergens.

Recurrent angioedema without urticaria, along with a familial history, points to hereditary angioedema. Decreased serum levels of C4 and C1 esterase inhibitor confirm this diagnosis.

Treatment. Treatment aims to prevent or limit contact with triggering factors or, if this is impossible, to desensitize the patient to them and to relieve symptoms. Once the triggering stimulus has been removed, urticaria usually subsides in a few days—except for drug reactions, which may persist as long as the drug is in the bloodstream.

Nursing interventions. Diphenhydramine or another antihistamine can ease itching and swelling with every kind of urticaria.

Patient education. If food or drugs cause urticaria and angioedema, advise the patient to avoid the allergen. If environmental factors are the cause, advise him to avoid heat, sunlight, or cold. If infection is implicated, encourage treatment.

Evaluation. The recovered patient will be free from dermal wheals and associated pruritus. He'll be able to identify the cause of his condition and measures to ensure safety when using antihistamines.

Graft-versus-host disease

GVH disease may occur when an immunologically impaired recipient receives a graft from an immunocompetent donor. If donor and recipient cells aren't histocompatible, the foreign cells may launch an attack against the host cells, which can't reject them. This happens when graft cells become sensitized to the recipient's class II antigens.

Acute GVH disease occurs 30 to 70 days after transplantation; it nearly always indicates the development of chronic GVH disease. This autoimmune disease produces severe immunodeficiency leading to recurrent and life-threatening infections.

GVH disease usually affects the skin, liver, and GI tract; it may affect the bone marrow. Onset may occur from 7 to 20 days after infusion of the viable lymphocytes. It proves fatal in about one-third of patients.

Causes. GVH disease usually develops after a patient with impaired immune function receives a bone marrow transplant from an incompatible donor. However, it may also result from the transfusion of any blood product containing viable lymphocytes. This means that patients may develop GVH disease during the transfusion of whole blood or transplantation of fetal thymus, liver, or bone marrow. The risk of transmission also exists during maternal-fetal blood transfusions and intrauterine transfusions.

Assessment findings. Signs of acute GVH disease include skin rash, severe diarrhea, and jaundice. Skin rash usually develops 10 to 28 days after transplantation. It typically begins as a diffuse erythematous macular rash on the palms, soles, and scalp and may spread to the trunk and possibly the extremities. In severe GVH disease, the rash can become desquamative. Abdominal cramps and, in severe cases, GI bleeding may accompany watery diarrhea. Jaundice results from the hyperbilirubinemia caused by inflammation of the small bile ducts, possibly accompanied by elevated levels of serum alkaline phosphatase, alanine aminotransferase, and aspartate aminotransferase. Skin, intestine, and liver biopsies reveal immunocompetent T cells.

Diagnostic tests. Although graft survival commonly hinges on early detection of transplant rejection, no single test or combination of tests proves definitive. Tests reveal only nonspecific evidence, which may be attributed to other causes, especially infection. Diagnosis becomes a matter of exclusion and depends on careful evaluation of signs and symptoms along with results from specific organ function tests, standard laboratory studies, and tissue biopsy.

Tissue biopsy provides the most reliable diagnostic information, especially in heart, liver, and kidney transplants. Biopsy usually involves obtaining several tissue samples and examining them to determine the extent of tissue damage.

Repeat biopsies may help identify early histologic changes characteristic of rejection, determine the degree of change from previous biopsies, and monitor the course and success of treatment. The frequency of biopsies and the specific procedures employed vary.

Treatment. Because patients may die from GVH disease, initial interventions must focus on prevention. Most patients receive immunosuppressive drug therapy with methotrexate, cyclosporine, or cyclophosphamide for the first 3 to 12 months after transplantation. Treatment with prednisone, alone or with azathioprine, reverses many effects of chronic GVH disease.

Other strategies to decrease the incidence of GVH disease attempt to deplete donor marrow of T cells. One method is to incubate donor bone marrow in vitro with anti–T cell monoclonal antibodies plus complement or similar antibodies coupled with toxins. Another technique for depleting marrow of T cells employs soybean lectin agglutination and sheep RBC rosette formation.

Culturing of bone marrow cells. Researchers are investigating the potential for autogenetic transplants of cultured bone marrow cells. Growing cultures of hematopoietic stem cells in the presence of marrow-derived stromal cells promotes growth of normal stem cells but suppresses production of leukemic cells. The marrow can then be reinfused to the patient, thereby reducing the risk of GVH disease.

Thalidomide. This drug binds to lymphocytes at the same intracellular receptors as cyclosporine and helps the immune system recognize both host and donor tissues as "self," thus reducing the risk of GVH disease.

Nursing interventions. Assess the patient's level of pain and give anal-gesics as needed. Provide meticulous skin care to minimize skin breakdown. Note the quantity and character of stools.

Patient education. If the patient has chronic GVH disease, discuss ways he can protect himself against infection. Urge him to keep regular follow-up appointments.

Evaluation. The patient should have no rash or jaundice and no abdominal cramping or diarrhea.

Autoimmune disorders
This section covers SLE.

Systemic lupus erythematosus
A chronic inflammatory disorder of the connective tissue, SLE affects multiple organ systems (as well as the skin) and can be fatal. It's characterized by recurring remissions and exacerbations. The prognosis improves with early detection but remains poor for patients who develop cardiovascular, renal, or neurologic complications or severe bacterial infections.

Causes. Evidence points to interrelated immunologic, environmental, hormonal, and genetic factors as possible causes of SLE. Possible risk factors include genetic predisposition, stress, streptococcal or viral infections, exposure to sunlight or ultraviolet light, immunization, pregnancy, and abnormal estrogen metabolism. Medications, such as procainamide, hydralazine, anticonvulsants and, less frequently, penicillins, sulfa drugs, and oral contraceptives, also increase the risk of SLE.

Assessment findings. Characteristic findings in SLE include facial erythema (butterfly rash), nonerosive arthritis, and photosensitivity. (See *Recognizing butterfly rash,* page 614.) The patient may also exhibit discoid rash, oral or nasopharyngeal ulcerations, pleuritis, pericarditis, seizures, psychoses, and patchy alopecia. In addition, she may have some combination of these systemic signs and symptoms: aching, malaise, fatigue, low-grade or spiking fever, chills, anorexia, weight loss, lymph node enlargement, abdominal pain, nausea and vomiting, diarrhea or constipation, and irregular menstrual periods or amenorrhea.

Diagnostic tests. Antinuclear antibody, anti-DNA, and lupus erythematosus cell tests are the most specific tests for SLE. CBC with differential may show anemia and decreased WBC count. Platelet count may be decreased. ESR may be elevated. Serum electrophoresis may show hypergammaglobulinemia.

Urine studies may show RBCs and WBCs, urine casts and sediment, and protein loss (more than 3.5 g/24 hours). Blood studies showing decreased serum complement (C3 and C4) levels indicate active disease. Chest X-ray may show pleurisy or lupus pneumonitis. An electrocardiogram may reveal a conduction defect with cardiac involvement or pericarditis. Kidney biopsy determines disease stage and extent of renal involvement.

Treatment. Patients with mild disease require little or no medication. Nonsteroidal anti-inflammatory drugs, including aspirin, commonly control arthritis symptoms. Skin lesions need topical treatment. Corticosteroid creams such as flurandrenolide are recommended for acute lesions.

Refractory skin lesions are treated with intralesional corticosteroids or antimalarials, such as hydroxychloroquine and chloroquine. Because these two drugs can cause retinal damage, such treatment requires ophthalmologic examination every 6 months.

Corticosteroids remain the treatment of choice for systemic symptoms of SLE, for acute generalized exacerbations, and for associated pleuritis, pericarditis, lupus nephritis, vasculitis, and central nervous system (CNS) involvement. Initial doses equivalent to 60 mg or more of prednisone usually bring noticeable improvement within 48 hours. When symptoms are under control, steroid dosage is tapered slowly. Diffuse proliferative glomerulonephritis, a major complication of SLE, requires treatment with large doses of steroids. If renal failure occurs, dialysis or kidney transplant may be necessary. In some patients, cytotoxic drugs—such as azathioprine and cyclophosphamide—may prevent deteriorating renal status. Antihypertensive drugs and dietary changes may also be warranted in renal disease.

Recognizing butterfly rash

In classic butterfly rash, lesions appear on the cheeks and the bridge of the nose, creating a characteristic butterfly pattern. The rash may vary in severity from malar erythema to discoid lesions (plaque).

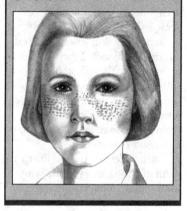

Nursing interventions. Careful assessment, supportive measures, emotional support, and patient education are all important parts of the plan of care for patients with SLE. (See *Treating a patient with SLE.*) Watch for constitutional symptoms: joint pain or stiffness, weakness, fever, fatigue, and chills. Observe for dyspnea, chest pain, and edema of the extremities. Note the size, type, and location of skin lesions. Check urine for hematuria, scalp for hair loss, and skin and mucous membranes for petechiae, bleeding, ulceration, and bruising.

Monitor vital signs, intake and output, weight, and laboratory reports closely. Check pulse rates regularly, and observe for orthopnea. Check stools and GI secretions for blood. Observe for hypertension, weight gain, and other signs of renal involvement. Assess for signs of neurologic damage: personality change, paranoid or psychotic behavior, ptosis, or diplopia. Take seizure precautions.

Patient education. Urge the patient to get plenty of rest. Teach ROM exercises as well as body alignment and postural techniques.

Explain the expected benefit of prescribed medications, and watch for adverse effects, especially with high-dose corticosteroids.

Tell the photosensitive patient to wear protective clothing (hat, sunglasses, long sleeves, pants) and use a sunscreen containing para-aminobenzoic acid when in the sun.

Evaluation. The patient should be free from pain and stiffness. Vital signs should be normal.

Immunodeficiency disorders

These disorders may involve deficiencies in cell-mediated immunity, humoral immunity, or both, plus complement deficiencies.

Severe combined immunodeficiency

In severe combined immunodeficiency (SCID), both cell-mediated (T cell) and humoral (B cell) immunity are deficient or absent, resulting in susceptibility to infection from all classes of microorganisms during infancy. At least three types of SCID exist: reticular dysgenesis, the most severe type; Swiss type agammaglobulinemia; and enzyme deficiency such as adenosine deaminase deficiency.

Causes. SCID is usually transmitted as an autosomal recessive trait, although it may be X-linked. In most cases, the genetic defect seems associated with failure of the stem cell to differentiate into T and B lymphocytes. Less commonly, it results from enzyme deficiency.

Assessment findings. An extreme susceptibility to infection becomes obvious in the infant with SCID in the first few months of life. Commonly, such an infant fails to thrive and develops chronic otitis; sepsis; watery diarrhea (associated with *Salmonella* or *Escherichia coli*); recurrent pulmonary infections (usually caused by *Pseudomonas*, cytomegalovirus, or *Pneumocystis carinii*); persistent oral candidiasis, sometimes with esophageal erosions; and common viral infections (such as chickenpox) that may be fatal.

P. carinii pneumonia usually strikes a severely immunodeficient infant in the first 3 to 5 weeks of life. Onset is typically insidious, with gradually worsening cough, low-grade fever, tachypnea, and respiratory distress. Chest X-ray characteristically shows bilateral pulmonary infiltrates.

Gram-negative infections don't usually appear until the infant is about 6 months old.

FOCUS ON CARING

Treating a patient with SLE

The patient with systemic lupus erythematosus (SLE) needs your emotional support. You can support the female patient's self-image by offering helpful cosmetic tips, such as the use of hypoallergenic makeup and the name of a hairdresser who specializes in scalp disorders.

Never downplay her feelings of unattractiveness. Accept any expressions of negative self-image before you offer specific advice.

Diagnostic tests. Diagnosis is usually made clinically because most SCID infants suffer recurrent overwhelming infections within 1 year of birth. Some infants are diagnosed after a severe reaction to vaccination.

Before 5 months of age, even normal infants have very small amounts of serum immunoglobulins IgM and IgA, and normal IgG levels merely reflect maternal IgG. However, severely diminished or absent T-cell number and function, and lymph node biopsy showing absence of lymphocytes can confirm the diagnosis of SCID.

Treatment. Treatment aims to restore the immune response and prevent infection. Histocompatible bone marrow transplantation is the only satisfactory treatment. Because bone marrow cells must be human leukocyte antigen (HLA)– and mixed leukocyte culture–matched, the most common donors are histocompatible siblings. Newer methods of bone marrow transplantation that eliminate GVH disease are being evaluated.

Fetal thymus and liver transplants have achieved limited success. Administration of immune globulin may also play a role in treatment. Some SCID infants have received long-term protection by being isolated in a sterile environment. However, this approach isn't effective if the infant already has had recurring infections.

Nursing interventions. Patient care is primarily preventive and supportive. Constantly monitor the infant for early signs of infection; if infection develops, provide prompt and aggressive drug therapy, as ordered. Watch for adverse reactions to medications. Avoid vaccinations, and give only irradiated blood products if transfusion is ordered.

Patient education. Explain all procedures, medications, and precautions to the parents. Because parents will have questions about the vulnerability of future offspring, refer them for genetic counseling.

Evaluation. The patient should be free from infection. Physical and emotional development should proceed at a normal rate.

Complement deficiencies

Complement is a series of circulating enzymatic serum proteins with nine functional components, labeled C1 through C9. When IgG or IgM reacts with antigens as part of an immune response, it activates C1, which then combines with C4, initiating the complement pathway or cascade. Complement then combines with the antigen-antibody complex and undergoes a sequence of complicated reactions that amplifies the immune response. This complex process is called complement fixation.

Complement deficiency or dysfunction may increase susceptibility to infection and also seems related to certain autoimmune disorders.

Causes. Primary complement deficiencies (rare) are inherited. Secondary complement deficiencies may follow complement-fixing (complement-consuming) immunologic reactions, such as drug-induced serum sickness, acute streptococcal glomerulonephritis, and acute active SLE.

Assessment findings. C2 and C3 deficiencies and C5 familial dysfunction increase susceptibility to bacterial infection (which may involve several body systems simultaneously). C5 dysfunction, which occurs in infants, causes failure to thrive, diarrhea, and seborrheic dermatitis. C1 esterase inhibitor deficiency (hereditary angioedema) may cause periodic swelling in the face, hands, abdomen, or throat, with potentially fatal laryngeal edema.

Diagnostic tests. Total serum complement level (CH_{50}) is low in various complement deficiencies. Specific assays may be done to confirm deficiency of specific complement components.

Treatment. Primary complement deficiencies have no known cure. Associated infection, collagen vascular disease, or renal disease requires prompt, appropriate treatment. Transfusion of fresh frozen plasma to provide replacement of complement components is controversial because replacement therapy doesn't cure complement deficiencies and any beneficial effects are transient. Bone marrow transplant may be helpful but can cause potentially fatal GVH disease. Anabolic steroids and antifibrinolytic agents are commonly used to reduce acute swelling in patients with C1 esterase inhibitor deficiency.

Nursing interventions. After bone marrow transplant, monitor the patient closely for signs of transfusion reaction and GVH disease. Meticulous patient care can speed recovery and prevent complications. For example, a patient with renal infection needs careful monitoring of intake and output, tests for serum electrolyte levels and acid-base balance, and observation for signs of renal failure. When caring for a patient with hereditary angioedema, watch for laryngeal edema, and keep airway equipment on hand.

Patient education. Teach the patient (or his family, if he's a child) how to recognize and avoid infection and the need for prompt treatment if it occurs.

Evaluation. The patient should be free from infection. He (or his parents) should be able to state early signs of infection and preventive measures.

Acquired immunodeficiency syndrome

Characterized by progressive weakening of cell-mediated (T-cell) immunity, AIDS heightens susceptibility to opportunistic infections and unusual cancers. Diagnosis depends on careful correlation of the patient's history and clinical features with CD4 T-cell counts. (See *Classifying HIV infection and AIDS,* pages 619 and 620.) The time between probable exposure to the causative human immunodeficiency virus (HIV) and diagnosis averages 1 to 3 years. In children, incubation time appears to be shorter, with a mean of 8 months.

Causes. The retrovirus HIV causes AIDS. This virus appears in body fluids, such as blood and semen. Modes of transmission include sexual contact, especially associated with trauma to the rectal or vaginal mucosa; transfusion of contaminated blood or blood products; and use of contaminated needles. The virus can also be transmitted perinatally from mother to fetus.

Risk factors include multiple sexual contacts with homosexual and bisexual men, heterosexual contact with someone who has AIDS or is at risk for it, present or past abuse of I.V. drugs, and transfusions of blood or blood products. Prenatal and perinatal exposure to AIDS also increases the risk of AIDS in infants.

So does breast-feeding if the mother has AIDS or is at risk for it.

Assessment findings. Signs and symptoms of AIDS vary widely, and nonspecific ones may include fatigue, afternoon fevers, night sweats, weight loss, diarrhea, and cough. Children present a different clinical profile than adults. For instance, they don't usually develop hepatitis B or peripheral lymphopenia, and they rarely develop Kaposi's sarcoma, B-cell lymphoma, or acute mononucleosis-like symptoms; however, they may have diseases that are uncommon or milder in affected adults. These include hypergammaglobulinemia, lymphoid interstitial pneumonitis, serious bacterial infection, and progressive neurologic disease caused by CNS infection. Patients may be asymptomatic until the abrupt onset of such complications as opportunistic infections, Kaposi's sarcoma, and HIV encephalopathy (dementia), which is marked by confusion, apathy, and paranoia.

Kaposi's sarcoma is characterized by purple or blue patches, plaques, or nodular skin lesions that spread widely. The lesions occur most commonly in the skin, oral mucosa, lymph nodes, GI tract, lungs, and visceral organs. GI lesions are associated with GI symptoms, lung lesions with congestion and difficulty breathing, and lymphatic system lesions with severe facial and extremity swelling and secondary pain.

Diagnostic tests. The Centers for Disease Control and Prevention defines AIDS as an illness characterized by laboratory evidence of HIV infection coexisting with one or more indicator diseases. Most patients are diagnosed by these criteria.

Laboratory evidence of seroconversion occurs 8 to 12 weeks after HIV exposure. Antibody tests, the most commonly performed studies, indirectly indicate infection by revealing HIV antibodies. The recommended protocol calls for initial screening with an enzyme-linked immunosorbent assay (ELISA). If results are positive, the ELISA test is repeated. If still positive, the findings are confirmed by an alternative method, usually the Western blot or an immunofluorescence assay.

Antibody testing isn't always reliable. An infected patient can test normal anywhere from a few weeks to as long as 35 months. Transferred maternal antibodies, lasting for up to 10 months, make neonatal antibody tests unreliable.

Direct testing is more reliable because it detects HIV itself. Direct tests include antigen tests (p24 antigen), HIV cultures, nucleic acid probes of peripheral blood lymphocytes, and the polymerase chain reaction tests.

Further blood tests help evaluate the severity of immunosuppression: CD4 and CD8 T-cell subset counts, ESR, CBC, serum beta$_2$-microglobulin, p24 antigen, neopterin levels, and anergy testing. Patients are tested for syphilis, hepatitis B, tuberculosis, toxoplasmosis, or histoplasmosis.

Classifying HIV infection and AIDS

In 1993, the Centers for Disease Control and Prevention (CDC) revised its classification system for human immunodeficiency virus (HIV) infection and expanded its surveillance case definition for acquired immunodeficiency syndrome (AIDS). The new classification groups HIV-infected patients according to three ranges of CD4 T-cell counts and three clinical categories, and it includes three new AIDS-indicator conditions. The chart below shows the nine mutually exclusive subgroups.

CD4 cell categories	Clinical categories		
	A	**B**	**C**
≥500/µl	A1	B1	C1
200 to 499/µl	A2	B2	C2
<200/µl AIDS-indicator cell count	A3	B3	C3

KEY: A = Asymptomatic or persistent generalized lymphadenopathy (PGL)
   B = Symptomatic, not A or C conditions
   C = AIDS-indicator conditions

CD4 T-cell categories

These CD4 T-cell ranges are considered positive markers for HIV infection:
• *Category 1:* 500 or more cells/µl of blood
• *Category 2:* 200 to 499 cells/µl of blood
• *Category 3:* less than 200 cells/µl of blood

Disease categories

The CDC defines three related disease categories as follows:
• *Category A:* Patients without symptoms, with PGL, or with acute primary HIV infection. Conditions in categories B and C must not have occurred.
• *Category B:* HIV-infected patients with symptoms or diseases not included in category C, such as bacillary angiomatosis, oropharyngeal or persistent vulvovaginal candidiasis, fever or diarrhea lasting more than 1 month, idiopathic thrombocytopenic purpura, pelvic inflammatory disease (particularly if complicated by tubo-ovarian abscess), and peripheral neuropathy.
• *Category C:* HIV-infected patients with disorders defined by the CDC as AIDS-indicator conditions.

AIDS-indicator conditions

The CDC recognizes the following AIDS-indicator conditions:
• candidiasis of the bronchi, trachea, or lungs
• candidiasis of the esophagus
• cervical cancer, invasive

(continued)

Classifying HIV infection and AIDS *(continued)*

- coccidioidomycosis, disseminated or extrapulmonary
- cryptococcosis, extrapulmonary
- cryptosporidiosis, chronic intestinal (persisting more than 1 month)
- cytomegalovirus (CMV) disease affecting organs other than the liver, spleen, or lymph nodes
- CMV retinitis with vision loss
- encephalopathy related to HIV
- herpes simplex, involving chronic ulcers (persisting more than 1 month) or herpetic bronchitis, pneumonitis, or esophagitis
- histoplasmosis, disseminated or extrapulmonary
- isosporiasis, chronic intestinal (persisting more than 1 month)
- Kaposi's sarcoma
- lymphoma, Burkitt's (or its equivalent)
- lymphoma, immunoblastic (or its equivalent)
- lymphoma of the brain, primary
- *Mycobacterium avium* complex or *Mycobacterium kansasii*, disseminated or extrapulmonary
- *Mycobacterium tuberculosis* at any site (pulmonary or extrapulmonary)
- *Mycobacterium*, any other species, disseminated or extrapulmonary
- *Pneumocystis carinii* pneumonia
- pneumonia, recurrent
- progressive multifocal leukoencephalopathy
- *Salmonella* septicemia, recurrent
- toxoplasmosis of the brain
- wasting syndrome caused by HIV.

To diagnose AIDS dementia, you must confirm HIV infection; identify signs of dementia; and rule out other possible causes, such as hypoxia, hypoglycemia, CNS tumors, and brain atrophy.

Treatment. No cure has yet been found for AIDS. However, several antiretroviral treatments can inhibit or temporarily inactivate HIV. Immunomodulatory drugs strengthen the immune system and anti-infective and antineoplastic drugs combat opportunistic infections and associated cancers. Some anti-infectives also serve as prophylaxis against opportunistic infections. New protocols combine two or more of these drugs to produce the maximum benefit with the fewest adverse reactions. Combination therapy also helps inhibit the production of mutant HIV strains resistant to a particular drug.

Although many opportunistic infections respond to anti-infective drugs, they tend to recur. Therefore, the patient usually requires continued prophylaxis until the drug loses its efficacy or can't be tolerated.

A new group of antivirals called protease inhibitors has greatly increased the life expectancy of HIV-infected individuals. Saquinavin mesylate, which inhibits the activity of HIV protease, is usually administered in combination with a nucleoside analogue such as zalcitabine.

Zidovudine (AZT) effectively slows the progression of HIV infection, decreasing the number of opportunistic infections, prolonging survival, and slowing the progress of associated dementia. However, the drug produces severe adverse effects and toxicities. Initially, the zidovudine regimen consisted of 200 mg every 4 hours; however, this regimen is giving way to a lower-dose one that calls for 100 mg every 4 hours. The lower-dose regimen appears to be as effective but causes fewer adverse effects and less toxicity.

Because of the significant risk of toxicity, only symptomatic patients or patients with a CD4 T-cell count of 200 or less receive the higher-dose regimen. Asymptomatic patients with a CD4 T-cell count at or below 500 may receive the lower-dose regimen.

Didanosine (ddI), an antiretroviral drug, is used only in patients who can't tolerate zidovudine because of its more severe effects, including life-threatening pancreatitis. Supportive treatment helps maintain nutrition and relieve pain and other symptoms.

Zidovudine, didanosine, and dideoxycytidine (ddC) treat the virus itself. These three drugs inhibit replication of the virus through inhibition of reverse transcriptase. Didanosine has been approved for use after failure of zidovudine, and dideoxycytidine has been approved for use in combination with zidovudine. Using two agents restricts viral replication, minimizes the toxicity of each drug, and decreases the emergence of resistant strains. Alternating the drugs at 12-week intervals may be the most successful protocol. Research is ongoing, so it's important to keep informed about new advances in AIDS treatment.

Because treatment can be administered simultaneously with anticancer chemotherapy and radiation, the ensuing immunosuppression and adverse reactions must be treated symptomatically.

Alpha interferon, a natural human protein, can boost the immune system and interfere with the assembly of HIV particles.

Nursing interventions. Monitor the patient for fever, noting its pattern. Assess for tender, swollen lymph nodes, and check laboratory values regularly. Watch for signs and symptoms of infection, such as skin breakdown, cough, sore throat, and diarrhea.

Follow universal precautions as directed by your facility, depending on the patient's stage and condition.

If Kaposi's sarcoma is present, monitor the progression of lesions. Provide meticulous skin care, especially in the debilitated patient.

Recognize that diagnosis of AIDS is typically emotionally charged.

If your patient is a child, note that he needs special care, and that his parents may be infected or dead.

Patient education. Tell the patient how AIDS increases his susceptibility to opportunistic infection. Discuss ways to prevent infection.

Urge the patient to avoid use of recreational drugs and alcohol. Explain to him that these substances may increase his vulnerability.

Review safe sex practices to prevent transmission of HIV infection.

Evaluation. The patient should be able to state the early signs of infection. He should also be able to explain how HIV is transmitted and how to practice safe sex. His nutritional status will be optimally maintained.

Anemias

Anemias are marked by abnormally low numbers of RBCs, a deficiency of hemoglobin, or a low volume of packed RBCs per 100 ml of blood. Such disorders include aplastic anemia, sickle cell anemia, and pernicious anemia.

Aplastic anemia

Also called hypoplastic anemia, aplastic anemia results from a deficiency of all of the blood's formed elements, caused by the bone marrow's failure to generate an adequate supply of new cells. This disorder usually develops when damaged or destroyed stem cells inhibit RBC production.

Although commonly used interchangeably with other terms for bone marrow failure, aplastic anemia properly refers to pancytopenia resulting from the decreased functional capacity of a hypoplastic, fatty bone marrow. Two forms of idiopathic aplastic anemia are known: congenital hypoplastic anemia (Blackfan-Diamond anemia), which develops between ages 2 months and 3 months, and Fanconi's syndrome, in which chromosomal abnormalities are usually associated with multiple congenital anomalies. Death may result from bleeding or infection.

Causes. Aplastic anemia may result from drug use; toxic agents, such as benzene and chloramphenicol; radiation; (unconfirmed) immunologic factors; severe disease, especially hepatitis; preleukemia and neoplastic infiltration of bone marrow; congenital abnormalities (a possible cause of idiopathic anemias); or induced change in fetal development.

Assessment findings. Clinical features of aplastic anemia vary with the severity of pancytopenia, develop insidiously, and may include the following signs and symptoms: progressive weakness, fatigue, shortness of breath, headache, pallor, ultimately tachycardia and heart failure; ecchymoses, petechiae; hemorrhage, especially from the mucous membranes (nose, gums, rectum, vagina) or into the retina or CNS; or infection (fever, oral and rectal ulcers, sore throat) but without characteristic inflammation.

Diagnostic tests. Confirmation of aplastic anemia requires a series of laboratory tests. RBCs are usually normochromic and normocytic (although macrocytosis [larger than normal erythrocytes] and anisocytosis [excessive variation in erythrocyte size] may exist), with a total count of 1,000,000/mm³ or less. Absolute reticulocyte count is very low. Serum iron level is elevated (unless bleeding occurs), but total iron-binding capacity is normal or slightly reduced. Hemosiderin is present, and tissue iron storage is visible microscopically. Platelet and

WBC counts fall. Lower platelet count is reflected in abnormal coagulation tests (bleeding time).

Bone marrow biopsies taken from several sites may yield a "dry tap" or show severely hypocellular or aplastic marrow; absence of tagged iron and megakaryocytes; and depression of erythroid elements.

Treatment. Effective treatment must eliminate any identifiable cause and provide vigorous supportive measures, such as packed RBC, platelet, and experimental HLA-matched leukocyte transfusions. Even then, recovery can take months. Bone marrow transplantation is the preferred treatment for anemia stemming from severe aplasia and for patients needing constant RBC transfusions.

Patients with low WBC levels may need reverse isolation to avoid infection. Antibiotics may be given but prophylactic use encourages resistant strains of organisms. Patients with low hemoglobin counts may need oxygen therapy and blood transfusions.

Other treatments include corticosteroids to stimulate erythroid production (successful in children, but not in adults), marrow-stimulating agents such as androgens (which are controversial), and immunosuppressant agents (if the patient doesn't respond to other therapy). Colony-stimulating factors are used for patients who have had chemotherapy or radiation therapy. These agents include granulocyte colony-stimulating factor, granulocyte-macrophage colony-stimulating factor, and erythropoietic stimulating factor.

Nursing interventions. If the patient's platelet count is low (less than 20,000/mm^3), take steps to prevent hemorrhage by avoiding I.M. injections, suggesting the use of an electric razor and a soft toothbrush, humidifying oxygen to prevent drying of mucous membranes, and promoting regular bowel movements with stool softeners and a proper diet. Also, apply pressure to venipuncture sites until bleeding stops. Detect bleeding early by checking for blood in urine and stool and assessing skin for petechiae. Monitor blood studies carefully in the patient receiving anemia-inducing drugs.

Patient education. Teach the patient to recognize and immediately report signs of infection.

Encourage the patient who does not require hospitalization to continue his normal lifestyle, with appropriate restrictions, until remission occurs.

Evaluation. The patient should have fewer infections, his blood cell counts should return to normal, he should breathe easily, and he should no longer experience trauma-induced hemorrhagic episodes. He and his family should understand energy-saving strategies.

Sickle cell anemia

A congenital hemolytic anemia that occurs primarily in African-Americans, sickle cell anemia results from a defective hemoglobin molecule (hemoglobin S) that causes RBCs to roughen and become sickle shaped. These cells impair circulation, resulting in chronic ill health, periodic crises, long-term complications, and premature death.

Causes. Sickle cell anemia may stem from homozygous inheritance of the hemoglobin S–producing gene, which causes the amino acid valine to replace glutamic acid in the B hemoglobin chain. (See *Sickle cell trait.*)

Blood vessel obstruction by rigid, tangled cells causes tissue anoxia and possible necrosis, which in turn cause painful vaso-occlusive crisis, a hallmark of the disease. Bone marrow depression results in aplastic (megaloblastic) crisis.

Assessment findings. Clinical features of sickle cell anemia include tachycardia, cardiomegaly, systolic and diastolic murmurs, chronic fatigue, unexplained dyspnea or dyspnea on exertion, hepatomegaly, splenomegaly during early childhood, jaundice, pallor, joint swelling, aching bones, chest pains, ischemic leg ulcers, and increased susceptibility to infection.

A patient with painful vaso-occlusive crisis may manifest severe abdominal, thoracic, muscular, or bone pain; possible increased jaundice and dark urine; low-grade fever; and, in long-term disease, spleen shrinkage.

Diagnostic tests. Stained blood smear showing sickle-shaped cells and hemoglobin electrophoresis showing hemoglobin S confirm the diagnosis.

CBC shows low RBC and elevated WBC and platelet counts; the hemoglobin level may be low or normal. ESR and RBC survival time are decreased; serum iron and reticulocyte counts are increased.

Treatment. Treatment can alleviate symptoms and prevent painful crises. Vaccines such as polyvalent pneumococcal and *Haemophilus influenzae* B, anti-infectives such as low-dose oral penicillin, and chelating agents such as deferoxamine can minimize complications. The most commonly used antisickling agent, sodium cyanate, produces many adverse effects.

Treatment begins before age 4 months with prophylactic penicillin. If the patient's hemoglobin level drops suddenly or if his condition deteriorates rapidly, he'll need transfusion of packed RBCs.

In an acute sequestration crisis, treatment may include sedation, analgesia, blood transfusion, oxygen therapy, and large amounts of oral or I.V. fluids.

Nursing interventions. Suspect a crisis in a sickle cell anemia patient with pale lips, tongue, palms, or nail beds; lethargy; listlessness; difficulty awakening; irritability; severe pain; temperature over 104° F (40° C) or a fever of 100° F (37.8° C) lasting at least 2 days.

During a painful crisis, apply warm compresses to painful areas and cover the patient with a blanket. (Never use cold compresses, which aggravate the condition.) Give an analgesic-antipyretic, such as aspirin or acetaminophen. Encourage bed rest, and place the patient in a sitting position. If dehydration or severe pain occurs, he may be hospitalized.

Patient education. During remission, help the patient prevent exacerbation. Advise him to avoid tight clothing that restricts circulation. Warn against strenuous exercise, vasoconstricting medications, cold temperatures, unpressurized aircraft, high altitudes, and other conditions that provoke hypoxia.

Emphasize the need for prevention and prompt treatment for infection. Stress the need to increase fluid intake to prevent dehydration.

Refer parents of children with sickle cell anemia for genetic counseling. Recommend screening of family members to determine if they're heterozygote carriers.

Evaluation. The patient should be free from pain and infection. He and his family should understand how to avoid exacerbations.

Pernicious anemia

Also called Addison's anemia, pernicious anemia is a progressive, megaloblastic, macrocytic anemia. The disorder causes neurologic, gastric, and intestinal abnormalities. Untreated, it may lead to permanent neurologic disability and death.

Sickle cell trait

Sickle cell trait is a relatively benign condition that results from heterozygous inheritance of the abnormal hemoglobin S–producing gene. Like sickle cell anemia, this condition is most common in African-Americans. Sickle cell trait *never* progresses to sickle cell anemia.

In persons with sickle cell trait (also called carriers), 20% to 40% of their total hemoglobin is hemoglobin S; the rest is normal. Such persons usually have no symptoms. They have a normal hemoglobin level and normal hematocrit and can expect a normal life span. Nevertheless, they must avoid situations that provoke hypoxia because these occasionally cause a sickling crisis similar to that in sickle cell anemia.

Genetic counseling is essential for sickle cell carriers. If two sickle cell carriers marry, each of their children has a 25% chance of inheriting sickle cell anemia.

Causes. This disorder results from a deficiency of vitamin B_{12}, which may be due to a genetic predisposition or an inherited autoimmune response.

Assessment findings. Characteristically, pernicious anemia has an insidious onset but eventually causes an unmistakable triad of symptoms including weakness, sore tongue, and numbness and tingling in the extremities. Pale lips, gums, and tongue and faintly jaundiced sclerae also occur. Systemic signs may include pale to bright yellow skin and indications of infection, especially of the genitourinary tract.

Other signs and symptoms include:

- GI—nausea, vomiting, anorexia, weight loss, flatulence, diarrhea, and constipation. Gingival bleeding and tongue inflammation may hinder eating and intensify anorexia.
- CNS—neuritis; weakness in extremities; peripheral numbness and paresthesias; disturbed position sense; lack of coordination; ataxia; impaired fine finger movement; positive Babinski's and Romberg's signs; light-headedness; altered vision (diplopia, blurred vision), taste, and hearing (tinnitus); optic muscle atrophy; loss of bowel and bladder control; irritability, poor memory, headache, depression, and delirium; and, in males, impotence. Irreversible CNS changes may have occurred before treatment.
- Cardiovascular—weakness, fatigue, light-headedness, palpitations, wide pulse pressure, dyspnea, orthopnea, tachycardia, premature beats and, eventually, heart failure.

Diagnostic tests. The Schilling test provides definitive diagnosis of pernicious anemia. Hemoglobin level and RBC count are decreased. Mean corpuscular volume is increased (greater than 120 mm³/red cell) and, because larger-than-normal RBCs contain increased amounts of hemoglobin, mean corpuscular hemoglobin level is also increased. WBC and platelet counts are commonly low, and large, malformed platelets may be present. Serum vitamin B_{12} assay levels may be less than 0.1 µg/ml.

Treatment. Early parenteral vitamin B_{12} replacement can reverse pernicious anemia and minimize complications and may prevent permanent neurologic damage. An initial high dose of parenteral vitamin B_{12} stimulates rapid RBC regeneration. Within 2 weeks, the hemoglobin level should rise to normal, and the patient's condition should improve markedly. Because rapid cell regeneration increases the patient's iron requirements, concomitant iron replacement is necessary. After the patient's condition improves, vitamin B_{12} doses can be decreased to maintenance levels and given monthly. The patient should learn to perform self-injection.

Nursing interventions. Supportive measures minimize the risk of complications and speed recovery. Patient and family teaching can promote compliance with lifelong vitamin B_{12} replacement.

Patient education. Warn the patient to guard against infections. Tell him to report signs of infection promptly, especially of pulmonary and urinary tract infections. Warn the patient with a sensory deficit not to use a heating pad because it may cause burns. Stress that vitamin B_{12} replacement is not a permanent cure and that these injections must be continued for life.

Evaluation. The patient should have minimal oral discomfort and should use energy-saving strategies.

Polycythemias

Polycythemias are marked by an excess of RBCs.

Polycythemia vera

Polycythemia vera is a chronic, myeloproliferative disorder marked by increased RBC mass, leukocytosis, thrombocytosis, and increased hemoglobin level, with normal or decreased plasma volume. Mortality is high if polycythemia is untreated or is associated with leukemia or myeloid metaplasia.

Cause. Uncontrolled and rapid cellular reproduction and maturation cause proliferation or hyperplasia of all bone marrow cells (panmyelosis). The cause is unknown, but it probably results from a multipotential stem cell defect.

Assessment findings. Clinical features of affected body systems are as follows:
• Eye, ear, nose, and throat—visual disturbances and congestion of conjunctiva, retina, retinal veins, and oral mucous membranes.
• CNS—headache, lethargy, syncope, and paresthesia of digits.
• Cardiovascular system—hypertension, dyspnea, intermittent claudication, thrombosis, angina, and hemorrhage.
• Skin—pruritus, urticaria, and ruddy cyanosis.

• GI system—epigastric distress, early satiety and fullness, peptic ulcer pain, and hepatosplenomegaly.
• Musculoskeletal—joint symptoms.

Diagnostic tests. Laboratory studies confirm polycythemia vera by showing increased RBC mass and normal arterial oxygen saturation in association with splenomegaly or two of the following: thrombocytosis, leukocytosis, elevated leukocyte alkaline phosphatase level, or elevated serum vitamin B_{12} or unbound B_{12}-binding capacity. Other studies may reveal increased serum uric acid, increased blood histamine, decreased serum iron concentration, and decreased or absent urinary erythropoietin. Bone marrow biopsy reveals panmyelosis.

Treatment. Phlebotomy, the primary treatment, can be performed repeatedly and can promptly reduce RBC mass. Typically, 350 to 500 ml of blood can be removed every other day until the patient's hematocrit falls to the low-normal range. After repeated phlebotomies, the patient develops iron deficiency, which stabilizes RBC production and reduces the need for this treatment. However, phlebotomy doesn't reduce the WBC or platelet count and won't control the hyperuricemia associated with marrow cell proliferation.

Myelosuppressive therapy may be used for patients with severe symptoms, such as extreme thrombocytosis, a rapidly enlarging spleen, and hypermetabolism. It's also used for elderly patients who have difficulty tolerating the procedure. Radioactive phosphorus (^{32}P) or chemotherapeutic agents, such as melphalan, busulfan, or chlorambucil can satisfactorily control the disease. However, these agents may cause leukemia and should be reserved for older patients and those with serious problems not controlled by phlebotomy.

Pheresis technology allows removal of RBCs, WBCs, and platelets individually or collectively. Pheresis also permits the return of plasma to the patient, thereby diluting the blood and reducing hypovolemic symptoms.

As appropriate, additional treatments include administration of cyproheptadine (12 to 16 mg/day) and allopurinol (300 mg/day) to reduce serum uric acid levels. Treatment usually improves symptomatic splenomegaly; rarely splenectomy may be performed.

Nursing interventions. Keep the patient active and ambulatory to prevent thrombosis. If bed rest is necessary, prescribe a daily program of both active and passive ROM exercises.

Watch for complications, such as hypervolemia, thrombocytosis, and signs of an impending cerebrovascular accident. Regularly examine the patient closely for bleeding.

To compensate for increased uric acid production, give the patient additional fluids; administer allopurinol, as ordered; and alkalinize the urine to prevent uric acid calculi. Report acute abdominal pain immediately; it may signal splenic infarction, renal calculi, or abdominal organ thrombosis.

Patient education. If the patient has symptomatic splenomegaly, suggest or provide small, frequent meals, followed by a rest period, to prevent nausea and vomiting. Tell him to watch for and report any signs and symptoms of iron deficiency (pallor, weight loss, asthenia, and glossitis). Advise him to report any abnormal bleeding promptly.

Evaluation. Look for an optimum activity level. The patient should have no bleeding episodes or joint discomfort.

Hemorrhagic disorders

Hemorrhagic disorders include DIC, thrombocytopenia, idiopathic thrombocytopenic purpura, and hemophilia.

Disseminated intravascular coagulation

A grave coagulopathy that occurs as a complication of conditions that accelerate clotting, DIC causes small blood vessel occlusion, organ necrosis, depletion of circulating clotting factors and platelets, and activation of the fibrinolytic system. These processes, in turn, can provoke severe hemorrhage. Clotting in the microcirculation usually affects the kidneys and extremities but may occur in the brain, lungs, pituitary and adrenal glands, and GI mucosa. Usually acute, DIC may be chronic in cancer patients.

Causes. DIC can result from *infection* (gram-negative or gram-positive septicemia; viral, fungal, or rickettsial infection; or protozoal infection [falciparum malaria]), *obstetric complications* (abruptio placentae, amniotic fluid embolism, or retained dead fetus), *neoplastic disease* (acute leukemia or metastatic carcinoma), and *tissue necrosis* (extensive burns and trauma, brain tissue destruction, transplant rejection, or hepatic necrosis).

Other causes of DIC include heatstroke, shock, poisonous snakebite, cirrhosis, fat embolism, incompatible blood transfusion, cardiac arrest, intraoperative cardiopulmonary bypass, giant hemangioma, severe venous thrombosis, or purpura fulminans.

Assessment findings. Abnormal bleeding, without a history of a serious hemorrhagic disorder, can signal DIC. Principal signs of such bleeding include cutaneous oozing, petechiae, ecchymoses, hematomas, bleeding from sites of surgical or invasive procedures, and bleeding from the GI tract.

Also assess for acrocyanosis and signs of acute tubular necrosis. Related or possible signs and symptoms include nausea, vomiting, dyspnea, oliguria, convulsions, coma, shock, failure of major organ systems, and severe muscle, back, and abdominal pain.

Diagnostic tests. Initial laboratory findings that support a tentative diagnosis of DIC include prolonged prothrombin time (PT) (> 15 seconds), prolonged activated partial thromboplastin time (APTT) (> 60 to 80 seconds), decreased fibrinogen levels (< 150 mg/dl), decreased platelet count (< 100,000/mm³), and increased fibrin degradation products (commonly > 100 µg/ml).

Supportive data may include positive fibrin monomers, diminished levels of factors V and VIII, fragmentation of RBCs, and decreased hemoglobin (< 10 g/dl). Assessment of renal status demonstrates reduced urine output (< 30 ml/hour), and elevated blood urea nitrogen (> 25 mg/dl) and serum creatinine (> 1.3 mg/dl) levels.

Additional diagnostic measures may be required to determine the underlying disorder.

Treatment. Effective treatment for DIC requires prompt recognition and treatment for the underlying disorder. Treatment may be supportive (when the underlying disorder is self-limiting) or highly specific. If the patient isn't actively bleeding, supportive care alone may reverse DIC. However, active bleeding may require heparin I.V. and administration of blood, fresh frozen plasma, platelets, or packed RBCs to support hemostasis.

Nursing interventions. Focus your patient care on early recognition of principal signs of abnormal bleeding, prompt treatment for the underlying disorders, and prevention of further bleeding. To prevent clots from dislodging, don't scrub bleeding areas. Use pressure, cold compresses, and topical hemostatic agents to control bleeding. Protect the patient from injury. Enforce complete bed rest during bleeding episodes. If the patient is agitated, pad the side rails. Check all I.V. and venipuncture sites frequently. Apply pressure to injection sites for at least 10 minutes.

Monitor intake and output hourly in acute DIC, especially when administering blood products. For suspected intra-abdominal bleeding, measure the patient's vital signs and abdomen at least every 4 hours, and monitor closely for signs of shock. Monitor the results of serial blood studies (especially hematocrit, hemoglobin level, and coagulation times).

Patient education. Explain all diagnostic tests and procedures.

Evaluation. The patient should be free from bleeding, and tests should show that coagulation parameters and renal status are normal.

Thrombocytopenia

A deficiency of circulating platelets signals thrombocytopenia, the most common hemorrhagic disorder. Platelets play a vital role in coagulation, so this disorder seriously threatens hemostasis. It may be congenital or acquired.

Causes. Platelet count may be reduced in several ways:
• *diminished or defective platelet production.* Congenital causes include Wiskott-Aldrich syndrome, maternal ingestion of thiazides, neonatal rubella, and thrombopoietin defi-

ciency. Acquired causes include aplastic anemia, marrow infiltration (acute and chronic leukemias, tumor), nutritional deficiency (B_{12}, folic acid), myelosuppressive agents, chemotherapeutic agents, drugs that directly influence platelet production (thiazides, alcohol, antibiotics such as co-trimoxazole, hormones), radiation, and viral infections (measles, dengue).
• *increased peripheral platelet destruction.* Congenital causes may be nonimmune (prematurity, erythroblastosis fetalis, infection) or immune (drug sensitivity, maternal idiopathic thrombocytopenic purpura [ITP]). Acquired causes may be nonimmune (infection, DIC, thrombotic thrombocytopenic purpura) or immune (drug-induced, especially with quinine and quinidine; posttransfusion purpura; ITP; sepsis; alcohol).
• *platelet sequestration.* Causes include hypersplenism and hypothermia.
• *platelet loss.* Causes include hemorrhage and extracorporeal perfusion.

Assessment findings. Watch for these signs and symptoms: abnormal bleeding (typically sudden onset; petechiae or ecchymoses in the skin or bleeding into any mucous membrane), malaise, fatigue, general weakness, lethargy, and large blood-filled bullae in mouth (a characteristic sign in adults).

Diagnostic tests. Coagulation tests show diminished platelet count, and bleeding time is prolonged. Bone marrow studies may reveal a greater number of megakaryocytes and shortened platelet survival.

Treatment. Removal of the causative agents in drug-induced thrombocytopenia or proper treatment for the underlying cause, when possible, is essential. Treatment includes splenectomy for hypersplenism; chemotherapy for acute or chronic leukemia; steroids, danazol, or I.V. immune globulin for ITP; and corticosteroids to enhance vascular integrity. Platelet transfusions may be given when platelet counts fall below 20,000/mm³.

Nursing interventions. When caring for the patient with thrombocytopenia, take every possible precaution against bleeding.

Protect the patient from trauma. When venipuncture is unavoidable, be sure to exert pressure on the puncture site for at least 20 minutes or until the bleeding stops. Don't take rectal temperatures.

Monitor platelet count daily. Test stool for occult blood; also test urine and emesis for blood. Watch for bleeding (petechiae, ecchymoses, surgical or GI bleeding, menorrhagia).

When the patient is bleeding, keep him on strict bed rest, if necessary. During platelet transfusion, monitor for febrile reaction (flushing, chills, fever, headache, tachycardia, hypertension). If he has a history of minor reactions, he may benefit from acetaminophen and diphenhydramine before the transfusion.

Patient education. Warn the patient to avoid taking aspirin in any form as well as other drugs that impair coagulation. Promote the use of an electric razor and a soft toothbrush.

Advise the patient to take a stool softener to avoid straining, which could possibly cause cerebral hemorrhage. Tell him to avoid enemas and rectal suppositories.

Evaluation. The patient should have neither gross nor microscopic bleeding. He and his family should know how to reduce bleeding risks.

Idiopathic thrombocytopenic purpura

Idiopathic thrombocytopenic purpura results from immunologic platelet destruction. It may be acute (postviral thrombocytopenia) or chronic (Werlhof's disease, purpura hemorrhagica, essential thrombocytopenia, or autoimmune thrombocytopenia). Acute ITP usually affects children between ages 2 and 6; chronic ITP mainly affects women between ages 20 and 40.

Causes. Acute ITP usually follows a viral infection, such as rubella or chickenpox. It may also be drug-induced or associated with lupus erythematosus or pregnancy. ITP may be an autoimmune disorder.

Assessment findings. ITP produces clinical features that are common to all forms of thrombocytopenia: petechiae, ecchymoses, and mucosal bleeding from the mouth, nose, or GI tract. Generally, hemorrhage is the only abnormal physical finding. Purpuric lesions may occur in vital organs such as the brain and may prove fatal. In acute ITP, which commonly occurs in children, onset is usually sudden and without warning, causing easy bruising, epistaxis, and bleeding gums. Onset of chronic ITP is insidious.

Diagnostic tests. A platelet count less than 20,000/mm³ and prolonged bleeding time suggest ITP. Platelets may be abnormal in size and shape; anemia may be present if bleeding has occurred. As in thrombocytopenia, bone marrow studies show an abundance of megakaryocytes (platelet precursors) and a shortened circulating platelet survival time.

Treatment. Treatment for ITP begins with corticosteroids to promote capillary integrity; however, the drugs are only temporarily effective in chronic ITP.

This includes immunosuppression (with vincristine, for instance), danazol, high-dose I.V. gamma globulin, and splenectomy in adults (85% successful). Before splenectomy, the patient may require blood, blood components, and vitamin K to correct anemia and coagulation defects. After splenectomy, he may need blood and component replacement, and platelet concentrate. Normally, however, platelets multiply spontaneously after splenectomy.

Nursing interventions. Patient care for ITP is essentially the same as for thrombocytopenia.

Patient education. Teach the patient to observe for petechiae, ecchymoses, and other signs of recurrence, especially following acute ITP. Also advise him to restrict activity and avoid trauma (especially important in children).

Closely monitor patients receiving immunosuppressives (commonly given before splenectomy) for signs of bone marrow depression, infection, mucositis, GI tract ulceration, and severe diarrhea or vomiting.

Evaluation. The patient should be free from bleeding and infection. He and his family should recognize signs of recurring ITP.

Hemophilia

Hemophilia is a hereditary bleeding disorder that results from a lack of specific clotting factors. Hemophilia A (classic hemophilia), which affects more than 80% of all persons with hemophilia, results from deficient (or nonfunctional) factor VIII. Hemophilia B (Christmas disease), which affects 15% of persons with hemophilia, results from deficient (or nonfunctional) factor IX.

Cause. Hemophilia A and B are inherited as X-linked recessive traits. Female carriers have a 50% chance of transmitting the gene to each son or daughter. Daughters who received the gene would be carriers; sons who received it would be born with hemophilia.

Assessment findings. In *mild hemophilia,* bleeding does not occur spontaneously or after minor trauma. Prolonged bleeding occurs after major trauma or surgery. In *moderate hemophilia,* spontaneous bleeding occurs occasionally. Bleeding is excessive after surgery or trauma. In *severe hemophilia,* bleeding occurs spontaneously and possibly severely after minor trauma. This may produce large subcutaneous and deep intramuscular hematomas.

Bleeding into joints and muscles may also occur. This causes pain, swelling, extreme tenderness, and possibly permanent deformity.

Diagnostic tests. Characteristic findings in hemophilia A include factor VIII assay 0% to 30% of normal, prolonged APTT, normal platelet count and function, bleeding time, and PT.

In hemophilia B, an assay of factor IX is characteristically deficient. Baseline coagulation results are similar to hemophilia A, with normal factor VIII.

In hemophilia A or B, the degree of factor deficiency determines severity. In mild hemophilia, factor levels are 5% to 40% of normal. In moderate hemophilia, factor levels are 1% to 5% of normal, while in severe hemophilia, factor levels are less than 1% of normal.

Treatment. Hemophilia isn't curable, but treatment can prevent crippling deformities and prolong life expectancy. Correct treatment stops bleeding by increasing plasma levels of deficient clotting factors.

In hemophilia A, cryoprecipitated antihemophilic factor (AHF), lyophilized AHF, or both, given in doses large enough to raise clotting factor levels above 25% of normal can support normal hemostasis. Before surgery, AHF is administered to raise clotting factors to hemostatic levels. Levels are then kept within a normal range until the wound has completely healed. Fresh-frozen plasma can also be given.

After multiple transfusions, 10% to 20% of patients with severe hemophilia become resistant to factor VIII infusions. Desmopressin may be given to stimulate the release of stored factor VIII, raising the level in the blood. In hemophilia B, administration of factor IX concentrate during bleeding episodes increases factor IX levels.

Nursing interventions. During bleeding episodes, give clotting factor or plasma, as ordered. The body uses up AHF in 48 to 72 hours, so repeat infusions, as ordered, until bleeding stops. Apply cold compresses or ice bags and raise the injured part. To prevent recurrent bleeding, restrict the patient's activity for 48 hours after bleeding is under control. If bleeding into a joint occurs, immediately elevate the joint.

After bleeding episodes and surgery, watch closely for signs of further bleeding, such as increased pain and swelling, fever, or symptoms of shock. Closely monitor APTT. To restore mobility in an affected joint, begin ROM exercises, if ordered, at least 48 hours after the bleeding is controlled. Tell the patient to avoid placing weight on the joint until bleeding stops and swelling subsides.

Patient education. Teach parents how to prevent bleeding episodes and how to handle them when they do occur.

Refer new patients or those in whom hemophilia is suspected to a hemophilia treatment center for evaluation.

Evaluation. The patient should be free from bleeding. He and his family should understand how to minimize bleeding risks and know what to do if bleeding occurs.

Cancers of blood and lymph

Important malignancies of these systems include Hodgkin's disease, malignant lymphomas, acute leukemia, chronic myelogenous leukemia, and multiple myeloma.

Hodgkin's disease

Hodgkin's disease is a lymphatic cancer, marked by painless, progressive enlargement of lymph nodes, the spleen, and other lymphoid tissue. Reed-Sternberg cells are characteristic of this disease. Left untreated, Hodgkin's disease follows a variable but relentlessly progressive and ultimately fatal course. Recent advances in therapy make Hodgkin's disease potentially curable.

Cause. The cause of Hodgkin's disease is unknown but may be related to a viral infectious process.

Assessment findings. Painless swelling in the cervical or supraclavicular lymph nodes is usually the first sign. Occasionally, this early sign appears in lymph nodes in the axillary or inguinal area. Pruritus may also occur.

Persistent fever, night sweats, fatigue, weight loss, and malaise may occur first in older patients. Episodes of high fever become increasingly frequent over time until they're nearly continuous (Pel-Ebstein fever pattern).

Late-stage signs and symptoms include edema of the face and neck, possible jaundice, nerve pain, enlargement of retroperitoneal nodes, and nodular infiltration of the spleen, liver, and bones.

Diagnostic tests. The same tests are used for diagnosis and for staging.

Stage I disease is limited to a single lymph node region or to a single extralymphatic organ. In stage II disease, two or more nodes on the same side of the diaphragm are involved as well as an extralymphatic organ and one or more node regions or the spleen. Stage III disease involves nodes on both sides of the diaphragm as well as the spleen. And stage IV disease is marked by diffuse or disseminated involvement of one or more extralymphatic organs or tissues, with or without associated lymph node involvement.

Lymph node biopsy checks for abnormal histiocyte proliferation and nodular fibrosis and necrosis. Other appropriate tests include bone marrow, liver, and spleen biopsies and routine chest X-ray, abdominal computed tomography (CT) scan, lung scan, bone scan, and lymphangiography.

Hematologic tests show mild to severe normocytic anemia; normochromic anemia (in 50% of cases); elevated, normal, or reduced WBC count; and WBC differential showing any combination of neutrophilia, lymphocytopenia, monocytosis, and eosinophilia.

A staging laparotomy is necessary for patients under age 55 or those without obvious stage III or stage IV disease, lymphocyte predominance subtype histology, or medical contraindications.

Treatment. Appropriate therapy includes chemotherapy, radiation, or both, varying with the stage of the disease. Radiation therapy may be used alone for stage I and stage II and in combination with chemotherapy for stage III. Chemotherapy is used for stage IV, sometimes inducing a complete remission. The most commonly used combination regimens are MOPP (mechlorethamine, Oncovin [vincristine], procarbazine, prednisone) and ABVD (Adriamycin [doxorubicin], bleomycin, vinblastine, dacarbazine).

Nursing interventions. Because the patient with Hodgkin's disease is usually healthy when therapy begins, he'll need emotional support. Offer appropriate counseling and reassurance.

Patient education. Make sure the patient and his family know that local chapters of the American Cancer Society (ACS) and Leukemia Society of America are available for information, financial assistance, and supportive counseling.

Evaluation. The patient should understand and comply with the self-care regimen for radiation and chemotherapy. He should know the adverse effects of treatment and when to notify the doctor. He should control his weight loss and remain free from infection.

Malignant lymphomas

The Rappaport histologic classification categorizes lymphomas according to the degree of cellular differentiation and the presence or absence of nodularity. Nodular lymphomas yield a better prognosis than diffuse forms, but prognosis is less hopeful in both than in Hodgkin's disease.

Cause. The cause of malignant lymphomas is unknown, but a viral etiology is strongly suspected. Both human T-cell leukemia/lymphoma virus and Epstein-Barr virus have been implicated in the development of adult T-cell leukemia/lymphoma and Burkitt's lymphoma, respectively.

Assessment findings. Clinical features of malignant lymphomas include swollen lymph glands, enlarged tonsils and adenoids, and painless rubbery nodes in the cervical supraclavicular area, with possible dyspnea and coughing. As the disease progresses, the patient may report fatigue, malaise, weight loss, fever, and night sweats.

Diagnostic tests. Diagnosis is confirmed by histologic evaluation of biopsied lymph nodes; of tonsils, bone marrow, liver, bowel, or skin; or, as needed, of tissue removed during exploratory laparotomy.

Other relevant tests include bone and chest X-rays, lymphangiography, liver and spleen scan, CT scan of the abdomen, and intravenous pyelography (IVP).

Laboratory tests include CBC (may show anemia), uric acid (elevated or normal), serum calcium (elevated if bone lesions are present), serum protein (normal), and liver function studies.

Treatment. Treatment for malignant lymphomas may include radiotherapy or chemotherapy. Radiotherapy is used mainly against early localized disease. Total body irradiation is effective for both nodular and diffuse lymphomas.

Chemotherapy is most effective with multiple combinations of antineoplastic agents. Numerous drug combinations are used, including doxorubicin, cyclophosphamide, etoposide, bleomycin, vincristine, methotrexate, nitrogen mustard, and prednisone. The goal is to expose the patient to as many effective agents in full doses as early in the treatment plan as possible.

High-dose therapy with autologous bone marrow transplant can induce second remissions in patients who relapse.

Nursing interventions. Provide emotional support by informing the patient and the family about the prognosis and by listening to their concerns.

Patient education. If needed, refer the patient and his family to the local chapter of the ACS or Leukemia Society of America for information and counseling. Stress the need for continued treatment and follow-up care.

Evaluation. The patient should understand and comply with the self-care regimen for radiation and chemotherapy. He should know potential adverse effects and when to notify the doctor. He should control his weight loss and remain free from infection.

Acute leukemia

With acute leukemia, WBC precursors (blasts) proliferate malignantly in bone marrow or lymph tissue and accumulate in peripheral blood, bone marrow, and body tissues. Its most common forms include acute lymphoblastic (lymphocytic) leukemia (ALL); acute myeloblastic (myelogenous) leukemia (AML); and acute monoblastic (monocytic) leukemia. Other variants include acute myelomonocytic leukemia and acute erythroleukemia.

Causes. The cause of acute leukemia is unknown. Risk factors are thought to include some combination of viruses, genetic and immunologic factors, and exposure to radiation and certain chemicals.

Assessment findings. Typical features include sudden onset of high fever, abnormal bleeding (for example, nosebleeds, gingival bleeding, purpura, ecchymoses, petechiae), easy bruising after minor trauma, recurrent infections, and prolonged menses. Nonspecific symptoms include low-grade fever, pallor, and weakness and lassitude that may persist for months before appearance of other symptoms.

Possible signs and symptoms of ALL, AML, and acute monoblastic leukemia include dyspnea, fatigue, malaise, tachycardia, palpitations, systolic ejection murmur, and abdominal or bone pain. Meningeal leukemia may be heralded by confusion, lethargy, and headache.

Diagnostic tests. Bone marrow aspiration typically shows a proliferation of immature WBCs and confirms the diagnosis. Bone marrow biopsy is performed in a patient with typical clinical findings but whose aspirate is dry or free from leukemic cells. Chromosomal analysis confirms the diagnosis and helps to classify the leukemia.

CBC shows thrombocytopenia and neutropenia. Differential leukocyte count determines cell type. Lumbar puncture detects meningeal involvement.

Treatment. Systemic chemotherapy aims to eradicate leukemic cells and induce remission, restoring bone marrow function. Chemotherapy varies with the specific disorder:

• meningeal leukemia—intrathecal instillation of methotrexate or cytarabine with cranial radiation
• vincristine and/or prednisone with intrathecal methotrexate or cytarabine; I.V. asparaginase, daunorubicin, and doxorubicin; maintenance with mercaptopurine and methotrexate. Bone marrow transplant is used in younger patients with an HLA-matched donor in the first relapse.
• AML—a combination of I.V. daunorubicin or doxorubicin, cytarabine, and oral thioguanine; or, if these fail to induce remission, a combination of cyclophosphamide, vincristine, prednisone, or methotrexate; high-dose cytarabine alone or with other drugs; amsacrine; azacitidine and mitoxantrone (both investigational); maintenance with additional chemotherapy
• acute monoblastic leukemia—cytarabine and thioguanine with daunorubicin or doxorubicin.

Nursing interventions. Control infection by placing the patient in a private room and imposing reverse isolation, if necessary. Watch for and report any signs of infection. Monitor temperature every 4 hours; patients with a temperature over 101° F (38° C) and decreased WBC counts should receive prompt antibiotic therapy.

Watch for bleeding; if it occurs, apply ice compresses and pressure, and elevate the extremity. Avoid giving aspirin and aspirin-containing drugs. Don't take rectal temperatures, give rectal suppositories, or do digital examinations.

Watch for signs of meningeal leukemia. If these occur, provide care after intrathecal chemotherapy. If the patient receives cranial radiation, teach him about potential adverse effects, and do what you can to minimize them.

Prevent hyperuricemia. Force fluids to about 2 qt (2 L) daily, and give acetazolamide, sodium bicarbonate tablets, and allopurinol. Check urine pH often—it should be above 7.5. Watch for rash or other hypersensitivity reaction to allopurinol.

Patient education. Teach the patient and his family how to recognize and avoid infection (fever, chills, cough, sore throat) and abnormal bleeding (bruising, petechiae) and how to stop bleeding (pressure, application of ice).

Evaluation. The patient should understand chemotherapy and its potential complications. He should also recognize signs of infection and notify the doctor if these occur. He should discuss treatment options and concerns about prognosis.

Chronic myelogenous leukemia

Also known as chronic granulocytic leukemia, chronic myelogenous (or myelocytic) leukemia (CML) produces abnormal overgrowth of granulocyte precursors in bone marrow, peripheral blood, and body tissues.

CML progresses in three distinct phases: the insidious chronic phase, with anemia and bleeding abnormalities; an accelerated phase; and, eventually, the acute phase (blastic crisis), in which myeloblasts, the most primitive granulocyte precursors, proliferate rapidly.

Causes. Almost 90% of patients with CML have the Philadelphia (Ph[1]) chromosome. Radiation and carcinogenic chemicals may induce this chromosome abnormality. Myeloproliferative diseases also seem to increase the incidence of CML, and some doctors suspect that an unidentified virus causes this disease.

Assessment findings. Typically, CML induces the following effects: anemia (fatigue, weakness, decreased exercise tolerance, pallor, dyspnea, tachycardia, and headache), thrombocytopenia (resulting in bleeding and clotting disorders), and splenomegaly, with abdominal discomfort and pain.

Other signs and symptoms include sternal and rib tenderness; low-grade fever; weight loss; anorexia; pain associated with renal calculi or gouty arthritis; occasionally, prolonged infection and ankle edema; and, rarely, priapism and symptoms of vascular insufficiency.

Diagnostic tests. Chromosomal analysis of peripheral blood or bone marrow showing the Ph[1] chromosome and low leukocyte alkaline phosphatase levels confirm CML in patients with typical clinical changes.

WBC abnormalities include leukocytosis (leukocytes more than 50,000/mm³, ranging as high as 250,000/mm³), occasional leukopenia (leukocytes less than 5,000/mm³), neutropenia (neutrophils less than 1,500/mm³) despite a high leukocyte count, and increased circulating myeloblasts.

Hemoglobin is commonly below 20 g. Hematocrit is low (less than 30%). Thrombocytopenia is common (less than 50,000/mm³), but platelet levels may be normal or elevated. Serum uric acid may be more than 8 mg. Bone marrow aspirate or biopsy shows hypercellular bone marrow infiltration by increased numbers of myeloid elements. In the acute phase, myeloblasts predominate.

Treatment. CML can only be cured with the complete ablation of the leukemic cells and the Ph¹ chromosome. This is accomplished with high-dose chemotherapy followed by allogenic (matched donor) bone marrow transplant. Chemotherapy usually includes busulfan and, occasionally, melphalan, other nitrogen mustards, thioguanine, and hydroxyurea.

During the acute phase, treatment is the same as for AML and emphasizes supportive measures and chemotherapy with doxorubicin or daunorubicin, thioguanine, cyclophosphamide, vincristine, methotrexate, cytarabine, or daunorubicin with prednisone. CML is rapidly fatal after onset of the acute phase.

Nursing interventions. Throughout the chronic phase of CML, follow these guidelines when the patient is hospitalized.

If the patient has persistent anemia, plan your care to help avoid exhaustion. Schedule lab tests and physical care to allow frequent rest periods, and help the patient ambulate, if necessary. Regularly check his skin and mucous membranes for pallor, petechiae, and bruising.

To reduce the abdominal discomfort of splenomegaly, provide small, frequent meals. Give a stool softener or laxative, as needed. Maintain adequate fluid intake, and ask the dietitian to provide a high-bulk diet. Stress the need for coughing and deep-breathing exercises.

Patient education. To minimize bleeding, suggest a soft-bristle toothbrush, an electric razor, and other safety precautions. Because many patients with CML receive outpatient chemotherapy throughout the chronic phase, sound patient education is essential.

Evaluation. The patient should understand the treatment and potential complications. He should also know the signs of infection and when to call the doctor. Fatigue, bleeding, fever, and weight loss should be under control.

Multiple myeloma

In multiple myeloma, malignant plasma cells infiltrate bone to produce osteolytic lesions throughout the skeleton; in late stages, it infiltrates the internal organs. Prognosis is usually poor because the diagnosis typically follows widespread skeletal destruction.

Cause. The cause of multiple myeloma is unknown.

Assessment findings. Constant severe back pain that increases with exercise is the earliest symptom. Other signs and symptoms include achiness, joint swelling and tenderness, fever, and malaise; slight evidence of peripheral neuropathy such as paresthesias; and pathologic fractures. In advanced disease, anemia, weight loss, thoracic deformities, and loss of height are evident.

Diagnostic tests. CBC shows moderate or severe anemia. The WBC differential may show 40% to 50% lymphocytes but seldom more than 3% plasma cells. Rouleaux formation seen on differential smear results from ESR elevation. This is often the first clue to the disease.

Urine studies may show Bence Jones protein and hypercalciuria. Absence of Bence Jones protein doesn't rule out multiple myeloma; however, its presence almost invariably confirms the disease.

Bone marrow aspiration detects myelomatous cells (abnormal number of immature plasma cells).

Serum electrophoresis shows an elevated globulin spike that is electrophoretically and immunologically abnormal.

X-rays during early stages may show only diffuse osteoporosis. Eventually, they show characteristic multiple, sharply circumscribed osteolytic (punched out) lesions, particularly on the skull, pelvis, and spine. IVP can assess renal involvement.

Treatment. Long-term treatment for multiple myeloma consists mainly of chemotherapy to suppress plasma cell growth and control pain. The therapy uses combinations of melphalan and prednisone or of cyclophosphamide and prednisone. Adjuvant local radiation reduces acute lesions such as collapsed vertebrae and relieves localized pain. Other treatment usually includes a melphalan-prednisone combination in high intermittent doses or low continuous daily doses or a combination of vincristine, doxorubicin, and decadron as well as analgesics for pain. If the patient develops spinal cord compression, he may require a laminectomy; if he has renal complications, he may need dialysis.

Because the patient may have bone demineralization and may lose large amounts of calcium into blood and urine, he becomes a prime candidate for kidney stones, nephrocalcinosis and, eventually, renal failure from hypercalcemia.

Nursing interventions. Prevent complications by watching for fever or malaise, which may signal the onset of infection, and for signs of other problems, such as severe anemia and fractures.

If needed, refer the family to an appropriate community resource such as a local chapter of the

Leukemia Society of America for additional support.

Patient education. Encourage the patient to drink 3 to 4 qt (3 to 4 L) of fluids daily, particularly before IVP. Monitor fluid intake and output (daily output should not be less than 1,500 ml).

Encourage the patient to walk.

Evaluation. The patient should have no pathologic fractures. He should understand the importance of maintaining hydration, nutrition, and activity. He should express his feelings about his condition and its prognosis to staff, friends, or family.

TREATMENTS

Immunologic and hematologic treatments include drug therapy, transfusion, bone marrow transplantation, and surgery.

Drug therapy

For some disorders such as asthma, drugs are the primary treatment. For other immune disorders, drugs are prescribed to treat associated symptoms. Cancer drug therapy includes cytotoxic drugs.

Hematologic drugs include hematinics, which help arrest anemia; anticoagulants and heparin antagonists, which impede clotting; hemostatics, which arrest blood flow or reduce capillary bleeding; blood derivatives, which replace blood loss; thrombolytic enzymes, which treat thrombotic disorders; and vitamins, which correct deficiencies of vitamins (such as vitamin B_{12}).

Transfusion

Transfusion procedures allow administration of a wide range of blood products such as RBCs, which can revive oxygen-starved tissues; leukocytes, which can combat infections beyond the reach of antibiotics; and clotting factors, plasma, and platelets, which can help patients with hemophilia live virtually normal lives.

Factor replacement

I.V. infusion of deficient clotting elements is a major part of treatment for coagulation disorders. Factor replacement typically corrects clotting factor deficiencies, thereby stopping or preventing hemorrhage.

The blood products used depend on the specific disorder being treated. *Fresh frozen plasma* (FFP), for instance, helps treat clotting disorders whose causes aren't known, clotting factor deficiencies resulting from hepatic disease or blood dilution, consumed clotting factors secondary to DIC, and deficiencies of clotting factors for which no specific replacement product exists.

Cryoprecipitate, which forms when FFP thaws slowly, helps treat von Willebrand's disease, fibrinogen deficiencies, and factor XIII deficiencies. In addition, it's used for hemophilia patients who are young or whose disease is mild.

AHF concentrate is the long-term treatment of choice for hemophilia A because the amount of factor VIII that it contains is less variable than with cryoprecipitate. It's given I.V. whenever the hemophilia patient has sustained an injury.

Prothrombin complex, which contains factors II, VII, IX, and X, can be given to treat hemophilia B, severe liver disease, and acquired deficiencies of the factors it contains.

Patient preparation. Explain the procedure to the patient, then assemble the equipment: a standard blood administration set for administering FFP or prothrombin complex, a component syringe or drip set for giving cryoprecipitate, a plastic syringe for I.V. injection of factor VIII, or a plastic syringe and infusion set for I.V. infusion.

Then obtain the plasma fraction from the blood bank or pharmacy. Check the expiration date and carefully inspect the plasma fraction for cloudiness and turbidity. If you'll be transfusing FFP, do so within 4 hours because it has no preservatives.

Take the patient's vital signs. If an I.V. line isn't in place, perform a venipuncture and infuse normal saline solution at a keep-vein-open rate.

Monitoring and aftercare. During and after administration of clotting factors, watch for signs of anaphylaxis, other allergic reactions, and fluid overload. Also monitor the patient for bleeding, increased pain or swelling at the transfusion site, and fever. Closely monitor partial thromboplastin time. Alert the doctor if adverse reactions occur or if you suspect bleeding.

Patient education. Increasingly, the patient or his family can administer factor replacement therapy at home. In fact, children as young as age 9 can do it. If ordered, demonstrate correct venipuncture and infusion techniques to the family or patient. Tell them to keep the factor replacement and infusion equipment at hand and to begin treatment immediately if the patient experiences a bleeding episode.

The patient and his family should watch for signs of anaphylaxis, allergic reactions, and fluid overload. Instruct them to call the doctor immediately if such reactions occur. Also tell them to watch for signs of hepatitis, which may appear 3 weeks to 6 months after treatment with blood components.

Bone marrow transplantation

Bone marrow transplantation refers to the collection of marrow cells from either the patient or another donor and the subsequent administration of these cells to the patient. The treatment of choice for aplastic anemia and SCID, it's also used to treat leukemia patients who are at high risk for relapse or who have undergone high-dose chemotherapy and total body radiation therapy. Bone marrow transplantation is used as a treatment for other hematologic disorders and for oncologic disorders, such as multiple myeloma and some solid tumors.

The three types of bone marrow transplants are autologous, syngeneic, and allogeneic. In an *autolo-*

gous transplant, marrow tissue is harvested from the patient before treatment or while he's in remission and is frozen for later use. A *syngeneic* transplant refers to the transplantation of marrow between identical twins. An *allogeneic* transplant, the most common type, uses bone marrow tissue from a histocompatible individual, usually a sibling.

Bone marrow harvesting is performed in the operating room. In contrast, bone marrow administration is done at bedside using a peripheral I.V. line or a central venous catheter. The bone marrow stem cells eventually enter the marrow spaces, where they begin forming new cells. This may take as long as 10 to 23 days.

Patient preparation. Inform the patient that his WBC count will be depleted, putting him at high risk for infection. He will be placed in reverse isolation and contact with his family will be limited for several weeks after the procedure.

Before the procedure, make sure that diphenhydramine and epinephrine are on hand to manage transfusion reactions. Start an I.V. line for hydration and record vital signs. Obtain an administration set (without a filter, which can trap marrow cells) and, if ordered, insert a central venous catheter for infusion of the bone marrow.

Monitoring and aftercare. Once the transfusion has begun, take the patient's vital signs at least every 15 minutes for an hour, every 30 minutes for the next 2 hours, and then every hour for another 4 hours. This will help you to promptly recognize such reactions as fever, dyspnea, and hypotension. Treat other reactions symptomatically. Monitor closely for signs of infection.

Patient education. Tell the patient to protect himself from infection—especially if he has chronic GVH disease. Warn him that he may remain vulnerable to infection for up to a year after the transplant.

Surgery

Surgical removal of the spleen is sometimes used to treat various immunologic and hematologic disorders.

Splenectomy

The spleen may be removed to reduce the rate of RBC and platelet destruction, to remove a ruptured spleen, or to stage Hodgkin's disease. It's also done as an emergency procedure after traumatic splenic rupture. Splenectomy is the treatment of choice for such diseases as hereditary spherocytosis and chronic ITP when patients fail to respond to steroids or danazol.

Patient preparation. Explain to the patient that splenectomy involves removal of the spleen under general anesthesia. Inform him that he'll be able to lead a normal life without it, but will be more prone to infection.

Obtain the results of blood studies, including coagulation tests and CBC, and report them to the doctor. If ordered, transfuse blood to correct anemia or hemorrhagic loss.

Similarly, give vitamin K to correct clotting factor deficiencies.

Take the patient's vital signs and perform a baseline respiratory assessment. Note signs and symptoms of respiratory infection, such as fever, chills, crackles, rhonchi, and a cough. Notify the doctor if you suspect respiratory infection; he may delay surgery. Teach coughing and deep-breathing techniques.

Monitoring and aftercare. During the early postoperative period, watch carefully, especially if the patient has a bleeding disorder, for bleeding from the wound or drain and for signs of internal bleeding, such as hematuria or hematochezia.

Leukocytosis and thrombocytosis occur after splenectomy and may persist for years. Because thrombocytosis may predispose the patient to thromboembolism, help the patient exercise and walk as soon as possible after surgery. Encourage him to perform coughing and deep-breathing exercises to reduce the risk of pulmonary complications.

Watch for signs of infection and monitor hematologic studies.

Patient education. Inform the patient that he's at an increased risk for infection and urge him to report any of its telltale signs. Teach him measures to help prevent infection.

REFERENCES AND READINGS

Clancy, J. *Basic Concepts in Immunology: A Student's Survival Guide.* New York: McGraw-Hill Book Co., 1996.

Nursing TimeSavers: Immune & Infectious Disorders. Springhouse, Pa.: Springhouse Corp., 1994.

Schiffman, F. *Hematologic Pathophysiology.* Philadelphia: Lippincott-Raven Pubs., 1997.

Sigal, R. *Immunology & Inflammation: Basic Mechanisms & Clinical Consequences.* New York: McGraw-Hill Book Co., 1994.

Tizard, I.R., *Immunology: An Introduction,* 3rd ed. Philadelphia: W.B. Saunders Co., 1992.

Workman, M.L., et al. *Nursing Care of the Immunocompromised Patient.* Philadelphia: W.B. Saunders Co., 1993.

12

REPRODUCTIVE
CARE

Because misinformation and cultural taboos surround the reproductive system, reproductive disorders present a formidable nursing challenge. Patients with such disorders as impotence, abnormal uterine bleeding, and infertility require sensitive counseling and straightforward teaching. You'll have to help many of the patients overcome feelings of vulnerability, guilt, and embarrassment.

ASSESSMENT

Assessing the reproductive system is an essential—but potentially uncomfortable—part of a health assessment. Performed with sensitivity and tact, your assessment may uncover important information and concerns that the patient was previously unwilling to share.

Physical examination

For the male patient, physical assessment involves inspecting and palpating the groin, penis, and scrotum. If the patient is over age 40 or has a high likelihood of having prostate problems, you will also palpate the prostate gland. For the female patient, assessment may involve only the external genitalia or a complete gynecologic examination.

Examining the male patient

Instruct the patient to urinate before the examination and to undress and don a gown.

Explain each step before performing it, and expose only the necessary areas.

Inspection. To begin physical assessment of the male reproductive system, inspect the patient's genitals and inguinal area. Don gloves before starting.

Penis. Evaluate the color and integrity of the penile skin. This should appear loose and wrinkled over the shaft, and taut and smooth over the glans penis. The skin should be pink to light brown in whites and light to dark brown in blacks, and free from scars, lesions, ulcers, or breaks of any kind.

Ask an uncircumcised patient to retract his prepuce to expose the glans penis. The urethral meatus, a slitlike opening, should be located at the tip of the glans. The urethral meatus should have no discharge.

Scrotum. Evaluate the amount, distribution, color, and texture of pubic hair. Inspect the scrotal skin for obvious lesions, ulcerations, induration, or reddened areas, and evaluate the scrotal sac for symmetry and size. It should be coarse and more deeply pigmented than the body skin. The left testis usually hangs slightly lower than the right.

Inguinal area. Check this area for obvious bulges—a sign of hernias. Then ask the patient to bear down as you inspect again. Also check for enlarged lymph nodes, a sign of infection.

Palpation. After inspection, palpate the penis and scrotum for structural abnormalities; then palpate the inguinal area for hernias.

Penis. To palpate this organ, gently grasp the shaft between the thumb and first two fingers and palpate along its entire length, noting any indurated, tender, or lumpy areas. The flaccid penis should feel soft and have no nodules.

Scrotum. Palpate the scrotum, also using the thumb and first two fingers. Begin by feeling the scrotal skin for nodules, lesions, or ulcers.

Next, palpate the scrotal sac. Normally, the right and left halves of the sac have identical contents and feel the same. Their surface should feel smooth and even in contour. Slight compression of the testes should elicit a dull, aching sensation that radiates to the patient's lower abdomen. This pressure-pain sensation should not occur when the other structures are compressed. No other pain or tenderness should be present.

The absence of a testis may result from temporary migration. This contraction is normal and may occur at any time during the assessment.

Palpate the epididymis on the posterolateral surface by grasping each testis between the thumb and forefinger and feeling from the epididymis to the spermatic cord or vas deferens up to the inguinal ring. The epididymis should feel like a ridge of tissue lying vertically on the testicular surface. The vas deferens should feel like a smooth cord and be freely movable. The arteries, veins, lymph vessels, and nerves may feel like indefinite threads.

Transilluminate any swellings, lumps, or nodular areas. If the swollen area contains serous fluid, it will glow orange-red; if it contains blood or tissue, it won't. Describe a lump or mass anywhere in the scrotal sac according to its placement, size, shape, consistency, tenderness, and response to transillumination.

Inguinal area. Palpate this area for hernias. (See *Palpating the inguinal area*, pages 648 and 649.)

Examining the female patient

You may either assist a doctor or nurse practitioner with a gynecologic assessment or perform the assessment yourself.

Preparing for the assessment. Before beginning the assessment, gather the necessary equipment and supplies.

If this is the patient's first gynecologic assessment, explain the procedure so she knows what to expect. Tell her to empty her bladder before the examination begins.

Positioning. The patient usually must assume the lithotomy position for the assessment. Her heels should be secure in the stirrups and her knees comfortably placed in the knee supports if they are used. Adjust the foot or knee supports so that the legs are comfortably separated and balanced.

The patient's buttocks must extend about 1/2" (1.3 cm) over the table end. The hips and knees will be flexed and the thighs abducted. She should place her feet (or knees) in the stirrups and inch down to the proper position. A pillow placed beneath her head may help her to relax the abdominal muscles. Raising the head of the examination table helps maintain eye contact and doesn't hinder the examination.

Beginning the assessment. Describe what she will feel. Show the patient how to relax by inhaling slowly and deeply through the nose, exhaling through the mouth, and concentrating on breathing regularly to relax the muscle. If the patient begins to tense up, remind her to breathe and relax. Assure the patient that the assessment takes little time and that she'll be told what to expect before each new step. (See *Avoiding embarrassment,* page 650.)

If the examiner is male, a female assistant should attend the examination for the patient's comfort and the examiner's legal protection.

Inspection. Sometimes only the patient's external genitalia need be inspected to determine the origin of sores or itching. Wash your hands, don gloves, then follow these steps.

Place the patient in a supine position with the pubic area uncovered, and begin the assessment by determining sexual maturity. Inspect pubic hair for amount and pattern. It's usually thick and appears on the mons pubis as well as the inner aspects of the upper thighs. Using a gloved index finger and thumb, gently spread the labia majora and look for the labia minora. The labia should be pink and moist with no lesions. Normal cervical discharge varies in color and consistency; it's clear and stretchy before ovulation, white and opaque after ovulation, and usually odorless and nonirritating to the mucosa. No other discharge should be present. Specimens of all discharges should be cultured or examined microscopically in the laboratory.

Gynecologic assessment. In some facilities, you may perform complete gynecologic assessments. As part of this assessment, obtain a Papanicolaou (Pap) smear after inspecting the cervix. (Obtain the smear before touching the cervix in any manner.) Also obtain other specimens if an abnormal cervical or vaginal discharge indicates infection.

Palpating the inguinal area

Palpate the inguinal area to assess for inguinal and femoral hernias.

Inguinal hernias

To palpate for an inguinal hernia, first place the index and middle finger of each hand over each external inguinal ring and ask the patient to bear down or cough to increase intra-abdominal pressure momentarily. Then, with the patient relaxed, proceed as follows: Gently insert the middle or index finger (if the patient is an adult) or the little finger (if the patient is a young child) into the scrotal sac and follow the spermatic cord upward to the external inguinal ring, to an opening just above and lateral to the pubic tubercle known as Hesselbach's triangle. Holding the finger at this spot, ask the patient to bear down or cough again. A hernia will feel like a mass or bulge.

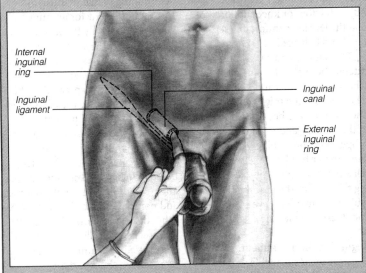

Internal inguinal ring

Inguinal ligament

Inguinal canal

External inguinal ring

DIAGNOSTIC TESTS

Diagnostic testing may help to assess reproductive organs and associated structures for abnormalities, detect cancers, or determine the cause of infertility or sexual dysfunction. Diagnostic procedures include tissue analyses, endoscopy, colposcopy, radiography, ultrasonography, and blood and urine tests. (See *Diagnostic tests for reproductive disorders*, pages 651 and 652.)

NURSING DIAGNOSES

When caring for patients with reproductive disorders, you'll find that several nursing diagnoses are commonly used. These diagnoses appear

Femoral hernias

To palpate for a femoral hernia, place your right hand on the patient's thigh with the index finger over the femoral artery. The femoral canal is then under the ring finger in an adult patient and between the index and ring finger in a child. A hernia here will feel like a soft bulge or mass.

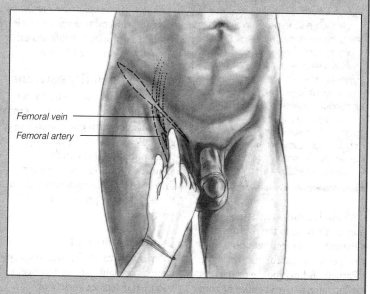

Femoral vein

Femoral artery

below, along with appropriate nursing interventions and rationales. (Rationales appear in italic type.)

Sexual dysfunction

Related to altered body structure or psychological stress, the diagnosis of sexual dysfunction can be applied to such conditions as endometriosis, pelvic inflammatory disease, arousal and orgasmic dysfunction, dyspareunia, vaginismus, impotence, or premature ejaculation.

Expected outcomes

• Patient acknowledges a problem in sexual dysfunction.
• Patient states reason for dysfunction.

• Patient identifies any stressors that may contribute to the dysfunction.
• Patient voices feelings about changes in sexual function.
• Patient and his spouse or partner explore alternative avenues of communication or sexual expression.
• Patient expresses understanding of limitations caused by illness or injury.

Nursing interventions and rationales

• Encourage the patient to ask about personal sexuality. *This permits the patient to ask pertinent questions.*
• Provide time for privacy. *This allows time for introspection.*
• Suggest that the patient discuss concerns with spouse or significant other. *This relieves stress and strengthens relationships.*
• Provide support for the patient's spouse or significant other. *Active listening communicates concern.*
• Educate the patient and spouse or significant other about limitations imposed by the patient's present physical condition. *This helps the patient avoid complications or injury.*
• Suggest referral to a sex counselor or other appropriate professional *to provide the patient with support.*

Altered sexuality patterns

Related to illness or medical treatment, altered sexuality patterns may be associated with genitourinary or gynecologic disorders; sexually transmitted diseases, such as acquired immunodeficiency syndrome (AIDS), herpes, gonorrhea, and syphilis; or pregnancy and postpartum.

Expected outcomes

• Patient expresses feelings associated with sexuality and self-concept.
• Patient discusses variety of options involved in maintaining intimacy throughout their life.
• Patient expresses an understanding of normal physiologic changes that occur with aging.
• Patient expresses understanding of options available to relieve discomfort associated with menopause or hysterectomy.

Nursing interventions and rationales

• Allow a specific amount of uninterrupted time to talk with the patient. *This reassures the patient*

Diagnostic tests for reproductive disorders

Tests	Purpose	Nursing considerations
Pap test	Early detection of cervical cancer	• Explain the procedure and that the best time is a week before or after menses. • Instruct patient not to douche or insert vaginal medications for 72 hours before the test. • Just before the test, have patient empty her bladder. • Have patient disrobe from waist down and drape herself. • Ask her to lie on examining table with feet in stirrups. • After obtaining specimen, preserve the slides immediately. • Upon completion of the exam, assist patient to an upright position and instruct her to dress.
Semen analysis	Evaluates male fertility	• Inform the patient that the most desirable specimen requires masturbation, ideally in a doctor's office or laboratory. • If the patient prefers to collect the specimen at home, emphasize the importance of delivering it to the laboratory within 3 hours after collection. • Warn him not to expose the specimen to temperature extremes or direct sunlight.
Colposcopy	Evaluates abnormal cytologic specimens and to examine cervix and vagina	• Explain the procedure. • Instruct the patient to refrain from using vaginal creams or gels beforehand. • Advise her that a biopsy may be performed and that it may cause cramping and pain for a short time and minimal bleeding. • After biopsy, instruct her to abstain from intercourse until healing of biopsy site. • Instruct her to call the doctor if she begins to bleed more heavily than during a period, or has discharge, pain, or fever.

(continued)

Diagnostic tests for reproductive disorders *(continued)*

Tests	Purpose	Nursing considerations
Laparoscopy	Helps detect endometriosis and ectopic pregnancy, evaluate pelvic masses, and identify cause of pelvic pain	• Explain the 15- to 30-minute procedure and check for allergies. • Instruct the patient to fast for at least 8 hours before the test. • Assure her that she'll receive a local or general anesthetic. • Warn her that she may experience pain at the puncture site and in the shoulder. • During the procedure, check for proper drainage of the catheter and monitor vital signs and observe for allergic reactions. • After recovery, have her ambulate as ordered. • Instruct her to restrict activity for 2 to 7 days, as ordered. • Reassure her that some abdominal and shoulder pain is normal and should disappear within 24 to 36 hours. Provide analgesia as ordered.
Hysterosalpingography	Helps to confirm tubal abnormalities, uterine abnormalities, and presence of fistulas or peritubal adhesions	• Explain the procedure. • Advise the patient that she may experience moderate cramping, but she may receive a sedative. • Assure her that cramps and a vagal reaction are transient. • Monitor the patient for an allergic reaction to the contrast medium.
Pelvic ultrasonography	Evaluates symptoms that suggest pelvic disease, confirms a tentative diagnosis, and determines fetal viability	• Explain the procedure. • Instruct the patient to drink liquids and not to void before the test as it requires a full bladder. • Allow the patient to empty her bladder immediately after the test.
Prostate-specific antigen	Helps confirm prostate cancer along with a digital rectal exam	• Explain the procedure. • After the test, observe the venipunctive site for bleeding.

that sexuality issues are acceptable for discussion.

• Provide a nonthreatening, non-judgmental atmosphere *to encourage the patient to express feelings about perceived changes in sexual identity and behaviors.*

• Provide the patient and spouse with information about the illness and its treatment. Clarify any misconceptions they may have. *This helps avoid misunderstandings.*

• Provide time for privacy. *This gives the patient control over time spent interacting with others.*

• Encourage social interaction and communication between the patient and spouse or significant other. *This strengthens relationships.*

• Offer referral to counselors or support persons, such as a mental health professional, sex counselor, or illness-related support groups (such as "I Can Cope," Reach for Recovery, and the Ostomy Association) *to provide the patient with additional resources.*

Self-esteem disturbance

Related to feelings of shame or guilt, self-esteem disturbance may occur with sexually transmitted diseases, congenital anomalies, infertility, menopause, sexual dysfunction, and other reproductive disorders.

Expected outcomes

• Patient discusses accomplishments and meaningful events in his life.
• Patient discusses chronic illness and its impact on lifestyle.
• Patient states that he feels more independent.

Nursing interventions and rationales

• Allow a specific amount of uninterrupted, non-care-related time to engage the patient in conversation. *This helps the patient to open up.*

• Assess the patient's mental status through interview and observation at least once daily. *This helps reveal abnormal feelings and behaviors.*

• Involve the patient in the decision-making process *to reduce feelings of dependence on others.*

• Encourage social interaction between the patient and others *to help restore self-confidence.*

• Refer the patient to a mental health professional if indicated. *Consultation can enhance patient care.*

Social isolation

Related to altered state of wellness, social isolation may be associated with sexually transmitted diseases, such as AIDS and genital herpes, which make patients liable to social isolation.

Expected outcomes

• Patient expresses desire to increase social activity.
• Patient shows understanding of the disorder and other circumstances that may limit social activity.
• Patient interacts with members of the health team.
• Patient and members of the health care team explore ways to increase social activity.
• Patient contacts appropriate resources for developing social relationships.

• Patient notes an improvement in social relationships.

Nursing interventions and rationales

• Assign a primary nurse to this patient if possible. *Primary nursing provides consistency and decreases the potential for fragmented care.*
• Provide honest and immediate feedback about the patient's behavior *to modify, verify, or correct his perceptions.*
• Involve the patient and family or significant other in setting goals and planning care. *This decreases feelings of helplessness and isolation.*
• Depending on the patient's physical condition, encourage him to perform self-care activities *to foster independent action.*
• Spend at least 15 minutes each shift with the patient. Sit with the patient and listen. *Active listening reduces stress.*
• Arrange with the patient for specific periods of planned diversionary activity. *Diversionary activities decrease self-absorption.*
• Allow ample private time for the patient to spend with family or friends. *This demonstrates respect for the patient and for his relationships.*
• Provide referral to an appropriate social agency *to ensure a comprehensive approach to the patient's care.*

DISORDERS

This section discusses common female and male reproductive disorders, including sexually transmitted diseases. For each disorder, you'll find information on causes, assessment findings, diagnostic tests, treatments, nursing interventions, patient education, and evaluation criteria.

Female reproductive disorders

This section covers common gynecologic disorders, including premenstrual syndrome (PMS), ovarian cysts, endometriosis, uterine leiomyomas, breast cancer, cervical cancer, endometrial cancer, ovarian cancer, female infertility, and pelvic inflammatory disease.

Premenstrual syndrome

Effects of PMS range from minimal discomfort to severe, disruptive behavioral and somatic changes. Symptoms appear 7 to 14 days before menses and usually subside with its onset. Incidence seems to rise with age and parity.

Causes. Although its direct cause is unknown, PMS may result from a progesterone deficiency in the secretory phase of the menstrual cycle or from an increased estrogen-progesterone ratio. (See *Understanding the menstrual cycle.*) Other hypotheses include fluid imbalance, vitamin deficiencies, altered responses to prostaglandins, and alterations in glucose metabolism.

Assessment findings. Behavioral changes in PMS include mild to severe personality changes, nervousness, hostility, irritability, agitation, sleep disturbances, fatigue, lethargy, and depression.

Understanding the menstrual cycle

The menstrual cycle is divided into three distinct phases.

• During the menstrual phase, which starts on the first day of menstruation, the top layer of the endometrium breaks down and flows out of the body. This flow, the menses, consists of blood, mucus, and unneeded tissue.
• During the proliferation phase, the endometrium begins to thicken, and the level of estrogen in the blood rises.
• During the secretory (luteal) phase, the endometrium continues to thicken to nourish an embryo should fertilization occur. Without fertilization, the top layer of the endometrium breaks down, and the menstrual phase of the cycle begins again.

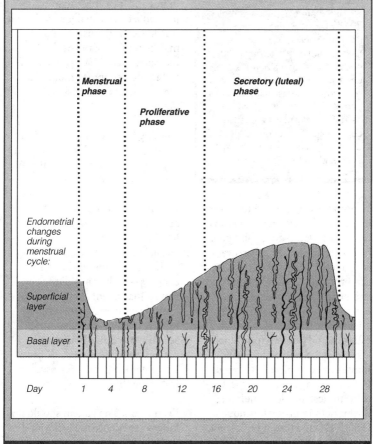

ALTERNATIVE THERAPY

Chinese herbal therapy

For centuries Chinese herbal therapy has been used to treat dysmenorrhea. Herbal therapy is an important part of traditional Chinese medicine, which is based on a philosophy that strives for balance and harmony between ying and yang.

Herbs are classified according to their taste, which signifies their medicinal action and commonly their natural affinity to particular body organs. Some herbs are used to treat common menstrual problems, such as water retention and uterine cramping. Chinese herbal therapy may be used in combination with acupuncture, depending on the patient's symptoms and preferences.

Somatic changes include breast tenderness or swelling, abdominal tenderness or bloating, joint pain, headache, edema, and diarrhea or constipation. The patient may have exacerbations of skin, respiratory, and neurologic problems.

Diagnostic tests. Evaluation of estrogen and progesterone blood levels may help rule out hormonal imbalance; complete blood count (CBC), fasting blood glucose, thyroid studies, follicle-stimulating hormone/luteinizing hormone (FSH/LH), and serum prolactin levels may help to rule out underlying disorders. Psychological evaluation may rule out or detect an underlying psychiatric disorder.

Treatment. Primarily symptomatic, treatment may include tranquilizers, sedatives, antidepressants, nonsteroidal anti-inflammatory drugs (NSAIDs), vitamins, and progestins. It may also require a diet that is low in simple sugars, caffeine, and salt, with adequate amounts of protein, high amounts of complex carbohydrates and, possibly, vitamin supplements formulated for PMS. (Salt restriction or the use of diuretics may be unnecessary.) Self-help measures include stress reduction techniques, support groups, and exercise. (See *Chinese herbal therapy.*)

Nursing interventions. Obtain a complete patient history to identify any emotional problems that may contribute to PMS.

Patient education. Inform the patient that self-help groups exist for women with PMS. If appropriate, help her contact such a group.

If possible, discuss lifestyle changes—such as avoiding stimulants—that might alleviate symptoms by reducing anxiety. Advise further medical consultation if severe symptoms disrupt the patient's normal lifestyle. If necessary, refer the patient for psychological counseling.

Evaluation. The patient should no longer experience the behavioral and somatic signs and symptoms of PMS.

Ovarian cysts

Usually, ovarian cysts are nonneoplastic sacs that contain fluid or semisolid material. They should be thoroughly investigated as possible sites of malignant change. Common types include follicular cysts, which are usually small, semitransparent, and fluid-filled; and lutein cysts, including corpus luteum cysts, which are functional, nonneoplastic enlargements of the ovaries; and theca-lutein cysts, which are commonly bilateral and filled with clear, straw-colored fluid. Polycystic (or sclerocystic) ovary disease is part of the Stein-Leventhal syndrome.

Ovarian cysts can develop any time between puberty and menopause. Corpus luteum cysts occur infrequently, usually during early pregnancy.

Causes. Follicular cysts arise from follicles that overdistend instead of going through the atretic stage of the menstrual cycle. Corpus luteum cysts are caused by excessive accumulation of blood during the hemorrhagic phase of the menstrual cycle. Theca-lutein cysts are commonly associated with hydatidiform mole, choriocarcinoma, or hormone therapy (with human chorionic gonadotropin [HCG] or clomiphene). Polycystic ovary disease results from endocrine abnormalities.

Assessment findings. Small cysts usually produce no symptoms, unless torsion or rupture causes acute pain. General signs and symptoms include mild pelvic discomfort, low back pain, dyspareunia, abnormal uterine bleeding, and acute abdominal pain similar to that of appendicitis (in ovarian cysts with torsion).

In corpus luteum cysts appearing early in pregnancy, the patient may develop unilateral pelvic discomfort and (with rupture) massive intraperitoneal hemorrhage.

In polycystic ovary disease, the patient may develop amenorrhea, oligomenorrhea, or infertility secondary to the disorder as well as bilaterally enlarged ovaries.

Diagnostic tests. Visualization of the ovary through ultrasonography, laparoscopy, or surgery (commonly for another condition) confirms ovarian cysts.

Laboratory tests may show slightly elevated urine 17-ketosteroid concentrations. Extremely elevated HCG titers strongly suggest theca-lutein cysts. Basal body temperature graphs and endometrial biopsy results may show anovulation.

Treatment. Follicular cysts usually don't require treatment because they tend to disappear spontaneously within 60 days. However, if they interfere with daily activities, clomiphene by mouth for 5 days or progesterone I.M. (also for 5 days) reestablishes the ovarian hormonal cycle and induces ovulation. Oral contraceptives may also accelerate involution of functional cysts.

Treatment for corpus luteum cysts that occur during pregnancy is symptomatic because these cysts diminish during the third trimester and rarely require surgery. Theca-lutein cysts disappear spontaneously after elimination of hydatidiform mole or choriocarcinoma or discontinuation of HCG or clomiphene therapy.

Treatment for polycystic ovary disease may include drugs, such as clomiphene to induce ovulation or, if drug therapy fails to induce ovulation, surgical wedge resection of one-half to one-third of the ovary.

Surgery may become necessary for both diagnosis and treatment. Pathologic studies confirm the diagnosis.

Nursing interventions. Preoperatively, watch for signs and symptoms of cyst rupture—which occurs suddenly and can be life-threatening—such as increasing abdominal pain, distention, and rigidity. Monitor vital signs for fever, shock, tachypnea, or hypotension, a sign of possible peritonitis or intraperitoneal hemorrhage.

Postoperatively, encourage frequent movement in bed and early ambulation, as ordered, to prevent pulmonary embolism. Offer appropriate reassurance if the patient fears cancer or infertility.

Patient education. Explain the nature of the particular cyst and, if appropriate, the type of discomfort the patient will probably experience. Also discuss how long the condition is expected to last. Assure her that recurrence is unlikely.

Before discharge, advise the patient to increase her activity gradually—over 4 to 6 weeks. Urge her to abstain from having intercourse, using tampons, and douching during this time.

Evaluation. The patient should be asymptomatic and experience no postoperative complications.

Endometriosis

In endometriosis, endometrial tissue appears outside the lining of the uterine cavity. This ectopic tissue usually remains in the pelvic area, most commonly around the ovaries, uterovesical peritoneum, uterosacral ligaments, and the cul-de-sac, but it can appear anywhere in the body. Severe symptoms of endometriosis may occur abruptly or develop slowly over many years. Infertility is the primary complication. Spontaneous abortion may also occur.

Causes. The direct cause is unknown, but familial susceptibility or recent surgery that required opening the uterus (such as a cesarean section) may predispose a woman to endometriosis.

Assessment findings. The classic symptom of this disorder, acquired dysmenorrhea may produce constant pain in the lower abdomen and in the vagina, posterior pelvis, and back. Pain usually begins 5 to 7 days before menses reaches its peak and lasts for 2 to 3 days. It's less cramping and less concentrated in the abdominal midline than primary dysmenorrheal pain. The severity of pain doesn't necessarily indicate the extent of the disease.

Multiple tender nodules occur on uterosacral ligaments or in the rectovaginal system. They enlarge and become more tender during menses. Ovarian enlargement may also be evident.

Diagnostic tests. Laparoscopy may confirm the diagnosis and determine the stage of the disease. Barium enema rules out malignant or inflammatory bowel disease.

Treatment. Conservative therapy for young women who want to have children includes androgens such as danazol, which produce a temporary remission in stages I and II. Progestins and oral contraceptives also relieve symptoms.

When ovarian masses are present (stages III and IV), they should be removed to rule out cancer. The treatment of choice for women who don't want to bear children or who have extensive disease (stages III and IV) is a total abdominal hysterectomy performed with bilateral salpingo-oophorectomy.

Nursing interventions. Minor gynecologic procedures are contraindicated immediately before and during menstruation.

Patient education. Explain laparoscopy or other scheduled procedures or surgeries to the patient, including their impact on childbearing. Advise adolescents to use sanitary napkins instead of tampons.

Because infertility is a possible complication, advise the patient who wants children not to postpone childbearing. Also stress the importance of treatment to prevent or postpone complications.

Teach the patient how to recognize endometrioma rupture and what to do if it occurs. Also teach her how to relieve dyspareunia and how to recognize and prevent symptoms of anemia.

Encourage the patient to contact the Endometriosis Association for further information and counseling. Remind her to have an annual pelvic examination and Pap smear.

Evaluation. The patient should be free from pain (or at least able to manage symptoms) and have no postoperative complications. She should understand the importance of frequent gynecologic examinations and the possible consequences of delaying surgery, if applicable.

Uterine leiomyomas

Also known as myomas, fibromyomas, and fibroids, uterine leiomyomas are the most common benign tumors in women. They usually occur in the uterine corpus, although they may appear on the cervix or on the round or broad ligament.

Cause. The cause of uterine leiomyomas is unknown, but excessive levels of estrogen and human growth hormone (HGH) probably influence tumor formation by stimulating susceptible fibromuscular elements. Large doses of estrogen and the later stages of pregnancy increase both tumor size and HGH levels. Conversely, uterine leiomyomas usually shrink or disappear after menopause.

Assessment findings. Clinical signs and symptoms include submucosal hypermenorrhea (the cardinal sign) and possibly other forms of abnormal endometrial bleeding, dysmenorrhea, and pain.

If the tumor is large, the patient may develop a feeling of heaviness in the abdomen, pain, intestinal obstruction, constipation, urinary frequency or urgency, and irregular uterine enlargement.

Diagnostic tests. Blood studies showing anemia support the diagnosis. Dilatation and curettage (D&C) or submucosal hysterosalpingography detects submucosal leiomyomas, and laparoscopy visualizes subserous leiomyomas on the uterine surface.

Treatment. Appropriate intervention depends on the severity of symptoms, the size and location of the tumors, and the patient's age, parity, pregnancy status, desire to have children, and general health.

A surgeon may remove small leiomyomas that have caused problems in the past or that may threaten a future pregnancy. This is the treatment of choice for a young woman who wants to have children.

Tumors that twist or cause intestinal obstruction require a hysterectomy, with preservation of the ovaries if possible.

If a pregnant woman has a leiomyomatous uterus the size of a 5- to 6-month normal uterus by the 9th week of pregnancy, spontaneous abortion will probably occur, especially with a cervical leiomyoma. If surgery is necessary, a hysterectomy is usually performed 5 to 6 months after delivery (when involution is complete), with preservation of the ovaries if possible.

Nursing interventions. In a patient with severe anemia due to excessive bleeding, administer iron and blood transfusions, as ordered.

Patient education. Tell the patient to report any abnormal bleeding or pelvic pain immediately.

If a hysterectomy or an oophorectomy is indicated, explain the effects of the operation on menstruation, menopause, and sexual activity. Reassure the patient that she won't experience premature menopause if her ovaries are left intact. If she must undergo a multiple myomectomy, make sure she understands that pregnancy is still possible. However, if the surgeon must enter the uterine cavity, explain that a cesarean delivery may be necessary.

Evaluation. The patient should experience no bleeding, pain, or postoperative complications.

Female infertility

Approximately 10% to 15% of all couples in the United States can't conceive after regular intercourse for at least 1 year without contraception. About 40% to 50% of all infertility is attributed to the female.

After extensive investigation and treatment, approximately 50% of infertile couples achieve pregnancy.

Causes. Infertility may be caused by any defect or malfunction of the hypothalamic-pituitary-ovarian axis such as certain neurologic diseases. Other causes include the destruction of sperm by female antibodies; anovulation or oligo-ovulation; uterine abnormalities, leiomyomas, or Asherman's syndrome; tubal loss, impairment, or occlusion; cervical factors such as infection; and psychological problems.

Assessment findings. Diagnosis requires a complete physical examination and health history, including the patient's reproductive and sexual function, past diseases, mental state, previous surgery, types of contraception used in the past, and family history.

Diagnostic tests. The doctor may order tests to assess ovulation and the structural integrity of the fallopian tubes, the ovaries, and the uterus as well as male-female interaction studies.

Assessing ovulation. Basal body temperature graph shows a sustained elevation in body temperature after ovulation indicating the approximate time of ovulation. *Endometrial biopsy* provides histologic evidence that ovulation has occurred. *Progesterone blood levels* can show a luteal phase deficiency.

Assessing structural integrity. Hysterosalpingography provides radiologic evidence of tubal obstruction and abnormalities of the uterine cavity after injection of a radiopaque contrast medium through the cervix. *Endoscopy* confirms the results of hysterosalpingography and permits visualization of the endometrial cavity by hysteroscopy or explores the posterior surface of the uterus, fallopian tubes, and ovaries by culdoscopy. *Laparoscopy* allows visualization of the abdominal and pelvic areas.

Assessing male-female interaction. The *postcoital test* (Sims' test) examines the cervical mucus for motile sperm cells after midcycle intercourse (as close to ovulation as possible). *Immunologic* or *antibody testing* detects spermicidal antibodies in the female's sera.

Treatment. Intervention aims to correct the underlying abnormality or dysfunction within the hypothalamic-pituitary-ovarian axis. In hyperactivity or hypoactivity of the adrenal or thyroid gland, hormone therapy is necessary. Progesterone deficiency requires replacement.

Anovulation is treated with clomiphene, human menopausal gonadotropins, or HCG. Ovulation usually occurs several days after administration. If mucus production decreases (an adverse effect of clomiphene), small doses of estrogen may be given concomitantly to restore cervical mucus.

Surgical restoration may correct certain anatomic causes of infertility. Endometriosis requires drug therapy (danazol, medroxyprogesterone, or noncyclic administration of oral contraceptives), surgical

Understanding in vitro fertilization

When the patient's fallopian tubes are absent, blocked, or damaged, in vitro fertilization offers an alternative method to achieve pregnancy. Although certain religious groups oppose this practice, many couples see it as a last resort for having children. Here's how this controversial treatment works.

Inducing ovulation

In vitro fertilization begins with the administration of a hormone to stimulate the development of an ovarian follicle. Measurement of serum estradiol confirms this.

Next, ultrasonography determines the best time to administer human chorionic gonadotropin (HCG), used to induce ovulation.

Retrieving the ovum

Ovum retrieval can occur 36 hours after HCG administration. The doctor performs laparoscopy to visualize and aspirate the ovum. He then punctures the mature follicle with a needle and transfers the ovum and fluid into a sterile test tube.

Fertilizing the ova

The doctor places the aspirated ovum in a culture dish containing maternal serum and a culture medium that is a mixture of amino acids, carbohydrates, and vitamins. After the ovum incubates in this medium for 24 hours at 98.6° F (37° C), sperm is added to the dish. (The husband or a donor provides a semen sample 2 hours after ovum retrieval, and the sperm is frozen until needed.) After another incubation period, this time for 36 hours, the oocyte divides if fertilization has occurred.

Transferring the embryo

With the patient in the knee-chest position, the doctor uses a small catheter to transfer the embryo into the fundus of the cervix. Typically, this causes no cervical dilation or pain.

Immediately after the patient receives the embryo, she's given progesterone I.M. To prevent loss of the embryo, she must maintain the knee-chest position for at least 8 hours. Afterward, she may return home.

Educating the patient and her spouse

At home, the patient will need daily I.M. doses of progesterone to help implant the ovum in the uterine wall. Teach the patient's husband how to give this injection.

Tell the couple to return for a follow-up appointment after hormonal therapy has been completed. At that time, the patient will have a pregnancy test.

---

removal of areas of endometriosis, or a combination of both.

Artificial insemination and in vitro (test-tube) fertilization may aid conception.(See *Understanding in vitro fertilization*.)

For immune disorders, transfusing male white cells into the female has been effective in some women. The female then develops titers, which should prevent her immune system from destroying sperm.

Nursing interventions. An infertile couple may suffer from feelings of lost self-esteem, anger, guilt, or inadequacy. Encourage the patient and her partner to talk about their feelings.

Patient education. Diagnostic procedures for this disorder may intensify the anxiety and embarrassment of the patient and her partner. You can help by explaining these procedures thoroughly. Acknowledge their expressions of embarrassment. If the patient requires surgery, tell her what to expect postoperatively.

Refer the patient and her partner to support groups and private counseling.

Evaluation. After successful treatment, the patient should conceive.

Pelvic inflammatory disease

Pelvic inflammatory disease (PID) includes any acute, subacute, recurrent, or chronic infection of the oviducts and ovaries, with adjacent tissue involvement. PID may refer to inflammation of the cervix (cervicitis), uterus (endometritis), fallopian tubes (salpingitis), and ovaries (oophoritis), which can extend to the connective tissue lying between the broad ligaments (parametritis). (See *Three types of pelvic inflammatory disease*, page 664.) Early diagnosis and treatment prevent damage to the reproductive system. Complications of PID may include potentially fatal septicemia, pulmonary emboli, infertility, and shock. Untreated PID may be fatal.

Causes. PID can result from infection with aerobic or anaerobic organisms. About 60% of cases result from overgrowth of one or more of the common bacterial species found in cervical mucus, including staphylococci, streptococci, diphtheroids, chlamydiae, and such coliforms as *Pseudomonas* and *Escherichia coli*. PID also results from infection with *Neisseria gonorrhoeae*. Finally, multiplication of normally nonpathogenic bacteria in an altered endometrial environment can cause PID. This occurs most commonly during parturition.

Risk factors. Risk factors that increase the patient's chances of developing PID include any sexually transmitted infection, more than one sex partner, and conditions or procedures, such as conization or cauterization of the cervix, that alter or destroy cervical mucus. Any procedure that risks transfer of contaminated cervical mucus into the endometrial cavity by instrumentation, such as use of a biopsy curet or an irrigation catheter, tubal insufflation, abortion, or pelvic surgery is also of concern. Infection during or after pregnancy or infectious foci within the body—such as drainage from a chronically infected fallopian tube, a pelvic abscess, a ruptured appendix, or diverticulitis of the sigmoid colon—may also increase her chances.

Assessment findings. Clinical features vary with the affected area. They may include low-grade fever and malaise (especially if *N. gonorrhoeae* is the cause), lower abdomi-

Three types of pelvic inflammatory disease

Cause and clinical features	Diagnostic findings
Salpingo-oophoritis	
• *Acute:* sudden onset of lower abdominal and pelvic pain, usually after menses; increased vaginal discharge; fever; malaise; lower abdominal pressure and tenderness; tachycardia; pelvic peritonitis • *Chronic:* recurring acute episodes	• Elevated or normal white blood cell (WBC) count. • X-ray may show ileus. • Pelvic examination reveals extreme tenderness. • Smear of cervical or periurethral gland exudate shows gram-negative intracellular diplococci.
Cervicitis	
• *Acute:* purulent, foul-smelling vaginal discharge; vulvovaginitis, with itching or burning; red, edematous cervix; pelvic discomfort; sexual dysfunction; metrorrhagia; infertility; spontaneous abortion • *Chronic:* cervical dystocia, laceration or eversion of the cervix, ulcerative vesicular lesion (when cervicitis results from herpes simplex virus type 2)	• Cultures for *Neisseria gonorrhoeae* are positive. • In *chronic cervicitis,* causative organisms are usually *Staphylococcus* or *Streptococcus*. • Cytologic smears may reveal severe inflammation. • If cervicitis is not complicated by salpingitis, WBC count is normal or slightly elevated; erythrocyte sedimentation rate (ESR) is elevated. • *In acute cervicitis,* cervical palpation reveals tenderness.
Endometritis (usually postpartum or postabortion)	
• *Acute:* mucopurulent or purulent vaginal discharge oozing from cervix; edematous, hyperemic endometrium, possibly leading to ulceration and necrosis (with virulent organisms); lower abdominal pain and tenderness; fever; rebound pain; abdominal muscle spasm; thrombophlebitis of uterine and pelvic vessels • *Chronic:* recurring acute episodes (more common from multiple sexual partners and sexually transmitted infections)	• In severe infection, palpation may reveal boggy uterus. • Uterine and blood samples are positive for causative organism, usually *Staphylococcus*. • WBC count and ESR are elevated.

nal pain, and profuse, purulent vaginal discharge. The patient may also develop extreme pain on movement of the cervix or palpation of the adnexa.

Diagnostic tests. Gram stain of secretions from the endocervix or cul-de-sac helps identify the infecting organism. Culture and sensitivity testing aids selection of the appropriate antibiotic. Urethral and rectal secretions may also be cultured. Ultrasonography identifies an adnexal or uterine mass. Culdocentesis obtains peritoneal fluid or pus for culture and sensitivity testing.

Treatment. Effective management eradicates the infection, relieves symptoms, and avoids damaging the reproductive system. Aggressive therapy with multiple antibiotics begins immediately after culture specimens are obtained. Such therapy can be reevaluated as soon as laboratory results are available. Infection may become chronic if treated inadequately.

Treatment for PID resulting from gonorrhea consists of cefoxitin I.M. with probenecid; or ceftriaxone I.M., doxycycline by mouth for 14 days. Supplemental treatment of PID may include bed rest, analgesics, and inpatient or outpatient I.V. therapy.

A pelvic abscess requires adequate drainage. A ruptured pelvic abscess is a life-threatening condition. If this complication develops, the patient may need a total abdominal hysterectomy, with bilateral salpingo-oophorectomy.

NSAIDs are preferred for pain relief, but narcotics may be used.

Nursing interventions. After establishing that the patient has no drug allergies, give antibiotics and analgesics, as ordered. Check for elevated temperature. Watch for abdominal rigidity and distention, possible signs of peritonitis. Provide frequent perineal care if vaginal drainage occurs.

Patient education. Encourage compliance with treatment, and explain the nature and seriousness of PID. Because PID may cause painful intercourse, advise the patient to consult with her doctor about sexual activity. Stress the need for the patient's sexual partner to be examined and treated for infection.

To prevent infection after minor gynecologic procedures such as D&C, tell the patient to immediately report any fever, increased vaginal discharge, or pain. After such procedures, instruct her to avoid douching or intercourse for at least 7 days.

Evaluation. The patient should experience no pain, discharge, or fever. She should also remain free from any recurring infection. (Up to 25% of patients may become infertile after one episode of PID.)

Breast cancer
Breast cancer is the leading cause of death in women ages 40 to 44 and ranks second only to lung cancer as the leading cause of cancer death in women ages 35 to 54.

Causes. The cause of breast cancer is unknown. Risk factors include a family history of breast cancer, long menstrual cycles, early onset of menses or late onset of menopause, first pregnancy after age 35, endometrial or ovarian cancer, being white and middle or upper class, constant stress or unusual disturbances in home or work life.

At least two breast cancer genes have been discovered (BRCA-1 and BRCA-2).

Assessment findings. Clinical features of breast cancer include a lump or mass in the breast (a hard, stony mass is usually malignant); changes in breast symmetry or size; changes in breast skin, such as thickening, dimpling (peau d'orange), edema, or ulceration; changes in nipples, such as itching, burning, erosion, or retraction; and changes in skin temperature (a warm, hot, or pink area).

Suspect cancer in a nonlactating woman past childbearing age until proven otherwise. Investigate spontaneous discharge of any kind in a nonlactating woman as well as any discharge produced by breast manipulation (greenish black, white, creamy, serous, or bloody). If a nursing infant rejects one breast, this may suggest possible breast cancer.

Pain doesn't usually signal breast cancer, but it should be investigated. Other signs include bone metastasis, pathologic bone fractures, and hypercalcemia.

Diagnostic tests. A combination of monthly breast self-examination (BSE), a yearly clinical examination by a health care practitioner, and screening mammograms followed by immediate evaluation of any abnormality is the most reliable method of detection. (See *Teaching about breast self-examination* in Chapter 3.) Diagnostic mammograms, ultrasound, and magnetic resonance imaging (MRI) are diagnostic tests used to diagnose and localize breast cancer. Tissue samples are obtained by fine-needle aspiration biopsy, needle biopsy, open biopsy, or stereotactic biopsy.

Bone scan, computed tomography (CT) scan, measurement of alkaline phosphatase (ALP) levels, liver function studies, and liver biopsy can detect distant metastases.

Other parameters assessed to help determine prognosis include estrogen-progesterone receptor status, deoxyribonucleic acid (DNA) ploidy, nuclear grade, and invasiveness of the tumor; size of tumor; and status of the axillary lymph nodes.

Treatment. Breast cancer treatments are complex; therapy should consider the stage of the disease, the woman's age and menopausal status, and the disfiguring effects of the surgery. Treatment may include the following:

Surgery. Lumpectomy (complete excision of the tumor) may be the initial surgery. In many cases it's the only surgery some patients require, especially those with a small tumor and no evidence of axillary node involvement. For stages I and II breast cancers, lumpectomy (with clear margins) combined with radiation is effective.

In lumpectomy and dissection of the axillary lymph nodes, the tumor and the axillary lymph nodes are removed, leaving the breast intact. A simple mastectomy removes the breast but not the lymph nodes or pectoral muscles. Modified radical mastectomy removes the breast and the axillary lymph nodes. Radical mastectomy is in declining use.

Postmastectomy, reconstructive surgery can create a breast mound if the patient desires it and if she doesn't show evidence of advanced disease. Additional surgery to modify hormone production may include oophorectomy.

Chemotherapy. Various cytotoxic drug combinations are used, either as adjuvant or preoperative therapy. The use of chemotherapy before surgery permits evaluation of the tumor's response and may permit more conservative therapy.

Radiation therapy. Primary radiation therapy *after* lumpectomy is effective for small tumors in early stages with no evidence of distant metastasis. It's also used to prevent or treat local recurrence.

Other methods. Treatment may also include estrogen, progesterone, or androgen therapy; antiandrogen therapy with aminoglutethimide; or antiestrogen therapy, specifically tamoxifen, a drug with few adverse effects that inhibits DNA synthesis. Tamoxifen, used in postmenopausal women, most effectively combats estrogen-receptor-positive tumors.

The success of these newer drug therapies has caused a decline in ablative surgery.

Nursing interventions. Obtain a thorough history. Preoperatively, learn what kind of surgery the patient will have, so you can prepare her properly.

Patient education. Teach female patients the importance of BSE, mammography, and follow-up. Postoperatively, patients should continue these practices to detect recurrences.

Your teaching should also include any female relatives of the patient, particularly if a positive family history exists.

Evaluation. With effective therapy, the patient recovers uneventfully from surgery, radiation, or chemotherapy. She performs appropriate exercises and understands postoperative safety precautions for the affected arm. She also correctly demonstrates BSE.

Cervical cancer

Cervical cancer is classified as either preinvasive or invasive carcinoma. Preinvasive changes are now commonly called cervical intraepithelial neoplasia (CIN). CIN is divided into three categories: CIN 1 is mild dysplasia, CIN 2 is moderate dysplasia, and CIN 3 is severe dysplasia or carcinoma in situ. The CIN classification also depends on depth of invasion of the epithelium.

Causes. The cause of cervical cancer is unknown. Risk factors include intercourse at a young age, multiple sexual partners, multiple pregnancies, and sexually transmitted infections, particularly herpes simplex virus type 2 (HSV2) and human papillomavirus.

Assessment findings. Preinvasive cervical cancer is asymptomatic. Abnormal vaginal bleeding, persistent vaginal discharge, or postcoital pain and bleeding may signal early invasive disease. Advanced disease may cause pelvic pain, foul-smelling vaginal discharge, vaginal leakage of urine and feces from a fistula, anorexia, weight loss, and fatigue.

Diagnostic tests. A cytologic examination (Pap smear) can detect cervical cancer before clinical evidence appears. Colposcopy can reveal the presence and extent of preclinical lesions. Biopsy and histologic examination confirm the diagnosis.

Additional studies—such as lymphangiography, cystography, and scans—can detect metastasis.

Treatment. Preinvasive lesions may require cryosurgery, total excisional biopsy, laser destruction, loop electrosurgical excision procedure, conization (and frequent Pap smear follow-up) or, rarely, hysterectomy. Treatment of invasive squamous cell carcinoma may require radical hysterectomy and radiation therapy and is based on age, extent of cancer and other complications.

Nursing interventions. Cancer patients require compassionate psychological support.

If the patient is to be treated with internal radiation, determine if the radioactive source will be inserted while the patient is in the operating room (preloaded) or at the bedside (afterloaded). Remember that safety precautions—time, distance, and shielding—begin as soon as the radioactive source is in place. Inform the patient that she'll require a private room.

Check vital signs every 4 hours; watch for skin reaction, vaginal bleeding, abdominal discomfort, or evidence of dehydration. Make sure the patient can reach everything she needs without stretching or straining. Assist her in range-of-motion arm exercises (leg exercises and other body movements could dislodge the source). If ordered, give a tranquilizer to relax the patient. Organize time spent with the patient to minimize your exposure to radiation. Inform visitors of safety precautions; hang a sign listing these precautions on the patient's door.

Patient education. If you assist with a biopsy, drape and prepare the patient as you would for a routine pelvic examination. Have a container of formaldehyde ready to preserve the specimen during transfer to the pathology laboratory. Explain to the patient that she may feel pressure, minor abdominal cramps, or a pinch from the punch forceps. Reassure her that pain will be minimal.

If you assist with cryosurgery, drape and prepare the patient as you would for a routine pelvic examination. Explain that the procedure takes approximately 15 minutes, during which time the doctor will use refrigerant to freeze the cervix. Warn the patient that she may experience abdominal cramps, headache, and sweating, but reassure her that she'll feel little, if any, pain.

If you assist with laser therapy, drape and prepare the patient as you would for a routine pelvic examination. Explain that the procedure takes approximately 30 minutes and may cause abdominal cramps.

After excisional biopsy, cryosurgery, or laser therapy, tell the patient to expect a discharge or spotting for about 1 week. Advise her not to douche, use tampons, or engage in sexual intercourse during this time. Tell her to watch for and report signs of infection. Stress the need for a follow-up Pap smear and a pelvic examination within 3 to 4 months and periodically thereafter.

Explain that external outpatient radiation therapy, when needed, continues for about 4 to 6 weeks. Tell the patient she may be hospitalized for a 2- to 3-day internal radiation treatment (an intracavitary implant of radium, cesium, or other radioactive material). Find out if she's to have internal or external therapy, or both. Usually, internal radiation therapy is the first procedure. (See *Internal radiation safety precautions*, page 670.)

Explain the preloaded internal radiation procedure, and answer the patient's questions. Tell her that internal radiation requires a 2- to 3-day stay, a bowel preparation, a povidone-iodine vaginal douche, a clear liquid diet, and nothing by mouth the night before the implantation; it also requires an indwelling catheter. Also tell her the procedure is performed in the operating room under a general anesthetic, during which time she will be placed in the lithotomy position and a radium applicator will be inserted.

If afterloaded radiation therapy is scheduled, explain that a member of the radiation team will implant the source after she returns to her room. Encourage the patient to lie flat and limit movement while the source is in place. If she prefers, elevate the head of the bed slightly.

Teach the patient to report uncomfortable adverse reactions. As radiation therapy may increase susceptibility to infection by lowering the white blood cell count, warn her during therapy to avoid persons with obvious infections. Reassure the patient that this disease and its treatment should not radically alter her lifestyle or prohibit sexual intimacy. Mention the availability of American Cancer Society (ACS) literature on sexual concerns.

Evaluation. Note the patient's tolerance of therapy. She should understand that it won't impair her ability to have sex. She should also understand the importance of complying with the treatment regimen.

Endometrial cancer

Also known as cancer of the uterus, endometrial cancer is the most

Internal radiation: Safety precautions

There are three cardinal safety rules in internal radiation therapy:

• *Time*. Wear a radiosensitive badge. Remember, your exposure increases with time, and the effects are cumulative. Therefore, carefully plan the time you spend with the patient to prevent overexposure. (However, don't rush procedures, ignore the patient's psychologic needs, or give the impression that you can't get out of the room fast enough.)
• *Distance*. Radiation loses its intensity with distance. Avoid standing at the foot of the patient's bed, where you're in line with the radiation.
• *Shield*. Lead shields reduce radiation exposure. Use them whenever possible.

   Also remember these additional points:
• The patient is radioactive while the radiation source is in place, usually 48 to 72 hours.
• Pregnant women should not be assigned to care for these patients.
• Check the position of the source applicator every 4 hours. If it appears dislodged, notify the doctor immediately. If it's completely dis-

lodged, remove the patient from the bed, pick up the applicator with long forceps and place it on a lead-shielded transport cart, and notify the doctor immediately. *Never* pick up the radiation source with your bare hands.
• Notify the doctor and the radiation safety officer whenever there's an accident, and keep a lead-shielded transport cart on the unit as long as the patient has a radiation source in place.

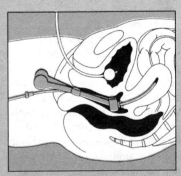

Positioning of internal radiation applicator for endometrial cancer

common gynecologic cancer. Usually, it affects postmenopausal women between ages 50 and 60. Most premenopausal women who develop endometrial cancer have a history of anovular menstrual cycles or other hormonal imbalance.

Causes. The cause of endometrial cancer is unknown. Risk factors for the development of this cancer

include low fertility index and anovulation; abnormal uterine bleeding; late menopause; history of breast or ovarian cancer; obesity, hypertension, or diabetes; familial tendency; history of uterine polyps or endometrial hyperplasia; and estrogen therapy (still controversial).

Assessment findings. Abnormal vaginal bleeding is the most common sign. Any vaginal bleeding in a postmenopausal woman should be evaluated. In premenopausal women the onset of irregular menses warrants attention.

Late signs and symptoms include pain and weight loss.

Diagnostic tests. Diagnosis of endometrial cancer requires endometrial, cervical, and endocervical biopsies. Negative biopsies call for a fractional D&C to determine diagnosis. Other tests include chest X-ray or CT scan, intravenous pyelography (IVP) and, possibly, cystoscopy, complete blood studies, electrocardiogram, and MRI may be used to evaluate the amount of myometrium involved.

Treatment. Treatment for endometrial cancer may require surgery, radiation, or hormonal therapy, or various combinations of these.

Surgery usually involves total abdominal hysterectomy, bilateral salpingo-oophorectomy, or possibly omentectomy with or without pelvic or para-aortic lymphadenectomy. Total exenteration removes all pelvic organs, including the vagina, and is done only when the disease is sufficiently contained to allow surgical removal of diseased parts. Partial exenteration may retain an unaffected colorectum or bladder.

Radiation therapy (intracavitary or external radiation, or both, given 6 weeks before surgery) may inhibit recurrence and lengthen survival time when the tumor isn't well differentiated.

Hormonal therapy isn't proven as an adjuvant treatment but is usually used in recurrent disease. Synthetic progestational agents are most commonly used. Chemotherapy isn't commonly used in the management of endometrial cancer.

Nursing interventions. Provide comprehensive patient teaching to help her cope with surgery, radiation, and chemotherapy. Provide good postoperative care and psychological support. Mention the availability of American Cancer Society (ACS) literature on sexual concerns.

Evaluation. Note the patient's tolerance of therapy. She should understand the importance of complying with the treatment regimen.

Ovarian cancer

The three main types of ovarian cancer are primary epithelial tumors (90% of all ovarian cancers), germ cell tumors, and sex cord (stromal) tumors. Ovarian tumors spread rapidly intraperitoneally and occasionally through the lymphatic system and the bloodstream. Generally, the tumor spreads extraperitoneally through the diaphragm into the chest cavity, which may cause pleural effusions. Other metastasis is rare.

Cause. The cause of ovarian cancer is unknown. Risk factors associated with the development of ovarian cancer include environmental, reproductive, menstrual, dietary, and hereditary factors.

Assessment findings. Unfortunately, ovarian cancer is seldom diagnosed early. Localized early-stage disease is usually asymptomatic. As the mass grows, vague abdominal discomfort, dyspepsia, and other mild GI disturbances occur. Other clinical features may include urinary frequency, constipation, pelvic discomfort, distention, weight loss, and pain (which can mimic appendicitis in young patients and results from tumor rupture, torsion, or infection).

In some types of tumors, signs and symptoms include bleeding between periods in premenopausal women and, in advanced ovarian cancer, ascites, postmenopausal bleeding (rarely), pain, and symptoms related to metastatic sites (most commonly pleural effusion).

Diagnostic tests. Routine pelvic examinations are still the most common method of detecting ovarian cancer early. Any palpable ovary in a woman 3 to 5 years postmenopause should be treated with suspicion.

Accurate diagnosis and staging are impossible without exploratory laparotomy, including lymph node evaluation and tumor resection. Preoperative evaluation involves the following tests:
• abdominal ultrasonography, CT scan, or X-ray (may delineate tumor size)
• CBC and blood chemistries
• IVP to assess renal function and possible urinary tract anomalies or obstruction
• chest X-ray to detect distant metastasis and pleural effusion
• barium enema (especially in patients with GI symptoms) to reveal obstruction and show its size
• lymphangiography to show lymph node involvement
• mammography to rule out primary breast cancer
• liver function studies or a liver scan in patients with ascites
• radioimmunoassay (RIA) for tumor markers (usually CA_{125}).

Treatment. Treatment of ovarian cancer requires varying combinations of surgery, chemotherapy and, in some cases, radiation. Occasionally, in girls or young women with a unilateral encapsulated tumor who wish to maintain fertility, conservative approaches may be appropriate, including resection of the involved ovary, biopsies of the omentum and the uninvolved ovary, peritoneal washings for cytologic examination of pelvic fluid, and careful follow-up, including periodic chest X-rays to rule out lung metastasis.

However, ovarian cancer usually requires more aggressive treatment, including total abdominal hysterectomy and bilateral salpingo-oophorectomy with tumor resection, omentectomy, appendectomy, lymph node palpation with probable lymphadenectomy, tissue biopsies, and peritoneal washings. Complete tumor resection may be impossible. Bilateral salpingo-oophorectomy in a girl who hasn't reached puberty necessitates hormone replacement therapy.

Chemotherapy extends the length of survival time in most ovarian cancer patients but is largely palliative in advanced disease. However, prolonged remissions are being achieved in some patients. Chemotherapy may include various combinations of paclitaxel (Taxol), melphalan, chlorambucil, thiotepa, methotrexate, cyclophosphamide, doxorubicin, vincristine, vinblastine, actinomycin D, bleomycin, cisplatin, or carboplatin. Intraperitoneal (IP) chemotherapy may also be used to administer methotrexate, doxorubicin, 5-fluorouracil, cisplatin, mitomycin, mitoxantrone, cytarabine, and interferon through a Tenckhoff catheter directly into the abdominal cavity. IP administration of other biologic agents is being investigated.

In early-stage ovarian cancer, instillation of a radioisotope such as radioactive phosphorus 32 is occasionally useful when peritoneal washings are positive. Radiation treatment is likely to be more than merely palliative only if residual tumor size is $4/5''$ (2 cm) or less; if there's no evidence of ascites or no metastatic deposits on the peritoneum, the liver, or kidneys; and if there are no distant metastases and no history of abdominal radiation.

Nursing interventions. Provide psychological support for the patient and her family. Encourage open communication among family members, but discourage them from overcompensating or smothering the patient. If the patient is a young woman grieving for her lost fertility, support her (and her family). Enlist the help of a social worker, chaplain, and other members of the health care team.

Evaluation. The patient should tolerate the therapy well and understand its potential adverse effects, including ascites. She should realize the importance of complying with the treatment regimen and verbalize concerns about her lost fertility.

Male reproductive disorders

The disorders described in this section may all have a potentially devastating effect on male sexuality. They include impotence, infertility, prostate, and testicular cancer.

Impotence

Impotence is also known as erectile dysfunction. A man with this disorder can't attain or maintain penile erection sufficient to complete intercourse. The patient with primary impotence has never achieved a sufficient erection; secondary impotence, more common and less serious, implies that he has succeeded in completing intercourse in the past. Erectile dysfunction affects all age-groups but increases in frequency with age.

Causes. Psychogenic factors cause approximately 50% to 60% of erectile dysfunction; organic factors underlie the rest. In some patients, psychogenic and organic factors coexist, hampering isolation of the primary cause.

Psychogenic causes may be intrapersonal, reflecting personal sexual anxieties, or interpersonal, reflecting a disturbed sexual relationship. Intrapersonal factors usually involve guilt, fear, or depression, resulting from previous traumatic sexual experience, rejection by parents or peers, or other factors. Interpersonal factors may stem from differences in sexual preferences between partners, lack of communication, insufficient knowledge of sexual function, or nonsexual personal conflicts. Stress may cause temporary situational impotence.

Organic causes may include chronic disorders, such as cardiopulmonary disease, diabetes, multiple sclerosis, or renal failure; spinal cord trauma; complications of surgery; drug- or alcohol-induced dysfunction; and, rarely, genital anomalies or central nervous system (CNS) defects.

Assessment findings. Secondary erectile dysfunction is classified as follows:
• partial—the patient can't achieve a full erection
• intermittent—the patient is sometimes potent with the same partner
• selective—the patient is potent only with certain partners.

Some patients lose erectile function suddenly; others lose it gradually. If the cause isn't organic, erection may still be achieved through masturbation.

Patients with psychogenic impotence may appear anxious, with sweating and palpitations, or they may become totally disinterested in sexual activity. Patients with psychogenic or drug-induced impotence may suffer extreme depression, which may cause the impotence or result from it.

Diagnostic tests. Personal sexual history is the key in differentiating between organic and psychogenic factors and between primary and secondary impotence. Does the patient have intermittent, selective, nocturnal, or early-morning erections? Can he achieve erections through other sexual activity, such as masturbation or fantasizing? When did his dysfunction begin, and what was his life situation at that time? Did erectile problems occur suddenly or gradually? Is he taking large quantities of prescription or over-the-counter drugs? What is his alcohol intake?

Diagnosis also must rule out chronic disease, such as diabetes and other vascular, neurologic, or urogenital problems.

Treatment. Sex therapy, largely directed at reducing performance anxiety, may cure psychogenic impotence. Such therapy should include both partners. Alternatively, treatment for drug and alcohol abuse may solve the problem.

The course and content of sex therapy for impotence depend on the specific cause of the dysfunction and the nature of the male-female relationship. Usually, therapy includes sensate focus techniques.

Treatment of organic impotence focuses on reversing the cause, if possible. If not, psychological counseling may help the couple explore alternatives for sexual expression. Certain patients suffering from organic impotence may benefit from surgically inserted inflatable or noninflatable penile implants; others with low testosterone levels benefit from testosterone injections.

Nursing interventions. When you identify a patient with impotence or with a condition that may cause impotence, help him feel comfortable about discussing his sexuality. Assess his sexual health during your initial nursing history. When appropriate, refer him for further evaluation or treatment.

Patient education. After penile implant surgery, instruct the patient to avoid intercourse until the incision heals, usually in 6 weeks.

To help prevent impotence, provide information about resuming sexual activity as part of discharge instructions for any patient with a condition that requires modification of daily activities. Such patients include those with cardiac disease, diabetes, hypertension, or chronic obstructive pulmonary disease, and all postoperative patients.

Evaluation. The patient should report achieving and maintaining an erection and express satisfaction with his sexual relationships.

Male infertility

Male infertility may be indicated whenever a couple fails to achieve pregnancy after 1 year of regular unprotected intercourse. Approximately 40% to 50% of infertility problems in the United States are totally or partially attributed to the male. (See *What causes male infertility?* page 676.)

Assessment findings. Clinical features of male infertility include atrophied testes; empty scrotum; scrotal edema; varicocele or anteversion of the epididymis; inflamed seminal vesicles; beading or abnormal nodes on the spermatic cord and vas; penile nodes, warts, plaques, or hypospadias; and prostatic enlargement, nodules, swelling, or tenderness. In addition, infertility may cause feelings of anger, hurt, disgust, guilt, and loss of self-esteem.

Diagnostic tests. A detailed patient history may reveal abnormal sexual development, delayed puberty, infertility in previous relationships, and a medical history of prolonged fever, mumps, impaired nutritional status, previous surgery, or trauma to genitalia. After a thorough patient history and physical examination, the most conclusive test for male infertility is semen analysis. Other laboratory tests include gonadotropin assay to determine the integrity of the pituitary-gonadal axis, serum testosterone levels to determine end-organ response to LH, urine 17-ketosteroid levels to measure testicular function, and testicular biopsy to help clarify unexplained oligospermia or azoospermia. Vasography and seminal vesiculography may be necessary.

What causes male infertility?

Some factors that cause male infertility include:
• varicocele, a mass of dilated and tortuous varicose veins in the spermatic cord
• semen disorders, such as volume or motility disturbances or inadequate sperm density
• proliferation of abnormal or immature sperm, with variations in the size and shape of the head
• systemic diseases, such as diabetes mellitus, neoplasms, hepatic and renal diseases, and viral disturbances, especially mumps orchitis
• genital infection, such as gonorrhea, tuberculosis, and herpes
• disorders of the testes, such as cryptorchidism, Sertoli-cell–only syndrome, and ductal obstruction (caused by absence or ligation of vas deferens or infection)
• genetic defects, such as Klinefelter's syndrome (chromosomal pattern XXY, eunuchoidal habitus, gynecomastia, and small testes) or Reifenstein's syndrome (chromosomal pattern 46XY, reduced testosterone level, azoospermia, eunuchoidism, gynecomastia, and hypospadias)
• immunologic disorders such as autoimmune infertility
• endocrine imbalance (rare) that disrupts pituitary gonadotropins, inhibiting spermatogenesis, testosterone production, or both; such imbalances occur in Kallmann's syndrome, panhypopituitarism, hypothyroidism, and congenital adrenal hyperplasia
• chemicals and drugs that inhibit gonadotropins or interfere with spermatogenesis, such as arsenic, methotrexate, medroxyprogesterone, nitrofurantoin, monoamine oxidase inhibitors, and some antihypertensives
• sexual problems, such as erectile dysfunction, ejaculatory incompetence, or low libido.

Other causative factors include age, occupation, and trauma to the testes.

Treatment. When an anatomic dysfunction or an infection causes infertility, treatment seeks to correct the underlying problem. A varicocele requires surgical repair or removal. For patients with sexual dysfunction, treatment includes education, counseling or therapy, and proper nutrition with vitamin supplements. Decreased FSH levels may respond to vitamin B therapy; decreased LH levels, to HCG therapy. Elevated LH levels require low dosages of testosterone. Decreased testosterone levels, decreased semen motility, and volume disturbances may respond to HCG.

Patients with oligospermia who have a normal history and physical examination, normal hormonal assays, and no signs of systemic disease require emotional support and counseling, adequate nutrition, multivitamins, and selective therapeutic agents, such as clomiphene, HCG, and low dosages of testosterone. Alternatives to such treatment are adoption and artificial insemination.

Nursing interventions. Help prevent male infertility by encouraging patients to have regular physical examinations, to protect the testes during athletic activity, and to receive early treatment for sexually transmitted diseases and surgical correction for anatomic defects.

Patient education. Educate the couple regarding reproductive and sexual functions and about factors that may interfere with fertility, such as the use of lubricants and douches.

Urge men with oligospermia to avoid wearing tight underwear and athletic supporters or heavy work pants (especially in warm climates), taking hot tub baths, or habitually riding a bicycle. Explain that cool scrotal temperatures are essential for adequate spermatogenesis.

When possible, advise infertile couples to join support groups.

Evaluation. The patient and his partner should be able to express an understanding of infertility and demonstrate effective coping mechanisms. The couple should know alternatives to normal conception, such as artificial insemination and adoption.

If surgery was performed, assess for postoperative complications.

Prostate cancer

Prostate cancer most commonly occurs in men between the ages of 60 and 70. To detect this cancer early, all males over age 40 should undergo a rectal examination as well as have blood drawn for prostate-specific antigen (PSA) testing as part of their annual physical examination.

Cause. Although the cause of prostatic cancer is unknown, age, infectious agents, diet, family history and endocrine function may all play a role.

Assessment findings. Signs and symptoms of prostatic cancer may appear only in the advanced stages of the disease. Clinical effects include difficult urination, dribbling, urine retention, unexplained cystitis, and hematuria (rare). A hard nodule may appear on rectal examination. This may be felt before symptoms develop.

Diagnostic tests. In general, screening involves a digital rectal examination and PSA testing—although neither is diagnostic. Transrectal prostatic ultrasonography will detect a mass. Biopsy confirms this diagnosis. CT and MRI may also be used.

Serum acid phosphatase is elevated in 80% of patients with metastasized prostatic cancer. Successful therapy restores a normal enzyme level; a subsequent rise points to recurrence.

Increased ALP levels and a positive bone scan point to bone metastasis. However, routine bone X-rays don't always show evidence of metastasis.

Treatment. Therapy for prostatic cancer must be chosen carefully because the disease usually affects older men, who commonly have serious coexisting disorders.

Treatments vary but generally include radiation, surgery,

chemotherapy, and endocrine or hormone manipulation. Radical prostatectomy is usually effective for localized lesions with no evidence of metastasis. Radiation therapy is used in early stages, to relieve bone pain from metastatic skeletal involvement, or prophylactically for patients with tumors in regional lymph nodes. Alternatively, internal beam radiation focuses radiation on the prostate while minimizing exposure of surrounding tissue.

Hormone manipulation may be accomplished through surgical castration, medical castration (using diethylstilbestrol [DES], LH-releasing hormone analogs, such as leuprolide [Lupon], and goserelin [Zoladex]), adrenal suppression (surgical or medical), or antiandrogens (flutamide, oxymetholone [Anadrol], Casodex).

If hormone or radiation therapy and surgery can't be done or don't work, chemotherapy (using various combinations of cyclophosphamide, vinblastine, doxorubicin, mitomycin C, or 5-fluorouracil may be tried.

Nursing interventions. Your plan of care should include supportive care for the patient scheduled for prostatectomy as well as good postoperative care and symptomatic treatment of radiation adverse effects.

When a patient receives radiation or hormonal therapy, watch for and treat nausea, vomiting, dry skin, and alopecia. Also watch for adverse effects of DES (gynecomastia, fluid retention, nausea, and vomiting). Watch for thrombophlebitis (pain, tenderness, swelling, warmth, and redness in calf), which is always a possibility in patients receiving DES.

Evaluation. The patient should understand the treatment regimen and be aware of adverse effects that require immediate medical attention (such as thrombophlebitis). He should express his feelings about potential sexual dysfunction.

Testicular cancer

Testicular cancer is the leading cause of death from solid tumors in men between the ages of 15 and 34. Prognosis varies with the cancer cell type and staging. When treated with surgery and radiation, if the cancer has not metastasized beyond regional lymph nodes, 100% of patients with seminomas and 90% of those with nonseminomas survive beyond 5 years.

Causes. Whites and men with a history of cryptorchidism (with surgical correction performed after age 5) are at increased risk for testicular cancer, as are male children born to women given exogenous estrogens (birth control pills or DES) but its cause is unknown.

Assessment findings. Clinical features of testicular cancer include a firm, painless, smooth testicular mass, and testicular enlargement and heaviness. In later stages, ureteral obstruction, abdominal mass, cough, hemoptysis, shortness of breath, weight loss, fatigue, pallor, and lethargy, with lymph node involvement and distant metastases are possible.

Diagnostic tests. Used together, the following tests may confirm diagnosis: radical inguinal orchiectomy (as biopsy), IVP (detects ureteral deviation resulting from para-aortic node involvement), lymphangiography, and abdominal CT.

Treatment. Combinations of surgery, radiation, and chemotherapy are used, depending on tumor cell type and staging. Surgery includes orchiectomy and possibly retroperitoneal node dissection to prevent extension of the disease and to assist staging. Most surgeons remove the testis but preserve the scrotum for a possible low prosthetic testicular implant later.

Seminomas are treated with postoperative radiation to the retroperitoneal and homolateral iliac nodes and, in patients with retroperitoneal extension, prophylactic radiation to the mediastinal and supraclavicular nodes. In nonseminomas, postoperative radiation therapy has been replaced by postoperative chemotherapy using cisplatin, etoposide (VP-16), and bleomycin.

Chemotherapy is essential in patients with large abdominal or mediastinal nodes and frank distant metastases or in others at high risk for developing metastases. Combinations of cyclophosphamide, ifosfamide, vinblastine, doxorubicin, bleomycin, cisplatin, etoposide, and vincristine are used.

Nursing interventions. Your plan of care should emphasize dealing with the patient's psychological response to the disease, preventing postoperative complications, and minimizing and controlling the adverse effects of radiation and chemotherapy.

Before orchiectomy, encourage the patient to talk about his fears.

For the first day after surgery, apply an ice pack to the scrotum and provide analgesics, as ordered. Check for excessive bleeding, swelling, and signs of infection. Provide a scrotal athletic supporter to minimize pain.

Patient education. Reassure the patient that unilateral orchiectomy doesn't cause sterility and impotence, however, sperm count may be affected. Therefore, young men considering fathering a child should be counseled about sperm banking before surgery. Inform the patient that most surgeons don't remove the scrotum and that implant of a testicular prosthesis can correct disfigurement.

Instruct the patient on how to perform testicular self-examination. Mention the availability of ACS literature on sexual concerns of cancer patients.

Evaluation. The patient's concerns about possible sexual disfigurement should be resolved. He should understand how to do testicular self-examination and the importance of complying with the treatment regimen.

Sexually transmitted disorders

An important group of sexually related disorders results from infection transmitted through sexual contact. These disorders include gonorrhea, chlamydial infections, trichomoniasis, genital herpes, genital warts (condylomata acuminata), syphilis (including prenatal syphilis), and chancroid. (**Note:** AIDS is discussed in Chapter 11 "Immunologic and Hematologic Care.") (For assessment findings and treatment, see *Treatment of sexually transmitted disorders.*)

Gonorrhea

Gonorrhea is a common venereal disease that infects the genitourinary tract (especially the urethra and cervix) and may occasionally infect the rectum, pharynx, and even the eyes. After adequate treatment, the prognosis in both males and females is excellent, although reinfection is common.

Left untreated, gonorrhea can spread through the blood to the joints, tendons, meninges, and endocardium. Children and adults with gonorrhea can contract gonococcal conjunctivitis by touching their eyes with contaminated hands. Children born of infected mothers can contract gonococcal ophthalmia neonatorum during passage through the birth canal. Other possible results of untreated disease include gonococcal septicemia, sterility, corneal ulceration and blindness, and arthritis. (See *Documenting infectious diseases,* page 687.)

Diagnostic tests. Culture from the site of infection usually establishes the diagnosis by isolating the organism. A Gram stain showing gram-negative diplococci supports the diagnosis and may be sufficient to confirm gonorrhea in males.

Confirmation of gonococcal arthritis requires identification of gram-negative diplococci in smears of joint fluid and skin lesions. Complement fixation and immunofluorescent assays of serum reveal antibody titers four times higher than normal. Culture of conjunctival scrapings confirms gonococcal conjunctivitis.

Nursing interventions. Double-bag all soiled dressings and contaminated instruments; wear gloves when handling contaminated material and giving patient care. Isolate the patient with an eye infection.

Routinely instill two drops of 1% silver nitrate or erythromycin in the eyes of all neonates immediately after birth. Check the neonates of infected mothers for signs of infection. Take culture specimens from the infant's eyes, pharynx, and rectum.

To ease pain in the patient with gonococcal arthritis, apply moist heat to affected joints.

Urge the patient to inform sexual contacts of his infection so they can seek treatment also. Report all cases to public health authorities for follow-up on sexual contacts.

Patient education. Warn the patient that until cultures prove negative, he is still infectious and can transmit gonococcal infection. If the patient is being treated as an outpa-
(Text continues on page 686.)

Treatment of sexually transmitted disorders

Disease (causative agent)	Assessment findings	Treatment
Gonorrhea *Neisseria gonorrhoeae*	• Typically asymptomatic *Females:* • inflammation greenish yellow discharge from the cervix • severe pelvic and lower abdominal pain, muscle rigidity, tenderness, and abdominal distention; as infection spreads, nausea, vomiting, fever, and tachycardia in patients with salpingitis or pelvic inflammatory disease *Males:* • dysuria, purulent urethral discharge, redness and swelling, adult conjunctivitis *Newborns:* • gonococcal ophthalmia neonatorum	Uncomplicated gonorrhea (adults): • Ceftriaxone 250 mg I.M. in a single dose plus doxycycline hyclate 100 mg b.i.d., P.O. for 7 days. • Initially, tetracycline 1.5 g P.O., followed by 500 mg P.O. q 6 hours for 4 days (patients sensitive to penicillin). • Probenecid 1 g P.O. (to block penicillin excretion if suspected source of infection is non–penicillinase-producing gonorrhea) plus either a single dose of ampicillin 3.5 g P.O. or 4.8 million U of aqueous procaine penicillin G I.M. in at least two doses injected at different sites at one visit. • Disseminated gonococcal infection requires 1 g of ceftriaxone I.M. or I.V. every 24 hours for 7 days. • Adult gonococcal ophthalmia requires a single dose of 1 g of ceftriaxone I.M. • Follow-up cultures 4 to 7 days after treatment and again in 6 months. • Routine instillation of 1% silver nitrate or erythromycin ointment into neonates' eyes has greatly reduced the incidence of gonococcal ophthalmia neonatorum.
Chlamydial infections *C. trachomatis*	Lymphogranuloma venereum: • Painless vesicle or nonindurated ulcer, 2 to 3 mm in diameter	• 100 mg of doxycycline b.i.d. for 7 days. • 500 mg of erythromycin q.i.d. for 7 days. *(continued)*

Treatment of sexually transmitted disorders *(continued)*

Disease (causative agent)	Assessment findings	Treatment
Chlamydial infections *(continued)*	• Regional lymphadenopathy after 1 to 4 weeks and inguinal lymph node swelling about 2 weeks later • Myalgia, headache, fever, chills, backache, and weight loss *Proctitis:* • Diarrhea, tenesmus, pruritus, bloody or mucopurulent discharge, or diffuse or discrete ulceration in the rectosigmoid colon *Cervicitis:* • Cervical erosion, mucopurulent discharge, pelvic pain, or dyspareunia *Endometritis or salpingitis:* • Pain and tenderness of the abdomen, cervix, uterus, and lymph nodes; chills; fever; vaginal discharge; or dysuria *Urethral syndrome:* • Dysuria, pyuria, or urinary frequency *Epididymitis:* • Painful scrotal swelling and urethral discharge *Prostatitis:* • Lower back pain, urinary frequency, dysuria, nocturia, urethral discharge, or painful ejaculation *Urethritis:* • Dysuria, erythema and tenderness of the urethral meatus, urinary frequency, pruritus, or urethral discharge	• Azithromycin 1 g P.O. one time.
Trichomoniasis ***Trichomonas vaginalis***	• 70% of females and most males are asymptomatic *Acute infection (women):* • Vaginal discharge (gray or	• Oral metronidazole given simultaneously to both sexual partners cures trichomoniasis. The recommended

Treatment of sexually transmitted disorders *(continued)*

Disease (causative agent)	Assessment findings	Treatment
Trichomoniasis *(continued)*	greenish yellow and possibly profuse, frothy, and malodorous), "strawberry spots" on the cervix, severe itching, redness, swelling, tenderness, dyspareunia, dysuria, and urinary frequency • Postcoital spotting, menorrhagia, or dysmenorrhea *Men:* • Transient mild to severe urethritis, dysuria, or urinary frequency	dosage is 375 mg P.O. b.i.d. for 7 days. • A pregnant patient (second or third trimester): clotrimazole vaginal tablet h.s. for 7 days. Use during the first trimester only if clearly indicated.
Genital herpes *herpes simplex virus type 2*	• Fluid-filled, painless vesicles (women: cervix [the primary infection site] and possibly on the labia, perianal skin, vulva, or vagina; men: on the glans penis, foreskin, or penile shaft) • Extragenital lesions may occur in the mouth or anus. • In both men and women, vesicles rupture and develop into extensive, shallow, painful ulcers. • Edema and inguinal lymphadenopathy • Fever, malaise, dysuria and, in the female, leukorrhea	• Acyclovir (Zovirax) I.V. administration for patients who are hospitalized with severe genital herpes or who are immunocompromised and have potentially life-threatening herpes infections. • P.O. acyclovir for patients suffering from first-time infections or from recurrent outbreaks. • Patients experiencing outbreaks more often than every 6 weeks may require acyclovir 400 mg P.O. b.i.d. for up to 12 months..
Genital warts *human papilloma virus*	*Males:* • Genital warts develop on the subpreputial sac, within the urethral meatus and, less commonly, on the penile shaft *Females:* • On the vulva and on vaginal and cervical walls • Papillomas (painless warts that start as tiny red or pink swellings, grow [sometimes	• Warts may resolve spontaneously. • Topical 10% to 25% podophyllum in tincture of benzoin or trichloroacetic acid. • Warts larger than 1″ (2.5 cm) are usually removed by surgery, cryosurgery, or electrocautery. *(continued)*

Treatment of sexually transmitted disorders *(continued)*

Disease (causative agent)	Assessment findings	Treatment
Genital warts *(continued)*	to 4″ (10 cm)] and become pedunculated; multiple swellings give such warts a cauliflower appearance; malodorous) spread to the perineum and perianal area (in both sexes)	
Syphilis ***Treponema pallidum***	*Primary syphilis:* • Chancres—small, painless, fluid-filled lesions on genitalia, anus, fingers, lips, tongue, nipples, tonsils, or eyelids that eventually erode and develop indurated, raised edges and clear bases • Regional lymphadenopathy (unilateral or bilateral) *Secondary syphilis:* • Rash (macular, papular, pustular, or nodular) and for symmetrical mucocutaneous lesions • Macules commonly erupt between rolls of fat on the trunk and, proximally, on the arms, palms, soles, face, and scalp. In warm, moist areas (perineum, scrotum, vulva, between rolls of fat), the lesions enlarge and erode, producing highly contagious, pink or grayish white lesions (condylomata lata) • General lymphadenopathy • Headache, malaise, anorexia, weight loss, nausea, vomiting, and sore throat), brittle and pitted nails, possible low-grade fever, and possible alopecia *Latent syphilis:* • Absence of symptoms	• For early syphilis, treatment may consist of a single injection of penicillin G benzathine I.M. (2.4 million U). • For primary syphilis, erythromycin 30 to 40 g P.O. given in divided doses over a period of 10 to 15 days. • Syphilis of more than 1 year's duration should be treated with penicillin G benzathine I.M. (2.4 million U/ week for 3 weeks). • Patients allergic to penicillin may be treated successfully with erythromycin 500 mg P.O. four times a day for 15 days for early syphilis.

Treatment of sexually transmitted disorders *(continued)*

Disease (causative agent)	Assessment findings	Treatment
Syphilis *(continued)*	*Late syphilis (late benign syphilis, cardiovascular syphilis, and neurosyphilis)* • Any or all may be present • In *late benign syphilis,* the typical lesion is a gumma—a chronic, superficial nodule or deep, granulomatous lesion that is solitary, asymmetrical, painless, and indurated; other possible symptoms of this sub-type—liver involvement, causing epigastric pain, tenderness, enlarged spleen, and anemia; and upper respiratory involvement with potential perforation of the nasal septum or palate • In *cardiovascular syphilis,* the patient may develop aortitis, aortic regurgitation, or aortic aneurysm or may experience no symptoms at all • In *neurosyphilis,* meningitis and widespread central nervous system (CNS) damage typically occur; symptoms of CNS damage; general paresis, personality changes, and arm and leg weakness	
Chancroid ***Hemophilus ducreyi***	• Small papule appears at the site of entry, usually the groin or inner thigh; in the male, it may appear on the penis; in the female, on the vulva, vagina, or cervix (occasionally, may erupt on the tongue, lip, breast, or navel) • Papule rapidly ulcerates, becoming painful, soft, and malodorous; bleeds easily; and produces pus	• Co-trimoxazole usually cures chancroid within 2 weeks. • An alternative to sulfonamides, erythromycin may prevent detection of coexisting syphilis. • Aspiration of fluid-filled nodes helps prevent the infection from spreading. *(continued)*

Treatment of sexually transmitted disorders *(continued)*

Disease (causative agent)	Assessment findings	Treatment
Chancroid *(continued)*	• Gray and shallow, with irregular edges, and measures up to 1″ (2.5 cm) in diameter • Inguinal adenitis (within 2 to 3 weeks), creating suppurated, inflamed nodes that may rupture into large ulcers or buboes • Headache and malaise • Phimosis may develop during the healing stage	

tient, advise the family to take precautions against infection.

To prevent the spread of gonorrhea, tell the patient to avoid anyone suspected of being infected, to use condoms during intercourse, and to avoid sharing washcloths or douche equipment.

Evaluation. The patient should be free from infection and its symptoms.

Chlamydial infections

The most common sexually transmitted disorders in the United States, chlamydial infections include urethritis in men, cervicitis in women, and lymphogranuloma venereum (LGV) in both. Because many of these infections may produce no symptoms until late in their development, sexual transmission usually occurs unknowingly.

Left untreated, chlamydial infections can lead to such complications as acute epididymitis, salpingitis, PID and, eventually, sterility. In pregnant women, chlamydial infections are also associated with spontaneous abortion, premature delivery, and neonatal death, although a direct link with *Chlamydia trachomatis* hasn't been established. Children born of infected mothers may contract trachoma, otitis media, and pneumonia during passage through the birth canal.

Diagnostic tests. A swab culture from the infection site (urethra, cervix, or rectum) usually establishes the diagnosis of urethritis, cervicitis, salpingitis, endometritis, or proctitis.

Culture of aspirated blood, pus, or cerebrospinal fluid (CSF) establishes the diagnosis of epididymitis, prostatitis, or LGV.

Direct visualization of cell scrapings or exudate with Giemsa stain or fluorescein-conjugated monoclonal antibodies may be attempted, but tissue cell cultures are more sensitive and specific.

Serologic tests to determine previous exposure to *C. trachomatis* include complement fixation and microimmunofluorescence tests.

Nursing interventions. Take steps to prevent contracting a chlamydial infection by using standard precautions. Double-bag all soiled dressings and contaminated instruments. Wear gloves when handling contaminated material and giving patient care at the infection site.

Check neonates of infected mothers for signs of infection. Take specimens for culture from the infant's eyes, nasopharynx, and rectum. (Positive rectal cultures will peak by 5 to 6 weeks postpartum.)

Urge the patient to inform sexual contacts of his infection so they can seek treatment. Report all cases to local public health authorities for follow-up on sexual contacts.

Patient education. Make sure the patient understands dosage requirements of prescribed medications. Stress the importance of completing the course of drug therapy even after symptoms subside.

To prevent reinfection, urge the patient to abstain from intercourse or to use a condom. Advise the patient to continue condom use unless in a mutually monogamous relationship with a partner who has

CHARTING TIPS

Documenting infectious diseases

Various federal agencies require documentation of infections so that data can be assessed and used for preventing and controlling future infections. Also, proper documentation helps your health care facility meet national and local accreditation standards.

Typically you must report any culture result that shows a positive infection to your facility's infection control department. Additionally, with sexually transmitted diseases, local public health authorities must be contacted for follow-up on the patient's sexual contacts.

Document the signs and symptoms of the infection as well as the steps you take to prevent its spread. Always follow standard precautions and be sure to document that you've done so.

tested for *C. trachomatis* and has had a negative reaction.

Evaluation. The patient should be free from signs and symptoms including lesions, discharges, pain, fever, enlarged nodes, or recurrent infections.

Trichomoniasis

Trichomoniasis is a protozoal infection of the lower genitourinary tract. Most commonly spread by sexual contact, trichomoniasis may also be spread by contaminated douche equipment or moist washcloths or, if the mother is infected, by vaginal delivery. In females, the condition may be acute or chronic. Recurrence of trichomoniasis is minimized when sexual partners are treated concurrently.

Risk factors for infection include pregnancy, bacterial overgrowth, exudative vaginal or cervical lesions, frequent douching, and use of oral contraceptives.

Diagnostic tests. Direct microscopic examination of vaginal or seminal discharge is diagnostic when it reveals *Trichomonas vaginalis*. Urine specimens that are clear may also reveal *T. vaginalis*. A cytologic cervical smear may be abnormal in untreated trichomoniasis.

Nursing interventions. To prevent neonates from contracting trichomoniasis, make sure that pregnant females who are infected with this disease receive adequate treatment before delivery.

Patient education. Instruct the patient not to douche before being examined for trichomoniasis. To help prevent reinfection during treatment, urge abstinence from intercourse, or encourage the use of condoms.

Warn the patient to abstain from alcoholic beverages while taking metronidazole because alcohol consumption may cause confusion, headache, cramps, vomiting, and convulsions. Also, tell the patient that this drug may turn urine dark brown.

Caution the female patient to avoid reinfection by contaminated douche equipment. Advise the patient that chronic douching can alter vaginal pH. Tell her she can reduce the risk of genitourinary bacterial growth by wearing loose-fitting, cotton underwear that allows ventilation.

Evaluation. The patient should remain free from vaginal discharge, urinary symptoms, recurrent infection, and any local itching, tenderness, swelling, or redness.

Genital herpes

Also known as HSV2 or venereal herpes, genital herpes is an acute, inflammatory infection that is one of the most common recurring disorders of the genitalia. Primary genital herpes is usually self-limiting but may cause painful local or systemic disease. In neonates, in patients with a weak immune system, and in those with disseminated disease, genital herpes is commonly severe, with complications and a high mortality.

Pregnant women may transmit the infection to their neonates during vaginal delivery. Such transmitted infection may be localized (for instance, in the eyes) or disseminated and may be associated with CNS involvement.

Complications are rare and usually arise from extragenital lesions. These include hepatic keratitis, which may lead to blindness, and potentially fatal herpes simplex encephalitis.

Diagnostic tests. Demonstration of HSV2 in vesicular fluid, using tissue culture techniques, confirms genital herpes. Other helpful but nondiagnostic measures include laboratory data showing increased antibody titers and atypical cells in smears of genital lesions.

Nursing interventions. Encourage the patient to get adequate rest and nutrition and to keep the lesions dry, except for applying prescribed medications (using aseptic technique). Make sure the infected pregnant patient understands the risk to her neonate from vaginal delivery. Most doctors will perform cesarean section if cultures are positive at due date.

Patient education. Focus your teaching on helping the patient avoid subsequent infection and preventing the spread of disease. Encourage him to avoid sexual intercourse during the active stage of this disease (while lesions are present). Urge the patient to refer his sexual partners for medical examination. Advise the female patient to have a Pap smear taken every 6 months. Also encourage good nutrition, adequate rest, and stress reduction to help reduce subsequent outbreaks. Finally, refer the patient to the Herpes Resource Center, an American Social Health Association group, for support.

Evaluation. Note whether the patient can effectively manage symptoms and if he takes steps to prevent the spread of infection.

Genital warts

Also known as condylomata acuminata, genital warts consist of papillomas with fibrous tissue overgrowth from the dermis and thickened epithelial coverings.

Diagnostic tests. Dark-field examination of scrapings from wart cells shows marked vascularization of epidermal cells, which helps differentiate genital warts from condylomata lata of secondary syphilis.

Nursing interventions. Nursing care consists primarily of careful patient teaching after treatment.

Patient education. Tell the patient to wash off podophyllum with soap and water 4 to 6 hours after applying it. Recommend use of a condom during intercourse until healing is complete. Advise the patient to protect the surrounding tissue with petrolatum before using trichloroacetic acid.

Emphasize other preventive measures, such as avoiding sex with an infected partner and regularly washing genitalia with soap and water. To prevent vaginal infection, advise the female patient to avoid feminine hygiene sprays, frequent douching, tight pants, nylon underpants, or pantyhose.

Encourage examination of the patient's sexual partners. Also advise female patients to have a Pap smear taken every 6 months.

Evaluation. The patient should be free from genital warts or associated infections. The patient should understand the need for careful hygiene and other preventive measures to avoid reinfection.

Syphilis

Syphilis is a chronic, infectious venereal disease that begins in the mucous membranes and quickly becomes systemic. The disorder spreads by sexual contact during the primary, secondary, and early latent stages of infection; it may also be spread to the neonate through the placenta.

Diagnostic tests. Culture of a lesion, identifying *Treponema pallidum,* confirms the diagnosis in primary, secondary, and prenatal syphilis.

The fluorescent treponemal antibody absorption test identifies antigens of *T. pallidum* in tissue, ocular fluid, CSF, tracheobronchial secretions, and exudates from lesions in all stages of syphilis.

The Venereal Disease Research Laboratory (VDRL) slide test and rapid plasma reagin test detect nonspecific antibodies.

CSF examination identifies neurosyphilis when the total protein level is above 40 mg/dl, the VDRL slide test is reactive, and the cell count exceeds 5 mononuclear cells/mm³.

Nursing interventions. Check any syphilis patient for a history of drug sensitivity before giving the first dose of medication. Make sure the patient clearly understands the dosage schedule. Promote rest and adequate nutrition.

In secondary syphilis, keep lesions clean and dry. If they're draining, dispose of contaminated materials properly. In late syphilis, provide symptomatic care during prolonged treatment.

In cardiovascular syphilis, check for signs and symptoms of decreased cardiac output (decreased urine output, hypoxia, or decreased sensorium) and pulmonary congestion. In neurosyphilis, regularly check level of consciousness, mood, and coherence. Watch for signs of ataxia.

Finally, be sure to report all cases of syphilis to local public health authorities.

Patient education. Stress the importance of completing the course of therapy even after symptoms subside. Urge the patient to seek VDRL testing after 3, 6, 12, and 24 months to detect a possible relapse. Patients treated for latent or late syphilis should receive blood tests at 6-month intervals for 2 years. Finally, urge the patient to inform sexual partners of his infection so they can receive treatment.

Evaluation. The patient should remain asymptomatic without any recurrent infections and should know how to prevent spreading the infection.

Chancroid

Chancroid, also called soft chancre, is a venereal disorder marked by painful genital ulcers and inguinal adenitis. Although it occurs worldwide, the infection is especially common in tropical countries.

Diagnostic tests. Gram stain smears of ulcer exudate or bubo aspirate are 50% reliable; blood agar cultures are 75% reliable. Biopsy confirms the diagnosis but is reserved for resistant cases or those in which cancer is suspected.

Dark-field examination and serologic testing rule out other venereal diseases (such as genital herpes, syphilis, or LGV), which cause similar ulcers.

Nursing interventions. Make sure the patient isn't allergic to sulfonamides or any other prescribed drug before giving the initial dose.

Patient education. Instruct the patient not to apply creams, lotions, or oils on or near genitalia or on other lesion sites. Tell the patient to abstain from sexual contact until healing is complete (usually about 2 weeks after treatment begins) and to wash the genitalia daily with soap and water. Instruct uncircumcised males to retract the foreskin to thoroughly clean the glans penis.

To prevent chancroid, advise patients to avoid sexual contact with infected persons, to use condoms during sexual activity, and to wash the genitalia with soap and water after sexual activity.

Evaluation. The patient should be rid of his chancroid and free from other symptoms, such as headache or malaise. Infection should not recur. The patient should know how to avoid transmitting this disorder.

TREATMENTS

To provide effective care for a patient with a reproductive disorder, you'll need a working knowledge of current drug therapy, surgery, and related treatments. Keep in mind that these disorders commonly place your patient under enormous social and psychological stress. Your ability to maintain a caring, nonjudgmental attitude will prove especially valuable.

Drug therapy

Drugs represent the treatment of choice for many reproductive disorders. For example, estrogens such as dienestrol and DES treat many disorders associated with estrogen deficiency. Gonadotropins such as menotropins and gonadotropin treat certain forms of infertility. And fertility agents such as clomiphene may help childless couples conceive successfully.

Surgery

Women with gynecologic disorders must commonly undergo surgery. Types of gynecologic surgery include D&C, hysterectomy, and laparoscopy and laparotomy.

Dilatation and curettage or evacuation

In these most common gynecologic procedures, the doctor expands or dilates the cervix to access the endocervix and uterus. In D&C, he uses a curette to scrape endometrial tissue; in dilatation and evacuation (D&E), he applies suction to extract the uterine contents.

D&C provides treatment for an incomplete abortion, controls abnormal uterine bleeding, and can secure an endometrial or endocervical tissue sample for cytologic study. D&E can also be used for an incomplete or a therapeutic abortion, usually up to 12 weeks of gestation but occasionally as late as 16 weeks.

Potential complications of these surgeries include uterine perforation, hemorrhage, and infection. If cervical trauma occurs during these procedures, it may affect subsequent pregnancies. Rarely, such trauma can lead to spontaneous abortion, cervical incompetence, or premature birth. These surgeries should be avoided in acute infection.

Patient preparation. Be sure that the patient has followed preoperative directions for fasting and has used an enema to empty the colon before admission. Remind her that she'll be groggy after the procedure and won't be able to drive. Make sure that she has arranged transportation.

Ask the patient to void before you administer any preoperative medications, such as meperidine or diazepam. Start I.V. fluids, as ordered (either dextrose 5% in water or normal saline solution), to facilitate administration of the anesthetic. For D&C or D&E, the patient may receive a general anesthetic, a regional paracervical block, or a local anesthetic.

Monitoring and aftercare. After surgery, give analgesics, as ordered. Expect the patient to have moderate cramping and pelvic and low back pain, but be sure to report any continuous, sharp abdominal pain that doesn't respond to analgesics; this may indicate perforation of the uterus.

Monitor the patient for hemorrhage and signs of infection such as purulent, foul-smelling vaginal drainage. Also monitor the color and volume of urine; hematuria indicates infection. Report any of these signs immediately.

Administer fluids as tolerated, and allow food if the patient requests it. Keep the bed rails raised, and help the patient walk to the bathroom if appropriate.

Patient education. Instruct the patient to report any signs of infection. She should avoid using tampons and bathing in a tub because these increase the infection risk. Tell her to use analgesics to control pain but to report any unrelenting sharp pain. Spotting and discharge may last a week or longer (up to 4 weeks after an abortion). Tell her to report any bright red blood.

Advise the patient to schedule an appointment with the doctor for a routine checkup. Tell her to resume activity as tolerated, but remind her to follow her doctor's instructions for vigorous exercise and sexual intercourse. They're usually discouraged until 2 weeks after the follow-up visit. Encourage her to seek birth control counseling, if needed, and refer her to an appropriate center.

Hysterectomy

Hysterectomy involves removal of the uterus. Although it can be performed using a vaginal or an abdominal approach, the latter approach allows better visualization of the pelvic organs and a larger operating field. The vaginal approach may be used to repair relaxed pelvic structures, such as cystocele or rectocele, at the same time as hysterectomy. (See *Managing total abdominal hysterectomy,* pages 694 to 697.)

Hysterectomy may be classified as total, subtotal, or radical. A *total* hysterectomy (panhysterectomy) involves removal of the entire uterus, whereas a *subtotal* one removes only a portion of the uterus, leaving the cervical stump intact. (See *Types of hysterectomy,* page 698.) Both surgeries are commonly performed for uterine myomas or endometrial disease. They may also be performed postpartum if the placenta fails to separate from the uterus after a cesarean delivery or if amnionitis is present. A *radical* hysterectomy, the treatment of choice for cervical carcinoma, removes all the reproductive organs.

Complications of hysterectomy commonly reflect the surgical approach. With a vaginal hysterectomy, complications are few, although perineal infection is possible. More serious complications may occur with the abdominal approach, including infection, urine retention, abdominal distention, thrombophlebitis, atelectasis, and pneumonia. Major complications of a radical hysterectomy include the formation of ureteral fistulas and cystic lymphangiomas, pelvic infection, and hemorrhage.

Patient preparation. The patient may enter the health care facility on the day of surgery or 1 day before. Take this opportunity to discuss with the patient her expectations about her menstrual and reproductive status after surgery.

Review the surgical approach and the extent of the excision. To prepare the patient for an abdominal hysterectomy, tell her to expect a cleansing enema and a douche the evening before surgery, a shower with an antibacterial soap, and a shave prep. Explain that urine retention commonly occurs after surgery, requiring an indwelling urinary catheter. If the patient develops abdominal distention, she may have a nasogastric (NG) or rectal tube inserted. Explain that temporary abdominal cramping and pelvic and low back pain occur normally after the procedure.

Tell the patient scheduled for a vaginal hysterectomy that she may experience abdominal cramping and moderate amounts of drainage postoperatively and that she'll have a perineal pad in place.

Inform the patient that after surgery, she'll lie in a supine or a low to mid-Fowler's position. Demonstrate the exercises that she'll need to do to prevent venous stasis.

Monitoring and aftercare. If the patient has had a vaginal hysterecto-
(Text continues on page 696.)

Managing total abdominal hysterectomy

REPRODUCTIVE CARE LOS: 3 days DRG:	Date of surgery:
	Date: Day of surgery
Transition	• Report from recovery room nurse • Review of medical history • Orientation to unit
Consults	As requested _____ _____ _____
Tests	• Complete blood count (CBC) ordered for postoperative Day 1 _____ OR • Hemoglobin and hematocrit postoperative Day 1_____ • Other _____(as ordered)
Treatments	• Compression stockings ordered as needed (p.r.n.) _____ • Abdominal binder p.r.n. • Heating pad p.r.n. • Intake and output (I & O) • Indwelling urinary catheter
Assessment	• Check vaginal bleeding every 2 to 4 hrs. • Check dressing on admission and every shift. • Check vital signs (VS) every 4 hrs for 24 hrs. • Check bowel sounds every shift. • Check breath sounds every shift.
Activity	• Bedrest
Nutrition	• Nothing by mouth (NPO) if ordered_____. OR • Clear liquids as allowed and tolerated_____.
Medications and I.V.s	I.V.s _____ • Patient-controlled analgesia or I.M. medications for pain. • Medications for nausea and vomiting p.r.n.

Date: Postoperative Day 1	Date: Postoperative Day 2
• Continue unit orientation.	• Discharge
• Blood work done. Report results to doctor.	
• Compression stockings p.r.n.; discontinue when ambulating _____. • Continue abdominal binder p.r.n. if ordered. • Continue heating pad p.r.n. if ordered. • Discontinue I & O 24 hrs after I.V. and indwelling urinary discontinued. • Rectal tube if ordered _____	• Discontinue compression stockings prior to discharge (PTD). • Discontinue abdominal binder PTD. • Discontinue heating pad PTD. • Voiding adequate PTD. • Discontinue rectal tube PTD.
• Check vaginal bleeding every shift. • Check dressing every shift. Remove dressing. Redress if necessary. • Check VS every shift. • Check bowel sounds every shift. • Check breath sounds every shift.	• No excessive bleeding at discharge • Assess the incision PTD. Notify doctor of any problems. • Afebrile (100° F or less) • VS within expected parameters • Expelling flatus • Bowel sounds PTD • Clear breath sounds PTD
• Out of bed with help. Encourage to resume self-care. • Shower if incision dry.	• Resume self-care by discharge. • Shower PTD.
• Clear liquids to house diet as tolerated	• House diet at discharge
• I.V.s discontinued • Pain medications as needed • Other medications as needed	• Pain controlled at discharge • Discharge prescriptions given p.r.n. PTD • Dulcolax suppository PTD (if no bowel movement)

	Date: Day of surgery:
Medications and I.V.s *(continued)*	• Antibiotics if ordered
Family interactions	• Evaluate patient's psychosocial needs. • Verify advance directive.
Patient teaching	• Unit orientation • Daily care routines • Evaluate patient's teaching needs.
Discharge planning	Preoperative • Assess discharge needs, including home care follow-up. • Continue discharge planning postoperatively.

Adapted with permission from Holy Redeemer Hospital and Medical Center, Huntingdon Valley, Pa.

my, change her perineal pad frequently. Provide analgesics to relieve cramps.

If the patient has had an abdominal hysterectomy, tell her to remain in a supine or a low to mid-Fowler's position. Encourage her to perform the prescribed exercises and to ambulate early and frequently to prevent venous stasis. Monitor her urine output because retention commonly occurs.

If abdominal distention develops, relieve it by inserting an NG or rectal tube, as ordered. Note bowel sounds during routine assessment.

Patient education. If the patient has had a vaginal hysterectomy, instruct her to report severe cramping, heavy bleeding, or hot flashes (common with oophorectomy) to her doctor immediately.

If she has had an abdominal procedure, tell her to avoid heavy lifting, rapid walking, or dancing, which can cause pelvic congestion. Encourage her to walk a little more each day and to avoid sitting for a prolonged period. Tell her that swimming is permissible.

Advise any patient who's had a hysterectomy to eat a high-protein, high-residue diet to avoid constipation, which may increase abdominal pressure. Her doctor may also order increased fluid intake (3 qt [3 L]/day).

Advise the patient to express her feelings about her altered body image and to contact the doctor if she has questions. Mention that the

Date: Postoperative Day 1	Date: Postoperative Day 2
• Prophylactic antibiotics discontinued after 24 hr. • Dulcolax suppository p.r.n.	
• Patient expresses adaptive responses to surgery.	• Patient expresses adaptive responses to surgery.
Continue teaching: • Hydration: • Nutrition: • Activity: • Independence: • Other:	• Patient verbalizes understanding of all instructions. • Give doctor discharge booklets.
Continue discharge plans for follow-up care.	• Finalize home care plans. • Appointment for follow-up visit

doctor will inform her when she can resume sexual activity (usually 6 weeks after surgery). Explain to the patient and her family that abrupt hormonal fluctuations may cause her to feel depressed or irritable for a little while. She may also experience feelings of loss or depression for up to a year after the surgery. If her ovaries have been removed, the patient will receive hormone replacement therapy, which requires monitoring. Encourage family members to respond calmly and with understanding.

Laparoscopy and laparotomy

Laparoscopy lets the doctor visualize pelvic and upper abdominal organs and peritoneal surfaces. The doctor can also use the laparoscope to insert surgical instruments to remove small lesions with a laser beam or a cryosurgical or an electrocautery device.

If endometrial lesions are too large for removal by laparoscopy, a laparotomy may be performed. Laparotomy also allows the doctor to remove ovarian cysts containing endometrial tissue, thereby averting the risk of rupture.

Possible complications of laparoscopic procedures include excessive bleeding, abdominal cramps, and shoulder pain. Complications of laparotomy may include infection or other complications associated with abdominal surgery.

Patient preparation. Explain laparotomy or the specific laparo-

Types of hysterectomy

There are three types of hysterectomy: subtotal hysterectomy, total hysterectomy, and radical hysterectomy with a salpingo-oophorectomy. The excised portion (shaded in the illustrations below) varies in each one. However, the external genitalia and the vagina are left intact in each procedure, and the woman is able to resume sexual relations.

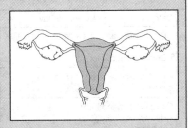

In a total hysterectomy, the entire uterus and the cervix are removed. The woman will no longer menstruate.

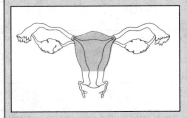

In a subtotal hysterectomy, the uterus is removed except for the distal portion. The woman will continue to menstruate.

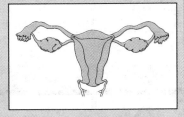

In a radical hysterectomy with a salpingo-oophorectomy, the uterus, the cervix, the fallopian tubes, and the ovaries are removed. The woman will no longer menstruate.

scopic procedure to the patient, and answer any questions she may have. If she'll be undergoing laparoscopic surgery, mention that she'll be discharged the same day, after she recovers from the procedure. If she'll be undergoing laparotomy, prepare her as you would for abdominal surgery. If she'll be having an ovarian cyst resected, determine if she has followed the prescribed preoperative regimen. She may have been given danazol to promote endometrial atrophy, thereby reducing the extent of resection required.

Monitoring and aftercare. After laparoscopy, check for excessive vaginal bleeding, which may indicate hemorrhage; minor bleeding is normal. Ask the patient about abdominal cramps or shoulder pain and provide analgesics, as ordered. If she complains of bloating or abdominal fullness, explain that the feeling will subside as the gas in her abdomen is absorbed into the bloodstream, exchanged in the lungs, and exhaled.

After laparotomy, provide care as you would for a patient who has undergone abdominal surgery. (See *Treating postsurgical pain*, page 700.)

Patient education. If the patient has undergone laparoscopy, emphasize the importance of reporting bright red vaginal bleeding. If she has undergone laparotomy, tell her about activity restrictions. Urge all patients to return for follow-up visits because endometrial implants tend to recur.

Artificial insemination

This section reviews in vivo fertilization, commonly used to achieve conception in cases of infertility.

In vivo fertilization

For in vivo fertilization, the doctor instills seminal fluid into the vaginal canal or cervix. This treatment for infertility may be attempted in obstruction of the male genital tract or in oligospermia. It may also be used if an abnormality in the female reproductive tract keeps sperm from reaching the ovum.

The in vivo technique achieves fertilization differently than the in vitro technique, which uses a culture medium in a laboratory to bond ovum and sperm.

The in vivo technique can use the husband's sperm (if he's fertile) or a donor's. If the husband's sperm is of poor quality or motility, the doctor will collect several samples from him. The spermatozoa-rich first portion from a split ejaculate is used. These samples are frozen, using liquid nitrogen, and later pooled to increase the sperm count.

The in vivo technique achieves conception in about 70% of patients when the husband's sperm is used. When donor sperm is used, the success rate stands at about 50% after 2 months and almost 90% after 6 months. However, multiple trials may be necessary before correctly timing insemination and ovulation.

In vivo fertilization causes few complications. Multiple births are possible but are usually welcomed by a childless couple. Donor semen should be used cautiously because of the risk of spreading AIDS. To help reduce this risk, sperm banks now screen for the human immunodeficiency virus antibody.

Patient preparation. Provide a supportive environment as the couple approaches this treatment. Emotions may run high; the couple has probably been disappointed and frustrated over their inability to have a child. They may have already undergone many tests and procedures. Make it clear that this technique usually makes pregnancy possible but doesn't guarantee it.

Point out that the woman may need several inseminations to achieve conception and that these will be coordinated with ovulation. Teach the patient how to track her basal body temperature and cervical

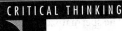

Treating postsurgical pain

Your patient has returned from the postanesthesia recovery care unit and is complaining of pain. You assume that she is referring to abdominal pain from the procedure. After questioning her further, you assess that the location of her pain is in her shoulder. Why is she experiencing shoulder pain from an abdominal procedure?

Suggested response
Laparoscopic surgery requires the instillation of carbon dioxide into the pelvic cavity to separate pelvic organs for better visualization. Because the carbon dioxide cannot be removed from the abdomen, the gas creates pressure in the abdomen, which irritates a branch of the phrenic nerve and causes deferred pain in the shoulder.

Encourage her to engage in mild activity, such as turning from side to side in bed or walking around early in the day to aid in the absorption of the carbon dioxide by the bloodstream. This will also promote a reduction in postoperative abdominal pain and shoulder pain.

mucus or how to use an ovulatory predictor test kit.

Explain to the patient that she may have to remain in the knee-chest position for several hours after the procedure. Inform her that the doctor may apply a cervical cap to prevent leakage of the instilled semen into the vagina. Be supportive to allay any embarrassment and anxiety she may have.

Monitoring and aftercare. Instruct the patient to remain in the knee-chest position for the prescribed period, which may be several hours.

Provide support for the couple as they go through artificial insemination. Keep in mind that they may feel that this treatment represents their last chance to have a child of their own.

Patient education. Encourage counseling for couples who are having difficulty communicating their feelings or who express uncontrollable anger or grief. Remind them to return for follow-up appointments, as necessary.

Prosthetic and mechanical aids

This section covers penile prosthesis implantation.

Penile prosthesis

The penile prosthesis consists of a pair of semirigid rods or inflatable cylinders surgically implanted in the corpora cavernosa of the penis. It's helpful in treating both organic and psychogenic erectile dysfunction. For patients with organic dysfunction, a prosthesis may be the only possible treatment. For those with psychogenic dysfunction, though, it's usually a last resort. Organic dysfunction may result from diabetes, arteriosclerosis, multiple sclerosis, spinal cord injury, or use of alcohol or drugs, such as antihypertensives. Psychogenic dysfunction may result from sexual performance anxiety, low self-esteem, or past failures in sustaining an erection.

A semirigid prosthesis helps the patient with limited hand or finger function because it doesn't demand manual dexterity. However, it's always semi-erect, which may embarrass the patient. Also, some couples complain that the semirigid prosthesis produces an erection that isn't sufficiently stiff to be sexually satisfying.

Compared with the semirigid device, the inflatable prosthesis provides a more natural erection. The patient or partner controls erection by squeezing a small pump in the scrotum that releases radiopaque fluid from a reservoir into the implanted cylinders. However, this device is contraindicated in patients with iodine sensitivity.

Both types of prostheses place the patient at risk for infection, although the incidence ranges from only 1% to 4%. Rarely, the inflatable prosthesis may also leak fluid, or the tubing connecting the pump, reservoir, and cylinders may become kinked.

Patient preparation. Reinforce the doctor's explanation of the surgery and answer any questions. Mention that the prosthesis won't affect ejaculation or orgasmic pleasure; if the patient experienced either before surgery, he'll remain capable after it. Recognize that the patient and his partner are likely to be anxious before surgery, so provide emotional support.

Instruct the patient to shower the evening before and the morning of the surgery, using an antimicrobial soap. Tell him that he'll be shaved in the operating room to reduce the risk of infection. If ordered, begin antibiotic therapy.

Monitoring and aftercare. Apply ice packs to the patient's penis for 24 hours after surgery. Empty the surgical drain when it's full, or as ordered, to reduce the risk of infection. If the patient has an inflatable prosthesis, tell him to pull the scrotal pump downward to ensure proper alignment. With the doctor's approval, encourage the patient to practice inflating and deflating the prosthesis when the pain subsides. Pumping promotes healing of the tissue sheath around the reservoir and the pump.

Patient education. Instruct the patient to wash the incision daily with an antimicrobial soap. Tell him to watch for signs of infection and to report them immediately to the doctor. Scrotal swelling and discoloration may last up to 3 weeks. Stress the importance of returning for all follow-up appointments to ensure that the incision is healing properly.

Warn the couple that they may experience dyspareunia when they're permitted to resume sexual activity—usually about 6 weeks after surgery. This may result from an inability to have intercourse for a prolonged period before surgery. Advise them to use a water-soluble gel to minimize or avoid discomfort. Also, emphasize the need for gentleness and prolonged foreplay to allow for sufficient vaginal lubrication, especially in older women whose lubrication normally decreases with age.

REFERENCES AND READINGS

Diseases, 2nd ed. Springhouse, Pa.: Springhouse Corp., 1997.

Guyton, A. *Textbook of Medical Physiology,* 9th ed. Philadelphia: W.B. Saunders Co., 1996.

McCourty, M.K. "Vaginal Infections: Keys to Treatment," *Contemporary Nurse Practitioner* 7(3):18-23, May/June 1995.

Nursing98 Drug Handbook. Springhouse, Pa.: Springhouse Corp., 1998.

Scarbo-DeHaan, M. "Management Strategies for Hormonal Replacement Therapy," *Contemporary Nurse Practitioner* 19(12):47-57, December 1994.

Taylor, C., et al. *Nursing Diagnosis Pocket Manual.* Springhouse, Pa.: Springhouse Corp., 1996.

13

SKIN CARE

The skin and its appendages (the hair, nails, and certain glands) protect the inner organs, bones, muscles, and blood vessels. They help to regulate body temperature and provide sensory information. What's more, they prevent body fluids from escaping and eliminate body wastes through more than 2 million pores.

This chapter will help you develop expert skin care skills.

ASSESSMENT

Assessment begins with a complete patient history. Remember that skin disorders may involve or stem from other disorders in other body systems. Don't discount minor symptoms or systemic complaints.

Physical examination

Physical assessment of the skin, hair, and nails requires inspection and palpation.

Preparing for skin assessment

Wash your hands and gather the necessary equipment: a bright, even light source; a penlight and tongue blade; centimeter rule; glass slide; flashlight with transilluminator; Wood's lamp (ultraviolet light); and gloves for palpating moist lesions or mucous membranes. (See *Keeping your patient comfortable,* page 704.) Expose areas for inspection and palpation sequentially.

Assessing appearance

Systematically assess all of the skin, hair, nails, and mucous membranes, even if the patient reports only a local lesion. Failure to assess the entire skin surface can lead to incorrect diagnosis.

Be alert for any variations in lesion color, vascular supply, and pattern compared to other lesions. Also check for lesion distribution over the whole body.

Inspection

Begin by observing the patient's overall appearance from a distance of 3' to 6' (0.9 to 1.8 m), noting complexion, general color, color variations, and general appearance.

Note disturbances in pigmentation (light or dark areas compared to the rest of the skin), freckles, moles (nevi), and tanning (usually considered normal variations). Though usually benign, nevi that occur in large numbers (over 40) and are irregular in size, shape, and color may be precursors to melanoma.

Next, note the color of healthy skin as well as problem areas. Rashes or lesions may range from red to brown to hypopigmented (as in vitiligo).

Alterations in skin vasculature usually appear as red or purple pigmented lesions. Some vascular lesions occur in persons in good health. For example, blood vessel hypertrophy (enlargement) may result in hemangiomas, which vary from bright red to purple. Press on the lesion with the lucite rule or glass slide, and observe and note the color change. Ecchymotic areas will remain unchanged when pressure is applied, while areas of dilated blood vessels will blanch (lose color or fade) when compressed. Permanently dilated superficial blood vessels (telangiectasia or spider veins) can indicate disease, but are in many cases normal.

Skin lesions. Carefully observe and document lesion morphology, distribution, and configuration.

Morphology. Note the lesion's size (measure and record its dimensions), shape or configuration, color, elevation or depression, pedunculation (connection to the skin by a stem or stalk), and texture. Note odor, color, consistency, and amount of exudate. Use a flashlight to assess the color of the lesion and elevation of its borders. Use a transilluminator to assess fluid in a lesion by darkening the room and placing the tip of the transilluminator against the side of the lesion; a fluid-filled lesion glows red, whereas a solid lesion does not. Use a Wood's lamp to assess pigmented or depigmented lesions.

Primary skin lesions appear on previously healthy skin in response to disease or external irritation. Modified lesions are described as secondary lesions. (See *Recognizing skin lesions.*)

Distribution. Assessment of distribution includes the extent and pattern of involvement. Is the pattern of lesions local (in one small

Recognizing skin lesions

The illustrations below depict the most common primary and secondary lesions.

Primary lesions

Bulla
Fluid-filled lesion greater than 3/4″ (2 cm) in diameter (also called a blister)—for example, severe poison oak or ivy dermatitis, bullous pemphigoid, second-degree burn

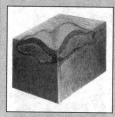

Macule
Flat, pigmented, circumscribed area less than 3/8″ (1 cm) in diameter—for example, a freckle, rubella

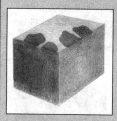

Nodule
Firm, raised lesion; deeper than a papule, extending into dermal layer; 1/4″ to 3/4″ (6 mm to 2 cm) in diameter—for example, intradermal nevus

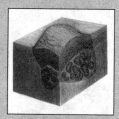

Papule
Firm, inflammatory, raised lesion up to 1/4″ (6 mm) in diameter; may be same color as skin or pigmented—for example, acne papule, lichen planus

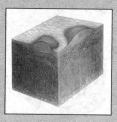

Patch
Flat, pigmented, circumscribed area greater than 3/8″ (1 cm) in diameter—for example, herald patch

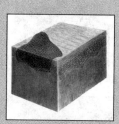

Plaque
Circumscribed, solid, elevated lesion greater than 3/8″ (1 cm) in diameter. Elevation above skin surface occupies larger surface area in comparison with height—for example, psoriasis

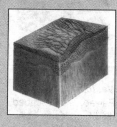

Pustule
Raised, circumscribed lesion usually less than 3/8″ (1 cm) in diameter; contains purulent material, making it a yellow-white color—for example, acne pustule, impetigo, furuncle

(continued)

Recognizing skin lesions *(continued)*

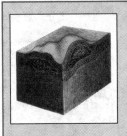

Secondary lesions
Crust
Dried sebum, serous, sanguineous, or purulent exudate, overlying an erosion or weeping vesicle, bulla, or pustule—for example, impetigo

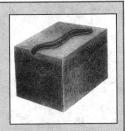

Tumor
Elevated solid lesion larger than 3/4″ (2 cm) in diameter, extending into dermal and subcutaneous layers—for example, dermatofibroma

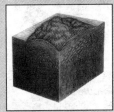

Fissure
Linear cracking of the skin extending into the dermal layer—for example, hand dermatitis (chapped skin)

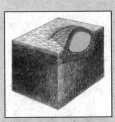

Erosion
Circumscribed lesion involving loss of superficial epidermis—for example, rug burn, abrasion

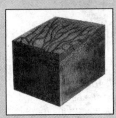

Lichenification
Thickened, prominent skin markings caused by constant rubbing—for example, chronic atopic dermatitis

Vesicle
Raised, circumscribed, fluid-filled lesion less than 1/4″ (0.5 cm) in diameter—for example, herpes simplex

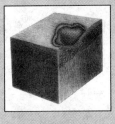

Excoriation
Linear scratched or abraded areas, often self-induced—for example, abraded acne lesions, eczema

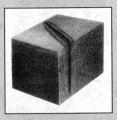

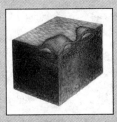

Recognizing skin lesions (continued)

Scale
Thin, dry flakes of shedding skin—for example, psoriasis, dry skin, newborn desquamation

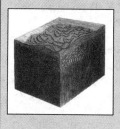

Scar
Fibrous tissue caused by trauma, deep inflammation, or surgical incision; red and raised (recent), pink and flat (6 weeks), or pale and depressed (old)—for example, a healed surgical incision

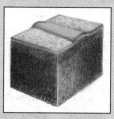

Ulcer
Epidermal and dermal destruction, may extend into subcutaneous tissue; usually heals with scarring—for example, pressure sore or stasis ulcer

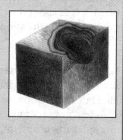

area), regional (in one large area), or general (over the entire body)? Also note characteristic locations, such as dermatomes (along cutaneous nerve endings), flexor or extensor surfaces, intertriginous areas, clothing or jewelry lines, or palms or soles, or if they appear randomly.

Configuration. Is the pattern of lesions discrete (separate), grouped, linear, annular (circular), or arciform (arranged in a curve or arc)? Also note polycyclic (two or more circles of lesions) and herpetiform (along the course of cutaneous nerves) configurations.

Palpation

Assess skin texture, consistency, temperature, moisture, and turgor. Also use palpation to evaluate changes or tenderness of particular lesions.

Texture and consistency. Skin texture refers to smoothness or coarseness; consistency refers to changes in skin thickness or firmness and relates more to changes associated with lesions.

While assessing texture and consistency, lightly rub the patient's skin. If it sloughs, leaving a moist base, this is a positive Nikolsky's sign, which characterizes staphylococcal scalded skin syndrome and other blistering conditions.

Temperature. The skin should feel warm to cool, and areas should feel the same bilaterally. A localized area of warmth may indicate a bacterial infection such as cellulitis.

Turgor. Assess turgor by gently grasping and pulling up a fold of skin, releasing it, and observing how quickly it returns to normal shape. Normal skin usually resumes its flat shape immediately. Poor turgor may indicate dehydration and connective tissue disorders.

Lesions. Palpate skin lesions to obtain details about their morphology, distribution, location, and configuration.

Hair and scalp. Note the quantity, texture, color, and distribution of hair. Hair distribution varies greatly. Rub a few strands of hair between your index finger and thumb. Feel for dryness, brittleness, oiliness, and thickness.

Nails. Inspect the nails for color, consistency, smoothness, symmetry, and freedom from ridges and cracks as well as for length, jagged or bitten edges, and cleanliness.

Assess the nail base for firmness and the nail for firm adherence to the nail bed; sponginess and swelling accompany infection.

DIAGNOSTIC TESTS

Several studies may help differentiate various integumentary disorders. These studies include the patch test, skin biopsy, Gram stain and culture, potassium hydroxide (KOH) preparation, Tzanck test, and phototesting. (For more information, see *Diagnostic tests for skin disorders.*)

NURSING DIAGNOSES

When caring for patients with skin disorders, you'll find that several nursing diagnoses are commonly used. These diagnoses appear below, along with expected outcomes, appropriate nursing interventions and rationales. (Rationales appear in italic type.)

Impaired skin integrity

Related to illness, impaired skin integrity can be associated with bacterial and fungal infections, parasitic infestations, follicular and glandular disorders, inflammatory reactions, and other skin disorders.

Expected outcomes

• Patient's skin condition is assessed and findings are documented.
• Patient's skin integrity improves in response to treatment and supportive measures—for example, pressure ulcer decreases in size (specify).
• Patient communicates understanding of skin protective measures.
• Patient demonstrates skill in care of wound, burn, or incision.
• Patient performs skin care routine.

Nursing interventions and rationales

• Inspect the patient's skin daily and document findings. *Early detection prevents or minimizes skin breakdown.*
• Perform prescribed treatment regimen and monitor progress. Report responses to treatment regimen *to maintain or modify current therapies as needed.*
• Apply bed cradle *to protect lesions from bedcovers.*

Diagnostic tests for skin disorders

Tests	Purpose	Nursing considerations
Patch test	To identify the cause of allergic contact sensitization	• Explain the procedure. • Make applications to normal, hairless skin on the back or ventral surface of the forearm. • Apply potential allergens to a small disk of filter paper attached to aluminum and coated with plastic and tape to the skin. • Apply liquids and ointments to the disk. Apply volatile liquids to the skin and allow to dry before covering. Powder solids and moisten before applying them. • Alternatively, you can use a ready-to-use patch for testing 24 of the most common allergens and allergen mixes. • Patches should remain in place for 48 hours. However, remove immediately if pain, pruritus, or irritation develops. • Check findings 72 to 96 hours after patch application for the possibility of a delayed reaction.
Skin biopsy	To provide differential diagnosis among skin carcinomas and benign growth; diagnose chronic bacterial or fungal skin infections	• Explain the procedure. • Position the patient and cleanse the biopsy site. • Explain that he'll receive a local anesthetic. • After the procedure, apply pressure to the site to stop bleeding, if necessary, and apply a dressing. • Advise the patient with sutures to keep the area as clean and dry as possible. • Advise the patient with adhesive strips to leave them in place for 14 to 21 days.
Gram stain and cultures	Gram stain: to separate bacteria into classification according to the composition of cell walls; cultures: to provide firm identification of the organisms	• Explain the procedure. • To obtain a specimen, roll a cotton-tipped applicator over a lesion or exudate, from the center outward. • If lesions are vesicular, aspirate fluid from the vesicle with a 25G needle. • Transport the culture to the laboratory immediately. *(continued)*

Diagnostic tests for skin disorders *(continued)*

Test	Purpose	Nursing considerations
KOH preparation	To help identify fungal skin infections	• Explain the procedure and the need to remain still. • Gently scrape the border of a rash or skin lesion with a sterile scalpel blade. • After scraping, inspect the area for bleeding and apply light pressure if necessary.
Tzanck test	To help confirm herpes virus infection	• Explain the procedure and the need to remain still. • Unroof intact vesicle, using a sterile blade, scraping the base of the lesion to obtain fluid and skin cells. • Apply the specimen to a glass slide and stain.
Phototesting	To help evaluate a patient's photosensitivity with compounds on his skin	• Explain the procedure and that he should expect to see minimal erythema 24 hours after exposure to phototesting. • Tell the patient to notify the doctor immediately if a generalized reaction occurs, such as general erythema, fever or nausea. • Encourage the patient to follow through with the full course of testing, as necessary. • Instruct him to avoid additional sun exposure during phototesting and to apply sunscreen to any exposed skin.

• Discuss precipitating factors, if known. *This helps patients reduce the occurrence and severity of skin reactions.*

• Instruct the patient and family in skin care regimen *to ensure compliance.*

• Supervise the patient and family in skin care regimen. Provide feedback. *Practice helps improve skill in managing skin care regimen.*

Risk for infection

Related to impaired skin integrity, risk for infection may also apply to any condition that impairs the skin's ability to protect against invasion by microorganisms.

Expected outcomes

• Patient's temperature stays within normal range.

• White blood cell count and differential stay within normal range.

• No pathogens appear in cultures.
• Patient maintains good personal and oral hygiene.
• Wounds and incisions appear clean, pink, and free from purulent drainage.
• I.V. sites show no signs of inflammation.
• Patient shows no evidence of skin breakdown.
• Patient receives the prescribed amount of fluid and protein daily.
• Patient identifies risk factors and signs and symptoms of infection.

Nursing interventions and rationales

• Minimize the patient's risk of infection by using proper hand washing and universal precautions when providing direct care. *Hand washing is the single best way to avoid spreading pathogens.*
• Monitor the patient's temperature at least every 4 hours, and record it on graph paper. Report elevations immediately. *Sustained postoperative fever may signal onset of pulmonary complications, wound infection or dehiscence, urinary infection, or thrombophlebitis.*
• Culture urine, respiratory secretions, wound drainage, or blood according to policy and doctor's orders. *This procedure identifies pathogens and guides antibiotic therapy.*
• Use strict aseptic technique when providing wound care *to avoid spreading pathogens.*
• Help the patient turn every 2 hours. Provide skin care, particularly over bony prominences, *to help*

prevent venous stasis and skin breakdown.
• Ensure adequate nutritional intake. Offer high-protein supplements unless contraindicated *to aid healing, help stabilize weight, and improve muscle tone and mass.*
• Educate the patient regarding good hand-washing technique, factors that increase infection risk, and infection signs and symptoms. *These measures help modify the patient's lifestyle to maintain optimum health level.*

Altered protection

Altered protection relates to itching, perspiring, pressure sores, immobility, or impaired healing or immunity.

Expected outcomes

• Patient has no chills, fever, or other signs and symptoms of illness.
• Patient demonstrates personal cleanliness.
• Patient uses protective measures, including conservation of energy, balanced diet, and adequate rest.
• Patient demonstrates increased strength and resistance.
• Patient's immunity improves.

Nursing interventions and rationales

• Assess patients at risk for decubitus ulcer formation *to prevent skin breakdown.*
• Employ universal precautions *to protect caregivers and patients from infection.*
• Administer antipruritic medications; use emollients and mild soaps and shampoo *to prevent skin breakdown and to reduce itching.*

• Encourage patients not to scratch *to avoid skin injury.*
• Change wet or soiled clothing or linen *to prevent skin maceration, irritation, and infection.*
• Turn patients every 2 hours and encourage activity and frequent changes of position *to promote circulation and healing and to prevent sores.*
• Maintain a comfortable environmental temperature *to prevent perspiring.*

Body image disturbance

Related to dermatologic condition, body image disturbance is extremely important when caring for patients with skin conditions. Unlike internal disorders, a skin condition is usually obvious and disfiguring. Such disorders can create tremendous psychological problems.

Expected outcomes

• Patient acknowledges change in body image.
• Patient participates in aspects of care and decisions about care.
• Patient communicates feelings regarding change in body image.
• Patient participates in a rehabilitation program and counseling.
• Patient identifies limitations and develops strategies to compensate for loss.
• Patient demonstrates ability to use new coping mechanisms.
• Patient engages in social interactions and can discuss deficit if confronted in a social setting.

Nursing interventions and rationales

• Encourage patients to express their feelings. *Active listening is the most basic therapeutic skill.*
• Emphasize any improvements in condition *to help improve the patient's outlook and self-esteem.*
• Encourage the patient to meet others with similar conditions. Refer him to a support group, if available. *This encourages more effective coping.*

DISORDERS

This section covers common skin disorders and includes information on causes, assessment findings, treatment, nursing interventions, patient education, and evaluation criteria.

Bacterial infections

Bacterial infections include impetigo, folliculitis, furunculosis, carbunculosis, and cellulitis.

Impetigo

Impetigo is a contagious, superficial, vesiculopustular eruptive disorder, which occurs in nonbullous and bullous forms. It can complicate skin conditions marked by open lesions such as chickenpox.

Causes. Beta-hemolytic streptococcus produces nonbullous impetigo. Coagulase-positive *Staphylococcus aureus* causes bullous impetigo.

Poor hygiene, anemia, malnutrition, and impaired skin integrity increase the risk of developing this disease.

Assessment findings. Streptococcal impetigo usually begins with a small red macule that turns into a vesicle, becoming pustular in a few hours. When the vesicle breaks, a thick, honey-colored crust forms from the exudate. Autoinoculation may cause satellite lesions. Other symptoms are pruritus, burning, and regional lymphadenopathy.

In staphylococcal impetigo, a thin-walled vesicle opens and a thin, clear crust forms from the exudate. The lesion consists of a central clearing circumscribed by an outer rim and commonly appears on the face or other exposed areas. It causes painless pruritus.

Diagnostic tests. Characteristic lesions suggest impetigo. Microscopic visualization of the causative organism in a Gram stain of vesicle fluid usually confirms infection.

Culture and sensitivity testing of fluid or denuded skin may indicate the most appropriate antibiotic, but therapy should not be delayed for laboratory results.

Treatment. Mupirocin applied three times a day for 7 to 10 days is usually effective. Widespread or recalcitrant impetigo should be treated with 10 days of a penicillinase-resistant penicillin or erythromycin. Lesions should be soaked 3 to 4 times a day with warm tap water, saline, or soap solution to remove crusts.

Nursing interventions. If this infection is present in a school-age child, notify his school. In addition, check the patient's family members for impetigo. Give medications, as ordered; check for penicillin allergy.

Patient education. Focus your teaching on helping the patient or family learn to care for impetiginous lesions. Urge the patient not to scratch because this exacerbates impetigo. Have parents cut the child's fingernails. Stress the need for the patient to continue taking the prescribed medications 7 to 10 days after lesions have healed.

Encourage frequent bathing using an antiseptic soap. Tell the patient not to share linens with family members. Emphasize the importance of proper handwashing techniques.

Evaluation. Assess whether the patient has completed the prescribed course of antibiotics and if any of his family members or other contacts have developed skin lesions. Evaluate whether skin lesions have resolved.

Folliculitis, furunculosis, and carbunculosis

A bacterial infection of the hair follicle, folliculitis causes pustule formation. Folliculitis may lead to the development of furuncles (furunculosis), commonly known as boils, or carbuncles (carbunculosis), especially if exacerbated by irritation, pressure, friction, or perspiration. Prognosis depends on the infection's severity and on the patient's condition and ability to resist infection. (See *Bacterial skin infection: A question of degree*, page 714.)

Bacterial skin infection: A question of degree

Degree of hair follicle involvement in bacterial skin infection ranges from superficial folliculitis (erythema and pustule in a single follicle), to deep folliculitis (extensive follicular involvement), to furuncles (red, tender nodules surrounding follicles with single draining points) and, finally, to carbuncles (deep abscesses involving several follicles with multiple draining points).

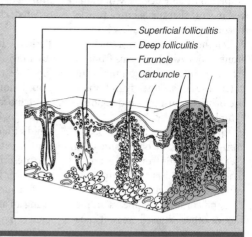

- Superficial folliculitis
- Deep folliculitis
- Furuncle
- Carbuncle

Cause. Coagulase-positive *S. aureus* is the most common cause. Risk factors include an infected wound elsewhere on the body, poor personal hygiene, debilitation, diabetes, exposure to chemicals (cutting oils), and management of skin lesions with tar or with occlusive therapy, using steroids.

Assessment findings. In folliculitis, pustules usually appear on the scalp, arms, and legs; on the faces of bearded men (sycosis barbae); and on the eyelids (styes). Pain may occur with deep folliculitis.

In furunculosis, the patient develops hard, painful nodules (furuncles), commonly appearing on the neck, face, axillae, and buttocks. After enlarging for several days, they rupture, discharging pus and necrotic material. Pain subsides after rupture. Erythema and edema may last several weeks.

In carbunculosis, the patient develops extremely painful, deep abscesses. These drain through multiple openings onto the skin surface, usually around several hair follicles. Associated findings include fever and malaise.

Diagnostic tests. Wound culture shows *S. aureus*.

Treatment. Folliculitis calls for cleaning the infected area thoroughly with soap and water; applying warm, wet compresses to promote vasodilation and drainage of infected material; cleaning with antibacterial soaps such as chlorhexidine; and, in recurrent infection, systemic antibiotics.

Furuncles may also require incision and drainage of ripe lesions after application of hot, wet compresses and topical antibiotics after drainage. Carbunculosis and furunculosis associated with a surrounding cellulitis requires systemic antibiotics.

Nursing interventions. Expect to provide supportive care with an emphasis on thorough patient education.

Patient education. Major topics should include scrupulous personal and family hygiene, and precautions to prevent spreading infection.

Caution the patient never to squeeze a boil because of possible rupture. To avoid spreading bacteria to family members, urge the patient not to share his towel and washcloth. Tell him that these items should be washed in hot water before being reused. Remind him to change dressings frequently and to discard them promptly in paper bags.

Evaluation. The patient's skin lesions should resolve. Erythema, pustules, and pain should be absent.

Cellulitis

An infection of the dermis and subcutaneous tissue, cellulitis commonly appears around a break in the skin—usually around fresh wounds or small puncture sites. Infection spreads rapidly through the lymphatic system.

Causes. This disorder usually results from infection by group A beta-hemolytic streptococci. It may also result from infection by other streptococci, *S. aureus,* or *Haemophilus influenzae.*

Assessment findings. Clinical signs include a tender, warm, erythematous, swollen area, which is usually well demarcated. A warm, red, tender streak that follows the course of a lymph vessel may appear. The patient may experience fever, chills, headache, and malaise.

Diagnostic tests. Although diagnosis is usually made on the basis of clinical presentation, the doctor may perform a Gram stain and culture of skin tissue. If the patient is acutely ill, the doctor may order blood cultures.

Treatment. Cellulitis must be treated aggressively with systemic antibiotics. The doctor may prescribe oral penicillin to treat small, localized areas of cellulitis on the legs or trunk.

Cellulitis of the face or hands, or that with lymphatic involvement, requires parenteral penicillin or a penicillinase-resistant antibiotic. Gangrene necessitates surgical debridement and incision and drainage of surrounding tissue.

Nursing interventions. Monitor the patient's vital signs, especially temperature, every 4 hours. Assess every 4 hours for an increase in size of the affected area or a worsening of pain. Administer antibiotics, analgesics, and warm soaks as ordered.

Patient education. Emphasize the importance of complying with treatment to prevent relapse.

Evaluation. Look for resolution of erythema, pain, and warmth. Assess the integrity of the patient's skin.

Fungal infections

This section covers dermatophytosis and candidiasis.

Dermatophytosis

Also called ringworm, dermatophytosis may affect the scalp (tinea capitis), body (tinea corporis), nails (tinea unguium), feet (tinea pedis), groin (tinea cruris), and bearded skin (tinea barbae).

Causes. Except for tinea versicolor, tinea infections result from dermatophytes (fungi) of the genera *Trichophyton, Microsporum,* and *Epidermophyton.* Infection may be transmitted either directly, through contact with infected lesions, or indirectly, through contact with contaminated articles, such as shoes, towels, or shower stalls.

Assessment findings. Lesions vary in appearance and duration. *Tinea capitis* is characterized by small, spreading papules on the scalp, causing patchy hair loss with scaling. Papules may progress to inflamed, pus-filled lesions (kerions). *Tinea corporis* produces slightly raised lesions on the skin at any site except the scalp, bearded skin, or feet. Lesions may be dry and scaly or moist and crusty. As they enlarge, their centers heal, causing the classic ring-shaped appearance. *Tinea unguium* (onychomycosis) usually starts at the tip of one or more toenails (fingernail infection

is less common) and produces gradual thickening, discoloration, and crumbling of the nail, with accumulation of subungual debris. Eventually, the nail may be destroyed completely.

Tinea pedis (athlete's foot) may take several forms: from mild to severe scaling and maceration with fissures between the toes. Severe infection may result in inflammation, with severe itching and pain on walking. A dry, squamous inflammation may affect the entire sole.

Tinea cruris (jock itch) produces red, raised, sharply defined, itchy lesions in the groin that may extend to buttocks, inner thighs, and external genitalia. *Tinea barbae* is an uncommon infection that affects the bearded facial area of men.

Diagnostic tests. Microscopic examination of lesion scrapings prepared in KOH solution usually confirms tinea infection. Identifying the infecting organism requires a culture of the lesion scrapings.

Treatment. Localized tinea infections usually respond to a topical antifungal agent, such as naftifine, terbinafine, or econazole. Tinea capitis and other persistent tinea infections require treatment with griseofulvin by mouth for 6 to 8 weeks. Tinea ungulum needs to be treated with systemic antifungals, either itraconazole or terbinafine for 3 months.

Supportive measures include open wet dressings, removal of scabs and scales, and application of keratolytics such as salicylic acid to soften and remove hyperkeratotic lesions of the heels or soles. The patient with tinea capitis should use selenium sulfide 2.5% shampoo during treatment and for 4 to 6 months after griseofulvin therapy to decrease fungal shedding and prevent recurrence.

Nursing interventions. Management of tinea infections requires application of topical agents, observation for sensitivity reactions, observation for secondary bacterial infections, and patient education.

Patient education. Teach the patient that topical treatment may require up to 2 weeks before showing improvement and that he must continue treatment another 4 or 5 days after the lesions clear. Instruct him to comply with oral treatment for the prescribed time.

Counsel the patient on preventing spread of infection. Tell him not to share clothing, hats, towels, or pillows with other family members and not to walk barefoot in shower rooms. He should keep the lesions covered. Finally, teach the patient to avoid scratching because scarring and secondary infection may occur.

Evaluation. Note if the patient's skin lesions and pruritus have resolved. Assess whether he recognizes signs of recurrence and whether any family members have become infected. Nails may take from 6 to 12 months to clear completely.

Candidiasis

Also called candidosis or moniliasis, this disorder usually occurs as a mild, superficial fungal infection of the skin, nails, or mucous membranes. Rarely, fungi enter the bloodstream, causing serious systemic infections.

Causes. Typically, candidiasis results from infection with *Candida albicans* and *Candida tropicalis.* Risk factors include broad-spectrum antibiotic therapy (most common), diabetes mellitus, cancer, immunosuppressant drug therapy, radiation therapy, and aging. Infants with diaper dermatitis commonly develop candidiasis.

Assessment findings. Superficial candidiasis produces signs in the skin, nails, and mouth.

Skin. The patient develops a scaly, erythematous, papular rash, sometimes covered with exudate. Itching and burning are severe. The rash may appear below the breast, between fingers, and at the axillae, groin, and umbilicus. Satellite erythematous papules or pustules are characteristic of candida infections.

Nails. Assess for thickened yellow-brown nail plate. Paronychia may develop displaying redness, swelling and tenderness of nail folds, with occasional purulent discharge and separation of a pruritic nail from the nail bed.

Mouth. Assess for white plaques loosely attached to mucous membranes; underlying mucosa is bright red and moist.

Diagnostic tests. Gram stain of skin gives evidence of *Candida*. Skin scrapings prepared in KOH solution can also diagnose superficial infection. To confirm diagnosis, fungal culture of skin specimen grows *C. albicans* in 48 to 72 hours.

Treatment. The doctor will first treat the underlying condition—for example, by controlling diabetes or discontinuing antibiotic therapy. The imidazoles and broader spectrum triazoles (ketoconazole, sulconazole, econazole) are most effective. Superficial skin infections are treated topically; nails are treated with systemic ketoconazole or itraconizole. Oral suspensions and tablets allow patients with oral candidiasis to swish and swallow.

Nursing interventions. Assess the patient with candidiasis for underlying systemic causes such as diabetes mellitus. When treating an obese patient, use dry padding in intertriginous areas.

Patient education. Focus on promoting comfort and preventing contagion. Encourage the patient to wear loose, nonocclusive cotton socks and clothing or canvas shoes over affected areas. He should dry affected areas well after washing. Counsel the patient that candidiasis isn't contagious by direct contact.

Evaluation. Assess whether skin lesions have resolved. A KOH preparation test should be normal.

Viral infections

This section covers herpes simplex virus (HSV) Type 1, herpes zoster, and warts.

Herpes simplex virus Type 1

HSV Type 1 primarily affects the skin and mucous membranes, commonly producing cold sores and fever blisters. After the first herpes simplex infection, a patient becomes susceptible to recurrent infections, which may be provoked by fever, menses, stress, heat, and cold.

Cause. This disorder results when *Herpesvirus hominis* is transmitted by oral and respiratory secretions and drainage from lesions.

Assessment findings. In primary infection, the patient experiences a brief period of prodromal tingling and itching, accompanied by fever and pharyngitis, followed by eruption of vesicles, erosions and maceration over the entire bucal mucosa. Vesicles form on an erythematous base, then rupture and leave a painful ulcer, followed by a yellowish crust. Other clinical findings may include submaxillary lymphadenopathy, increased salivation, halitosis, anorexia, conjunctivitis, and fever.

Usually, recurrent infection causes only characteristic vesicular eruptions on the lips or buccal mucosa.

Diagnostic tests. Appearance of characteristic lesions suggests HSV Type 1. Isolation of the virus from local lesions, histologic biopsy, and viral culture confirm the diagnosis.

The Tzanck test may show characteristic giant cells and inclusion bodies. A rise in antibody levels and moderate leukocytosis may support the diagnosis.

Treatment. Symptomatic and supportive therapy is essential. Generalized primary infection usually requires an analgesic-antipyretic to reduce fever and relieve pain. Anesthetic mouthwashes such as viscous lidocaine may reduce the pain of gingivostomatitis. Drying agents such as calamine lotion make skin lesions less painful.

Treatment with acyclovir, an antiviral agent, should begin within 3 days of onset of primary episode.

Nursing interventions. Watch immunosuppressed patients closely for signs of a nervous system infection. Because herpesviruses are extremely contagious, use universal precautions.

Patient education. Discuss steps to prevent contagion. Advise patients with cold sores to avoid kissing anyone, but especially infants and people with eczema. Also instruct patients to use good hygiene. Make it clear that the patient should use caution with close contacts. Tell him to see an ophthalmologist immediately if eye lesions develop.

Teach the patient methods to minimize pain. Teach the patient with painful oral lesions to use a soft toothbrush, eat a soft diet, and rinse with a saline solution.

Evaluation. Look for resolution of skin lesions. The patient should understand the possibility of recurrence and precipitating factors.

Herpes zoster

Also called shingles, herpes zoster is an acute unilateral and segmental inflammation of the dorsal root ganglia caused by infection with the herpesvirus varicella-zoster (V-Z), the same virus that causes chickenpox. Herpes zoster produces localized vesicular skin lesions confined to a dermatome and severe neuralgic pain in peripheral areas innervated by the nerves arising in the inflamed ganglia.

Cause. Shingles is caused by reactivation of the herpesvirus V-Z that has lain dormant in the ganglia.

Assessment findings. Onset of herpes zoster is characterized by fever and malaise. Within 2 to 4 days, severe deep pain, pruritus, and paresthesia or hyperesthesia develop, usually on the trunk and occasionally on the arms and legs. Pain may be continuous or intermittent. Small, red, nodular skin lesions then usually erupt on the painful areas and commonly spread unilaterally around the thorax or vertically over the arms or legs. They quickly become vesicles filled with clear fluid or pus. About 10 days after they appear, the vesicles dry and form scabs. (See *Looking at herpes zoster,* page 720.)

Diagnostic tests. Usually, the dermatomic distribution of lesions is

Looking at herpes zoster

This illustration shows vesicles characteristic of herpes zoster, which have erupted along a peripheral nerve in the torso.

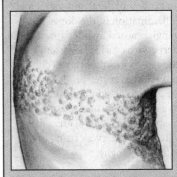

This illustration shows lesions about 10 days later—after they have begun to form scabs.

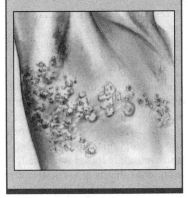

sufficient to confirm diagnosis. In unusual cases, confirmation may require a Tzanck smear, biopsy, and viral culture.

Treatment. Relieving itching and neuralgic pain may require calamine lotion or another topical antipruritic; aspirin, possibly with codeine or another analgesic; and application of Burrow's compresses to help dry lesions. If bacteria have infected ruptured vesicles, treatment includes a systemic antibiotic.

Trigeminal zoster with corneal involvement calls for instillation of idoxuridine ointment or another antiviral agent and a referral to an ophthalmologist.

If started within the first 24 to 48 hours, acyclovir, valacyclovir, or famciclovir can hasten lesion crusting, healing, and cessation of pain.

To treat postherpetic neuralgia, the doctor may order systemic corticosteroids to reduce inflammation, or tranquilizers, sedatives, or tricyclic antidepressants with phenothiazines.

Nursing interventions. Take steps to promote patient comfort. If calamine lotion has been ordered, apply it liberally to the lesions. If lesions are severe and widespread, apply a wet dressing. If vesicles rupture, apply a cold compress, as ordered. To minimize severe neuralgic pain, give analgesics exactly on schedule. Consider splinting the area of pain with an occlusive dressing.

Watch immunosuppressed patients closely for signs of dissemination and central nervous system infection (headache, weakness, fever, and stiff neck).

Patient education. Instruct the patient to avoid scratching the lesions. Repeatedly reassure him that herpetic pain will eventually subside. Provide diversionary activity to take his mind off the pain and pruritus. Finally, warn the patient to avoid close contact with individuals who haven't had chickenpox until the eruption has resolved.

Evaluation. Look for resolution of all skin lesions. Assess whether patient has postherpetic neuralgia.

Warts

Also called verrucae, warts are common, benign infections that affect the skin and mucous membranes.

Cause. Warts result from infection with the human papillomavirus. They may be transmitted by direct contact or by autoinoculation.

Assessment findings. Clinical manifestations depend on the type of wart and location. *Flat* warts are common on the face, neck, chest, knees, dorsa of hands, wrists, and flexor surfaces of the forearms. *Plantar* warts appears slightly elevated or flat. *Acuminate* or genital warts are sexually transmitted and appear on the penis, scrotum, vulva, and anus.

The *common* or verruca vulgaris wart is a rough, elevated wart that usually appears on extremities, particularly hands and fingers. The *filiform* wart is a stalk-like horny projection that commonly occurs around the face and neck. The *periungual* wart is a rough wart that occurs around edges of fingernails and toenails.

Diagnostic tests. Visual examination usually confirms diagnosis. To rule out internal involvement, the doctor may order sigmoidoscopy for recurrent anal warts.

Treatment. Appropriate intervention varies according to location, size, number, pain level, history of therapy, patient's age, and compliance with treatment. Most warts eventually disappear spontaneously.

Treatment may include cryosurgery, acid therapy, electrodesiccation and curettage, or carbon dioxide (CO_2) laser surgery. Application of 25% podophyllum in compound with tincture of benzoin may treat genital warts. Researchers are investigating the use of antiviral drugs to treat warts.

Nursing interventions. When applying podophyllum treatment, apply protective petroleum jelly around the wart. Instruct the patient to wash off podophyllum after 4 hours.

Patient education. Discuss measures to prevent the spread of infection. Teach the patient with genital warts to avoid sexual intercourse or to use condoms for protection until warts are treated. Also remind him that his partner may need treatment. Encourage the patient to have follow-up treatment, as required.

Advise pregnant patients to discuss genital warts with their doctor because vaginal birth may transmit the infection to the neonate.

Evaluation. Look for the resolution of all skin lesions. The patient should know that warts may recur.

Parasitic infestations

Parasitic infestations include scabies and pediculosis.

Scabies

Scabies is a highly contagious skin infection that occurs worldwide.

Cause. Scabies results from infestation with *Sarcoptes scabiei* (itch mite). Transmission occurs through skin or sexual contact. Risk factors include overcrowded conditions and poor hygiene.

Assessment findings. The patient experiences itching that intensifies at night. Characteristic lesions (called burrows), approximately ³/₈″ (1 cm) long, usually appear between fingers, on flexor surfaces of the wrists, on elbows, in axillary folds, at the waistline; on nipples in females, on genitalia in males, and possibly on head and neck in infants. These lesions are usually excoriated and may appear as erythematous nodules.

Diagnostic tests. Visual examination of the contents of the scabietic burrow may reveal the mite, eggs, or feces. A drop of mineral oil is placed over the burrow, followed by superficial scraping and examination of expressed material under a low-power microscope. If scabies is strongly suspected but diagnostic tests are unclear, the doctor may order skin clearing with a therapeutic trial of a pediculicide to confirm the diagnosis.

Treatment. Permethrin (Nix) 5% dermal cream is applied to the entire body from the neck down, left on, and then washed off after 8 to 12 hours. If treatment fails, repeat application 1 week later. Permethrin is safe for pregnant women and infants. (See *Caring for the patient with persistent pruritus.*)

Nursing interventions. If a hospitalized patient has scabies, prevent transmission to other patients. Practice good hand-washing technique, and wear gloves when touching the patient. Observe wound and skin precautions for 24 hours after treatment with a pediculicide.

Patient education. Instruct the patient in the proper use of medication. After applying permethrin cream, he must wait about 15 minutes before dressing and must avoid bathing for 8 to 12 hours. If a second application is needed, tell the patient he must wait at least 1 week. Contaminated clothing and linens must be washed in hot water or dry-cleaned.

Tell the patient not to apply lindane cream if his skin is raw or inflamed. Advise him to notify the doctor immediately if skin irritation or hypersensitivity reaction develops, and wash cream off his skin thoroughly. Family members and other close contacts of the patient must be treated simultaneously.

Evaluation. Look for resolution of the patient's skin lesions and pruritus. The patient's contacts should also remain free from symptoms.

Pediculosis

Pediculosis results from infestation with blood-sucking lice. These lice lay their eggs (nits) in body hairs or clothing fibers. After the nits hatch, the lice must feed within 24 hours or die. This causes pruritus, hypersensitivity reaction, and inflammation.

Assessment findings. Signs and symptoms of pediculosis capitis include itching, excoriation (with severe itching) and, in severe cases, matted, foul-smelling, lusterless hair. The patient may also experience occipital and cervical lymphadenopathy.

Oval, gray-white nits may appear on hair shafts. These cannot be shaken loose like dandruff.

Signs and symptoms of pediculosis corporis include excoriations, eczematous changes, urticaria and erythematous papules, most noticeable on the back. Secondary infection can develop if left untreated.

Signs and symptoms of pediculosis pubis may include skin irritation from scratching, small gray-blue spots on the thighs or upper body, and nits on pubic hairs, which feel coarse and grainy to the touch.

Treatment. Treatment for pediculosis capitas or pubis consists of application of pyrethrin with piperonyl (RID, A-200) or permethrin, or lastly lindane. In less severe cases,

FOCUS ON CARING

Caring for the patient with persistent pruritus

Persistent pruritus may develop from repeated use of pediculicides. An antipruritic emollient or topical steroid can reduce itching. Tell the patient to apply it immediately after a 15-minute bath in tepid water, if possible.

Assure the patient that the pruritus can be treated successfully. Encourage him not to scratch his skin to prevent further injury.

pediculosis corporis may require only bathing with soap and water and thorough washing of clothes.

Nursing interventions. Ask the patient with pediculosis pubis for a history of recent sexual contacts, so that they can be examined and treated. To prevent the spread of pediculosis to other hospitalized persons, examine all high-risk patients on admission, especially elderly persons who depend on others for care, those admitted from nursing homes, or persons living in crowded conditions. Avoid prolonged contact with the patient's hair, clothing, and bed sheets.

Patient education. Advise the patient how to eliminate lice, including creams, ointments, powders, and shampoos. The only certain way to remove dead nits is with a fine-tooth comb or forceps. Advise soaking combs, brushes, and hair accessories in pediculicide for 1 hour or boiling them in water for 10 minutes.

In addition, lice may be removed from clothes by washing, ironing, or dry-cleaning. Storing clothes for more than 30 days or placing them in dry heat of 140° F (60° C) kills lice. If clothes cannot be washed or changed, application of 10% dichlorodiphenyltrichloroethane (DDT) or 10% lindane powder is effective. Sheets should also be laundered.

Family members and other close contacts must be examined for lice and nits and treated simultaneously.

Evaluation. Look for resolution of pruritus and skin irritation as well as evidence that nits are gone.

Papulosquamous conditions

Disorders in the papulosquamous group produce raised, dry, scaling lesions. Such disorders include atopic dermatitis, seborrheic dermatitis, and psoriasis.

Atopic dermatitis

Also known as atopic or infantile eczema, atopic dermatitis refers to a chronic inflammatory skin response.

Atopic dermatitis usually develops in infants between ages 1 month and 1 year, commonly in those with strong family histories of atopic disease. Many of these children acquire other atopic disorders as they grow older. Usually, dermatitis subsides spontaneously by age 3, then flares up at prepuberty (ages 10 to 12).

Causes. The cause of atopic dermatitis is still unknown.

Exacerbating factors of atopic dermatitis include irritants, infections (commonly by *S. aureus*), and some allergens, including pollen, wool, silk, fur, ointments, detergent, and certain foods, particularly wheat, milk, and eggs. Flare-ups may occur in response to extremes in temperature and humidity, sweating, and stress.

Assessment findings. The patient develops an intensely pruritic, commonly excoriated, maculopapular eruption, usually on the face and antecubital and popliteal areas.

Diagnostic tests. Laboratory tests may reveal eosinophilia and elevated serum IgE levels.

Treatment. Effective measures against atopic lesions include eliminating allergens and avoiding irritants, extreme temperature changes, and other precipitating factors. Local and systemic treatment may relieve itching and inflammation. Topical application of a corticosteroid cream or ointment, especially after bathing, usually alleviates inflammation. Between steroid doses, application of petroleum jelly can help retain moisture. Systemic corticosteroid therapy should be used only during extreme exacerbations. Weak tar preparations and ultraviolet B light therapy are used to increase the thickness of the stratum corneum. If a bacterial agent has been cultured, the doctor may order an antibiotic.

Nursing interventions. Complement medical treatment by helping the patient plan for daily skin care.

Patient education. Instruct the patient to bathe daily by soaking in plain water for 10 to 20 minutes. Tell him to bathe with a special nonfatty soap and tepid water but to use soap only on areas that need cleaning when bathing is finished. Patients should apply lubricants immediately after bathing to lock in moisture, apply corticosteroid creams as prescribed, and keep fingernails short to limit excoriations.

Tell him to avoid irritants, such as detergents, wool, and emotional stress.

Evaluation. Assess whether treatment controls skin eruptions and pruritus. The patient should be aware of aggravating factors.

Seborrheic dermatitis

Seborrheic dermatitis occurs in areas with a high concentration of sebaceous glands, such as the scalp, trunk, and face.

Cause. The cause remains unknown. Predisposing factors may include heredity, physical or emotional stress, neurologic conditions, and acquired immunodeficiency syndrome.

Assessment findings. The patient may develop itching of affected areas. Lesions are distributed in sebaceous gland areas and appear as erythematous, scaly and, in many cases, yellowish greasy plaques.

Diagnostic tests. Patient history and physical findings confirm seborrheic dermatitis.

Treatment. Measures include removing scales with ketoconazole shampoo, washing and shampooing with selenium sulfide suspension, zinc pyrithione, or tar and salicylic acid shampoo. Topical steroids and ketoconazole cream may reduce inflammation.

Nursing interventions. Explore with the patient ways to reduce stress.

Patient education. Tell the patient that the disease's course will wax and wane and to expect exacerbations during cold weather.

Evaluation. Assess whether skin eruptions are well controlled and erythema and scaling have resolved. Determine if the patient understands the possibility of recurrence.

Psoriasis

A chronic disorder, psoriasis is marked by epidermal proliferation and recurring remissions and exacerbations. Its lesions, which appear as erythematous papules and plaques covered with silvery scales, vary widely in severity and distribution.

Causes. The tendency to develop psoriasis is genetically determined,

Psoriasis: Examining the effects

In this patient with psoriasis, plaques consisting of silver scales cover a large area of the face.

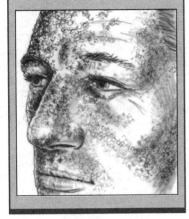

possibly resulting from an autoimmune deficiency.

Assessment findings. The initial sign is usually small erythematous papules. These enlarge or coalesce to form red, elevated plaques with silver scales on the scalp, face, chest, elbows, knees, back, buttocks, and genitals. Other features include pruritus and possible nail pitting and joint stiffness. (See *Psoriasis: Examining the effects.*)

Diagnostic tests. Establishing the diagnosis may require skin biopsy, though patient history and appearance of the lesions may be sufficient. Laboratory tests may reveal elevated serum uric acid levels and the presence of HLA 13 and 17.

Treatment. All methods of treatment are merely palliative. Lukewarm baths and the application of occlusive ointment bases (petroleum jelly or urea preparations) or salicylic acid preparations may soften and remove psoriatic scales. Steroid creams are also useful.

Methods to retard rapid cell proliferation include exposure to ultraviolet light (wavelength B [UVB] or natural sunlight) to the point of minimal erythema.

Anthralin, combined with a paste mixture, may be used for well-defined plaques but mustn't be applied to unaffected areas because it may cause inflammation. Anthralin irritates and stains the skin. It also stains clothing and the bathtub.

In a patient with severe chronic psoriasis, the Goeckerman treatment—which combines tar application and UVB treatments—may help achieve remission and clear the skin. The Ingram technique, a variation of this treatment, uses anthralin instead of tar.

A program called psoralens plus ultraviolet A (PUVA) combines administration of methoxsalen (a psoralen derivative) with exposure to ultraviolet light, wavelength A (UVA). Methotrexate may help severe, refractory psoriasis. As a last resort, the doctor may prescribe etretinate. (See *Tanning treatment for psoriasis.*)

Low-dosage antihistamines, oatmeal baths, emollients (with phenol and methol), and open wet dressings may help relieve pruritus. Aspirin and local heat help alleviate the pain of psoriatic arthritis; severe cases may require nonsteroidal anti-inflammatory drugs such as indomethacin.

Therapy for psoriasis of the scalp usually consists of a tar shampoo, followed by application of a steroid lotion while the hair is wet.

Nursing interventions. Monitor for adverse reactions to therapy. The patient may develop allergic reactions to anthralin, atrophy and acne from steroids, and burning, itching, nausea, and skin cancer from PUVA. The patient on methotrexate may develop hepatic or bone marrow toxicity.

Patient education. Discuss directions for using medications, an explanation of flare-ups, and cautions for the patient on PUVA therapy.

Teach the patient how to apply prescribed creams and lotions. A steroid cream, for example, should be applied in a thin film using the palm of the hand. Tell the patient using the Goeckerman treatment to apply tar with a downward motion to avoid rubbing it into the follicles.

Instruct the patient to apply anthralin only to psoriatic plaques. He should wear gloves because anthralin stains the skin. After application, the patient may dust himself with powder to prevent anthralin from rubbing off on his clothes. Warn the patient never to put an occlusive dressing over anthralin. Suggest use of mineral oil, then soap and water, to remove

ALTERNATIVE THERAPY

Tanning treatment for psoriasis

Exposing the skin to natural sunlight can improve the condition of psoriasis. When natural sunlight isn't available, treatment can continue with careful use of tanning beds.

The use of tanning beds to treat a patient with psoriasis is based on the therapeutic exposure to ultraviolet light that's used in psoralens plus ultraviolet A therapy on patients with severe chronic psoriasis.

anthralin. Caution the patient to avoid scrubbing his skin vigorously.

Tell the patient that flare-ups are commonly related to specific systemic and environmental factors, such as infection, pregnancy, cold weather, and emotional stress, but they may be unpredictable. They can usually be controlled with therapy.

Evaluation. Skin eruptions should be controlled. The patient should be able to demonstrate proper care of skin. He should keep follow-up appointments.

Follicular and glandular conditions

Follicular and glandular disorders include acne vulgaris and alopecia.

Acne vulgaris

Acne vulgaris is an inflammatory disease of the sebaceous follicles that primarily affects adolescents.

Causes. Research now centers on hormonal dysfunction and over-secretion of sebum as possible primary causes.

Factors that increase an individual's risk of developing acne vulgaris include use of oral contraceptives; cobalt irradiation; hyperalimentation therapy; exposure to heavy oils, greases, or tars; trauma or rubbing from tight clothing; family history; and cosmetics.

Certain medications may cause acne. These include corticosteroids, corticotropin, androgens, iodides, bromides, trimethadione, phenytoin, isoniazid, lithium, and halothane.

Assessment findings. The appearance of acne will vary. If the acne plug doesn't protrude from the follicle and is covered by the epidermis it may appear as a closed comedo, or whitehead. If the acne plug protrudes and is not covered by the epidermis, it may appear as an open comedo, or blackhead. The patient may develop characteristic acne pustules, papules or, in severe forms, acne cysts or abscesses. Cystic acne produces scars.

Treatment. Therapy is chosen depending on the type of acne lesions present and their severity. Tretinoin, a keratolytic (retinoic acid or topical vitamin A [Retin-A]) is effective against blackheads.

These agents may be used in combination; both may irritate the skin. Topical antibiotics, such as tetracycline, erythromycin, and clindamycin, may help reduce the effects of acne.

Systemic therapy consists primarily of antibiotics, usually tetracycline, erythromycin, or minocycline to decrease bacterial growth until the patient is in remission; then a lower dosage is used for long-term maintenance.

Oral isotretinoin (Accutane) combats acne by inhibiting sebaceous gland function and keratinization. Because of severe adverse effects, the usual 16- to 20-week course of isotretinoin is limited to those patients with severe cystic acne who don't respond to conventional therapy. Severe fetal abnormalities may occur if isotretinoin is used during pregnancy. Extreme caution must be used when administering the drug to women of childbearing age.

Other treatments for acne vulgaris include intralesional corticosteroid injections, estrogen therapy, cryotherapy, and surgery.

Nursing interventions. You can help the patient by seeking to identify predisposing factors that he can eliminate or modify. Pay special attention to the patient's perception of his physical appearance and offer emotional support.

Patient education. Explain the possible causes of acne to the patient and family. Emphasize that prescribed treatment is more likely to improve acne than are strict diet and fanatic scrubbing. Overzealous washing can worsen lesions.

• Instruct the patient receiving tretinoin to apply it at least 30 minutes after washing the face and at least 1 hour before bedtime. Warn against using this medication around the eyes or lips. If skin appears red or starts to peel, the preparation may have to be weakened or applied less often. Advise the patient to avoid exposure to sunlight or to use a sunscreening agent.

• Instruct the patient to take tetracycline on an empty stomach and not with antacids or milk.

• Tell the patient taking isotretinoin to avoid vitamin A supplements, which can worsen any adverse effects. Teach him to use a moisturizer to prevent dryness.

• Because of the danger of birth defects, advise the sexually active female patient that isotretinoin can't be prescribed unless she uses contraception. Tetracycline also carries some risk of birth defects if used during pregnancy.

• Tell the patient that acne is a chronic condition and long-term treatment is necessary.

• Instruct female patients to wear only noncomedogenic makeup.

Evaluation. Assess whether treatment successfully controls skin lesions. Look for the patient to demonstrate proper skin care.

Alopecia

Also known as hair loss, alopecia usually affects the scalp. It is rarer and less conspicuous elsewhere on the body. In the nonscarring form of this disorder (noncicatricial alopecia), the hair follicle can generally regrow hair. But scarring alopecia usually causes irreversible hair loss.

Causes. The most common form of nonscarring alopecia, male-pattern alopecia, appears to be related to androgen levels, aging, or genetic predisposition.

Other forms of nonscarring alopecia include physiologic alopecia, alopecia areata, and trichotillomania.

Scarring alopecia may result from physical or chemical trauma or chronic tension on a hair shaft, such as braiding or rolling the hair. Diseases that produce scarring alopecia include destructive skin tumors, granulomas, lupus erythematosus, scleroderma, lichen planus follicularis, and severe bacterial or viral infections, such as folliculitis or herpes simplex.

Assessment findings. In male-pattern alopecia, hair loss is gradual and usually affects the thinner, shorter, and less pigmented hairs of the scalp's frontal and parietal portions. In women, hair loss is generally diffuse; completely bald areas are uncommon but may occur.

Alopecia areata affects small patches of the scalp but may involve the entire scalp or the entire body. Although mild erythema may occur initially, affected areas of scalp or skin appear normal. "Exclamation point" hairs occur at the periphery of new patches. Regrowth initially appears as fine, white, downy hair, which is replaced by normal hair.

In trichotillomania (compulsive pulling out of one's own hair), patchy, incomplete areas of hair loss with many broken hairs appear on the scalp but may occur on other areas such as the eyebrows.

Diagnostic tests. Physical examination is usually sufficient to confirm alopecia.

Treatment. Topical application of minoxidil, a peripheral vasodilator more typically used as an oral antihypertensive, has some success in treating male-pattern alopecia. An alternative treatment is surgical redistribution of hair follicles by autografting.

In alopecia areata, treatment may be unnecessary because spontaneous regrowth is common. Intralesional corticosteroid injections are beneficial for small patches and may produce regrowth in 4 to 6 weeks. Hair loss that persists for over a year has a poor prognosis for regrowth. In trichotillomania, an occlusive dressing prevents hair loss. Treatment of other types of alopecia varies according to the underlying cause.

Nursing interventions. Take a thorough history to help identify underlying causes of alopecia.

Patient education. Provide reassurance to the patient without instilling false hopes. Reassure a woman with female-pattern alopecia that it doesn't lead to total baldness. Suggest wearing a wig. If the patient has alopecia areata, explain the disorder and emphasize that complete regrowth is possible, but progression may occur.

Evaluation. Assess response to treatment. Evaluate how well the patient understands the causes of hair loss and whether he accepts the prospect that hair loss may recur.

Skin cancers

The most common skin cancers are malignant melanoma, basal cell carcinoma, and squamous cell carcinoma.

Malignant melanoma

Malignant melanoma arises from melanocytes. The four types of melanoma are superficial spreading melanoma, nodular melanoma, lentigo melanoma, and acral-lentiginous melanoma.

Melanoma spreads through the lymphatic and vascular systems. Usually, superficial lesions are curable, while deeper lesions tend to metastasize.

Causes. The cause of malignant melanoma is unknown. Risk factors include familial tendency, a history of melanoma or dysplastic nevi, history of severe sunburns, and skin type.

Assessment findings. Suspect melanoma when any skin lesion or nevous enlarges, changes color, becomes inflamed or sore, itches, ulcerates, bleeds, changes texture, or shows surrounding pigment regression (halo nevus or vitiligo).

Diagnostic tests. A skin biopsy with histologic examination can distinguish malignant melanoma from a benign nevus, seborrheic keratosis, and pigmented basal cell carcinoma and can also evaluate tumor thickness. Physical examination, focusing on lymph nodes, can determine metastatic involvement.

Treatment. Wide surgical resection is imperative for malignant melanoma. The extent of resection and adjuvant chemotherapy depends on the size and location of the primary lesion. Radiation therapy is usually reserved for metastatic disease.

Nursing interventions. After surgery, take steps to prevent infection. If surgery included lymphadenectomy, minimize lymphedema by applying a compression stocking, and instruct the patient to keep the extremity elevated.

During chemotherapy, know what adverse effects to expect and what you can do to minimize them. Provide psychological support to help the patient cope with anxiety.

Patient education. Review the doctor's explanation of treatment alternatives. Tell the patient what to expect before and after surgery, what the wound will look like, and what type of dressing will be used.

For all types of skin cancers, emphasize the need for close follow-up to detect recurrences early. Stress the hazards of sun exposure, and recommend the use of a sunblock or sunscreen. Teach the patient and his family to conduct monthly skin self-examinations.

Evaluation. The patient recovers uneventfully from surgery. He also demonstrates understanding of sun protection methods and the importance of follow-up care.

Basal cell carcinoma

Basal cell carcinoma is a slow-growing destructive skin tumor, mostly occurring on sun-exposed skin. Three types include nodulo-ulcerative, superficial, and sclerosing (morphealike).

Causes. The cause is unknown, but precipitating factors include prolonged sun exposure (most common), arsenic ingestion; radiation exposure, burns and, rarely, vaccinations.

Assessment findings. *Nodulo-ulcerative basal cell carcinomas* occur mostly on the face. Early-stage lesions are small, smooth, pinkish translucent papules with telangiectatic vessels on the surface and occasional pigmentation. Late-stage lesions are enlarged, with depressed centers, firm and elevated borders.

Superficial basal cell carcinomas occur mostly on the chest and back and appear as oval or irregularly shaped, lightly pigmented plaques with sharply defined, slightly elevated threadlike borders.

Sclerosing basal cell carcinomas occur on the head and neck. They appear as waxy, sclerotic, yellow to white plaques without distinct borders and commonly resemble small patches of scleroderma.

Diagnostic tests. Basal cell carcinomas are diagnosed by clinical appearance and by incisional or excisional biopsy and histologic studies.

Treatment. Depending on the size, location, and depth of the lesion, treatment may include curettage and electrodesiccation for small lesions; chemotherapy with topical 5-fluorouracil (5-FU); or surgical excision, irradiation, or Mohs' technique (microsurgery).

Nursing interventions. Advise the patient to relieve local inflammation from 5-FU with cool compresses or with corticosteroid treatment, as prescribed by his doctor. Also advise him to eat frequent small meals that are high in protein. Suggest eggnogs or liquid protein supplements if the lesion has invaded the oral cavity and caused eating problems.

Patient education. Review the doctor's explanation of treatment alternatives. Tell the patient what to expect before and after surgery.

Emphasize the need for close follow-up. Recommend the use of a sunblock or sunscreen. Teach the patient and his family to conduct monthly skin self-examinations.

Evaluation. The patient recovers uneventfully from surgery, and the treated area heals without deformi-

ty. He demonstrates understanding of sun protection methods and the importance of follow-up care.

Squamous cell carcinoma

Squamous cell carcinoma is an invasive tumor with metastatic potential that arises from the keratinizing epidermal cells. Squamous cell carcinoma commonly develops on sun-damaged areas of the skin.

Causes. Squamous cell carcinoma may be caused by overexposure to ultraviolet rays, X-ray therapy, chronic skin irritation and inflammation, ingestion of herbicides containing arsenic, and exposure to local carcinogens (such as tar).

Assessment findings. In normal skin, this carcinoma typically appears as a nodule growing on a firm indurated base; some ulceration may appear at the lesion site.

A premalignant, preexisting lesion may be inflamed and indurated. Metastasis to regional lymph nodes may cause pain, malaise, fatigue, weakness, and anorexia.

Diagnostic tests, treatment, nursing interventions, patient education, and evaluation are generally the same as in basal cell carcinoma above.

Miscellaneous disorders

This section covers cutaneous ulcers. The two types of cutaneous ulcers are pressure sores (bedsores) and stasis ulcers.

Cutaneous ulcers

Cutaneous ulcers are localized areas of cellular necrosis that occur mostly in areas of inadequate circulation. Cutaneous ulcers may be superficial or deep.

Causes. *Pressure sores* result from pressure that interrupts normal circulatory function. The pressure's intensity and duration govern the sore's severity.

Conditions that increase the risk of developing pressure sores include altered mobility, inadequate nutrition, and breakdown in skin or subcutaneous tissue (as a result of edema or incontinence). Other predisposing factors include fever, pathologic conditions, and obesity.

Stasis ulcers result from chronic venous stasis caused by varicose veins or venous thrombosis. Risk factors include prolonged standing in one position and obesity.

Assessment findings. Pressure sores commonly develop over bony prominences. Early features of superficial lesions are shiny, erythematous changes over the compressed area, caused by localized vasodilation when pressure is relieved. Superficial erythema progresses ultimately to necrosis and ulceration.

An inflamed area on the skin's surface may be the first sign of underlying damage. Bacteria in a compressed site cause infection, which leads to further necrosis. A foul-smelling, purulent discharge may seep from a lesion that penetrates the skin from beneath. Infected, necrotic tissue prevents healthy granulation of scar tissue; a black eschar may develop around and over the lesion.

Stasis ulcers appear on the skin of the lower legs (usually over the medial malleolus). The skin may be patchy brown from chronic venous stasis, then erythematous and pruritic.

Diagnostic tests. Wound culture and sensitivity testing of the exudate in the ulcer identify infecting organisms and help to determine whether antibiotics are needed.

Treatment. Treatment for both types of ulcers involves debridement, wound cleaning, and application of dressings. Debridement removes devitalized tissue. Debridement may be sharp (using scalpel or scissors), mechanical (employing wet to dry dressing, wound irrigation, hydrotherapy, and dextranomers), enzymatic (using collagenase), or autolytic (using synthetic dressings).

Wound cleaning should be accomplished with a minimum of chemical and mechanical trauma. Don't clean ulcer wounds with antiseptic agents (for example, povidone-iodine or hydrogen peroxide) because they're cytotoxic. Normal saline adequately cleans most wounds and is the preferred cleaning agent.

Use a dressing that will keep the ulcer tissue moist and the surrounding intact skin dry. (See *Types of occlusive dressings,* page 734.)

Types of occlusive dressings

Five basic types of occlusive dressings are available. Use your best clinical judgment to select the type of dressing suitable for the ulcer. Avoid these dressings in cases involving cellulitis or infection.

Category	Advantages	Disadvantages
Films (Bioclusive, Tegaderm, Opsite)	• Permits wound visualization • Forms bacterial barrier • Adherent • Waterproof • Inexpensive	• Fluid collection under dressing • Difficult to apply • Adhesive can tear new epithelium • Can cause contact dermatitis
Hydrogels (Vigilon, Aquasorb)	• Comfortable and soothing • Debrides wound • Absorbs exudate	• Need secondary dressing • May cause maceration of skin around the wound • Expensive
Hydrocolloids (Duoderm, Comfeel, Cutinova hydro)	• Easy to apply • Impermeable to fluid and bacteria • Waterproof	• Has an offensive odor • Can stimulate excess granulation tissue • May cause maceration of skin around the wound • Difficult to use in cavities
Alginates (Kaltostat, Sorbsan)	• Absorbent • Useful in sinuses • Hemolytic properties	• Difficult to remove fibers from wound • Requires frequent dressing changes • Not useful for dry wounds
Foams (Allevyn, Mitraflex)	• Absorbent • Comfortable and protective • Conforms to body contours	• Requires secondary dressing • Adheres and dehydrates wound base if exudate dries

Nursing interventions. Change bed linens frequently for patients who are diaphoretic or incontinent. All individuals at risk should have systematic skin inspections at least once a day, paying special attention to bony prominences:

• Turn and reposition the patient every 1 to 2 hours unless contraindicated. For patients who can't turn themselves or who are turned on a schedule, use pressure-relieving and pressure-reducing devices, such as a 4″ (10-cm) convoluted foam mattress or a low-air-loss or

Clinitron therapy bed. Implement active or passive range-of-motion exercises to relieve pressure and promote circulation. (Combine them with bathing if applicable.)
• When turning the patient, lift rather than slide him.
• Use pillows to position your patient.
• Post a turning schedule at the patient's bedside.
• Except for brief periods, avoid raising the head of the bed more than 30 degrees.
• Provide patients in wheelchairs with pressure-relieving cushions as appropriate, but don't seat them on rubber or plastic doughnuts.
• Adjust or pad appliances, casts, or splints as needed.
• Ensure adequate dietary intake of protein and calories. Therapy may involve nutritional consultation, food supplements, enteral feeding, or total parenteral nutrition.
• If diarrhea develops or if the patient is incontinent, clean and dry soiled skin. Then, apply a protective moisture barrier.
• Avoid using elbow and heel protectors that fasten with a single narrow strap, which may impair neurovascular function.
• Use pressure reduction devices for protection.

Patient education. Recommend a diet that includes adequate calories, protein, and vitamins. Teach patients with venous stasis to avoid prolonged standing, to elevate their legs frequently to promote venous return, and to wear compression stockings during the day.

Emphasize the importance of regular position changes to the patient and his family. Encourage their participation in treatment and pressure ulcer prevention by teaching them how to change positions correctly.

Tell the patient to avoid heat lamps and harsh soaps. Treat dry skin with moisturizers after bathing. Also tell him to avoid vigorous massage.

Direct the patient who is confined to a chair or who uses a wheelchair to shift his weight every 30 minutes. Show a paraplegic patient how to shift his weight by doing push-ups in the wheelchair. If the patient needs your help, sit next to him and help him shift his weight to one buttock for 60 seconds, then repeat the procedure on the other side.

Evaluation. Assess whether the ulcer has reepithelialized. Note whether the patient and caretakers are taking adequate measures to prevent recurrence. (See *Documenting pressure ulcers,* page 736.)

TREATMENTS

With new skin treatments and with traditional ones, you play a key role. For example, you're responsible for carrying out or directly assisting with many treatments. And because therapy commonly depends on the patient's compliance with home care regimens that can last for months or even years, your patient education and monitoring are vitally important.

Documenting pressure ulcers

Because many patients are susceptible to pressure ulcers, you should always document findings related to skin condition. Clearly note in the medical record whether a patient had a pressure ulcer upon admission or whether the ulcer developed in the health care facility.

By documenting that skin care is given according to facility protocol, you can ensure that the patient receives adequate reimbursement. This is important, because many skin care treatments are very expensive.

Drug therapy

Drugs used to treat skin disorders include local anti-infectives, topical corticosteroids, keratolytics, astringents, and emollients, demulcents, and protectants.

Surgery

Surgical techniques for treating skin dysfunction include laser surgery, cryosurgery, skin grafting, and Mohs' micrographic surgery.

Laser surgery

The highly focused light of lasers proves effective in treating many types of dermatologic lesions. Laser surgery spares normal tissue, promotes faster healing, and helps prevent postsurgical infection.

Several types of lasers are used in dermatology and include: argon lasers, CO_2 lasers, tunable dye lasers, copper vapor and ruby lasers.

Patient preparation. If present, keep shades or blinds closed. Cover reflective surfaces and remove flammable materials.

Position the patient comfortably, drape him, and place protective gauze around the operative site. Make sure that everyone in the room—including the patient—is wearing safety goggles.

Monitoring and aftercare. The doctor uses the laser beam to cut away the lesion. After the procedure, apply direct pressure over any bleeding wound for 20 minutes.

Initial wound care varies, depending on the procedure. Areas treated with CO_2 laser require a surgical dressing. Vascular lesions treated with argon, tunable dye, or copper vapor laser need minimal postoperative care.

Patient education. Tell the patient to dress his wound daily, following the same procedure that you used. Permit him to take showers but advise him not to immerse the wound site in water.

If bleeding occurs, the patient should apply direct pressure on the site with clean gauze or a washcloth for 20 minutes. If pressure doesn't control the bleeding, he should call the doctor immediately. To avoid changes in pigmentation, warn the patient to protect the wound from exposure to the sun.

Cryosurgery

Cryosurgery is a common dermatologic procedure, in which the application of extreme cold leads to tissue destruction. It can be performed quite simply, using nothing more than a cotton-tipped applicator dipped into liquid nitrogen and applied to the skin, or it may involve a complex cryosurgical unit (CSU).

Patient preparation. Ask the patient if he has any known allergies or hypersensitivities, especially to iodine or cold. Tell the patient that he'll initially feel cold, followed by a burning sensation, during the procedure. Caution him to remain as still as possible to prevent inadvertent freezing of unaffected tissue.

The surgeon uses the cotton-tipped applicator or the CSU to freeze the lesion. He may refreeze a tumor several times to ensure its destruction.

Monitoring and aftercare. After cryosurgery, apply an adhesive bandage if needed or requested by the patient. Give analgesics to relieve pain if needed.

Patient education. Tell the patient to expect pain, redness, and swelling and that a blister may form within 24 hours of treatment. Ordinarily, it will flatten within a few days and slough off in 2 to 3 weeks. Serous exudation may follow during the first week, accompanied by the development of a crust or eschar. This blister may be large and it may bleed. To promote healing and prevent infection, warn the patient not to touch it. Tell him that if the blister becomes uncomfortable or interferes with daily activities, he should call the doctor, who can decompress it with a sterile blade or pin.

Tell the patient to clean the area gently with soap and water as ordered.

Skin grafts

Grafting may cover defects caused by burns, trauma, or surgery. It's indicated when primary closure isn't possible or cosmetically acceptable, when primary closure would interfere with functioning, when the defect is on a weight-bearing surface, or when a skin tumor is excised and the site needs to be monitored for recurrence.

Types of skin grafts include *split-thickness* grafts, which consist of the epidermis and a small portion of dermis; *full-thickness* grafts, which include all of the dermis as well as the epidermis; and *composite* grafts, which also include underlying tissues, such as muscle, cartilage, or bone.

Patient preparation. Because successful skin grafting begins with a good graft, take steps to preserve potential donor sites by providing meticulous skin care.

Prepare the donor and recipient sites for surgery. Prepare the skin while the anesthetic takes effect.

Monitoring and aftercare. After the procedure, your role is to ensure the graft survival. Position the patient so that he's not lying on the graft and, if possible, keep the graft area elevated and immobilized. Modify your nursing routine to protect the graft; for example, never use a blood pressure cuff over a graft site. For burn patients, omit hydrotherapy while the graft heals. Give analgesics as necessary, and help the patient use nonpharmacologic pain-reduction techniques.

Use sterile technique when changing a dressing, and work gently to avoid dislodging the graft. Clean the graft site with warm saline solution and cotton-tipped applicators, leaving the fine-mesh gauze intact. Aspirate any serous pockets. Change the gauze and apply the prescribed topical agent as needed. Then, cover the area with a bandage. Care for the donor site.

Patient education. Counsel the patient not to disturb the dressings on the graft or donor sites for any reason. If they need to be changed, instruct him to call the doctor. If grafting is done as an outpatient procedure, emphasize to him that the graft site must be immobilized to promote proper healing.

Instruct him to apply cream to the site several times a day—once the graft has healed—to keep the skin pliable and aid scar maturation. Because sun exposure can affect graft pigmentation, advise the patient to limit his time in the sun and to use a sunblock on all grafted areas.

Mohs' micrographic surgery

Mohs' micrographic surgery involves serial excision and histologic analysis of cancerous or suspected cancerous tissues. By allowing step-by-step excision of tumors, Mohs' surgery minimizes the size of the scar and helps prevent recurrence. This surgery is especially effective against basal cell carcinomas.

Patient preparation. Review the patient's history, noting allergies and hypersensitivities (especially to epinephrine and lidocaine), cardiac disease, or ongoing anticoagulant therapy. Emphasize that the procedure takes many hours, most of which will be spent waiting for histologic results. Reassure him that a long wait does not mean his cancer is grave.

Explain that the doctor will use electrocauterization to control bleeding and that a grounding plate will be affixed to the patient's leg or arm. Reassure the patient that he won't feel anything from the ground. Warn him, however, to expect a burning odor.

After the anesthetic takes effect, position the patient comfortably and place the grounding pad on his leg or arm. Then drape the surgical area and adjust the lights.

Monitoring and aftercare. During the procedure, be alert for any signs or symptoms of distress. Assess the patient's pain level and provide ordered analgesics. Periodically check for excessive bleeding. If it occurs, remove the dressing and apply pressure over the site for 20 minutes.

Patient education. Tell the patient to leave the dressing in place for 24 hours and to change the dressing daily afterward. However, if the site bleeds, he should reinforce the bandage and apply direct pressure to the wound for 20 minutes, using clean gauze or a clean washcloth. If this doesn't control bleeding, he should call the doctor.

Instruct the patient to report signs of infection. Advise him to refrain from alcohol, aspirin, or excessive exercise for 48 hours to prevent bleeding and promote healing. Recommend acetaminophen for discomfort.

Debridement, baths, and phototherapy

Expect to play a key role in debridement, administering therapeutic baths, and phototherapy.

Debridement

Debridement may call for mechanical, chemical, or surgical techniques to remove necrotic tissue from a wound. Although it can be extremely painful, it prevents infection and promotes healing of burns and skin ulcers.

Mechanical debridement. This technique includes wet-to-dry dressings, irrigation, hydrotherapy, and bedside debridement. Wet-to-dry dressings are appropriate for partially healed wounds with only slight amounts of necrotic tissue and minimal drainage. The nurse or doctor places a wet dressing on the lesion and covers it with an outer layer of bandaging. As the dressing dries, it sticks to the wound. When the dried dressing is removed, the necrotic tissue comes off with it.

Hydrotherapy (also known as tubbing or tanking) involves immersion of the patient in a tank of warm water and intermittent agitation of the water. It's usually performed on burn patients.

Bedside debridement of a burn wound involves careful prying and cutting of loosened eschar (burned tissue) with forceps and scissors to separate it from viable tissue beneath. Although painful, it may be the only practical means of removing necrotic tissue from a severely burned patient.

Chemical debridement. This procedure uses dextranomer (Debrisan) hydrophilic wound-cleaning beads or topical debriders to absorb exudate and particulate debris. These agents also absorb bacteria and thus reduce the risk of infection.

Surgical debridement. Done under general or regional anesthesia, surgical debridement is usually reserved for burn patients or those with extremely deep or large ulcers. In many cases, it's performed with skin grafting.

Patient preparation. Explain to the patient that debridement will remove dead tissue from his burn or ulcer. Discuss the type of debridement he'll undergo and reassure him that analgesics will be given, if needed.

Gather equipment and, if ordered, give an analgesic 20 minutes before the procedure. Then position the patient comfortably, providing maximum access to the site.

Monitoring and aftercare. For all the procedures, assess the patient's pain, using his own reports and such signs and symptoms as restlessness, increased muscle tension, and rapid respirations. Provide analgesics, as ordered.

During dressing changes, note the amount of granulation tissue, necrotic debris, and drainage. Be alert for signs of wound infection. If the patient's limb was debrided, keep it elevated to promote venous return—especially for stasis ulcers. Assess fluid and electrolyte status, especially if he has burns.

Patient education. If patients are sent home on wet-to-dry dressings, teach them or their caregivers how to perform the procedure. Make sure they have enough dressings and solution. Instruct them to recognize and report to the doctor any signs and symptoms of infection or poor healing.

Therapeutic baths

Therapeutic baths, also known as balneotherapy, may help psoriasis, atopic eczema, exfoliative dermatitis, bullous diseases, and pyodermas. Four types of baths are commonly used: antibacterial, colloidal, emollient, and tar. They permit treatment of large areas. Because they can cause dry skin, pruritus, scaling, and fissures, they should be limited to 20 or 30 minutes.

Patient preparation. Place the bath mat in the tub and run the bath. Use a bath thermometer to ensure that the water temperature is about 97° F (36° C). Then measure and add the medication to the water to achieve the prescribed dilution. Mix the water and medication well to prevent a sensitivity reaction.

Monitoring and aftercare. After the bath, apply ordered topical medications immediately because they're absorbed better when the skin is damp. Assess the skin and note any improvement or reaction. If necessary, help the patient dress and escort him back to his room.

Patient education. Provide the patient with instructions and outline safety precautions. Explain that the therapeutic agents may make the tub slippery and that a bath mat is a necessity. Tell him that overly hot water can increase pruritus.

The average bathtub holds 150 to 200 gallons of water; the patient should measure his medication accordingly and mix it thoroughly into the water. Mention that soap dries skin and that he can bathe every other day, applying soap only to the underarms, groin, and soles of feet.

Remind the patient that friction during or after a bath can damage his skin. Instruct him to wash himself with his bare hands instead of using a washcloth. Tell the patient with psoriasis to use a washcloth to gently loosen crusts, but only after he has soaked for 15 to 20 minutes. Instruct all patients to gently pat themselves dry with a clean towel, leaving the skin slightly damp. Finally, tell the patient to report any increase in pruritus, oozing, erythema, or scaling to the doctor.

Phototherapy

Used to help treat psoriasis, mycosis fungoides, atopic dermatitis, and uremic pruritus, phototherapy retards epidermal cell proliferation. Two different ultraviolet light wavelengths, A and B, are used therapeutically. The drug psoralen creates artificial sensitivity to UVA. The combination of psoralen with UVA is known as PUVA therapy, or photochemotherapy.

Patient preparation. Explain to the patient that UVB therapy may produce a mild sunburn that will help clear up skin lesions. Erythema appears within 6 hours after therapy. Sunburn may also occur within 72 hours.

Perform a thorough skin examination. If the patient will be undergoing PUVA therapy, tell him to take psoralen with food 1½ hours before treatment.

Monitoring and aftercare. Look for marked erythema, blistering, peeling, or other signs of overexposure 4 to 6 hours after UVB and 24 to 48 hours after UVA. If overexposure occurs, notify the doctor.

Patient education. Encourage the patient to use emollients and drink plenty of fluids. Warn him to avoid hot baths or showers and to curb his use of soap. Tell him to notify his doctor before taking any drug, including aspirin, to prevent heightened photosensitivity. Also tell him to limit natural light exposure, to use a sunblock when outdoors, and to notify his doctor if he discovers suspicious lesions.

If the patient is undergoing PUVA treatments, review his schedule for taking psoralen. Explain that any deviation from it could lead to burns or ineffective treatment. Stress the need to wear UV-opaque sunglasses when outdoors for at least 24 hours after taking psoralen. Similarly, patients who undergo frequent treatment need yearly eye exams to detect possible cataracts.

If the patient is using a sunlamp at home, tell him to let the lamp warm up for 5 minutes and then to limit exposure to the prescribed time. Instruct him to protect his eyes with goggles and to use a dependable timer or have someone in the room during therapy. Above all, *tell him never to use the sunlamp when he's tired;* falling asleep during therapy may lead to severe burns.

Tell the patient that he can help relieve a local burn by applying cool water soaks for 20 minutes or until skin temperature is cool. For larger burns, tepid tap water baths may be used, but have him check with the doctor. After the bath, he can apply oil-in-water moisturizing lotion; he shouldn't use a petroleum jelly–based product because it can trap heat. A severe PUVA burn may call for prednisone.

REFERENCES AND READINGS

"Application Techniques and Guidelines for Interpretation," *Dermatology Nursing,* February 1995, supplement.

Arndt, K.A., *Manual of Dermatologic Therapeutics,* 5th ed. Boston: Little, Brown & Co., 1995.

Chang, H., et al. "Moist Wound Healing," *Dermatology Nursing* 8(3):174-76, June 1996.

Diseases, 2nd ed. Springhouse, Pa.: Springhouse Corp., 1997.

Fiaklov, J.A., and McDougal, E.P. "Warmed Local Anesthetic Reduces Pain of Infiltration" *Annals of Plastic Surgery* 36:11-13, 1996.

Illustrated Guide to Diagnostic Tests, 2nd ed. Springhouse, Pa.: Springhouse Corp., 1997.

Phillips, T.J., "Leg Ulcer Management," *Dermatology Nursing* 8(5):333-40, October 1996.

Ruszkowski, A.M., et al., "Patch Testing Basics: Patient Selection, Application Techniques and Guidelines for Interpretation," *Dermatology Nursing,* February, 1995 supplement.

U.S. Department of Health and Human Services, Public Health Service, Agency for Health Care Policy and Research. *Treatment of Pressure Ulcers.* Clinical Practice Guideline. No. 15 (AHCHR Pub. No. 95-0653). Rockville, Md.: December 1994.

14

EYE, EAR, NOSE, AND THROAT CARE

Ear, nose, and throat (ENT) conditions require careful nursing assessment and, in many cases, recommendations for follow-up treatment. A patient may mention an eye problem during your assessment of another complaint or during routine care.

ASSESSMENT

Assessment of the eye includes testing the patient's vision and extraocular muscle function, inspecting the external ocular structures, and inspecting internal structures with an ophthalmoscope.

You'll use inspection and palpation to assess the ears, nose, and throat.

Assessing the eyes

For a basic eye assessment, obtain a Snellen eye chart, a piece of newsprint, an eye occluder or an opaque 3″ × 5″ card, a penlight, a wisp of cotton, a pencil or other narrow cylindrical article, and an ophthal-

moscope. The patient who normally wears corrective lenses should wear them for the distance- and near-vision tests.

Distance vision

To test the distance vision of a patient who can read English, use the Snellen alphabet chart containing various-sized letters. For patients who are illiterate or unable to speak English, use the Snellen E chart, which displays the letter in varying sizes and positions. The patient indicates the position of the E by duplicating the position with his fingers. Picture charts can be used for children.

Be certain to position the patient 20′ (6 m) from the chart. The denominator, which ranges from 10 to 200, indicates from what distance a normal eye can read the chart. For example, if he can only read a line identified by the numbers 20/100, this means that he can read from 20′ what a person with normal vision can read from 100′ (31 m).

Test each eye separately by covering the left eye first, and then the right, with an opaque 3″ × 5″ card or an eye occluder. Afterward, test binocular vision by having the patient read the chart with both eyes uncovered. Start with the line marked 20/40. Continue down the chart until the patient can read a line correctly with no more than two errors. That line indicates the patient's distance visual acuity. If he reads the 20/20 line correctly, this is considered "normal" visual acuity.

Near vision

Test the patient's near vision by holding either a Snellen chart or a card with newsprint 12″ to 14″ (30.5 to 35.5 cm) in front of the patient's eyes. As with distance vision, test each eye separately and then together. Any patient who complains of blurring with the card at 12″ to 14″ or who is unable to read it accurately needs retesting and then referral to an ophthalmologist if necessary. Keep in mind that a patient who is illiterate may be too embarrassed to say so. If a patient seems to be struggling to read the type or stares at it without attempting to read, change to the Snellen E chart.

Color perception

People with color blindness can't distinguish among red, green, and blue. The most common test to detect color blindness involves asking a patient to identify patterns of colored dots on colored plates. The patient who can't discern colors will miss the patterns.

Extraocular muscle function

To assess extraocular muscle function, first inspect the eyes for position and alignment, making sure they're parallel. Next, perform the following tests: the six cardinal positions of gaze test, the cover-uncover test, and the corneal light reflex test.

To perform the six cardinal positions of gaze test, sit directly in front of the patient, and ask him to remain still while you hold a cylindrical object such as a penlight directly in front of, and about 18″ (46 cm) away from, the patient's nose. Ask the patient to hold his head still and to watch the object as you move it from straight ahead to up and to the right, to the right side, down and to the right, straight down, down and to the left, to the left side, and up and to the left. Throughout the test, the patient's eyes should remain parallel as they move.

To perform the cover-uncover test, have the patient stare at an object on a distant wall directly opposite. Cover the patient's left eye with an opaque card and observe the uncovered right eye for movement or wandering. Next, remove the card from the left eye. The left eye should remain steady, without moving or wandering. Repeat the procedure on the right eye. This assesses the fusion reflex, which makes binocular vision possible.

To perform the corneal light reflex test, ask the patient to stare straight ahead while you shine a penlight on the bridge of his nose from a distance of 12″ to 15″ (30.5 to 38 cm). Check to make sure that the cornea reflects the light in exactly the same place in both eyes.

Peripheral vision

Assessment of peripheral vision tests the optic nerve (cranial nerve II) and measures the retina's ability to receive stimuli from the periphery of its field. You can grossly evaluate peripheral vision by assessing visual fields, which compares the patient's peripheral vision with your own. However, because this assumes you have normal vision, the test can be subjective and inaccurate. (See *Testing peripheral vision*, page 746.)

Inspection

Next inspect the eyelids, eyelashes, and lacrimal apparatus. Then inspect the eyeball, the conjunctiva, sclera, cornea, anterior chamber, iris, and pupil. Using an ophthalmoscope, inspect the vitreous humor and retina.

Eyelids, eyelashes, eyeball, and lacrimal apparatus. Inspect these structures for general appearance. The eyes are normally bright and clear. The eyelids should close completely over the sclera, and when opened, the margins of the upper eyelids should fall between the superior pupil margin and the superior limbus, covering a small portion of the iris. The eyelids should be free from edema, scaling, or lesions, and the eyelashes should curve outward and be equally distributed along the upper and lower eyelid margins. Inspect the palpebral folds for symmetry and the eyes for nystagmus (involuntary oscilla-

tions of the eyes) and lid lag (unequal eyelid movement). Further inspect the eyes for excessive tearing or dryness and the puncta for inflammation and swelling.

Conjunctiva and sclera. View the white sclera through the bulbar portion of the conjunctiva. The conjunctiva should be free from engorged blood vessels and mucus.

Inspect the color of the sclera, which is normally white. However, it's not unusual for patients with dark complexions, such as Blacks and those from the Middle East, to have small, darkly pigmented spots on the sclera.

Cornea, anterior chamber, and iris. To inspect the cornea and anterior chamber, shine a penlight into the patient's eye from several side angles (tangentially). Normally, the cornea and anterior chamber are clear and transparent. Calculate the depth of the anterior chamber from the side by figuring the distance between the cornea and the iris. The iris should illuminate with the side lighting.

The surface of the cornea normally appears shiny and bright without any scars or irregularities. The lids of both eyes should close when you touch either cornea.

Inspect the iris for shape and color. The iris should have a rather flat appearance when it's viewed from the side.

Pupil. Examine the pupil of each eye for equality of size, shape, reaction to light, and accommodation. To test for accommodation, ask the

Testing peripheral vision

To test peripheral visual fields, follow this procedure. Sit facing the patient, about 2' (61 cm) away, with your eyes at the same level as the patient's (see below). Have the patient stare straight ahead. Cover one of your eyes with an opaque cover or your hand and ask the patient to cover the eye directly opposite your covered eye. Next, bring an object such as a penlight from the periphery of the superior field toward the center of the field of vision, as shown in the illustration below. The object should be equidistant between you and the patient. Ask the patient to tell you the moment the object appears. If your peripheral vision is intact, you and the patient should see the object at the same time.

visual fields, as shown in the diagram below. When testing the temporal field, you will have difficulty moving the penlight far enough out so that neither person can see it. So test the temporal field by placing the penlight somewhat behind the patient and out of the patient's visual field. Slowly bring the penlight around until the patient can see it.

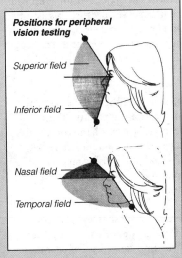

Positions for peripheral vision testing

Superior field

Inferior field

Nasal field

Temporal field

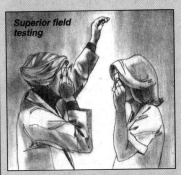

Superior field testing

Repeat the procedure clockwise at 45-degree angles, checking the superior, inferior, temporal, and nasal

The normal field of vision is about 50 degrees upward, 60 degrees medially, 70 degrees downward, and 110 degrees laterally. Remember that this test discovers only large peripheral vision defects such as blindness in one-quarter to one-half of the visual field.

patient to stare at an object across the room. Normally, the pupils should dilate. Then ask him to stare at your index finger or at a pencil held about 14″ (35.5 cm) away. The

pupils should constrict and converge equally on the object. (See *Documenting with PERRLA.*)

Palpation

After inspection, palpate the eye and related structures. Begin by gently palpating the eyelids for swelling and tenderness. Next, palpate the eyeball by placing the tips of both index fingers on the eyelids over the sclera while the patient looks down. The eyeballs should feel equally firm. However, never do this when you suspect traumatic eye injury.

Next, palpate the lacrimal sac by pressing the index finger against the patient's lower orbital rim on the side closest to his nose. While pressing, observe the punctum for any abnormal regurgitation of purulent material or excessive tears, which could indicate blockage of the nasolacrimal duct.

Ophthalmoscopic examination

Before beginning, practice holding and using the ophthalmoscope until you feel comfortable with it. The "0" lens is glass without any refraction. Set the lens at 0 and then slowly move toward a positive number, such as 6 or 8, or until the patient's optic disk becomes sharply focused.

An ophthalmoscopic examination can detect many disorders of the optic disk and retina, but the technique and the interpretation of abnormalities require skill, experience, and knowledge. (See *Performing an ophthalmoscopic examination*, pages 748 and 749.)

Assessing the ears, nose, and throat

You'll primarily use inspection and palpation to assess the ears, nose, and throat. If appropriate, you'll

also use a head mirror, postnasal mirrors, and an otoscopic and nasal speculum.

Inspecting and palpating the ears

Examine ear color and size. The ears should be similarly shaped, colored the same as the face, and sized in proportion to the head. Look for drainage, nodules, or lesions. Some ears normally drain large amounts of cerumen. Check behind the ear for inflammation, masses, or lesions.

Palpate the external ear and the mastoid process to discover any areas of tenderness, swelling, nodules, or lesions, and then gently pull the helix of the ear backward to detect pain or tenderness.

Otoscopic examination

Before examining the auditory canal and the tympanic membrane, become familiar with the function of the otoscope. (See *Performing an otoscopic examination,* page 750.)

Performing an ophthalmoscopic examination

An ophthalmoscope can help identify inner eye abnormalities. Place the patient in a darkened or semidarkened room, with neither you nor the patient wearing glasses unless you're very myopic or astigmatic. You or the patient may wear contact lenses.

1. Sit or stand in front of the patient with your head about 1½′ (46 cm) in front of and about 15 degrees to the right of the patient's line of vision in the right eye. Hold the ophthalmoscope in your right hand with the viewing aperture as close to your right eye as possible. Place your left thumb on the patient's right eyebrow to prevent hitting the patient with the ophthalmoscope as you move in close. Keep your right index finger on the lens selector to adjust the lens as necessary, as shown here. To examine the left eye, perform these steps on the patient's left side.

reflex indicates that the lens is free from opacity and clouding.

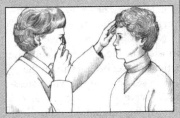

3. Move closer to the patient, changing the lens with your forefinger to keep the retinal structures in focus, as shown below.

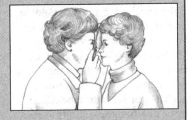

4. Change to a positive diopter to view the vitreous humor, observing for any opacity.

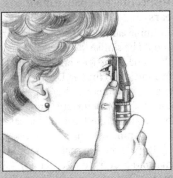

2. Instruct the patient to look straight ahead at a fixed point on the wall at eye level. Next, approaching from an oblique angle about 15″ (38 cm) out and with the diopter at 0, focus a small circle of light on the pupil. Look for the orange-red glow of the red reflex, which should be sharp and distinct through the pupil. The red

5. Next, view the retina, using a strong negative lens. Look for a retinal blood vessel, and follow that vessel toward the patient's nose, rotating the lens selector to keep the vessel in focus. Examine all the retinal structures, including the retinal vessels, the optic disc, the retinal background, the macula, and the fovea.

6. Examine the vessels for their color, the size ratio of arterioles to veins, the arteriole light reflex, and the arteriovenous (AV) crossing. The crossing points should be smooth, without nicks or narrowings, and the vessels should be free from exudate, bleeding, and narrowing. Retinal vessels normally have an AV ratio of 2:3 or 4:5.

7. Evaluate the color of the retinal structures. The retina should be light yellow to orange and the background free from hemorrhages, aneurysms, and exudates. The optic disc, located on the nasal side of the retina, should be orange-red with distinct margins. The physiologic cup is about one-third the size of the optic disc and is normally yellow-white and readily visible.

8. Examine the macula last, and as briefly as possible, because it's very light-sensitive. The macula, which is darker than the rest of the retinal background, is free from vessels and located temporally to the optic disc. The fovea centralis is a slight depression in the center of the macula.

Assessing the temporomandibular joints

Inspect and palpate the temporomandibular joints, which are located anterior to and slightly below the auricle. To palpate these joints, place the middle three fingers of each hand bilaterally over each joint. Then gently press on the joints as the patient opens and closes his mouth. Evaluate the joints for movability, approximation (drawing of bones together), and discomfort. Normally, this process should be smooth and painless for the patient.

Assessing the nose

Inspect the nose for symmetry and contour, noting any foreign bodies, unusual or foul odors, and any areas of deformity, swelling, or discoloration. To assess nasal symmetry, ask the patient to tilt his head back and observe the position of the nasal septum. The septum should be aligned with the bridge of the nose. With the head in the same position, evaluate flaring of the nostrils. Some flaring during quiet breathing is normal, but marked flaring may indicate respiratory distress. The nose should be intact and symmetrical, with no edema or deformity. Note the character and amount of any drainage from the nostrils.

Next, palpate the nose, checking for any painful or tender areas, swelling, or deformities. Evaluate nostril patency by gently occluding one nostril with your finger and having the patient exhale through the other.

Assessing the sinuses

To assess the paranasal sinuses, inspect, palpate, and percuss the frontal and maxillary sinuses. To assess the frontal and maxillary sinuses, first inspect the external skin surfaces above and to the side

Performing an otoscopic examination

Have the patient sit in a comfortable position or lie down on the side opposite the ear you wish to examine. Hold the otoscope's handle in the space between your thumb and index finger.

Assist the patient to tilt her head toward the shoulder opposite the ear you're examining. Keeping in mind how the ear canal curves in an adult, gently grasp the auricle and pull it up and back to straighten the ear canal before inserting the speculum.

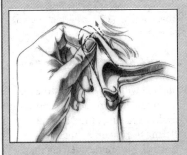

Keep in mind the sensitivity of the ear canal's skin. Improper technique at this point may cause the patient considerable discomfort or even pain.

If you're examining a child's ear, pull the auricle gently downward to straighten the ear canal before inserting the speculum.

Grasp the otoscope in your dominant hand with the handle parallel to the patient's head and the speculum at the patient's ear, as shown in the next column. Holding the otoscope

with the handle facing up allows you to brace your hand against the patient's head to stabilize the instrument. This helps to prevent injury if the patient moves her head quickly.

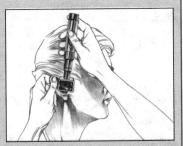

Inspect the auditory canal for cerumen, redness, or swelling. You'll see hairs and cerumen in the ear canal's distal two-thirds. Note if excessive cerumen obstructs your view; you may need to remove it to complete your inspection.

Inspect the tympanic membrane. Typically, middle ear problems will be evident by the tympanic membrane's appearance. Focus on the membrane's color and contour. It should be pearly gray and appear concave at the umbo. Then move the otoscope to identify landmarks on the tympanic membrane, including the umbo, handle of malleus, and cone of light. Be alert for perforations, bulging, missing landmarks, or a distorted cone of light.

of the nose for inflammation or edema. Then palpate and percuss the sinuses.

Assessing the mouth and oropharynx

Put on gloves and ask the patient to remove any partial or complete dentures.

When examining the oral mucosa, observe the gingivae and teeth. Gingival surfaces should appear pink, moist, and slightly irregular, with no spongy or edematous areas. The edges of the teeth should be clearly defined, with a shallow crevice visible between the gingivae and teeth. Note any missing, broken, loose, or repaired teeth.

The tongue should appear pink and slightly rough with a midline depression and a V-shaped division (sulcus terminalis) and should move freely.

Also inspect the hard and soft palates. They should appear pink to light red, with symmetrical lines. Normally, the hard palate is rougher and a lighter pink than the soft palate.

Examine the oropharynx, using a tongue blade and a flashlight, if necessary. Observe the position, size, and overall appearance of the uvula and the tonsils. Observe the tonsils for enlargement. Then place the tongue blade firmly on the midpoint of the tongue, almost far enough back to elicit the gag reflex, and ask the patient to say "ah." The soft palate and uvula should rise symmetrically.

DIAGNOSTIC TESTS

Tests to determine the presence of eye, ear, nose, or throat disorders should cause your patient little discomfort. For specific tests, see *Diagnostic tests for eye, ear, nose, and throat disorders,* pages 752 to 755.

NURSING DIAGNOSES

When caring for patients with eye and ENT disorders, you'll find that several nursing diagnoses are commonly used. These diagnoses appear below, along with appropriate nursing interventions and rationales. (Rationales appear in italic type.)

Impaired swallowing

Related to pain and inflammation, impaired swallowing may be associated with such conditions as pharyngitis, tonsillitis, and laryngitis.

Expected outcomes
• Patient shows no evidence of aspiration pneumonia.
• Patient achieves adequate nutrition.
• Patient maintains weight and oral hygiene.
• Patient (or caregiver) demonstrates correct eating (or feeding) techniques to maximize swallowing.

Nursing interventions and rationales
• Elevate the head of the bed at least 45 degrees at all times, and 90 degrees after food or fluid intake. Position the patient on his side while recumbent. Have suction equipment available in case aspiration occurs. Assess swallowing function frequently, especially before meals. *These measures prevent aspiration.*
• Monitor intake and output and weigh daily *to ensure adequate hydration and nutrition.*
• Provide a liquid to soft diet *to promote less painful swallowing.*

(Text continues on page 755.)

Diagnostic tests for eye, ear, nose, and throat disorders

Test	Purpose	Nursing considerations
Eye tests		
Fluorescein angiography	To allow evaluation of the entire retinal vascular bed, including retinal circulation	• Explain the procedure and that eyedrops will be instilled to dilate the patient's pupils. • Check history for hypersensitivity to contrast medium. • Remind the patient to maintain his position and fixation as the dye is injected. • Tell him his skin and urine will be colored yellow for 24 to 48 hours after the test and that his near vision will be blurred for up to 12 hours. • After the test, encourage fluids.
Orbital computed tomography	To allow visualization of abnormalities	• Explain the procedure. • If contrast enhancement is scheduled, withhold food and fluids for 4 hours before the test. • Check history for hypersensitivity to iodine, shellfish, and contrast medium. Warn the patient of possible adverse effects. • After the test, he may resume usual diet.
Orbital radiography	To help detect fractures and diagnose ocular and orbital pathology	• Explain the procedure. • Tell the patient that he'll be asked to turn his head from side to side to flex or extend his neck. • Instruct him to remove all metal and jewelry within the X-ray field.
Ocular ultrasonography	To evaluate eye structures and diagnose abnormalities	• Explain the procedure. • Inform the patient that he may be asked to move his eye or change his gaze during the test. • After the test, be sure to remove water-soluble jelly from patient's eyelids.
Refraction	To define the refractive error and determine the degree of correction required to improve visual acuity	• Explain the procedure. • Tell the patient that eyedrops may be instilled to dilate pupils. • Check history for hypersensitivity to eyedrops. • If corrective lenses are prescribed, advise the patient that it may take him a little time to adjust to the prescription.

Diagnostic tests for eye, ear, nose, and throat disorders

(continued)

Test	Purpose	Nursing considerations
Eye tests *(continued)*		
Slit-lamp examination	To allow visualization of the anterior segment of the eye; evaluate ocular fluids	• Explain the procedure. • If patient wears contact lenses, instruct him to remove them before the test. • Tell him that eyedrops may be instilled and that his near vision will be blurred for 40 minutes to 4 hours. • Advise him to wear dark glasses in bright sunlight until his pupils recover.
Tonometry	To allow indirect measurement of intraocular pressure	• Explain the procedure and that the patient must remain still. • Tell him an anesthetic will be instilled into his eyes, and that after the test he shouldn't rub his eyes for at least 20 minutes. • Instruct him that when the anesthetic wears off he may feel a scratching sensation that should disappear within 24 hours.
Audiologic tests		
Acoustic immittance test	To evaluate middle ear function and diagnose middle ear disorders, lesions, and eustachian tube dysfunctions	• Explain the procedure. • Instruct the patient not to move, speak, or swallow while immittance is being measured, and caution him not to startle during the loud tone. • Tell him to report any discomfort or dizziness.
Pure tone audiometry	To determine the presence, type, and degree of hearing loss	• Explain the procedure. • Advise the patient that he will hear tones at various intensities and that he will be instructed to give a signal each time he hears the tone. • Emphasize that he should respond even if the tone is very faint.
Rinne test	To compare bone conduction to air conduction	• Explain the procedure. • Place the base of a vibrating tuning fork on the mastoid process, noting how many *(continued)*

Diagnostic tests for eye, ear, nose, and throat disorders

(continued)

Test	Purpose	Nursing considerations
Audiologic tests *(continued)*		
Rinne test *(continued)*		seconds pass before the patient can no longer hear it. • Then quickly place the still-vibrating fork with the tines parallel to the ear canal, until the patient can no longer hear the tone. • Repeat the test on the other ear. • Record the results as a ratio of air to bone conduction.
Weber's test	To evaluate bone conduction	• Explain the procedure. • Place a vibrating tuning fork on top of the patient's head at midline. • Ask if he hears the tone in the left ear, right ear, or equally in both. • Record the results as Weber left, Weber right, or Weber midline, respectively.
Word recognition tests	To evaluate the clarity of speech reception, determine the need for and potential benefits from a hearing aid, and help locate auditory tract and central nervous system lesions	• Explain the procedure. • Tell the patient that he will hear a series of short words and that he should repeat each word after he hears it and should guess when unsure. • If the patient is wearing a hearing aid, ask him to remove it.
Nose and throat cultures		
Nasopharyngeal culture	To evaluate nasopharyngeal secretions for the presence of pathogens	• Explain the procedure and ask the patient to cough before collecting the specimen. • Position him with his head tilted back. • Gently pass the swab through the nostril and into the nasopharynx, keeping the swab near the septum and the floor of the nose. • Rotate the swab quickly and remove it. • If using a Pyrex tube, place it in the patient's nostril and carefully pass the

Diagnostic tests for eye, ear, nose, and throat disorders

(continued)

Test	Purpose	Nursing considerations
Nose and throat cultures *(continued)*		
Nasopharyn-geal culture *(continued)*		swab through the tube into the naso-pharynx. Rotate the swab for 5 seconds, then place it into the culture tube with the transport medium. Remove the Pyrex tube.
Throat culture	To isolate and identify group A hemolytic strepto-cocci	• Explain the procedure. • Obtain the specimen before beginning any ordered antibiotic therapy. • Tell the patient to tilt his head back and close his eyes. • Swab the tonsilar area from side to side. Include any inflamed or purulent sites. Don't touch the tongue, cheeks, or teeth with the swab. • Immediately place the swab into the culture tube. • Crush the ampule and force the swab into the medium.

• Provide mouth care frequently *to remove secretions and enhance comfort and appetite.*
• Teach the patient and family to maintain hydration with liquids (but avoid milk products) and to advance diet as tolerated on discharge. Notify doctor if patient can't swallow. *This allows the patient to resume normal intake as the swallowing function returns.*

Sensory/perceptual alteration: Auditory

Related to altered auditory reception or transmission, sensory/perceptual alteration, auditory, may be associated with such conditions as otitis media, otosclerosis, Ménière's disease, and labyrinthitis.

Expected outcomes
• Patient understands normal hearing changes that occur with age.
• Patient expresses feelings with regard to hearing deficits.
• Patient demonstrates correct use of hearing aids.
• Patient incorporates alternative communication techniques, such as lipreading, gestures, and written information, into daily activities.
• Patient expresses interest in attending community support groups.

Nursing interventions and rationales

• Determine how to communicate effectively with the patient, using gestures, lipreading, and written words as necessary, *to ensure adequate patient care.*

• When speaking to a partially hearing-impaired person, speak clearly and slowly in a normal to deep voice, and offer concise explanations of procedures, *to include the patient in his own care.*

• Provide sensory stimulation by using tactile and visual stimuli *to help compensate for hearing loss.*

• Encourage the patient to use his hearing aid as directed *to enhance auditory function.*

• Upon discharge, teach him to watch for visual cues in the environment, such as traffic lights and flashing lights on emergency vehicles, *to avoid injury.*

Sensory/perceptual alteration: Visual

Related to visual impairment, sensory/perceptual alteration, visual, represents the patient's deprivation of environmental stimuli.

Expected outcomes

• Patient's environment is enhanced to ensure safety.

• Patient openly expresses feelings regarding vision loss.

• Patient maintains orientation to time, place, and person.

• Patient regains visual functioning to the extent possible.

• Patient compensates for vision loss by use of adaptive devices.

• Patient plans to use appropriate resources.

Nursing interventions and rationales

• Allow the patient to express his feelings about vision loss. *This aids acceptance of vision loss.*

• Orient the patient to his surroundings. If appropriate, allow him to direct the arrangement of the room. *This allows him to maintain an optimal level of independence.*

• Always introduce yourself or announce when you're entering or leaving the patient's room. *Familiarizing the patient with the caregiver aids reality orientation.*

• Inform health care personnel of the patient's vision loss by recording information on the patient's Kardex and chart cover or by positioning it in the patient's room. *Nursing care is improved if the staff is aware of the patient's vision loss.*

• Refer the patient to the appropriate support groups or organizations. *This will help the patient and his family cope with vision loss.*

DISORDERS

This section discusses common eye, ear, nose, and throat disorders, including their causes, assessment findings, diagnostic tests, treatments, nursing interventions, patient education, and evaluation.

Eyelid and lacrimal duct disorders

The most common disorders of the eyelids and lacrimal ducts include blepharitis, dacryocystitis, and orbital cellulitis.

Blepharitis

A common inflammatory condition of the lash follicles and meibomian glands of the upper or lower eyelids, blepharitis in many cases occurs in children and is commonly bilateral. It usually occurs as seborrheic (nonulcerative) blepharitis or as staphylococcal (ulcerative) blepharitis. Both types may coexist. Blepharitis tends to recur and become chronic.

Causes. Seborrhea of the scalp, eyebrows, and ears generally causes seborrheic blepharitis. *Staphylococcus aureus* infection causes ulcerative blepharitis. Another cause is pediculosis of the brows and lashes (from *Phthirus pubis* or *Pediculus humanus capitis*), which irritates the lid margins.

Assessment findings. Signs and symptoms of blepharitis include redness of the eyelid margins, itching of affected eye(s), burning of affected eye(s), foreign-body sensation, and sticky, crusted eyelids on waking. Other indications are unconscious eye rubbing, continual blinking, greasy scales, flaky scales on lashes, loss of lashes, and ulcerated areas on lid margins. Nits on the lashes are a sign of pediculosis.

Diagnostic tests. Culture of ulcerated lid margins shows *S. aureus* in ulcerative blepharitis.

Treatment. Early treatment is essential to prevent recurrence or complications. Treatment depends on the type of blepharitis. In seborrheic blepharitis, warm compresses prior to daily shampooing (using a mild shampoo on a damp applicator stick or a washcloth) removes scales from the lid margins. The scalp and eyebrows should also be shampooed frequently.

In ulcerative blepharitis, sulfonamide eye ointment is applied or an appropriate antibiotic is given. In blepharitis caused by pediculosis, treatment requires removal of nits (with forceps) or application of ophthalmic physostigmine ointment.

Nursing interventions. If blepharitis results from pediculosis, be sure to check the patient's family and other contacts.

Patient education. Instruct the patient to remove scales from the lid margins daily with an applicator stick or a clean washcloth. Teach him the following method for applying warm compresses: First, run warm water into a clean bowl, and immerse a clean cloth in the water and wring it out. Then place the warm cloth against the closed eyelid (be careful not to burn the skin). Hold the compress in place until it cools. Continue this procedure for 15 minutes.

Evaluation. The patient should clean his eyelids and apply medication properly. The redness, irritation, and crusting of eyelids should be relieved.

Dacryocystitis

In adults, dacryocystitis is a common infection of the lacrimal sac, which results from an obstruction (dacryostenosis) of the nasolacrimal duct or from trauma. In infants, it results from congenital atresia of the nasolacrimal duct. Dacryocystitis can be acute or chronic and is usually unilateral.

Causes. The most common infecting organism in acute dacryocystitis is *S. aureus* or, occasionally, beta-hemolytic streptococcus. In chronic dacryocystitis, the causative organisms are *Streptococcus pneumoniae* and, sometimes, a fungus such as *Candida albicans.*

Assessment findings. The hallmark sign, which occurs in both forms, is constant tearing. In the acute form, the nasolacrimal sac becomes inflamed and swollen. With application of pressure, purulent discharge may ooze from the sac. In the chronic form, mucoid discharge may ooze.

Diagnostic tests. Culture of the discharged material demonstrates the causative organism. White blood cell (WBC) count may be elevated in the acute form. X-ray after injection of radiopaque medium (dacryocystography) locates the atresia in children.

Treatment. Application of warm compresses accompanies topical and systemic antibiotic therapy. Chronic dacryocystitis may eventually require dacryocystorhinostomy.

After surgery, apply ointment to the suture line.

Therapy for nasolacrimal duct obstruction in an infant consists of careful massage of the area over the lacrimal sac four times a day for 2 to 3 months. If this fails to open the duct, dilatation of the punctum and probing of the duct are necessary.

Nursing interventions. For care of the patient undergoing surgery for this condition, see "Orbitotomy and dacryocystorhinostomy," page 791.

Evaluation. The patient should apply warm compresses and medications as directed. If surgery has been performed, the condition should resolve without complication.

Orbital cellulitis

Orbital cellulitis is an acute infection of the orbital tissues and eyelids that doesn't involve the eyeball. It may be primary or secondary, with the primary form most common in young children. If cellulitis isn't treated, infection may spread to the cavernous sinus or the meninges.

Causes. Trauma such as an insect bite may cause a primary orbital cellulitis. Streptococcal, staphylococcal, or pneumococcal infections of nearby structures can cause secondary orbital cellulitis.

Assessment findings. Signs and symptoms include fever, unilateral eyelid edema, hyperemia of the orbital tissue, reddened eyelids, and matted eyelashes. Limitation of eye movement muscle may accompany proptosis because of edematous tissues within the bony confines of the orbit. Initially, the eyeball is unaffected. Other indications are extreme orbital pain, impaired eye movement, chemosis, and purulent discharge from indurated areas.

Diagnostic tests. Wound culture and sensitivity testing determine the causative organism and specific antibiotic therapy. WBC count is elevated. Ophthalmologic examination rules out cavernous sinus thrombosis.

Treatment. Prompt treatment prevents complications. Primary treatment consists of antibiotic therapy. Systemic antibiotics and eyedrops or ointment will be ordered. Supportive therapy consists of fluids; warm, moist compresses; and bed rest. Incision and drainage may also be necessary.

Nursing interventions. Have the patient apply compresses every 3 to 4 hours to relieve discomfort. Suggest analgesics, as ordered, after assessing pain level.

Patient education. Teach the patient to apply compresses. Urge early treatment, if the infection doesn't improve, to prevent infection from spreading.

Evaluation. The patient should comply with antibiotic therapy. Edema, redness, pain, proptosis, and discharge should resolve.

Conjunctival disorders

The most common disorder of the conjunctiva is conjunctivitis.

Conjunctivitis

An inflammation of the conjunctiva, conjunctivitis usually occurs as benign, self-limiting pinkeye. It may also be chronic, possibly indicating degenerative changes or damage from repeated acute attacks.

Causes. Causes include bacterial, viral, and chlamydial infection. Less common causes are allergy, parasitic disease and, rarely, fungal infection, or occupational irritants. Idiopathic causes are associated with certain systemic diseases, such as erythema multiforme and thyroid disease.

Assessment findings. Signs and symptoms include hyperemia of the conjunctiva, possible discharge, pain and photophobia with corneal involvement, itching and burning with allergy, and sensation of a foreign body in the eye with acute bacterial infection. An accompanying sore throat or fever is possible in children.

Diagnostic tests. Stained smears of conjunctival scrapings reveal if the cause is viral, bacterial, or an allergic response.

Treatment. Treatment of conjunctivitis varies with the cause. Bacterial conjunctivitis requires topical application of the appropriate antibiotic or sulfonamide. Viral conjunctivitis resists treatment, but sulfonamide or broad-spectrum antibiotic eyedrops may prevent secondary infection. Herpes simplex keratitis usually responds to treatment with trifluridine drops, but the infection may persist for 2 to 3 weeks. Treatment of vernal (allergic) conjunctivitis includes administration of vasoconstrictor antihistamine eyedrops such as naphazoline HCl 0.1%, cold compresses to relieve itching and, occasionally, oral antihistamines.

Nursing interventions. Notify public health authorities if cultures show *Neisseria gonorrhoeae*. Apply therapeutic ointment or drops, as ordered. Have the patient wash his hands before he uses the medication and use clean washcloths or towels so he doesn't infect his other eye.

Patient education. Teach proper hand-washing technique. Stress the risk of spreading infection to family members by sharing washcloths, towels, and pillows. Warn against rubbing the infected eye, which can spread the infection. Teach the patient to instill eyedrops and ointments correctly—without touching the bottle tip to his eye or lashes.

Stress the importance of safety glasses for the patient who works near chemical irritants.

Evaluation. The patient should use good hygiene measures and should apply medications as directed. Hyperemia, discharge, irritation, and photophobia should resolve.

Corneal disorders

Common disorders include keratitis and corneal abrasion.

Keratitis

An inflammation of the cornea, keratitis is usually unilateral. It may be acute or chronic, superficial or deep. Superficial keratitis is fairly common and may develop at any age. Untreated, recurrent keratitis may lead to blindness.

Causes. Type I infection by herpes simplex virus (dendritic keratitis) is the usual cause. Other causes include exposure of the cornea resulting from an inability to close eyelids, bacterial or fungal infection (less common), or congenital syphilis, which causes interstitial keratitis.

Assessment findings. Signs and symptoms may include opacities of the cornea, mild irritation, tearing, photophobia, and blurred vision.

Diagnostic tests. Keratitis can be confirmed on slit-lamp examination. If keratitis is caused by herpesvirus, staining the eye with a fluorescein strip reveals one or more small, branchlike (dendritic) lesions. Vision testing may show decreased acuity.

Treatment. For acute keratitis caused by herpesvirus, treatment consists of trifluridine eyedrops or oral acyclovir. Trifluridine is used to treat recurrent herpetic keratitis. Vidarabine (ointment) may be used. Fungal ulcers are treated with natamycin and in some cases amphotericin B.

Keratitis caused by exposure requires application of moisturizing ointment to the exposed cornea and of a plastic bubble eye shield or eye patch. Treatment of severe corneal scarring may include keratoplasty (cornea transplantation).

Nursing interventions. Protect the exposed corneas of unconscious patients by cleaning the eyes daily, applying moisturizing ointment, or covering the eyes with an eye shield or taping them shut.

Patient education. Explain that stress, trauma, fever, colds, and overexposure to the sun may trigger flare-ups of herpes keratitis.

Evaluation. The patient should apply medication as instructed and comply with therapy. Vision should improve as the cornea heals.

Corneal abrasion

The most common eye injury, corneal abrasion is a scratch on the surface epithelium of the cornea. A corneal scratch produced by a fingernail, a piece of paper, or other organic substance may cause a persistent lesion.

Causes. A foreign body causes corneal abrasion.

Assessment findings. Indications include redness, increased tearing, sensation of "something in the eye," pain disproportionate to the size of the injury, possible diminished visual acuity, and photophobia.

Diagnostic tests. Staining the cornea with fluorescein stain con-

firms the diagnosis. The injured area appears green when examined with a flashlight. Slit-lamp examination discloses the depth of the abrasion. Gross examination of the eye with a flashlight may reveal a foreign body on the cornea. The eyelid must be everted to check for a foreign body embedded under the lid. Visual acuity assessment provides a baseline before treatment.

Treatment. Removal of a superficial foreign body is done with a foreign body spud, after applying a topical anesthetic. A rust ring caused by a metallic foreign body on the cornea can be removed with an ophthalmic burr after applying a topical anesthetic. When only partial removal is possible, reepithelialization lifts the ring again to the surface and allows the doctor to remove it completely the following day.

Treatment also includes instillation of broad-spectrum antibiotic eyedrops in the affected eye every 3 to 4 hours, and cycloplegic eyedrops to allay the iridocyclitis that occurs with corneal damage.

Nursing interventions. Assist with examination of the eye. Check visual acuity before treatment. If a foreign body is visible, irrigate the eye with normal saline solution.

Patient education. Reassure the patient that the corneal epithelium usually heals in 24 to 48 hours. Teach the patient the proper way to instill eye medications.

Evaluation. The patient should apply medication and stop wearing contact lenses, as directed. The abrasion should heal without visual impairment. The patient should use eye safety precautions.

Lens, uveal tract, and retinal disorders

The most common disorders of these eye areas include cataracts, retinal detachment, uveitis, and vascular retinopathies.

Cataracts

A common cause of vision loss, a cataract is a gradually developing opacity of the lens or lens capsule of the eye. Cataracts commonly occur bilaterally, with each progressing independently.

Causes. Senile cataracts develop in the elderly, probably because of changes in the chemical state of lens proteins. Congenital cataracts occur in newborns as genetic defects or as a result of maternal rubella during the first trimester. Traumatic cataracts develop after a foreign body injures the lens with sufficient force to allow aqueous or vitreous humor to enter the lens capsule.

Complicated cataracts occur secondary to uveitis, glaucoma, retinitis pigmentosa, or detached retina. They may also occur in the course of a systemic disease, such as diabetes, hypoparathyroidism, or atopic dermatitis, and they can result from ionizing radiation or infrared rays. Toxic cataracts result from drug or chemical toxicity with ergot, dinitrophenol, naphthalene, phenothiazine or, in patients with galactosemia, from galactose.

Assessment findings. Signs and symptoms include painless, gradual blurring and loss of vision. With progression, the pupil whitens. Other possible symptoms include blinding glare from headlights at night, glare and poor vision in bright sunlight, and inability to recognize people at a distance.

Diagnostic tests. Shining a penlight on the pupil reveals the white area behind it (unnoticeable until the cataract is advanced) and suggests a cataract. Slit-lamp examination confirms the diagnosis by revealing an opacity of the normally clear lens.

Treatment. Treatment consists of surgically extracting the opaque lens and replacing it with an intraocular lens implant at the time of surgery. Surgery improves vision in 95% of affected persons. The current trend is to perform the surgery as a 1-day procedure.

Nursing interventions. For information on the care of the patient undergoing cataract removal surgery, see "Cataract removal," page 787.

Retinal detachment

In retinal detachment, the retinal layer splits, creating a subretinal space. Retinal detachment usually involves only one eye at first. Surgical reattachment is successful.

Causes. The most common causes are degenerative changes in the retina or vitreous humor. Other causes include trauma, inflammation, systemic diseases such as diabetes mellitus and, rarely, retinopathy of prematurity or tumors. Predisposing factors include high myopia and cataract surgery.

Assessment findings. Signs and symptoms include floaters, light flashes, and sudden, painless vision loss in a portion of the visual field.

Diagnostic tests. Ophthalmoscopic examination through a well-dilated pupil confirms the diagnosis. In severe detachment, examination reveals folds in the retina and a ballooning out of the area. Indirect ophthalmoscopy is also used to search the retina for tears and holes. Ocular ultrasonography may be necessary if the lens is opaque or the vitreous humor is cloudy.

Treatment. Measures depend on the location and severity of the detachment. They may include restricting eye movements through bed rest and sedation. If the patient's macula is threatened, positioning the head so the tear or hole is below the rest of the eye may be required prior to surgical intervention.

A hole in the peripheral retina can be treated with cryotherapy or diode laser; a hole in the posterior portion, with laser therapy. Retinal detachment rarely heals spontaneously. Surgery may be used to reattach the retina.

Nursing intervention. Provide emotional support because the patient may be understandably distraught. Position patient face down if gas has been injected.

Evaluation. The patient's vision should be restored and he should follow up as directed.

Uveitis

An inflammation of the uveal tract, uveitis occurs as anterior uveitis, which affects the iris (iritis) or both the iris and the ciliary body (iridocyclitis); as posterior uveitis, which affects the choroid (choroiditis) or both the choroid and the retina (chorioretinitis); or as panuveitis, which affects the entire uveal tract.

Causes. Typically, uveitis is idiopathic. It can result from allergy, bacteria, viruses, fungi, chemicals, trauma, surgery, or systemic diseases, such as rheumatoid arthritis, ankylosing spondylitis, toxoplasmosis, and sarcoidosis in African-Americans.

Assessment findings. Signs and symptoms of anterior uveitis include moderate-to-severe eye pain, ciliary injection, photophobia, tearing, a small pupil, and blurred vision. Patients will also complain of increased pain in the involved eye when light is shone in the uninvolved eye.

Signs and symptoms of posterior uveitis include slightly decreased or blurred vision, photophobia, floating spots, occasional redness, pain, and photophobia.

Diagnostic tests. Slit-lamp examination reveals a "flare and cell" pattern in the anterior chamber, which looks like light passing through smoke. Ophthalmoscopic examination or slit-lamp examination using a special lens reveals active inflammatory fundus lesions involving the retina and choroid. Clinical observation of a fundus lesion may be confirmed by serologic tests.

Treatment. Any known underlying cause receives treatment. Typically, treatment also includes application of a topical cycloplegic such as 1% atropine sulfate and topical corticosteroids. For severe uveitis, therapy includes oral systemic corticosteroids. Carefully monitor intraocular pressure (IOP) during acute inflammation. If IOP rises, therapy should include an antiglaucoma medication such as the beta blocker timolol, an oral carbonic anhydrase inhibitor such as acetazolamide, or a topical carbonic anhydrase inhibitor such as dorzolamide (Trusopt).

Nursing interventions. Provide thorough patient education.

Patient education. Encourage rest during the acute phase. Teach the patient the proper method of instilling eyedrops. Suggest dark glasses for photophobia. Instruct the patient to watch for and report adverse reactions to ocular medications, which should be tapered toward discontinuation. Stress the importance of follow-up care because of the strong likelihood of recurrence. Tell the patient to seek treatment at the first signs of iritis.

Evaluation. The patient should administer medications and perform follow-up procedures properly. His eye pain and vision should improve.

Vascular retinopathies

Vascular retinopathies are noninflammatory retinal disorders that result from disruption of the eye's blood supply. The four distinct types of vascular retinopathy are central retinal artery occlusion, central retinal vein occlusion, hypertensive retinopathy, and diabetic retinopathy. Diabetic retinopathy may be nonproliferative or proliferative.

Central retinal artery occlusion typically causes permanent blindness. Occasionally, with treatment, some patients experience resolution within hours and regain partial vision.

Causes. Central retinal artery occlusion may be idiopathic or result from embolism, atherosclerosis, infection (syphilis or rheumatic fever), or from conditions that retard blood flow, such as temporal arteritis, massive hemorrhage, or carotid occlusion.

Central retinal vein occlusion can be idiopathic as well as result from thrombosis or atherosclerosis. Other causes include glaucoma, polycythemia vera, and sickling hemoglobinopathies as well as vasculitis and diabetes.

Assessment findings. The signs and symptoms of central retinal artery occlusion include sudden painless, unilateral loss of vision (partial or complete). The condition may follow transient episodes of unilateral loss of vision.

Reduced visual acuity, allowing perception of only hand movement and light, indicates central retinal vein occlusion. This condition is painless, except when it results in secondary neovascular glaucoma (uncontrolled proliferation of blood vessels).

Diabetic retinopathy, in its non-proliferative form, may have no symptoms or may cause loss of central visual acuity.

Signs of the proliferative form may include sudden vision loss from vitreous hemorrhage, or macular distortion or retinal detachment from scar tissue formation.

Hypertensive retinopathy symptoms depend on the location of retinopathy (for example, blurred vision if located near the macula).

Diagnostic tests. Tests depend on the type of vascular retinopathy, and may include ophthalmoscopy, slit-lamp examination, ultrasonography, color Doppler imaging, and fluorescein angiography.

Treatment. No particular treatment has been shown to control central retinal artery occlusion, although the doctor may attempt to release the occlusion into the peripheral circulation. To reduce IOP, therapy includes acetazolamide 500 mg I.V. or I.M.; eyeball massage, using a Goldman-type gonioscope lens; and, possibly, anterior chamber paracentesis. The patient may receive inhalation therapy of carbogen (95% oxygen and 5% carbon dioxide) to improve retinal oxygenation. The patient may receive inhalation treatments hourly for 48 hours, so he should be hospitalized for careful monitoring.

Therapy for central retinal vein occlusion may include one aspirin per day. The doctor may also recommend focal laser photocoagulation for patients.

Therapy for diabetic retinopathy includes controlling the patient's blood glucose and laser photocoagulation. If a vitreous hemorrhage occurs and it isn't absorbed in 3 to 6 months, vitrectomy may be performed.

Therapy for hypertensive retinopathy involves controlling the patient's blood pressure.

Nursing interventions. Arrange for *immediate* ophthalmologic evaluation when a patient complains of sudden, unilateral loss of vision. Blindness may be permanent if treatment is delayed. Administer acetazolamide I.M. or I.V., as ordered. During inhalation therapy, monitor vital signs carefully. Discontinue this therapy if blood pressure fluctuates markedly or if the patient becomes arrhythmic or disoriented. Monitor a patient's blood pressure if he complains of occipital headache or blurred vision.

Patient education. Encourage diabetic patients to comply with prescribed diet, exercise, and medication regimens to prevent diabetic retinopathy. Recommend regular ophthalmologic examinations.

For patients with hypertensive retinopathy, stress the importance of complying with antihypertensive therapy.

Evaluation. The patient who has a chronic illness should receive follow-up care as directed and should comply with the treatment regimen. If vision worsens, the patient should seek immediate medical attention. He should follow safety precautions.

Miscellaneous disorders

Other common eye disorders include optic atrophy, strabismus, and glaucoma.

Optic atrophy

Optic atrophy is a degeneration of the optic nerve that can develop spontaneously (primary) or follow inflammation or edema of the nerve head (secondary). Some forms may subside without treatment, but optic nerve degeneration is irreversible.

Causes. Optic atrophy usually results from central nervous system (CNS) disorders, such as pressure on the optic nerve from aneurysms or intraorbital or intracranial tumors (descending optic atrophy). Optic neuritis in multiple sclerosis, retrobulbar neuritis, and tabes also can cause optic atrophy. Other causes include retinitis pigmentosa, chronic papilledema and papillitis, congenital syphilis, glaucoma, trauma, and ingestion of toxins, such as

methanol and quinine. Central retinal artery or vein occlusion that interrupts the blood supply to the optic nerve can cause degeneration of ganglion cells, a condition called ascending optic atrophy.

Assessment findings. Painless loss of either visual field or visual acuity, or both, can indicate optic atrophy. Loss of vision may be abrupt or gradual. Slit-lamp examination reveals a pupil that reacts sluggishly to direct light stimulation. Ophthalmoscopy shows pallor of the nerve head from loss of microvascular circulation in the disk and deposit of fibrous or glial tissue. Visual-field testing reveals a scotoma and, possibly, major visual field impairment.

Treatment. Optic atrophy is irreversible, so treatment usually consists of correcting the underlying cause to prevent further vision loss. Corticosteroids may be given to decrease inflammation and swelling, if a space-occupying lesion is the cause. In multiple sclerosis, resulting optic neuritis commonly subsides spontaneously.

Nursing interventions. Provide symptomatic care during diagnostic procedures and treatment.

Evaluation. The patient should retain independence despite vision loss. He should keep follow-up appointments as directed.

Strabismus

In strabismus, the absence of normal, parallel, or coordinated eye movement results in eye misalignment.

Causes. The cause of strabismus is unknown but may include congenital defect, trauma, high refractive errors, or anisometropia (unequal refractive power).

Assessment findings. An obvious indication is misalignment of the eyes—esotropia (eyes deviate inward), exotropia (eyes deviate outward), hypertropia (eyes deviate upward), or hypotropia (eyes deviate downward). This misalignment is evident upon assessment of the six cardinal positions of gaze, the cover-uncover test, or corneal light reflex testing. Diplopia, amblyopia, and other visual disturbances also can indicate strabismus.

Diagnostic tests. A physical exam reveals misalignment. Hirschberg's method also detects misalignment, while retinoscopy determines refractive error. A visual acuity test evaluates the degree of visual defect. The Maddox rods test assesses specific muscle involvement. Neurologic examination determines if the condition is muscular or neurologic in origin; it should be performed if the strabismus onset is sudden or if the CNS is involved.

Treatment. For strabismic amblyopia, therapy includes patching the normal eye or prescribing corrective glasses to keep the eye straight and to counteract farsightedness (especially in accommodative esotropia). Surgery is commonly necessary to correct strabismus from basic esotropia or residual accommodative esotropia after correction with glasses.

Surgical correction includes recession (moving the muscle posteriorly) or resection (shortening the muscle). Postoperative therapy may include applying antibiotic-steroid eyedrops. Corrective glasses may still be necessary. Surgery may have to be repeated.

Nursing interventions. If the patient is a child requiring surgery, gently wipe his tears, which will be serosanguineous, using universal precautions. Because the child may have temporary diplopia after surgery, ensure safety. Reassure parents that this is normal. Give antiemetics, if necessary. Apply antibiotic ointments or drops to the affected eye.

Patient education. Most children are discharged after they recover from anesthesia. Postoperatively, discourage a child from rubbing his eyes. Teach the parents how to administer eye medications and apply patches, if ordered.

Evaluation. The patient or a family member should properly administer medication.

Glaucoma

A group of disorders characterized by abnormally high IOP, glaucoma can damage the optic nerve. It occurs as congenital, open-angle (primary), and acute angle-closure glaucoma. It may also be secondary to other causes.

Causes. Chronic open-angle glaucoma results from overproduction of aqueous humor or obstruction of its outflow through the trabecular meshwork or the canal of Schlemm. This form of glaucoma is commonly familial. It affects 90% of all patients with glaucoma.

Acute angle-closure glaucoma, also called narrow-angle glaucoma, results from anatomic obstruction to the outflow of aqueous humor.

Congenital glaucoma is inherited as an autosomal recessive trait. Secondary glaucoma can result from uveitis, trauma, or drugs such as corticosteroids. Vein occlusion or diabetes can cause neovascularization in the angle.

Assessment findings. Chronic open-angle glaucoma is usually bilateral and slowly progressive. Its onset is insidious. Symptoms appear late in the disease. They include mild aching in the eyes, gradual loss of peripheral vision, seeing halos around lights, and reduced visual acuity, especially at night, that is uncorrectable with glasses.

The onset of acute angle-closure glaucoma is typically rapid, constituting an ophthalmic emergency. Unless treated promptly, this glaucoma produces permanent loss of or decreased vision in the affected eye. Symptoms may include unilateral inflammation and pain, pressure over the eye, moderate pupil dilation that's nonreactive to light, cloudy cornea, blurring and decreased visual acuity, photophobia, seeing halos around lights, nausea, and vomiting.

Diagnostic tests. Tonometry (using an applanation, Schiøtz, or pneumatic tonometer) measures the IOP and provides a baseline for reference. Slit-lamp examination is used to assess the anterior structures of the eye, including the cornea, iris, and lens.

Gonioscopy determines the angle of the eye's anterior chamber, enabling differentiation between chronic open-angle glaucoma and acute angle-closure glaucoma.

Ophthalmoscopy provides visualization of the fundus.

Perimetry establishes peripheral vision loss in chronic open-angle glaucoma. Fundus photography recordings are used to monitor the optic disk for any changes.

Treatment. For open-angle glaucoma, treatment initially decreases IOP through administration of beta blockers, such as timolol or betaxolol; epinephrine; or topical carbonic anhydrase inhibitors such as dorzolamide. Drug treatment also includes miotic eyedrops such as pilocarpine to facilitate outflow of aqueous humor.

Patients who are unresponsive to drug therapy may be candidates for argon laser trabeculoplasty or trabeculectomy.

In treating acute angle-closure glaucoma as an emergency, drug therapy may lower IOP. When pressure decreases, laser iridotomy or surgical peripheral iridectomy is performed. A prophylactic iridectomy is performed a few days later on the normal eye. Medical emergency drug therapy includes acetazolamide to lower IOP; timolol (Timoptic) and I.V. mannitol (20%) or oral glycerin (50%) to force fluid from the eye. Severe pain may necessitate narcotic analgesics.

Nursing interventions. For the patient with acute angle-closure glaucoma, give medications, as ordered, and prepare him psychologically for laser iridotomy or surgery. (For care of the surgical patient, see "Iridectomy," page 788, and "Trabeculectomy," page 789.)

Patient education. Stress the importance of meticulous compliance with prescribed drug therapy to prevent disk changes, loss of vision, and an increase in IOP.

Evaluation. The patient should follow the treatment regimen and obtain frequent IOP tests. He should recognize the symptoms of elevated IOP and know when to seek immediate medical attention.

Ear disorders

Ear disorders can cause pain, affect a patient's hearing, and interfere with his daily activities. They range from transient and treatable conditions such as acute otitis media to more severe ones such as Ménière's disease.

Otitis media

Otitis media, inflammation of the middle ear, may be suppurative or secretory, acute or chronic. Acute otitis media results from disruption of eustachian tube patency. In the suppurative form, respiratory tract infection or allergic reaction allows reflux of nasopharyngeal flora through the eustachian tube and colonization in the middle ear.

In secretory otitis media, obstruction of the eustachian tube results in negative pressure in the middle ear that promotes transudation of sterile serous fluid from blood vessels in the membrane of the middle ear.

Causes. Suppurative otitis media occurs as a result of pneumococci, beta-hemolytic streptococci, and gram-negative bacteria.

Chronic suppurative otitis media results from inadequate treatment of acute infection as well as infection by resistant strains of bacteria.

Secretory otitis media occurs as a result of a viral infection, allergy, or barotrauma (injury caused by an inability to equalize pressure).

The causes of chronic secretory otitis media are adenoidal tissue overgrowth, edema resulting from allergic rhinitis or chronic sinus infection, and inadequate treatment of acute suppurative otitis media.

Assessment findings. A patient with acute suppurative otitis media may be asymptomatic, but the usual clinical features include severe, deep, throbbing pain; signs of upper respiratory tract infection; mild to high fever; hearing loss, usually mild and conductive; dizziness; obscured or distorted bony landmarks of the tympanic membrane; and nausea and vomiting. Other possible effects include bulging of the tympanic membrane, with concomitant erythema, and purulent drainage in the ear canal from tympanic membrane rupture.

The patient with acute secretory otitis media is commonly asymptomatic but may develop severe conductive hearing loss ranging from 15 to 35 decibels (dB), depending on the thickness and amount of fluid in the middle ear cavity. Other signs and symptoms include a sensation of fullness in the ear; popping, crackling, or clicking sounds with swallowing or jaw movement; hearing an echo when speaking or experiencing a vague feeling of top-heaviness; and tympanic membrane retraction, which causes the bony landmarks to appear more prominent. Clear or amber fluid behind the tympanic membrane is seen on otoscopy. Some patients develop a blue-black tympanic membrane, seen on otoscopy if hemorrhage has occurred.

Chronic otitis media usually begins in childhood and persists into adulthood. Its effects include decreased or absent tympanic membrane mobility, cholesteatoma (a cystlike mass in the middle ear), and a painless, purulent discharge (in chronic suppurative otitis media). Conductive hearing loss varies with the size and type of tympanic membrane perforation and ossicular destruction. Some patients develop thickening and sometimes scarring of the tympanic membrane.

Diagnostic tests. Pneumatoscopy can show decreased tympanic membrane mobility, but this procedure is painful with the obviously bulging, erythematous tympanic membrane that occurs in acute suppurative otitis media.

Treatment. In acute suppurative otitis media, antibiotic therapy includes ampicillin or amoxicillin. For those who are allergic to penicillin derivatives, therapy may include cefaclor or co-trimoxazole. Aspirin or acetaminophen helps control pain and fever. Severe, painful bulging of the tympanic membrane usually necessitates myringotomy. Broad-spectrum antibiotics can help prevent acute suppurative otitis media in high-risk patients such as children with recurring episodes of otitis. However, in patients with recurring otitis, antibiotics must be used sparingly and with discretion to prevent development of resistant strains of bacteria.

In acute secretory otitis media, inflation of the eustachian tube by performing Valsalva's maneuver several times a day may be the only treatment required. Otherwise, nasopharyngeal decongestant therapy may be helpful. It should continue for at least 2 weeks and, sometimes, indefinitely, with periodic evaluation. If decongestant therapy fails, myringotomy and aspiration of middle ear fluid, followed by insertion of a polyethylene tube into the tympanic membrane, are necessary for immediate and prolonged equalization of pressure. The tube falls out spontaneously after 9 to 12 months. Concomitant treatment of the underlying cause (such as elimination of allergens) may also help.

Treatment of chronic otitis media includes antibiotics for exacerbations of acute infection, elimination of eustachian tube obstruction, and treatment of otitis externa (when present). If no resolution occurs after 90 days, then surgical intervention is likely. Types of procedures include myringoplasty (tympanic membrane graft) and tympanoplasty to reconstruct middle ear structures when thickening and scarring are present and, possibly, mastoidectomy. Cholesteatoma requires excision.

Nursing interventions. After myringotomy, maintain drainage flow. Don't place cotton or plugs deep in the ear canal; however, you may place sterile cotton loosely in the external ear to absorb drainage. To prevent infection, change the cotton whenever it gets damp, and wash your hands before and after providing ear care. Watch for and report headache, fever, severe pain, or disorientation.

After tympanoplasty, reinforce dressings, and observe for excessive bleeding from the ear canal. Administer analgesics as needed.

Patient education. Warn the patient against blowing his nose or getting the ear wet when bathing. If nasopharyngeal decongestants are ordered, teach correct instillation and risk of overuse.

Suggest applying heat to the ear to relieve pain. Advise the patient with acute secretory otitis media to watch for and immediately report pain and fever.

To promote eustachian tube patency, instruct the patient to perform Valsalva's maneuver several times daily. Urge prompt treatment of otitis media.

Instruct parents not to feed their infant in a supine position or put him to bed with a bottle. This prevents reflux of nasopharyngeal flora.

Evaluation. The patient should be free from pain and fever, and hearing should be completely restored.

Otosclerosis

The most common cause of conductive deafness, otosclerosis is an osseous dyscrasia of the temporal bone. In this disorder, resorption and replacement by sclerotic lesions deform the temporal bone. Spongy, vascular bone forms in the otic capsule at the oval window. With surgery, the prognosis is good.

Causes. Otosclerosis results from a genetic factor transmitted as an autosomal dominant trait. Many patients with this disorder report family histories of hearing loss (excluding presbycusis). Pregnancy may trigger onset.

Assessment findings. Several signs and symptoms can indicate otosclerosis. They include a slowly progressive unilateral hearing loss, which may advance to bilateral deafness; tinnitus (low and medium pitch); patient's own voice seeming louder; and paracusis of Willis (hearing conversation better in a noisy environment than in a quiet one). Disease can spread to the cochlea and cause sensorineural hearing loss. The patient may have a history of audiograms demonstrating air-bone gap and of successful use of a hearing aid.

Diagnostic tests. A Rinne test that shows bone conduction lasting longer than air conduction diagnoses otosclerosis. As the condition progresses, bone conduction also deteriorates. Weber's test detects sound lateralizing to the more affected ear. Radiologic imaging in the axial and coronal oblique views may confirm the diagnosis.

Treatment. Treatment depends on the patient, his disease state, and surgical eligibility. Some patients choose to do nothing. Surgical treatment consists of stapedectomy (removal of the stapes) and insertion of a prosthesis to restore partial or total hearing. This procedure is performed one ear at a time, beginning with the more damaged. Postoperative treatment includes antibiotics to prevent infection. If surgery is contraindicated, a hearing aid (air conduction aid with molded ear insert receiver) enables the patient to hear conversation in normal surroundings.

Evaluation. The patient's hearing should improve. No postsurgical infection should occur. He should understand the importance of antibiotic compliance and follow-up care postoperatively.

Ménière's disease

Also known as endolymphatic hydrops, Ménière's disease is a labyrinthine dysfunction. Violent paroxysmal attacks of severe vertigo last from 10 minutes to several hours. After multiple attacks over several years, this disorder leads to residual tinnitus and hearing loss.

Cause. The cause is unknown. Idiopathic causative theories suggest it may be an autoimmune, hereditary, viral, or environmental (noise-related) disorder.

Assessment findings. The patient has a history of increasing ear fullness and roaring tinnitus. Other characteristic effects may include rotary vertigo, with nausea and vomiting and autonomic sequelae during severe attacks. The patient reports two or more episodes lasting a minimum of 20 minutes.

Diagnostic tests. Audiometric studies indicate a loss of sensorineural hearing, discrimination, and recruitment. The examiner elicits nystagmus. The pneumatic otoscope is used to observe for Hennebert's sign or a fistula. Electronystagmography and X-rays of the internal meatus may be necessary.

Treatment. Atropine may stop an attack in 20 to 30 minutes. Epinephrine or diphenhydramine may be necessary in a severe attack. Dimenhydrinate, meclizine, diphenhydramine, or diazepam may relieve a milder attack.

Long-term management includes use of a diuretic or vasodilator and restricted sodium intake. Prophylactic antihistamines or mild sedatives (phenobarbital or diazepam) may also help. If the disease persists after more than 2 years of treatment or produces incapacitating vertigo, the patient may require surgical destruction of the affected labyrinth. This procedure permanently relieves symptoms but results in irreversible hearing loss.

Nursing interventions. After surgery, record intake and output carefully. Give prophylactic antibiotics and antiemetics, as ordered.

Patient education. During an attack of Ménière's disease, advise him against reading and exposure to glaring lights. Provide the patient and the family with a "falls protection" and activities of daily living plan. Tell him to expect dizziness and nausea for 1 to 2 days after surgery. Teach the adverse effects of antihistamine therapy (drowsiness and dry mouth).

Evaluation. The patient should no longer experience vertigo, tinnitus, nausea, or vomiting. He should observe safety precautions when he is dizzy.

Labyrinthitis

Labyrinthitis is an inflammation of the inner ear labyrinth, which commonly incapacitates the patient by producing severe vertigo that lasts for 3 to 5 days. Symptoms gradually subside over a 3- to 6-week period.

Viral labyrinthitis is commonly associated with upper respiratory tract infections. Labyrinthitis is called either serous, when toxins enter the labyrinth fluid compartment, or supportive, when destruction of membrane and ossification in the inner ear occur.

Causes. Labyrinthitis results from bacterial organisms that cause acute febrile diseases, such as pneumonia, influenza, and especially chronic otitis media. Toxic drugs can also be a cause.

Assessment findings. Severe vertigo from any movement of the head and sensorineural hearing loss both signal labyrinthitis. Other symptoms include possible spontaneous nystagmus, with jerking movements of the eyes toward the unaffected ear; nausea, vomiting, and giddiness; and, with severe bacterial infection, purulent drainage.

Diagnostic tests. Audiometric testing, culture and sensitivity testing, microscopic examination, and computed tomography (CT) scan of the temporal bone confirm labyrinthitis. Other tests include an intracranial CT scan to rule out a brain lesion or fistula and caloric testing to exclude Ménière's disease.

Treatment. Treatment includes drainage of toxins and administration of antibiotics with corticosteroids. Symptomatic treatment includes bed rest with the head immobilized between pillows, oral meclizine (Antivert) to control vertigo, and massive doses of antibiotics to combat diffuse purulent labyrinthitis. Oral fluids can prevent dehydration from vomiting. For severe nausea and vomiting, I.V. fluids may be necessary.

When conservative management fails, the patient may require surgical drainage of the infected areas of the middle and inner ear. Early and vigorous treatment of predisposing conditions, such as otitis media and local or systemic infection, can prevent this condition.

Nursing interventions. Keep the bed side rails up to prevent falls. For severe vomiting, give antiemetics, as ordered. Record intake and output, and give I.V. fluids, as ordered.

Patient education. Teach the patient to seek prompt treatment for otitis media. Tell him that hearing can take up to 6 weeks to return with serous labyrinthitis, and that activities should be limited because vertigo can make driving and handling heavy equipment hazardous. In supportive labyrinthitis, vertigo will improve with treatment but hearing loss will not.

Evaluation. The patient should no longer experience vertigo or nystagmus. His hearing should be restored (with serous labyrinthitis) and he should know the safety precautions to follow to avoid injury.

Hearing loss

Hearing loss results from a mechanical or nervous system impediment to the transmission of sound waves.

It's classified as conductive, sensorineural, and mixed. Conductive hearing loss is correctable in many cases, whereas sensorineural loss is not.

Causes. Sudden deafness refers to sudden hearing loss in a person with no prior hearing impairment. This condition is considered a medical emergency because prompt treatment may restore full hearing. Its causes and predisposing factors may include acute infections, other bacterial and viral infections (such as rubella, rubeola, influenza, herpes zoster, and infectious mononucleosis), and mycoplasma infections; metabolic disorders, such as diabetes mellitus, hypothyroidism, or hyperlipoproteinemia; vascular disorders, such as hypertension or arteriosclerosis; head trauma or brain tumors; ototoxic drugs, such as tobramycin, streptomycin, quinine, gentamicin, furosemide, or ethacrynic acid; neurologic disorders, such as multiple sclerosis or neurosyphilis; and blood dyscrasias, such as leukemia and hypercoagulation.

Noise-induced hearing loss, which may be transient or permanent, may follow prolonged exposure to loud noise (85 to 90 dB) or brief exposure to extremely loud noise (greater than 90 dB).

Presbycusis, an otologic effect of aging, results from a loss of hair cells in the organ of Corti. This disorder causes sensorineural hearing loss, usually of high-frequency tones.

Assessment findings. Noise-induced hearing loss causes sensorineural damage, the extent of which depends on the duration and intensity of the noise. Initially, the patient loses perception of certain frequencies but, with continued exposure, he eventually loses perception of all frequencies.

Presbycusis usually produces tinnitus and the inability to understand the spoken word.

Diagnostic tests. The patient, family, occupational histories, and a complete audiologic examination usually provide ample evidence of hearing loss and suggest possible causes or predisposing factors. Weber's test, the Rinne test, and specialized audiologic tests differentiate between conductive and sensorineural hearing loss.

Treatment. Therapy for congenital hearing loss that is refractory to surgery consists of teaching the patient to communicate through sign language, speech reading, or other effective means.

To treat sudden deafness, the underlying cause must be promptly identified.

In individuals whose hearing loss is induced by noise levels greater than 90 dB for several hours, overnight rest usually restores normal hearing. However, such hearing restoration doesn't occur if the person is exposed to such noise repeatedly. As the patient's hearing deteriorates, speech and hearing rehabilitation must be provided.

Presbycusis usually requires the use of a hearing aid.

Nursing interventions. When speaking to a patient with hearing loss who can read lips, stand directly in front of him, with the light on your face, and speak slowly and distinctly. Approach the patient within his visual range, and elicit his attention by raising your arm or waving; touching him may unnecessarily startle him.

Refer children with suspected hearing loss to an audiologist or otolaryngologist for further evaluation.

Watch for signs of hearing impairment in patients receiving ototoxic drugs.

Patient education. Teach the patient how a hearing aid works and how to maintain it.

Emphasize the danger of excessive exposure to noise and encourage the use of protective devices in a noisy environment. Stress the danger to pregnant women of exposure to drugs, chemicals, and infection (especially rubella).

Evaluation. The patient should be able to maintain communication with others. Both the patient and his family members should understand the importance of wearing protective devices while in a noisy environment.

Nasal disorders

Conditions of the nose and sinuses can interfere with the patient's breathing and cause congestion, discomfort, and headache.

Epistaxis

Epistaxis may be primary or secondary. Nose bleeding usually originates in the anterior nasal septum and tends to be mild. Epistaxis that originates in the posterior septum can be severe and more difficult to evaluate.

Causes. Epistaxis usually results from external causes (such as a blow to the nose, nose picking, insertion of a foreign body, or inhalation of irritating chemicals) or internal causes including polyps, nasal neoplasms, and acute or chronic infections, such as sinusitis or rhinitis, which cause congestion and eventual bleeding of the capillary blood vessels.

Assessment findings. Clinical effects depend on the severity of the bleeding. It can be local or systemic. Bleeding is considered severe if it persists longer than 10 minutes after pressure is applied; severe bleeding may cause blood loss as great as 1 qt (1 L)/hour in adults.

The patient bleeds unilaterally except when dyscrasia or severe traumatic injury causes epistaxis. Blood oozing from the nostrils usually originates in the anterior nose and is bright red. Blood from the back of the throat originates in the posterior area and may be dark or bright red. It's commonly mistaken for hemoptysis because of expectoration.

In severe epistaxis, blood seeps behind the nasal septum and may enter the middle ear and the corners of the eyes. Other symptoms include light-headedness, dizziness, slight respiratory distress, and shock. Severe hemorrhage causes a drop in blood pressure, rapid and bounding pulse, dyspnea, pallor, and other indications of progressive shock. (See *What's causing her epistaxis?*)

Diagnostic tests. Simple observation confirms epistaxis; inspection with a bright light and nasal speculum locates the site of bleeding.

Tests show a gradual reduction in hemoglobin levels and hematocrit; results are commonly inaccurate immediately after epistaxis because of hemoconcentration. A patient with blood dyscrasia has a decreased platelet count. Prothrombin time and activated partial thromboplastin time show a coagulation time twice that of normal because of a bleeding disorder or anticoagulant therapy.

Treatment. The goal is to remove the cause. For anterior bleeding, treatment may consist of the application of a cotton ball saturated with epinephrine to the bleeding site, external pressure, and cauterization by electrocautery or silver nitrate stick. If these measures don't control the bleeding, the patient may require petroleum gauze nasal packing.

For posterior bleeding, therapy includes gauze packing inserted through the nose or postnasal pack-

What's causing her epistaxis?

On the advice of a friend, Barbara, a 33-year-old office worker, came to the ambulatory center for evaluation of recurrent epistaxis.

A problem or not?

During the history phase of the examination you ascertain that Barbara began having the recurrent epistaxis episodes after she started her current job about six months ago. Although she was an office worker, she worked in a factory and was exposed to chemicals each time she entered or left her office. She initially had no difficulty controlling these occasional episodes, but then they began to occur daily. The episodes were also becoming more severe and disruptive to her work. She was becoming more and more fatigued and had headaches and rhinitis. Barbara had been self-treating it with over-the-counter allergy medications. Should you accept her self-diagnosis?

During the physical examination, she has an episode of epistaxis which doesn't stop within 8 minutes. Anterior nasal packing is put in place. You arrange for Barbara to return the same night for packing removal, and further assessment.

You draw blood for a complete blood count, prothrombin time, and partial thromboplastin time. You question the patient and are able to determine that the bleeding has always been in the left nares, and that she has a sensation of facial fullness and pressure. You have her scheduled for nose, sinus, and oropharyngeal X-rays and soft tissue films as well as an endoscopy, which will be performed the following day.

Suggested response

When Barbara returned for the packing removal, an otolaryologist examined her but could not definitively identify the site of bleeding. During the endoscopy procedure a nasal polyp was removed, biopsied, and found to be benign. It would have been easy to assume that Barbara was suffering from an allergic reaction to the chemicals at her work site. But you recognized the need for a definitive diagnosis to provide appropriate teaching and care.

ing inserted through the mouth, depending on the bleeding site. (Gauze packing usually remains in place for 24 to 48 hours; postnasal packing, 3 to 5 days.) An alternative method, the nasal balloon catheter, also controls bleeding effectively. Antibiotics may be appropriate. If local measures fail to control bleeding, treatment may include supplemental vitamin K and, for severe bleeding, blood transfusions and surgical ligation of a bleeding artery.

Nursing interventions. Have suction available at the bedside. To control epistaxis, apply firm pressure on the lateral wall of the involved nostril for 4 minutes, then check to see if the bleeding has stopped. If bleeding continues after 10 minutes of pressure, notify the doctor. Monitor vital signs and skin color; record blood loss.

Patient education. Instruct the patient to breathe through his mouth. Tell him not to swallow blood, talk, or blow his nose. Teach him to sit up and lean forward. To prevent recurrences, instruct the patient not to pick his nose or insert foreign objects in it. Emphasize the need for follow-up examinations and periodic blood studies.

Instruct the patient to keep vasoconstrictors such as phenylephrine handy. Reassure the patient and family.

Instruct patients with the following risk factors to be alert for epistaxis and seek medical care promptly for uncontrolled bleeding: anticoagulant therapy, hypertension, chronic use of aspirin, high altitudes and dry climates, sclerotic vessel disease, Hodgkin's disease, scurvy, vitamin K deficiency, rheumatic fever, and blood dyscrasias, such as hemophilia, purpura, leukemia, and some anemias.

Evaluation. The patient's bleeding should stop and shock, if any, should be controlled. He should understand methods to prevent epistaxis.

Sinusitis

Sinusitis results from interference with the natural outflow tract of the sinus. Acute sinusitis usually results from the common cold. Chronic sinusitis follows persistent bacterial infection. Allergic sinusitis accompanies allergic rhinitis. Hyperplastic sinusitis is a combination of purulent acute sinusitis and allergic sinusitis or rhinitis.

Causes. Sinusitis may result from a bacterial or viral infection or an allergy.

Assessment findings. Symptoms associated with sinusitis include nasal congestion, pressure, pain over the cheeks and upper teeth, pain over the eyes, pain over the eyebrows and, rarely, pain behind the eyes. Other signs and symptoms include fever (in acute sinusitis), nasal discharge, nasal stuffiness, and possible inflammation and pus on nasal examination. In the chronic form, the patient has decreased and diminishing pain with an increased feeling of pressure and fullness.

Diagnostic tests. Sinus X-rays reveal cloudiness in the affected sinus, air-fluid levels, or thickened mucosal lining. Endoscopy, CT scans, and magnetic resonance imaging may also be used in diagnosing sinus diseases. Antral puncture promotes drainage and removal of purulent material.

Treatment. Antibiotics are the primary treatment for acute sinusitis. Analgesics may relieve pain. Vasoconstrictors, such as epinephrine or phenylephrine, are used to decrease nasal secretions. Steam inhalation also promotes vasoconstriction and encourages drainage. Antibiotics combat persistent infection. Local applications of heat may relieve pain and congestion.

Antibiotic therapy also is the primary treatment for subacute sinusitis. Vasoconstrictors may lessen nasal secretions. Failure to resolve this condition after 3 to 4 weeks of treatment requires further evaluation.

Treatment of allergic sinusitis includes treatment of allergic rhinitis—administration of antihistamines, identification of allergens by skin testing, and desensitization by immunotherapy. Severe allergic symptoms may require corticosteroids and epinephrine.

In both chronic and hyperplastic sinusitis, antihistamines, antibiotics, and a steroid nasal spray may relieve pain and congestion. If irrigation fails to relieve symptoms, one or more sinuses may require surgery.

Nursing interventions. Enforce bed rest, and encourage the patient to drink plenty of fluids to promote drainage in the acute form. Don't elevate the head of the bed more than 30 degrees.

Apply warm compresses continuously or four times daily for 2-hour intervals. Also give analgesics as needed. Watch for and report complications, such as vomiting, chills, fever, edema of the forehead or eyelids, blurred or double vision, and personality changes.

Patient education. Instruct the patient on how to apply compresses.

Evaluation. The patient should be free from pain, congestion, and fever. He should maintain humidification and drainage of his sinuses, and should understand the importance of complying with the prescribed therapies.

Nasal polyps

Nasal polyps are normally benign and edematous growths, which are usually multiple, mobile, and bilateral. They may become large and numerous enough to cause nasal distention and enlargement of the bony framework, possibly occluding the airway. They tend to recur.

Cause. Nasal polyps usually develop as a result of continuous pressure resulting from a chronic allergy that causes mucous membrane edema in the nose and sinuses. They may also be the result of a sinus infection.

Assessment findings. Symptoms include nasal obstruction (primary indication), anosmia, a sensation of fullness in the face, nasal discharge, and shortness of breath. Associated clinical features usually indicate allergic rhinitis.

Diagnostic tests. X-rays of sinuses and nasal passages reveal soft tissue shadows over the affected areas. Examination with a nasal speculum shows a gray pendulous opalescent swelling. Those that prolapse have lost the opalescent appearance and have a dry and red surface. Large growths may resemble tumors.

Treatment. Treatment usually consists of corticosteroids, either by nose drops or sprays, to reduce the polyp temporarily. Treatment of the underlying cause may include antihistamines and antibiotic therapy. Local application of an astringent shrinks hypertrophied tissue.

Medical management alone is rarely effective, however. For this reason, the treatment of choice is polypectomy (intranasal removal of the nasal polyp with a wire snare), usually performed under local anesthesia. Continued recurrence may require surgical evacuation of diseased tissue.

Nursing interventions. Administer antihistamines, as ordered, for the patient with allergies. After surgery, monitor for excessive bleeding or other drainage, and promote patient comfort. Elevate the head of the bed. Change the mustache dressing or drip pad, as needed. Intermittently apply ice compresses over the nostrils to lessen swelling, prevent bleeding, and relieve pain.

If nasal bleeding occurs—most likely after packing is removed—have the patient sit up, monitor his vital signs, and advise him not to swallow blood. Compress the outside of the nose against the septum for 4 to 10 minutes. If bleeding persists, notify the doctor immediately; nasal packing may be necessary.

Patient education. Tell the patient what to expect postoperatively such as nasal packing for 1 to 2 days after surgery. Advise patients with chronic allergies, chronic rhinitis, chronic sinusitis, and recurrent nasal infections that they're at risk for developing nasal polyps.

Evaluation. Nasal obstruction and drainage should improve. After surgery, epistaxis should no longer recur. The patient should know that the polyps can recur and that he needs to treat episodes of allergic rhinitis promptly.

Throat disorders

You can significantly relieve throat disorders if you help the patient identify and eliminate irritants, suggest that he humidify his environment, and stress the importance of resting his voice.

Pharyngitis

Pharyngitis is an acute or chronic inflammation of the pharynx that occurs most commonly among adults who live or work in dusty or very dry environments, use their voices excessively, use tobacco or alcohol habitually, or suffer from chronic sinusitis, persistent coughs, or allergies. Acute pharyngitis may precede the common cold or other communicable diseases. Chronic pharyngitis is commonly an extension of nasopharyngeal obstruction or inflammation. Uncomplicated pharyngitis usually subsides in 3 to 10 days.

Causes. In 90% of cases, pharyngitis occurs as the result of a virus. In children, it's commonly caused by streptococcal bacteria.

Assessment findings. Symptoms include sore throat and slight difficulty swallowing (swallowing saliva is usually more painful than swallowing food); possible sensation of a lump in the throat; possible constant, aggravating urge to swallow; reddened, inflamed posterior pharyngeal wall; red, edematous mucous membranes studded with white and yellow follicles; and exudate, usually confined to the lymphoid areas of the throat, sparing the tonsillar pillars. Associated features may include mild fever, headache, rhinorrhea, and muscle and joint pain, especially in bacterial pharyngitis.

Diagnostic tests. Throat culture may identify bacterial organisms.

Treatment. Treatment is usually symptomatic, consisting mainly of rest, warm saline gargles, throat lozenges containing a mild anesthetic, plenty of fluids, and analgesics, as needed. If the patient cannot swallow fluids, hospitalization may be required for I.V. hydration.

Bacterial pharyngitis necessitates rigorous treatment with penicillin—or another broad-spectrum antibiotic if the patient is allergic to penicillin—because streptococci are the chief infecting organisms. Antibiotic therapy should continue for 48 hours after visible signs of infection have disappeared or for at least 7 to 10 days. Chronic pharyngitis requires the same supportive measures as acute pharyngitis but with greater emphasis on eliminating the underlying cause.

Nursing interventions. Administer analgesics and warm saline gargles, as ordered and as appropriate. Encourage the patient to drink plenty of fluids (up to $2^1/2$ qt [2.5 L]/day). Monitor intake and output scrupulously, and watch for signs of dehydration: cracked lips, dry mucous membranes, and low urine output. Provide adequate nutrition and meticulous mouth care to prevent dry lips and oral pyoderma.

Patient education. Teach the patient the nursing interventions stated above.

Evaluation. The patient should be free from pain, fever, and erythema.

Tonsillitis

Inflammation of the tonsils can be acute or chronic. The uncomplicated acute form usually lasts 4 to 6 days. Tonsils tend to hypertrophy during childhood and atrophy after puberty.

Causes. The most common cause of tonsillitis is beta-hemolytic streptococci. The condition can also result from other types of bacteria, viruses, and tubercular and immune deficiency diseases.

Assessment findings. The discomfort associated with acute tonsillitis usually subsides after 72 hours. Signs and symptoms include mild to severe sore throat (a very young child who can't express this complaint may stop eating), dysphagia, fever, swelling and tenderness of lymph glands in the submandibular area, muscle and joint pain, chills, malaise, headache, pain (commonly referred to ears), possible urge to swallow constantly, and a constricted feeling in the back of the throat.

Signs and symptoms associated with chronic tonsillitis are a recurrent sore throat, purulent drainage in tonsillar crypts, and frequent attacks of acute tonsillitis.

Diagnostic tests. Culture may determine the infecting organism. Erythrocyte sedimentation rate and WBC count may be elevated.

Treatment. Treatment of acute tonsillitis requires rest, adequate fluid intake, and administration of aspirin or acetaminophen and, for bacterial infection, antibiotics. When the causative organism is a group A beta-hemolytic streptococcus, penicillin is the drug of choice. To prevent complications, antibiotic therapy should continue for 10 days. Chronic tonsillitis or the development of complications may require a tonsillectomy.

Nursing interventions. Despite dysphagia, urge the patient to drink plenty of fluids, especially if he has a fever. Avoid dairy products but offer flavored nonacidic drinks and ices. Suggest gargling to soothe the throat, unless it exacerbates pain.

Patient education. Make sure the patient and parents understand the need for adequate fluid intake, and the importance of completing the prescribed antibiotic therapy.

Evaluation. The patient's fever and pain should subside. He should maintain hydration and understand the importance of completing his antibiotic regimen and increasing his oral fluid intake.

Throat abscesses

Throat abscesses may be peritonsillar (quinsy) or retropharyngeal.

Causes. Peritonsillar abscess occurs as a complication of acute tonsillitis, usually after a streptococcal or staphylococcal infection. Acute retropharyngeal abscess is caused by an infection in the retropharyngeal lymph glands, which may follow an upper respiratory tract bacterial infection. Chronic retropharyngeal abscess results from tuberculosis of the cervical spine.

Assessment findings. Key signs and symptoms include severe throat pain, occasional ear pain on the affected side, tenderness of the submandibular gland, dysphagia, drooling, and trismus. Other effects include high fever, chills, malaise, pressure sensation in the throat, dry cough, rancid breath, nausea, muffled speech, dehydration, cervical adenopathy, and localized or systemic sepsis.

When examining a patient for retropharyngeal abscess, look for pain, dysphagia, fever, nasal obstruction (when the abscess is in the upper pharynx), dyspnea, progressive inspiratory stridor, and neck hyperextension.

Diagnostic tests. A culture may reveal a streptococcal or staphylococcal infection. A retropharyngeal abscess can be diagnosed by X-rays that show the larynx pushed forward and a widened space between the posterior pharyngeal wall and vertebrae. In addition, culture and sensitivity tests can isolate the causative organism.

Treatment. For early-stage peritonsillar abscess, following needle aspiration of the abscess for culture and sensitivity, large doses of penicillin or another broad-spectrum antibiotic are necessary. For late-stage abscess, with cellulitis of the tonsillar space, primary treatment is usually incision and drainage under a local anesthetic, followed by antibiotic therapy for 7 to 10 days. Tonsillectomy, scheduled no sooner than 1 month after healing, prevents recurrence but is recommended only after several episodes.

In acute retropharyngeal abscess, the primary treatment is incision and drainage through the pharyngeal wall. In chronic retropharyngeal abscess, an external incision behind the sternomastoid muscle enables drainage. During incision and drainage, strong, continuous mouth suction prevents aspiration of pus. Postoperative drug therapy includes antibiotics (usually penicillin) and analgesics.

Nursing interventions. Be alert for signs of respiratory obstruction (inspiratory stridor, dyspnea, increasing restlessness, or cyanosis). Keep emergency airway equipment nearby.

Monitor vital signs, and report any significant changes or bleeding.

Provide meticulous mouth care. Apply petroleum jelly to the patient's lips. Promote healing with warm saline gargles or throat irrigations for 24 to 36 hours after incision and drainage.

Patient education. Explain the drainage procedure to the patient or his parents. Because the procedure is usually done under a local anesthetic, the patient may be anxious.

Evaluation. The patient should have no pain or fever. He should maintain airway patency and hydration. Also he should understand the importance of completing antibiotic therapy and getting enough rest.

Laryngitis
Acute laryngitis may occur as an isolated infection or as part of a generalized bacterial or viral upper respiratory tract infection. Repeated attacks of acute laryngitis cause inflammatory changes associated with chronic laryngitis.

Causes. Acute laryngitis results from infection, excessive use of the voice, inhalation of smoke or fumes, or aspiration of caustic chemicals. Chronic laryngitis results from upper respiratory tract disorders (sinusitis, bronchitis, nasal polyps, or allergy), mouth breathing, smoking, constant exposure to dust or other irritants, or alcohol abuse.

Assessment findings. Look for hoarseness, pain (especially when swallowing or speaking), a dry cough, fever, malaise, or laryngeal edema. Persistent hoarseness is a symptom of chronic laryngitis.

Diagnostic tests. Indirect laryngoscopy confirms the diagnosis by revealing exudate and red, inflamed, and occasionally hemorrhagic vocal cords, with rounded (not sharp) edges. Bilateral swelling, which restricts movement but doesn't cause paralysis, may be present.

Treatment. Primary treatment consists of resting the voice. For viral infection, symptomatic care includes analgesics and throat lozenges for pain relief. Bacterial infection requires antibiotic therapy; usually, 250 mg of cefuroxime twice a day is prescribed for adults. Severe, acute laryngitis may necessitate hospitalization. When laryngeal edema results in airway obstruction, tracheotomy may be necessary. In chronic laryngitis, treatment must eliminate the underlying cause.

Nursing interventions. Explain to the patient and family why he should not talk. Provide a pad and pencil or a slate for communication.

Patient education. Suggest that the patient maintain adequate humidification by using a home humidifier during the winter, by avoiding air conditioning during the summer (because it dehumidifies), by using medicated throat lozenges, and by not smoking. Instruct the family on the need to monitor the patient for an adequate airway. Encourage modification of predisposing habits.

Evaluation. The patient should no longer be hoarse or have pain or fever. He should not have to undergo tracheotomy. He should understand the need to stop smoking, maintain humidification, and complete his antibiotic therapy.

Laryngeal cancer

Squamous cell carcinoma is the most common form of laryngeal cancer, comprising 90% of cases.

Laryngeal cancer is classified according to its location: *supraglottic, glottic,* and *subglottic* (rare).

Causes. The cause of laryngeal cancer is unknown. A major risk factor is smoking.

Assessment findings. The earliest sign of a glottic tumor is hoarseness, lasting longer than 2 weeks. A supraglottic tumor has few early signs or symptoms. Patients may complain of a lump in the throat or of burning or pain in the throat when drinking citrus juice or hot liquid.

Diagnostic tests. Hoarseness lasting longer than 2 weeks is evaluated through indirect laryngoscopy utilizing direct laryngoscopy for biopsy. Xeroradiography, laryngeal tomography, CT scan, or laryngography helps define the borders of the lesion.

Treatment. The goal of treatment is to eliminate the cancer through surgery, radiation, or both, and to preserve speech. Surgical procedures vary with tumor stage.

Nursing interventions. Psychological support and good preoperative and postoperative care can minimize complications and speed recovery. Postoperatively, monitor for airway obstruction; ensure the patency of the laryngectomy tube. Keep the stoma area clean.

Patient education. Prepare the patient by helping him choose an alternative method of communication (such as pencil and paper, sign language, or alphabet board).

If you're preparing the patient for total laryngectomy, arrange for a laryngectomee to visit him. Explain postoperative procedures (suctioning, nasogastric feeding, care of laryngectomy tube) and their results (breathing through neck, speech alteration). Also prepare him for other functional losses.

You'll need to teach such a patient to remove, clean, and reinsert the prosthesis as needed to clear it of mucus.

Evaluation. The patient should understand and independently perform laryngectomy or stoma care. He should understand the need for good nutrition, know the signs and symptoms of infection that require immediate medical attention, and seek speech rehabilitation and follow up as directed.

Vocal cord nodules and polyps

Vocal cord *nodules,* which are hypertrophied fibrous tumors, form at the point where the cords come together forcibly. Vocal cord *polyps* are chronic, subepithelial, edema-tous masses. Both nodules and polyps have good prognoses, unless continued voice abuse causes recurrence, with subsequent scarring and permanent hoarseness. Most common in teachers, singers, and sports fans, polyps are also common in adults who smoke, live in dry climates, or have allergies.

Causes. Vocal cord nodules and polyps usually result from voice abuse, especially with concurrent infection.

Assessment findings. Painless hoarseness and, possibly, a breathy or husky sounding voice are signs that vocal cord nodules or polyps could be present.

Diagnostic tests. Indirect laryngoscopy confirms the diagnosis.

Treatment. Conservative management of small vocal cord nodules and polyps includes humidification, speech therapy (voice rest and training to reduce the intensity and duration of voice production), and treatment of underlying allergies.

When conservative treatment fails, nodules or polyps require removal under direct laryngoscopy. Microlaryngoscopy may be done for small lesions to avoid injuring the vocal cord surface. If nodules or polyps are bilateral, excision may be performed in two stages: One cord is allowed to heal before polyps on the other cord are excised. Two-stage excision prevents laryngeal web, which occurs when epithelial tissue is removed from adjacent cord surfaces and these surfaces grow together.

Nursing interventions. Provide an alternative means of communication—slate, pad and pencil, or alphabet board. Place a sign over the bed to remind visitors that the patient shouldn't talk. Minimize the need to speak by trying to anticipate the patient's needs. Humidify room air to decrease throat irritation. Make sure the patient receives speech therapy after healing, if necessary, because continued voice abuse causes recurrence of growths.

Patient education. Postoperatively, stress the importance of resting the voice for 10 to 14 days while the vocal cords heal. If the patient is a smoker, encourage him to stop smoking entirely or, at the very least, to refrain from smoking during recovery from surgery.

Evaluation. The patient should no longer be hoarse and should be able to communicate. He should comprehend the importance of changing the causative behavior.

TREATMENTS

This section provides practical information about the most common drugs, surgeries, and procedures used to treat eye and ENT conditions. Most procedures are performed as outpatient or same-day surgeries.

Drug therapy

Drugs used to treat eye disorders include anti-infectives, anti-inflammatory agents, miotics, mydriatics, and ophthalmic anesthetics. Drugs for ENT disorders include otic, nasal, and systemic drugs, such as antihistamines and decongestants.

Surgery

Surgical treatments for eye disorders include refractive surgery, cataract removal, corneal transplant, iridectomy, trabeculectomy, and other procedures. Surgical treatments for ENT disorders include myringotomy, stapedectomy, and septoplasty.

Refractory surgery

Refractory surgery includes methods of changing the shape of the cornea by radial keratotomy or photorefractive keratectomy using an excimer laser PRK or Lasik procedure. These methods are used to correct myopia when glasses and contact lenses are unsuccessful.

In radical keratotomy, radial cuts are made into the cornea to flatten it and bring light rays on to the retina. In photorefractive keratectomy, the stromal layer is vaporized. The Lasik procedure involves removing the epithelial and Bowman's corneal layers using a microkeratome, leaving one edge attached. The stroma is then ablated with the excimer laser, and the flap is replaced over the stromal head.

Patient preparation. Tell the patient that his face will be cleaned with an antiseptic and that a sedative will be given to help him relax. He'll also have a drape placed over his face, supplemental oxygen provided, and a local anesthetic instilled in the affected eye. Explain that the procedure takes 3 to 8 minutes and that he must remain still until it's over. Inform him that the doctor may cover the eye with a dressing after surgery.

Monitoring and aftercare. After the patient recovers from the topical anesthetic, he may experience considerable pain. Administer analgesics, as ordered. Warn the patient not to rub the eye, as this may damage the cornea. If his eye isn't patched, lower the lights, as brightness may aggravate his discomfort.

Patient education. If the doctor prescribes eyedrops, review their use with the patient. Emphasize the importance of instilling them as prescribed. Explain that photophobia commonly occurs after keratotomy but usually subsides in a month or two. Suggest that the patient wear dark sunglasses or glasses with polarizing lenses when he's in bright sunlight. Warn him to avoid night driving.

Because the patient's vision may fluctuate, advise him to avoid any activity that requires clear vision until symptoms subside. Instruct the patient to protect the affected eye from soap and water when showering and bathing and to avoid contact and water sports until the doctor gives permission. Also advise the female patient to refrain temporarily from wearing eye makeup.

Cataract removal

Cataracts can be removed by one of two techniques. In the first tech-

nique, *intracapsular cataract extraction*, the entire lens is removed, with either a cryoprobe or by expressing the lens with instruments.

In *extracapsular cataract extraction* (ECCE), the patient's anterior capsule, cortex, and nucleus are removed, leaving the posterior capsule intact. This technique may be carried out using phacoemulsification, manual extraction, irrigation, and aspiration. ECCE—the primary treatment for cataracts—is used to treat children and young adults because the posterior capsule adheres to the vitreous until about age 20. By leaving the posterior capsule undisturbed, ECCE avoids disruption and loss of vitreous.

Immediately after removal of the natural lens, many patients receive an intraocular lens implant. An implant is especially well suited for elderly patients because it eliminates the need for +10 cataract glasses (which can distort images), and doesn't require those suffering from arthritis or hand tremors to manipulate contact lenses.

Patient preparation. Inform the patient that after surgery he'll have to wear an eye patch temporarily to prevent traumatic injury and infection. If a collagen shield is inserted after surgery, no patch is worn, and the shield (similar to a contact lens) will dissolve after 24 hours.

Monitoring and aftercare. Notify the doctor if the patient has severe pain unrelieved by analgesics.

Assist him with ambulation and observe other safety precautions.

Maintain the eye patch until after discharge, and have the patient wear an eye shield, especially when sleeping.

Patient education. Give instructions on when the patient should remove the eye patch and begin his eyedrops. Teach the patient or a family member how to administer eyedrops and ointments. Warn the patient to contact the doctor immediately if sudden eye pain, red or watery eyes, photophobia, or sudden visual changes occur. Instruct him to avoid activities that raise IOP, including heavy lifting, straining during defecation, or vigorous coughing. Encourage gentle exercising to stimulate circulation.

If the patient will be wearing contact lenses, teach him how to insert, remove, and care for them.

Corneal transplant

In a corneal transplant, healthy corneal tissue from a human donor replaces a damaged part of the cornea. Corneal transplants help restore corneal clarity lost through injury, inflammation, ulceration, or chemical burns. They may also correct corneal dystrophies such as keratoconus.

A corneal transplant can take one of two forms: a full-thickness penetrating keratoplasty, involving excision and replacement of the entire cornea, or a lamellar keratoplasty, which removes and replaces a superficial layer of corneal tissue.

Patient preparation. Tell the patient that he may experience a dull aching and that analgesics will be available after surgery. Inform him that a bandage and protective shield will be placed over the eye. As ordered, administer a sedative or an osmotic agent to reduce IOP.

Monitoring and aftercare. After the patient recovers from the anesthetic, assess for and immediately report sudden, sharp, or excessive pain.

Patient education. Upon discharge, instruct the patient on correct use of corticosteroid eyedrops or application of topical antibiotics to prevent inflammation and graft rejection. Teach the patient and his family to recognize the signs and symptoms of graft rejection (inflammation, cloudiness, drainage, and pain at the graft site). Instruct them to notify the doctor immediately if any of these signs or symptoms occur, especially if pain is sharp and severe.

Instruct the patient to avoid rapid head movements, hard coughing or sneezing, and other activities that could increase IOP; likewise, he shouldn't rub his eyes. Remind him to ask for help in walking until he adjusts to changes in his vision.

Iridectomy

Performed by laser or standard surgery, an iridectomy reduces IOP by facilitating the drainage of aqueous humor from the posterior chamber to the anterior chamber through a hole in the iris, bypassing the pupil. Iridectomy is commonly used to treat acute angle-closure glaucoma.

It may also be indicated for a patient with an anatomically narrow angle between the cornea and iris. Iridectomy is also used in chronic angle-closure glaucoma, in excision of tissue for biopsy or treatment, and sometimes with other eye surgeries.

Patient preparation. Make it clear to the patient that an iridectomy can't restore vision loss caused by glaucoma but that it may prevent further loss. Before laser iridectomy, administer aproclonidine hydrochloride. Miotics, topical beta blockers, and oral or I.V. osmotic agents have been used to reduce IOP in the acute stages of angle-closure glaucoma.

Monitoring and aftercare. After an iridectomy, be alert for hyphema with sudden, sharp eye pain or the presence of a small half-moon-shaped blood speck in the anterior chamber. (Check with a flashlight.) If either occurs, have the patient rest quietly in bed, with his head elevated, and notify the doctor.

To decrease inflammation, administer topical corticosteroids and medication to dilate the pupil. And if the patient received osmotic therapy before iridectomy, encourage him to increase his fluid intake to restore normal hydration and electrolyte balance.

To prevent elevated IOP from increased venous pressure in the head, neck, and eyes, discourage patients from wearing tight clothing around the neck. Recommend stool softeners. Advise the patient to refrain from rubbing his eyes.

Patient education. Instruct the patient to report any sudden, sharp eye pain immediately, as it may indicate increased IOP. Discourage the patient from vigorous coughing, sneezing, or nose blowing, for they all raise venous pressure.

Trabeculectomy

A surgical filtering procedure, trabeculectomy removes part of the trabecular meshwork to allow aqueous humor to bypass blocked outflow channels and flow safely away from the eye. This helps treat glaucoma that doesn't respond to drug therapy. An iridectomy is performed to prevent the iris from prolapsing into the new opening and obstructing the flow of aqueous humor.

Patient preparation. Inform the patient that this procedure will probably prevent further visual impairment but that it can't restore vision that's already lost.

Monitoring and aftercare. After a trabeculectomy, observe for nausea and administer antiemetics because vomiting and pain can be symptomatic of increased IOP.

Administer eyedrops after surgery, and instill a cycloplegic such as atropine, a prophylactic antibiotic (such as Polytrim or ofloxacin), corticosteroids to reduce iritis, and analgesics to relieve pain.

Patient education. Instruct the patient to immediately report sudden onset of severe eye pain, photophobia, excessive lacrimation, inflammation, or vision loss.

Explain that glaucoma isn't curable but can be controlled. Stress that he must take prescribed drugs regularly to treat this condition.

To overcome the loss of peripheral vision, teach him to turn his head fully to view objects on his side. Remind him to avoid all activities that increase IOP.

Vitrectomy

This microsurgical procedure removes part or all of the vitreous humor—the transparent gelatinous substance that fills the cavity behind the lens. A vitrectomy is performed to remove a vitreous hemorrhage and other opacities, and to treat traction retinal detachment and vitreous contraction. It's also used for removal of foreign bodies and endophthalmitis (infection within the eye).

Patient preparation. Tell the patient that the procedure will be performed under local or general anesthesia and will last between 1 to 2 hours. The patient should be prepared to wear patches postoperatively. If no complications arise, he'll be able to go home upon recovery after local anesthesia, or the day after surgery if general anesthesia was used.

Monitoring and aftercare. If the patient received injections of air or gas during surgery, inform him that he'll need to assume a certain position, usually face down, to keep the gas bubble in place over the retina. Explain that he must maintain this position for several days, although

he'll be allowed to sit upright when eating meals or stand to use the bathroom. Suggest to the patient that it might be helpful to listen to a radio or have a family member read to him to help pass the time in this uncomfortable position.

As ordered, administer I.M. or oral analgesics, mydriatic and cycloplegic drops, and antibiotic and corticosteroid drops. Apply cold compresses to manage eyelid and conjunctival edema.

Patient education. If the patient has had a gas bubble injected into his eye, tell him to avoid air travel until the bubble is completely absorbed, usually about 4 to 8 days after surgery. Instruct him not to lift heavy objects or exercise strenuously. However, he may read, watch TV, go up and down stairs, and take walks. Suggest that he wear dark glasses if photosensitivity develops. Emphasize the importance of instilling eyedrops as prescribed for up to 6 weeks to prevent infection and inflammation. Remind the patient to schedule a follow-up appointment 1 week after discharge.

Scleral buckling

Used to repair retinal detachment, scleral buckling involves applying external pressure to the separated retinal layers, thus bringing the choroid into contact with the retina. Indenting (or buckling) brings the layers together so that an adhesion can form. It also prevents vitreous fluid from seeping between the detached layers of the retina and leading to further detachment and possible vision loss. When the break or tear is small enough, laser therapy, diathermy, or cryotherapy may be used to seal the retina. Another method of reattaching the retina involves sealing the tear or hole with endolaser or cryotherapy and introducing gas to tamponade the retina.

Patient preparation. Advise the patient whether he'll receive a local or general anesthetic.

Monitoring and aftercare. After scleral buckling, place the patient in the ordered position. Notify the doctor immediately if you observe any eye discharge or if the patient experiences fever or sudden, sharp, or severe pain. As ordered, administer mydriatic and cycloplegic eyedrops, antibiotics, and corticosteroids; apply ice packs to decrease eyelid swelling.

The patient's operative eye may have a patch on for 12 hours, during which time eyedrops and compresses are started. Advise him to avoid activities that increase IOP. If the patient feels nauseous, administer prescribed antiemetics.

Patient education. Instruct the patient to notify the doctor of any symptoms of recurring detachment, including floating spots, flashing lights, and progressive shadow. He should also report any fever, persistent excruciating eye pain, or drainage. Stress the importance of avoiding activity that risks eye injury. Warn against heavy lifting, straining, or any strenuous activity that increases IOP.

Show him how to use prescribed dilating, antibiotic, or corticosteroid drops. Stress the importance of meticulous cleanliness to avoid infection. Explain the importance of keeping follow-up appointments.

Laser surgery

The treatment of choice for a wide variety of ophthalmic disorders, laser surgery is relatively painless and especially useful for patients who are poor surgical risks.

Laser surgery can be used to treat retinal tears, diabetic retinopathy, macular degeneration, and glaucoma.

Patient preparation. Advise the patient that he will be awake and seated at a slit-lamp-like instrument for the procedure. Tell him that his chin will be supported and that a special contact lens will prevent him from closing his eye.

Monitoring and aftercare. Following the procedure, the patient may occasionally have pain. Give mild analgesics, as ordered, and apply ice packs as needed to help decrease the pain. The patient may be discharged after this office procedure.

Patient education. Instruct the patient to receive follow-up care as scheduled. Tell the patient that ice packs may ease discomfort.

Orbitotomy and dacryocystorhinostomy

Orbitotomy and dacryocystorhinostomy treat disorders of the lacrimal system. Orbitotomy is a surgical procedure for removing a lacrimal gland tumor. Dacryocystorhinostomy (DCR) establishes a new drainage path for tears. Before DCR surgery can be performed, any dacryocystitis must be controlled with hot compresses and antibiotics.

Patient preparation. Explain to the patient that he'll receive a general anesthetic. Tell him that he'll have bruising and swelling around his eyes and nose, and a small amount of drainage from the nares.

Monitoring and aftercare. In the immediate postoperative period, notify the doctor if you discover excessive bleeding or increased pain. Administer analgesics, as ordered, and apply cold compresses to the surgical site for the duration of the patient's stay (or 24 hours) to reduce swelling, bleeding, and pain.

Patient education. Instruct the patient to immediately contact the doctor if bleeding occurs or if discharge, redness, or swelling develops at the surgical site. Have him report increased bruising around his nose and eyes or a change in vision.

Tell the patient to use cold compresses at home, as ordered by the doctor, for 48 hours after surgery to relieve pain and decrease swelling. Advise him to avoid forcibly blowing his nose. Tell him to avoid hot drinks for 48 hours.

Remind the patient that he must schedule an appointment to have the skin sutures removed 5 to 7 days after surgery.

Eye muscle surgery

Eye muscle surgery corrects defects in the strength or placement of the eye muscles. These defects cause misalignment of the eye, disrupting the visual axis, and may cause diplopia or amblyopia. Eye muscle surgery realigns the visual axis and restores binocular vision.

Two types of eye muscle surgery may be performed: *resection* and *recession*. One or both techniques may be used to position the eye back into proper alignment.

Patient preparation. Inform the patient that the surgery will be performed under general anesthesia.

Monitoring and aftercare. Watch for and report any swelling or unresolved pain over the surgical site.

Patient education. If appropriate, teach the patient or his parents to instill antibiotic or corticosteroid eyedrops. Tell them that the conjunctiva will be red for 1 to 2 weeks. Stress the importance of notifying the doctor if increased redness, fever, or eye discharge occurs.

Explain that double vision may persist until the patient begins to focus his eyes. If it persists, notify the ophthalmologist.

Enucleation

When no other options exist, enucleation—the surgical removal of the eyeball—is indicated for intractable pain in a blind eye, intraocular malignant tumors, or marked intraocular inflammation following a ruptured globe or penetrating injury.

Patient preparation. Tell the patient to expect only mild pain and that he'll receive analgesics for any discomfort. He can also expect a large pressure bandage over the operative site for 12 to 24 hours to prevent swelling and bleeding.

Monitoring and aftercare. When the patient returns to his room, check for bleeding at the dressing site; if bleeding is evident, notify the doctor immediately.

Make sure the pressure dressing stays in position for 24 to 48 hours after surgery or until the doctor orders its removal. Warn the patient that the bandage is an important safeguard against swelling.

Patient education. Explain that a small plastic conformer is placed over the surface of the conjunctiva to maintain the integrity of the eyelids. This may dislodge after the swelling decreases. When this occurs, instruct the patient to clean the conformer with water, then slip it back between his eyelids, turning the point towards his nose. Eventually an ocular prosthesis will replace this. The patient should schedule a follow-up examination for 1 week after discharge from the hospital. Tell him also to make an appointment with an ocularist in 4 to 6 weeks to begin the fitting process for a permanent prosthesis.

Myringotomy

Myringotomy is a surgical incision of the tympanic membrane that relieves pain and prevents membrane rupture by allowing drainage of pus or fluid from the middle ear. It's most commonly performed on children with acute otitis media. If the tympanic membrane ruptures, the doctor may perform a myringoplasty.

After myringotomy, the doctor may insert a pressure-equalizing tube through the incision to allow fluid drainage. Usually, myringotomy provides almost instant symptomatic relief, and the incision typically heals in 2 to 3 weeks. (Tubes are usually expelled spontaneously after 6 to 12 months.)

Patient preparation. Explain whether surgery will be performed on one or both ears. Mention that the doctor may insert a tube through the incision to allow drainage until the inflammation subsides.

Monitoring and aftercare. Assess the condition of the patient's ear, and instruct the family to do so. Note the amount, type, color, and odor of any drainage. If you see bright red blood in the drainage, notify the doctor immediately; this may indicate injury to the ear canal.

If needed, cover the ear with a gauze pad or lay cotton fluff gently over the ear's orifice to absorb drainage. Apply petroleum jelly or zinc oxide to the external ear to protect it from excoriation by drainage, and change dressings as needed. If exudate cakes on the outer ear, remove it by gently swabbing with a cotton-tipped applicator dipped in hydrogen peroxide. Don't attempt to clean the ear canal or allow peroxide to run into the ear.

Patient education. Emphasize the need to notify the doctor if drainage lasts more than 1 week or changes in color or character—for example, from serous to purulent. Advise the patient to report any ear pain or fever, which may signal blocked tubing or reinfection.

Explain the importance of not allowing water to enter the ear canal until the tympanic membrane is intact. Show the patient or his parents how to roll absorbent cotton in petroleum jelly to form a plug and then how to insert the plug in the outer part of the ear before showering or washing hair. Tell the patient to expect considerable drainage through the tubes. Emphasize the need to return for follow-up examinations and to notify the doctor if the tubes are expelled.

Stapedectomy

Stapedectomy removes all or part of the stapes. Stapedectomy is the treatment of choice for otosclerosis. Because otosclerosis is usually bilateral, the doctor usually performs stapedectomy twice: first in the ear with the greatest hearing loss and then, a year or so later, in the second ear.

Laser stapedectomy, a popular technique, is easier to perform than conventional surgery but carries some risk that the laser beam will penetrate the bone.

Patient preparation. Mention that improved hearing may not be evident for several weeks after surgery, because ear packing and edema may mask any initial improvement. Tell the patient that the doctor usually removes the packing after a week.

Monitoring and aftercare. After surgery, position the patient as ordered. Advise the patient to move slowly without bending when he changes position. If he develops vertigo and nausea, administer antiemetic drugs, steroids, and vestibular suppressives, as ordered, and keep the bed's side rails up at all times. Help the patient when he first tries to walk because he may feel dizzy. Keep in mind that vertigo may also indicate labyrinthitis or an inner ear reaction. Provide pain medication, as ordered.

Patient education. Instruct the patient to call the doctor immediately if he develops fever, pain, changes in taste, prolonged vertigo, or a "sloshing" feeling in his ear. These symptoms may indicate infection or displacement of the prosthesis.

Instruct him to replace soiled or bloody pledgets in the ear canal as needed, and to keep the ear dry.

Tell him to protect his ear from cold drafts for 1 week and to avoid contact with people who have colds, influenza, or other contagious illnesses. Explain that he should take his prescribed antibiotics and report any respiratory infection to his doctor immediately.

Advise him to postpone washing his hair for 2 weeks. Then, for the next 4 weeks, he should avoid getting water in his ears when washing his hair. Instruct him not to swim for 6 weeks unless the doctor specifically allows it. To avoid prosthesis dislodgment, warn him to avoid blowing his nose for at least 1 week after surgery and traveling by airplane for 6 months.

Rhinoplasty and septoplasty

Rhinoplasty changes the nose's external appearance, correcting congenital or traumatic deformity. Septoplasty corrects a deviated septum, preventing nasal obstruction, thick discharge, and secondary pharyngeal, sinus, and ear problems. Usually, they're performed using local and topical anesthetics.

Patient preparation. With rhinoplasty, stress that changes may not be evident for up to several months. Point out that the facial swelling accompanying this surgery should subside in 3 to 4 weeks. For both rhinoplasty and septoplasty, tell the patient to expect nasal packing after surgery and that this, along with swelling, may give him an uncomfortable sensation of facial fullness. Warn him against trying to relieve this by manipulating the packing.

Monitoring and aftercare. For the patient with nasal packing in place, watch closely to make sure the packing doesn't slip and obstruct the airway. At first, assess airway patency

every hour and frequently check the nasal pack's position. If the patient becomes restless or starts to choke, notify the doctor—the nasal pack may have slipped. If needed, provide analgesics, as ordered, to relieve headache. Tell the patient that he will need to return to the doctor to remove the packing 24 to 48 hours after surgery.

Monitor vital signs and observe for hemorrhage, which may be immediate or delayed. Keep the patient on his side to prevent inhalation of blood, and periodically examine the back of his throat for fresh blood. Also check any sputum or vomitus for bleeding.

Help the patient rinse his mouth every 2 to 4 hours, and give him ice chips as needed. Offer fluids 4 hours after surgery. The patient should resume his normal diet the next day.

Patient education. After the nasal packing is removed, instruct the patient not to blow his nose for at least 10 days because it may precipitate bleeding. If he needs to clear his nose, tell him to sniff gently.

If the doctor prescribes inhalation treatments, instruct the patient to place a bowl of hot water before him and to drape a towel over his head, creating a tent. Then he should breathe in the warmed air.

If the doctor prescribes nose drops, tell the patient how to administer them. He should lie flat on his back, instill the drops, and remain supine for 5 minutes to facilitate absorption by swollen tissues. Then he should turn his head from side to side for 30 seconds to distribute the drops inside his nose.

Procedures

This section includes discussion of foreign body removal from the eye, emergency eye irrigation, ear irrigation, and insertion of nasal packing.

Foreign body removal

Typically, removal of a foreign body from the eye is a first-aid measure. However, if the object is embedded in the cornea, medical assistance is required for removal and a local anesthetic and an antibiotic need to be applied.

Patient preparation. If the foreign body is embedded in the cornea, apply anesthetic drops, as ordered, and check visual acuity.

If a foreign particle is lying on the surface of the conjunctiva, examine the particle by instructing the patient to tilt his head back and move his eyes away from the site of the particle. Hold the patient's eyelids open to prevent blinking.

If the particle is embedded in the conjunctiva in a place that requires better visualization during removal (such as the upper fornix), you may need to evert the eyelid.

Procedure. To remove a foreign body in the cornea, first visualize the particle and then gently touch it with the tip of a cotton swab moistened with sterile basic saline solution and lift it from the eye. Take care, however, not to drag the swab across the corneal surface.

If the particle is imbedded in the cornea, the doctor will examine the eye, using a slit lamp to determine the particle's location and depth. He'll administer a topical anesthetic and remove the foreign particle in the cornea. Then he'll apply an antibiotic ointment and an eye patch.

Monitoring and aftercare. After an embedded particle has been removed, instruct the patient to sit quietly for a few minutes with his eyes closed. Warn him not to rub the eye.

Patient education. Teach the patient how to correctly apply the antibiotic drops by pulling down the lower lid. Caution him to avoid touching the tip of the bottle to the eye or lid.

Apply an eye patch. Explain that the patch is a comfort measure and may only be necessary for 12 to 24 hours. Tell the patient to be sure to contact the doctor if his eye pain doesn't decrease in 24 hours or if his vision deteriorates.

Emergency eye irrigation

Irrigation is used to flush secretions, chemicals, and particulate matter such as foreign bodies from the eye. For emergency irrigation, tap water may be used.

The amount of solution needed to irrigate an eye depends on the contaminant. Secretions require only small amounts; major chemical burns need copious amounts. Use of I.V. tubing connected to an I.V. bottle or bag of normal saline solution ensures that enough solution is available for continuous irrigation of a chemical burn.

Patient preparation. Assist the patient into the supine position, with his head turned to the affected side, to prevent solution flowing over the nose and into the other eye. Place a towel under the patient's head and have him hold another towel against his affected side to catch excess solution.

If ordered, instill proparacaine eyedrops, a topical anesthetic, as a comfort measure. Use them only once because repeated use retards healing.

Procedure. Put on gloves. To irrigate the lower cul-de-sac, hold the eyelids apart with your thumb and index finger. To irrigate the upper lid, use a lid retractor.

To perform *moderate irrigation,* direct a constant stream of sterile ophthalmic irrigating solution at the inner canthus. Evert the lower eyelid and double-evert the upper lid to inspect for retained particles. Remove any particles by gently wiping the fornices of the conjunctiva with sterile, wet, cotton-tipped applicators. Resume the irrigation until the eye is clean.

To perform *copious irrigation,* open the control valve on the I.V. tubing and direct the stream at the inner canthus, so the normal saline flows across the cornea to the outer canthus. Periodically stop the flow and tell the patient to close his eye to help dislodge any particles.

Dry the patient's eyelids with cotton balls.

Monitoring and aftercare. Inspect the patient's eye thoroughly following irrigation to ensure foreign body removal. Notify the doctor of your findings. If the foreign body remains, continue irrigation until it dislodges or until the doctor orders other treatment.

Patient education. Teach the patient how to instill antibiotic ointment or drops, if ordered. Instruct him to notify the doctor if eye redness persists or if pain or a visual disturbance develops. If the patient has had a corneal injury, tell him to follow up with an ophthalmologist immediately.

Ear irrigation

Ear irrigation involves washing the external auditory canal with a stream of solution to clean the canal of discharges, to soften and remove impacted cerumen, or to dislodge a foreign body.

When performing ear irrigation, care must be taken to avoid causing discomfort, vertigo, or maceration of the canal skin, which may precipitate otitis externa, or damaging the tympanic membrane and causing otitis media. Because ear irrigation may contaminate the middle ear if the tympanic membrane is ruptured, the ear must be examined with an otoscope first.

Patient preparation. Select the appropriate syringe and obtain the prescribed irrigating solution.

Warm the solution to body temperature to avoid extreme temperature changes, which may affect inner ear fluids and cause nausea and dizziness. Then test the temperature by placing a few drops of the solution on the inner aspect of your wrist.

Procedure. If you haven't already done so, use the otoscope to check the auditory canal to be irrigated.

Assist the patient to a sitting position in an otoscopic exam chair. Tilt his head slightly forward and toward the affected side. Make sure you have adequate lighting.

If the patient is sitting, place a linen-saver pad—covered with a bath towel—on his shoulder and upper arm, under the affected ear. If he's lying down, cover his pillow and the area under the affected ear. Have the patient hold the emesis basin close to his head under the affected ear.

Clean the auricle and the meatus of the auditory canal with a cotton ball or cotton-tipped applicator moistened with normal saline or irrigating solution. Don't place the applicator into the canal. Draw up the irrigating solution into the syringe and expel any air.

Straighten the auditory canal by grasping the helix between the thumb and index finger of your nondominant hand and pulling upward and backward. Place the tip of the irrigating syringe at the meatus of the auditory canal. Make sure you don't occlude the meatus because this will prevent the solution from running back out the ear, causing increased pressure in the

canal. Point the tip of the syringe upward and toward the posterior ear canal.

Begin irrigation by directing a gentle flow of solution against the canal wall. This avoids damage to the tympanic membrane.

When the syringe is empty, remove it and inspect the return flow. Refill the syringe and continue the irrigation until the return flow is clear or until all the solution is used. Next, remove the syringe.

If you're using an irrigating catheter instead of a syringe, regulate the flow of solution to a steady, comfortable rate with the irrigation clamp. Don't raise the container above 6″ (15 cm). If the container is higher, the resulting pressure may damage the tympanic membrane.

Dry the patient's auricle and neck, and remove the bath towel and linen-saver pad. Help the seated patient lie on his affected side with the 4″ × 4″ gauze sponge under his ear to facilitate drainage of residual debris.

Monitoring and aftercare. Observe the patient for signs of pain or dizziness. If either occurs, stop the procedure immediately. Inspect the ear canal for cleanliness with the otoscope.

Patient education. If irrigation doesn't dislodge impacted cerumen, the doctor may order a ceruminolytic medication (glycerin, carbamide peroxide [Debrox], or a similar preparation.) Instruct the patient to instill the drops for 2 to 3 days, then to return for follow-up irrigation or to irrigate with a bulb syringe at home. Tell the patient to report ear pain, fever, or drainage after the procedure.

Nasal packing

When direct pressure or cautery fails to stop severe epistaxis, nasal packing may be used. An anterior pack consists of a strip of petroleum or iodoform gauze layered horizontally in the anterior nostrils, usually near the turbinates. A posterior pack consists of a rolled gauze pack secured with sutures and inserted into the nasopharynx. Insertion of a posterior pack requires sedation and hospitalization. Alternative methods to control posterior epistaxis include insertion of a Foley or nasal balloon catheter, or cautery.

Patient preparation. Before nasal packing, explain to the patient that he'll have to breathe through his mouth, but that mouthwashes will relieve dry mouth. Tell him pain medication will be available.

Procedure. To begin, have the patient lean forward to prevent blood from draining into his throat. Monitor his vital signs and watch for impending hypovolemic shock from blood loss. The doctor anesthetizes the patient's nasal passages with a vasoconstrictive agent. Then, as soon as the anesthetic takes effect, he suctions the patient's nose to remove any clots and locate the bleeding site. Then the doctor performs the nasal packing.

Monitoring and aftercare. Watch for signs and symptoms of hypoxia, such as tachycardia, confusion, and restlessness. Check arterial blood gas levels, as ordered, and monitor the patient's pulse rate and blood pressure. Keep emergency equipment (flashlight, scissors, and hemostat) at the patient's bedside, and place a call bell within his reach. If he has a posterior pack, check its placement frequently, and remove it immediately if it's visible at the back of his throat and he appears to be choking. Avoid tension on the sutures taped in place because this may dislodge the pack.

Monitor blood loss to help detect impending hypovolemia. Note the amount of bleeding on the dental rolls, and have the patient report any fresh blood in the back of his throat or blood he spits out. Also monitor fluid status. Note the patient's intake and output, and maintain an I.V. line if one is in place. Check the oral mucosa and skin turgor for signs of dehydration, and instruct the patient to report any nausea and vomiting.

Offer mouthwashes or ice chips, and provide sedation, as ordered. If he develops a headache, provide analgesics as ordered. Also monitor his temperature.

Patient education. When the nasal packs have been removed and the patient is ready for discharge, instruct him to avoid blowing his nose for 2 to 3 days because this may precipitate bleeding. Inform him that he can expect slight oozing of blood-stained fluid from his nose for the next few days but that he should report any frank bleeding.

Teach the patient how to use a steam inhaler at home to help prevent crusting inside the nose. Suggest using menthol and eucalyptus in the steam inhaler for a more soothing effect. Explain that he can start using the inhaler 6 hours after the packing is removed.

REFERENCES AND READINGS

Bowers, A.C., and Thompson, J. *Clinical Manual of Health Assessment,* 4th ed. St. Louis: Mosby–Year Book, Inc., 1992.

Consensus on Hearing. Agency for Health Care and Policy Research, July 1994.

Doane, J.F., et al. "A Comprehensive Approach to LASIK," *Journal of Ophthalmic Nursing and Technology* 15(5):144-47, July-August 1996.

Howard, B.J., et al. *Clinical and Pathogenic Microbiology,* 2nd ed. St. Louis: Mosby–Year Book, Inc., 1993.

Illustrated Guide to Diagnostic Tests, 2nd ed. Springhouse, Pa.: Springhouse Corp., 1997.

Nursing98 Drug Handbook. Springhouse, Pa.: Springhouse Corp., 1998.

Professional Guide to Diseases, 5th ed. Springhouse, Pa.: Springhouse Corp., 1995.

Reeves, W. "Surgical Experience of the Ophthalmic Patient," *Insight* 18(1): 16-19, 22, April 1993.

Selesnick, S.H., ed. "Diseases of the External Auditory Canal," *The Otolaryngology Clinics of North America* 29(5). W.B. Saunders Co., 1996.

Som, P.M., and Curtin, H.D. *Head and Neck Imaging,* vol. 1, 3rd ed. St. Louis: Mosby–Year Book, Inc., 1996.

"Standards of Ophthalmic Clinical Nursing Practice," *Insight* 18(1):23, April 1993.

Tasman, W., and Joeger, E. *The Wills Eye Hospital Atlas of Clinical Ophthalmology.* Philadelphia: Lippincott-Raven Pubs., 1996.

Yanagisawa, E. *Color Atlas of Diagnostic Endoscopy in Otolaryngology.* New York: Igaku-Shoin, 1997.

15

MATERNAL AND
NEONATAL CARE

During recent decades, infant and maternal mortality has progressively declined, even among women over age 35.

Nevertheless, improving maternal and neonatal health care is still a vital concern. Infant and maternal mortality remains high for the poor, minority groups, and teenage mothers largely because of a lack of good prenatal care. This chapter will help you to understand your role in promoting the well-being of mother and child.

ASSESSMENT

Assessment begins with the mother's first prenatal visit, and continues throughout labor and delivery and the postpartum period. It includes evaluation of fetal and neonatal well-being.

Keep in mind the interdependence of the mother and fetus. Changes in the mother's health may affect fetal health and changes in fetal health may affect the mother's physical and emotional health. (See *Assessing pregnancy by trimester,* pages 802 and 803.)

Fetal assessment

Assess the fetus prenatally by monitoring the fetal heart rate (FHR) and by using indirect and direct monitoring techniques. (For additional methods of evaluating fetal health, see *Diagnostic tests for maternal and neonatal disorders,* pages 815 to 817.)

Fetal heart rate

Placing a Doppler stethoscope on the mother's abdomen will enable you to count fetal heartbeats. Simultaneously palpating the mother's pulse will help you avoid confusion between maternal and fetal heartbeats. The Doppler stethoscope can detect fetal heartbeats as early as the 10th week of gestation.

Because the FHR usually ranges from 120 to 160 beats per minute, auscultation yields only an average rate at best. Auscultation is recommended in the uncomplicated preg-

Assessing pregnancy by trimester

The first trimester includes weeks 1 to 12. The second trimester begins at week 13 and ends at week 27; the third trimester begins at week 28.

Weeks 1 to 4
- Amenorrhea occurs.
- Breast changes begin.
- Immunologic pregnancy tests become positive: Radioimmunoassay test is positive a few days after implantation; urine human chorionic gonadotropin test is positive 10 to 14 days after occurrence of amenorrhea.
- Nausea and vomiting begin between the 4th and 6th week.

Weeks 5 to 8
- Goodell's sign occurs (softening of cervix).
- Ladin's sign occurs (softening of uterine isthmus).
- Hegar's sign occurs (softening of lower uterine segment).
- Chadwick's sign appears (purple-blue vagina and cervix).
- McDonald's sign appears (easy flexion of the fundus over the cervix).
- Braun von Fernwald's sign occurs (irregular softening and enlargement of the uterine fundus at the site of implantation).
- Piskacek's sign may occur (asymmetrical softening and enlargement of the uterus).
- Cervical mucus plug forms.
- Uterine shape changes from pear to globular.
- Urinary frequency and urgency occur.

Weeks 9 to 12
- Fetal heartbeat detected using ultrasonic stethoscope.
- Nausea, vomiting, and urinary frequency and urgency lessen.

- By 12 weeks, uterus palpable just above symphysis pubis.

Weeks 13 to 17
- Mother gains approximately 10 to 12 lb (4.5 to 5.5 kg) during second trimester.
- Uterine souffle heard on auscultation.
- Mother's heartbeat increases approximately 10 beats per minute between 14 and 30 weeks' gestation. Rate is maintained until 40 weeks' gestation.
- By the 16th week, the uterine fundus is palpable halfway between the symphysis pubis and the umbilicus.
- Maternal recognition of fetal movements, or quickening, occurs between 16 and 20 weeks' gestation.

Weeks 18 to 22
- Uterine fundus is palpable at the umbilicus.
- Fetal heartbeats are heard with fetoscope at 20 weeks' gestation.
- Fetal rebound or ballottement is possible.

Weeks 23 to 27
- Umbilicus appears level with abdominal skin.
- Uterine fundus is above the umbilicus.
- Shape of uterus changes from globular to ovoid.
- Braxton Hicks contractions start.

Weeks 28 to 31
- Mother gains approximately 8 to 10 lb (3.5 to 4.5 kg) in third trimester.

Assessing pregnancy by trimester *(continued)*

- Uterine wall feels soft and yielding.
- Uterine fundus is halfway between the umbilicus and xiphoid process.
- Fetal outline is palpable.
- Fetus is very mobile and may be found in any position.

Weeks 32 to 35
- Mother may experience heartburn.
- Uterine fundus palpable just below the xiphoid process.
- Braxton Hicks contractions increase in frequency and intensity.

- Mother may experience shortness of breath.

Weeks 36 to 40
- Varicosities, if present, become very pronounced.
- Ankle edema is evident.
- Urinary frequency recurs.
- Engagement, or lightening, occurs.
- Mucus plug is expelled.
- Cervix effacement and dilation begin.

---

nancy. For the high-risk pregnancy, indirect or direct electronic fetal monitoring provides more accurate information on fetal status.

To determine FHR of a fetus less than 20 weeks old, place the head of the Doppler stethoscope at the midline of the patient's abdomen above the pubic hairline. When fetal position can be determined, palpate for the back of the fetal thorax and position the instrument directly over it. It should be placed midway between the umbilicus and symphysis pubis for cephalic presentations, or above or at the level of the umbilicus for breech presentations. Locate the loudest heartbeats and palpate the maternal pulse.

Monitor maternal pulse and count fetal heartbeats for 60 seconds during the relaxation period between contractions to determine baseline FHR. Then count heartbeats for 60 seconds during a contraction and for 30 seconds immediately after it.

Notify the doctor or nurse-midwife immediately of marked changes in FHR from the baseline, especially during or immediately after a contraction. Remember that signs of fetal distress usually occur immediately after a contraction. If fetal distress develops, begin indirect or direct fetal monitoring. Repeat the procedure as ordered.

Indirect fetal monitoring

Indirect fetal monitoring is a noninvasive procedure that uses two devices strapped to the mother's abdomen to evaluate fetal well-being during labor. The ultrasound transducer records fetal heartbeats on a printout. The pressure-sensitive tocotransducer records the length and intensity of uterine contractions and traces this information on the same printout.

High-risk pregnancy, oxytocin-induced labor, and antepartum nonstress and contraction stress tests require indirect fetal monitoring.

Because fetal monitors are varied and complex, first familiarize yourself with the operator's manual. If the monitor has two paper speeds, set the monitor to 3 cm/minute to ensure a more readable tracing; a 1 cm/minute tracing is too condensed and can interfere with accurate interpretation of test results. Next, plug the tocotransducer into the uterine activity input jack and the ultrasound transducer into the phono/ultrasound jack. Attach the straps to the tocotransducer and the ultrasound transducer. Then take the following steps.

• Note the patient's name, the date, maternal vital signs and position, the paper speed, and the number of the strip on the printout paper to maintain consistent monitoring.

• Explain the procedure to the patient, and provide emotional support. Inform her that the monitor may make noise if the uterine tracing is above or below the strips on the printout paper and that this doesn't indicate fetal distress.

• After washing your hands and providing for the patient's privacy, help her assume a semi-Fowler's position with her abdomen exposed. The patient shouldn't be in a supine position to prevent maternal hypotension, decreased uterine perfusion, and fetal hypoxia. She may assume a left-lateral position once tracing is satisfactory.

• Palpate the patient's abdomen to locate the fundus—the area of greatest muscle density in the uterus. Then place the tocotransducer over the fundus and secure it with a strap. An elasticized body stocking may be used to secure the monitor to the mother's abdomen.

• Apply conduction gel to the ultrasound transducer crystals. Then, using Leopold's maneuvers, palpate the fetal back. (See *Performing Leopold's maneuvers,* pages 805 and 806.)

• After starting the monitor, place the ultrasound transducer directly over the site of strongest heart sounds and strap it in place. Press the record control to begin the printout. On the printout paper, note any coughing, position changes, drug administration, vaginal examinations, and blood pressure readings. Also note the frequency and duration of uterine contractions, and palpate the uterus to determine intensity of contractions.

• Teach the patient and her coach to time a contraction with the monitor. Inform them that the distance from one dark vertical line to the next on the printout paper represents a minute. The coach can use this information to prepare the patient for the onset of a contraction and to guide and slow her breathing as the contraction subsides.

Throughout monitoring, check the baseline FHR—the rate between contractions, which should be between 120 and 160 beats per minute. Assess periodic accelerations or decelerations from the baseline FHR. Note the shape of the FHR pattern in relation to that of the uterine contraction, the duration between the onset of an FHR deceleration and the onset of a uterine contraction, the duration of the lowest level of an FHR deceleration in relation to the peak of a uterine contraction, and the

Performing Leopold's maneuvers

Before auscultating the fetal heart rate, you'll need to determine fetal position. You will be able to hear fetal heartbeats most clearly through the fetal back. To determine fetal position, perform Leopold's maneuvers. Begin by having the patient empty her bladder. Position her supine, with her abdomen exposed. To perform the first three maneuvers, stand to either side of the patient and face her. For the fourth maneuver, reverse your position and face the patient's feet.

First maneuver
Place your hands on the patient's abdomen, curling your fingers around her uterine fundus. If the fetus is in a vertex position, you'll feel an irregularly shaped, firm object—the buttocks. If the fetus is in a breech position, you'll feel a hard, round, movable object—the head.

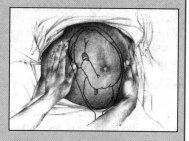

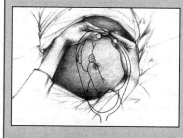

Second maneuver
Next, move your hands down the sides of the patient's abdomen and apply firm, even, inward pressure with the palms. Note whether you feel the fetal back on the patient's left side or right side and whether it's directed anteriorly, transversely, or posteriorly. If the fetus is vertex, you'll feel a smooth, hard surface on one side—the back. On the other side, you'll feel lumps and knobs—the knees, hands, feet, and elbows. If the fetus is breech, you may not be able to feel the back.

Third maneuver
Now spread apart your thumb and fingers of one hand and place them just above the patient's symphysis pubis. Bring your fingers together. If the fetus is vertex and hasn't descended, you'll feel the head; if the fetus has descended, you'll feel a less distinct mass.

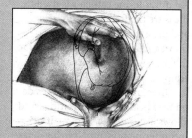

Fourth maneuver
Place your hands on both sides of her lower abdomen. Apply gentle pressure with the fingers of each hand, sliding your hands down toward the

(continued)

Performing Leopold's maneuvers *(continued)*

symphysis pubis. If the head presents, one hand's descent will be stopped by the cephalic prominence. The other hand will descend unobstructed more deeply. If the fetus is in the vertex position, you'll feel the cephalic prominence on the same side as the small parts. In face presentation, you'll feel the cephalic prominence on the same side as the back. If the fetus is engaged, you can't feel the cephalic prominence.

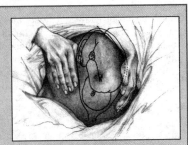

range of FHR deceleration. Move the tocotransducer and the ultrasound transducer to accommodate changes in maternal or fetal position.

Direct fetal monitoring

Also called internal fetal monitoring, direct fetal monitoring is a sterile invasive procedure, performed only after the amniotic sac ruptures and the cervix dilates about 3 cm. An intrauterine catheter is used to measure the frequency, duration, and pressure of uterine contractions, and an electrode is secured to the presenting fetal part, usually the scalp, to monitor FHR.

Direct monitoring furnishes data on true beat-to-beat variations and allows accurate measurement of intrauterine pressure. It helps determine the need for intervention. Direct fetal monitoring is usually performed by a doctor with a nurse assisting but can be performed by a specially instructed nurse.

Direct fetal monitoring is contraindicated in maternal blood dyscrasias, suspected fetal immune deficiency, and placenta previa; in face or brow presentations or when there's uncertainty as to the presenting part; or in the presence of cervical or vaginal herpes lesions.

Once a patient has an internal fetal monitor, note the frequency, duration, and intensity of uterine contractions. (Normal intrauterine pressure is between 8 and 12 mm Hg.) Also, check the baseline FHR (the rate between contractions), which should be between 120 and 160 beats per minute. Assess periodic accelerations or decelerations the baseline FHR. Track the FHR pattern in relation to that of the uterine contraction as you would for indirect fetal monitoring, page 803.

Assessment of labor and delivery

Your responsibilities may include palpating uterine contractions and assisting with vaginal examination.

Interpreting uterine contractions

When plotted on a graph, a uterine contraction forms a bell-shaped curve. The steepest slope of this curve, denoting the rapid rise in intra-amniotic pressure, marks the beginning of a contraction. The *duration* of a contraction measures in seconds the interval from the initial tightening of the uterus to the onset of relaxation. *Relaxation* gauges the time in minutes between the end of one contraction and the onset of the next. *Frequency* is the time between the onset of two consecutive contractions. *Intensity* describes the strength of a contraction, or the degree of uterine muscle tension, in millimeters of mercury. It varies considerably during labor and may be mild, moderate, or strong.

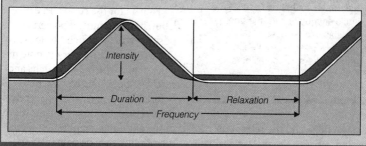

Palpating uterine contractions

Periodic, involuntary uterine contractions characterize normal labor and cause progressive cervical effacement and dilation and descent of the fetus. Palpation of the uterus evaluates the progress of labor by determining the frequency, duration, and intensity of contractions and the relaxation time between them. (See *Interpreting uterine contractions*.)

The character of contractions varies with the stage of labor. As labor advances, contractions usually become more frequent and intense and last longer. Regular contractions, which occur at 15- to 20-minute intervals and last 10 to 30 seconds, signal the onset of the first stage of labor. Contractions then become more regular, occurring every 3 to 5 minutes and lasting 45 to 60 seconds in the active phase of the first stage of labor. At the end of the first stage of labor, approaching complete cervical dilation, contractions occur every 2 minutes and last 60 to 90 seconds. In the second stage of labor, which culminates in childbirth, contractions space out to every 3 to 4 minutes but continue to last 60 to 90 seconds to complement pushing efforts of the uterus.

To assess contractions, first help the patient assume a comfortable position in semi- or high-Fowler's position. Next, place your fingertips on the fundus of the uterus, slightly above the umbilicus where you'll feel contractions most strongly. Time the duration and frequency of

Nutrition for the labor coach

During the average labor of 10 to 12 hours, the mother's labor coach may have little opportunity for adequate nourishment. A hungry coach can't provide the necessary emotional support. Order a hospital tray for your client and offer it to the coach so that he (or she) has sufficient nutrition for the energy that this role requires. If this isn't possible, offer tea, coffee, or juice and crackers, which all nursing units should stock.

contractions and the relaxation period between them. Also evaluate the intensity of contractions.

Meanwhile, assess the patient's breathing and relaxation techniques and provide emotional support. (See *Nutrition for the labor coach.*) Observe and note the patient's response to contractions to evaluate the need for pain relief.

Vaginal examination

Periodic vaginal examination during labor involves palpation of the cervix, the maternal pelvis, and the fetal presenting part. This sterile procedure monitors the progress of labor by determining cervical dilation and effacement, fetal presentation and station, and the status of the amniotic membranes. (See *Measuring cervical effacement and dilation.*)

First, have the patient empty her bladder. Next, assist the patient to the lithotomy position and drape her appropriately. Put a sterile glove on the hand to be used for the examination and apply sterile water-soluble lubricant to your index and middle fingers. Insert your lubricated fingers into the vagina, keeping your palm lateral to avoid placing discomforting pressure on the urinary meatus. Place your ungloved hand on the patient's abdomen to steady the fetus.

Palpate for the cervix. In early labor, it may assume a posterior position and be difficult to locate. Once you locate the cervix, note its consistency. The cervix softens and reaches a butterlike consistency before labor begins. During cervical palpation, determine the condition of the amniotic membranes. (The membranes may be palpable but may also be slick and well appressed to the presenting part and thus difficult to assess.) If you detect a small bulge at the cervix, the membranes are intact. However, if you express amniotic fluid, the membranes have ruptured. Confirm this by testing the exudate with nitrazine paper; a change from yellow to dark blue confirms membrane rupture.

Estimate cervical dilation by inserting your fingers inside the internal os (each fingerbreadth of dilation equals about 1.5 to 2 cm), and determine the percentage of effacement by palpating the ridge of tissue around the cervix.

Next, determine the fetal presenting part and its station by palpation. To determine station, first locate the ischial spines on the side walls of the pelvis. Then compare

Measuring cervical effacement and dilation

Dilation is measured in centimeters from 0 to 10; effacement is measured as a percentage from 0 to 100. Usually, a primigravida first experiences effacement and then dilation; a multigravida experiences both simultaneously.

Primigravida

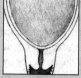
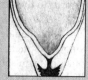

Before labor *Early effacement* *Complete efface-ment* *Complete dilation*

Multigravida

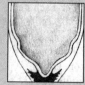
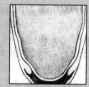

Before labor *Effacement and beginning dilation* *Dilation* *Complete dilation*

the location of the presenting part to the ischial spines. Note the station in centimeters with a plus sign for a station below the ischial spines or a minus sign for a station above the ischial spines. The number 0 reflects a station level with the ischial spines (engagement).

In early labor, perform the vaginal examination between contractions, focusing primarily on the extent of cervical dilation and effacement. At the end of the first stage, perform the examination and wait through the next contraction to determine the thrust of the contraction and the descent of the fetal presenting part.

If the amniotic membrane ruptures, observe and record the FHR.

Then note the time and describe the color, odor, and approximate amount of fluid. If the FHR decreases significantly below 120 beats per minute, suspect the possibility of umbilical cord prolapse and notify the doctor. After rupture, perform the vaginal examination only when labor changes significantly.

Neonatal assessment

The neonate's transition to extrauterine life is accompanied by rapid physiologic changes and numerous adaptations, all necessary for survival. Any threats to the neonate's well-being must be detected as quickly as possible.

During this initial examination, expect to calculate an Apgar score and make general observations about the neonate's appearance and behavior. Together with the maternal and fetal history, this information provides a baseline for use during subsequent examinations.

Apgar scoring

Apgar scoring evaluates neonatal heart rate, respiratory effort, muscle tone, reflex irritability, and color. Evaluation of each of the categories is performed 1 minute after birth and again 5 minutes later. Each item has a maximum score of 2 and a minimum score of 0. The final Apgar score is the total of the five items; a maximum score is 10.

Evaluation at 1 minute quickly indicates whether or not resuscitation is necessary. The 5-minute score gives a more accurate picture of the neonate's overall status. (See *Recording the Apgar score.*)

Assess *heart rate* first. If the umbilical cord still pulsates, you can palpate the neonate's heart rate by placing your fingertips at the junction of the umbilical cord and the skin. The neonate's cord stump is a good, easy place (next to the fetal abdomen) to check heart rate. Or place two fingers or a stethoscope over the neonate's chest at the fifth intercostal space to obtain an apical pulse.

Next, check the neonate's *respiratory effort.* Assess the neonate's cry, noting its volume and vigor. Then auscultate his lungs, using a stethoscope. Assess his respirations for depth and regularity. You may need to suction to clear the neonate's lower airway.

Determine *muscle tone* by evaluating the degree of flexion in his arms and legs and their resistance to straightening. Try to straighten an arm or leg and note how quickly it returns to the flexed position.

Assess *reflex irritability* by evaluating the neonate's cry for presence, vigor, and pitch. He may not cry at once, but you should elicit a cry by flicking his soles. A high-pitched or shrill cry is abnormal.

Finally, observe *skin color* for cyanosis. A white neonate usually has a pink body with blue extremities. When assessing a nonwhite neonate, observe for color changes in the mucous membranes of the mouth, conjunctivae, lips, palms, and soles.

The stable neonate may be weighed at this early stage. After this preliminary assessment, you'll usually take a neonate with an acceptable Apgar score to his mother for the first few minutes of bonding.

Closely observe the neonate whose mother has been heavily sedated just before delivery—because of secondary drug effects, he may score high at birth but may become unresponsive in the nursery. Indeed, some neonates "crash" in the delivery room after an initially stable evaluation.

Vital signs and other characteristics

Once the neonate is in the nursery, continue your assessment.

• Take the neonate's first temperature rectally, so you can also check

Recording the Apgar score

A score of 7 to 10 indicates that the neonate is in good condition; 4 to 6 indicates fair condition—the neonate may have moderate central nervous system depression, muscle flaccidity, cyanosis, and poor respirations; 0 to 3 indicates very poor condition—the neonate needs immediate resuscitation.

Apgar scoring system			
Sign	**0**	**1**	**2**
Heart rate	Absent	Slow (less than 100 beats/min)	More than 100 beats/min
Respiratory effort	Absent	Slow, irregular	Good crying
Muscle tone	Flaccid	Some flexion and resistance to extension of extremities	Active motion
Reflex irritability	No response	Grimace or weak cry	Vigorous cry
Color	Pallor, cyanosis	Pink body, blue extremities	Completely pink

for anal patency. Subsequent temperatures should be axillary, to avoid perforating the bowel. When taken for at least 3 minutes, an axillary temperature provides an approximate core temperature and reveals any heat or cold stress. Use a pediatric stethoscope to determine the neonate's heart rate apically. To ensure an accurate measurement, count the beats for 1 minute. Then assess his respiratory rate for at least 30 seconds. Note any signs of respiratory distress, such as cyanosis, tachypnea (respiratory rate greater than 60 breaths/minute), sternal retractions, grunting, nasal flaring,

or periods of apnea. Crackles may be heard until fetal lung fluid is absorbed. (See *Reviewing normal neonatal vital signs*, page 812.)
• Weigh the neonate again on admission to the nursery. Balance the scale, then weigh the naked neonate. Most newborns weigh between 6 and 9 lb (2,722 and 4,082 g); the average is 7 lb, 8 oz (3,402 g). Record weight in pounds and ounces as well as in grams.
• Measure the neonate's length, from the top of the head to the heel with the leg fully extended. Normal length is 18" to 22" (45.5 to 56 cm).

Reviewing normal neonatal vital signs

Respiration
30 to 50 breaths/min

Heart rate
(apical)
110 to 160 beats/min

Temperature
Rectal: 96° to 99.5° F (35.6° to 37.5° C)
Axillary: 97.7° to 98° F (36.5° to 36.7° C)

Blood pressure
(at birth)
Systolic: 60 to 80 mm Hg
Diastolic: 40 to 50 mm Hg

• Measure head circumference. Normal neonatal head circumference is 13″ to 14″ (33 to 35.5 cm). Remember, cranial molding or caput succedaneum from a vaginal delivery may affect this measurement, so repeat it daily until discharge. Measure his chest circumference at the nipple line; normal neonatal chest circumference is 12″ to 13″ (30.5 to 33 cm). Head circumference should be about 1″ (2.5 cm) larger than chest circumference.
• Observe the neonate's overall appearance, noting any obvious congenital defects or abnormalities.

Postpartum assessment

Your responsibilities include assessing the mother's uterus. Expect to provide perineal care and to teach her how to perform perineal care after discharge. (See *Reviewing postpartum perineal care.*)

Fundal checks

After delivery, the uterus gradually decreases in size and descends into its prepregnancy position in the pelvis—a process known as involution. Palpation of the uterine fundus evaluates this process by determining uterine size, degree of firmness, and rate of descent, which is measured in fingerbreadths above or below the umbilicus. Involution normally begins immediately after delivery, when the firmly contracted uterus lies midway between the umbilicus and the symphysis pubis. Soon the uterus rises to the umbilicus or slightly above it. After the second postpartum day, the uterus begins its descent into the pelvis at the rate of one fingerbreadth per day, or slightly less for the patient who has had a cesarean section. By the 10th postpartum day, the uterus lies deep in the pelvis, either at or below the symphysis pubis, and can't be palpated.

When the uterus fails to contract or remain firm during involution, uterine bleeding or hemorrhage can result. Fundal massage, the administration of synthetic oxytocin, or the release of natural oxytocin during breast-feeding helps to stimulate contraction and prevent uterine bleeding.

Unless the doctor orders otherwise, perform fundal checks every 15 minutes for 60 minutes; every 30 minutes for the next hour; every hour for the next 2 hours; and every 8 hours, if the patent is stable, until

Reviewing postpartum perineal care

A vaginal delivery stretches and sometimes tears the perineal muscles, resulting in postpartum edema and tenderness. What's more, an episiotomy can increase perineal discomfort. By providing postpartum perineal care, you can promote patient comfort and healing and prevent infection. Following elimination, you or the patient will assess the lochia, clean and dry the perineum, and apply a clean perineal pad.

Cleaning the perineum

Perineal cleaning may be performed with a handheld peri-bottle or a water-jet irrigation system. If you're using water-jet irrigation, first wash your hands and make sure the wall unit is turned off. Insert the prefilled cartridge of antiseptic or medicated solution into the handle, and push the disposable nozzle into the handle until it clicks into place. Instruct the patient to sit on the commode. Next, place the nozzle parallel to the perineum and turn on the unit. Rinse the perineum for at least 2 minutes from front to back. Then turn off the unit, remove the nozzle, and discard the cartridge. Have the patient stand up before you flush the commode to avoid spraying the perineum with contaminated water. Dry the nozzle and set it aside for subsequent use.

Teaching the ambulatory patient

Teach the ambulatory patient to perform perineal self-care with a peri-bottle or a water-jet irrigation system. Supervise her the first time she does it. Instruct her to count the number of perineal pads she uses, describe the discharge to you, and inform you of increased bleeding or the onset of bright red bleeding.

---

discharge. Give analgesics before fundal checks, if prescribed.

To perform a check, take the following steps.

• Help the patient urinate. You may need to catheterize her if she can't urinate by herself. This avoids bladder distention, which impairs uterine contraction. Next, lower the head of the bed so the patient is supine or her head is slightly elevated. Expose the abdomen for palpation and the perineum for observation.

• Place one hand on the lower portion of the uterus to provide stability and place your other hand flat on the abdomen, with your middle finger over the umbilicus and your thumb pointing toward the pubis. Gently palpate for the fundus. Once you've located it, count the number of fingerbreadths from the umbilicus to the fundus. One fingerbreadth equals about 1.3 cm.

• Cup your hands around the fundus to evaluate uterine firmness. If the uterus is soft and boggy, gently massage it with a circular motion until it becomes firm. Simply cupping the uterus between your hands may also stimulate contraction. If the uterus fails to contract and heavy bleeding occurs, notify the doctor immediately. If it becomes firm after massage, keep one hand on the lower uterus and apply gentle pressure toward the pubis to help expel any clots.

• Clean the perineal area, apply a clean pad, and help the patient assume a comfortable position.

Because incision pain makes fundal checks especially uncomfortable for the patient who has had a cesarean section, provide pain medication beforehand, as ordered. If the lochia isn't heavy after 4 hours, the doctor may permit fewer fundal checks than usual, especially if I.V. oxytocin is being administered. Be alert for the absence of lochia, which may indicate that a clot is blocking the cervical os. Sudden heavy bleeding could result if a change of position dislodges the clot.

DIAGNOSTIC TESTS

During pregnancy, diagnostic tests are ordered to assess the mother's health, to screen for maternal conditions that may endanger the fetus, and later to detect genetic defects and monitor fetal well-being. (See *Diagnostic tests for maternal and neonatal disorders.*)

Initial tests
Initial studies include blood type and rhesus (Rh) factor, a complete blood count (CBC) with differential, rubella titer, serologic test for syphilis, antibody screen, and a Papanicolaou test. Other tests include hemoglobin level, hematocrit, urinalysis and, if indicated,

blood glucose, alpha-fetoprotein, and gonorrhea culture.

If you suspect tuberculosis, administer the tuberculin skin test. Other possible tests include sickle cell trait testing, hepatitis screening, vaginal cultures, and postprandial blood sugar.

Fetal evaluation
Common tests include ultrasound studies, amniocentesis, chorionic villi sampling (CVS), percutaneous umbilical blood sampling, the antepartum nonstress test, the antepartum contraction stress test, and the nipple stimulation contraction stress test.

NURSING DIAGNOSES

When caring for pregnant women and neonates, you'll find that several nursing diagnoses are commonly used. These diagnoses appear below, along with appropriate nursing interventions and rationales. (Rationales appear in italic type.)

Altered parenting
Altered parenting is related to lack of knowledge about pregnancy and neonatal care.

Expected outcomes
• Parents ask for help in stopping abusive behavior.
• Parents have counseling to address abusive behavior.
• Parents describe appropriate ways to express and cope with anger.
• Parents participate in caring for the child and express their affection and concern for him.

Diagnostic tests for maternal and neonatal disorders

Test	Purpose	Nursing considerations
Ultrasonography	To help detect pregnancy; evaluate fetal viability, position, gestational age, and growth rate; detect anomalies in the placenta; detect fetal anomalies; and identify multiple gestation	• Explain the procedure. • Have the patient drink 1 qt (1 L) of fluid 1½ to 2 hours before the test. • Instruct her not to void before the test. • After the test, remove the conductive gel.
Triple screen (includes maternal serum alpha-fetoprotein, human chorionic gonadotropin, and unconjugated estriol)	To estimate the likelihood of occurrence of birth defects	• Explain the procedure. • This test requires no food or fluid restrictions. • After the test, observe venipuncture site for bleeding.
Amniocentesis	To detect open neural tube abnormalities, Down syndrome or other chromosomal defects, and certain metabolic disorders	• Explain the procedure. • Explain that the patient will feel a stinging sensation when the local anesthetic is injected. • Provide emotional support before and during the test and reassure her that adverse effects are rare. • Just before the test, ask her to void. • After the test, monitor fetal heart rate (FHR) and maternal vital signs every 15 minutes for at least 30 minutes. • If the patient feels faint or nauseous, or sweats profusely, position her on the left side to counteract uterine pressure on the vena cava. • Before the patient is discharged, instruct her to notify the doctor immediately if she experiences abdominal pain or cramping, chills, fever, vaginal bleeding or leakage of serous vaginal fluid, or fetal hyperactivity or unusual fetal lethargy.

(continued)

Diagnostic tests for maternal and neonatal disorders

(continued)

Test	Purpose	Nursing considerations
Chorionic villi sampling	To determine prenatal diagnosis of genetic disorders	• Explain the procedure. • Obtain preliminary blood work, as ordered. • Have the patient drink 1 qt (1 L) of water without voiding on the morning of the procedure. • If the patient is Rh negative, administer Rh_o immune globulin, as ordered. • After the test, advise her to notify the doctor immediately if cramping or bleeding occurs.
Percutaneous umbilical blood sampling	To assess and manage certain fetal disorders and allow direct access to the fetal circulation for obtaining blood samples or for administering transfusions	• Explain the procedure. • Clean the patient's abdomen with an iodine solution and cover with sterile drapes. • Maintain sterile technique, including operating room attire. • After the test, place the blood sample in an appropriate tube and transport it to the laboratory for analysis.
Antepartum non-stress test	To evaluate fetal well-being by measuring the fetal heart response to fetal movements	• Explain the procedure. • Place patient in a semi-Fowler's or lateral tilt position. Expose the abdomen. • Apply conductive gel and secure the tocotransducer and FHR transducer to the maternal abdomen. Obtain baseline vital signs. • Tell her to depress the test button when she feels the fetus move. • If you record two FHR accelerations that exceed baseline by at least 15 beats per minute, that last longer than 15 seconds, and that occur within a 10-minute period, conclude the test. • If you fail to record reactive results, monitor the fetus for an additional 40 minutes. If you still fail to obtain these results, perform the contraction stress test, as ordered.

Diagnostic tests for maternal and neonatal disorders
(continued)

Test	Purpose	Nursing considerations
Antepartum contraction stress test	To evaluate oxygen delivery by the placenta and identify when the fetus will be able to withstand the stress of labor	• Explain the procedure. • Assist the patient to a semi-Fowler's or a lateral tilt position. Drape the patient and expose the abdomen. • Secure the tocotransducer and the ultrasound transducer to the maternal abdomen. Obtain baseline maternal vital signs. • Record baseline measurements of uterine contractions, fetal movements, and FHR for 20 minutes. If testing fails to meet the specific criteria, prepare the oxytocin solutions, as ordered. • After recording three contractions, stop the oxytocin drip. • Continue to monitor the patient for 30 minutes or until the contraction rate returns to baseline. • Make sure the patient is comfortable while she waits for the results of the test.

• Parents identify and use a support system that includes family, friends, community resources, and appropriate health professionals.
• Parents understand normal childhood growth and development.

Nursing interventions and rationales

• Orient the expectant parents to the health care facility environment, visiting policies, and child care classes. *This helps allay anxiety.*
• Involve the parents in care of the neonate immediately. *This helps to establish bonding.*
• Allow the parents to share a room with the neonate or extend visitation periods. *This builds confidence in caretaking.*
• Educate parents in normal growth and development; feeding techniques (breast, bottle); neonatal care, such as bathing and dressing; signs and symptoms of illness; need for tactile and sensory stimulation; and routine medical follow-up. *This knowledge increases chances of successful parenting.*
• Encourage questions about caretaking and provide appropriate information. *This allays anxiety and monitors knowledge retention.*
• Refer the parents to a support group if difficulties in adapting are identified. *This enhances adaptation.*

• Encourage verbalization of the neonate's impact on family life. *Discussion helps family adapt to changes in plans and routines.*

Risk for altered body temperature

Risk for altered body temperature is related to possible neonatal heat loss during adjustment to the extrauterine environment.

Expected outcomes
• Patient's body temperature remains normal.
• Patient exhibits warm, dry skin.
• Patient shows no signs of hypothermia or hyperthermia.
• Mother or caregiver identifies warning signs of hypothermia and hyperthermia.
• Mother or caregiver expresses understanding of factors that cause hypothermia or hyperthermia.

Nursing interventions and rationales
• Use warm blankets at birth to keep the neonate dry.
• Cover the neonate's head.
• Wash the neonate with sterile cotton pads soaked in warm water, uncovering only small areas of the body at a time. Don't immerse the neonate in a tub of water. *These measures all prevent heat loss.*

Bathing/hygiene self-care deficit

Bathing/hygiene self-care deficit is related to the mother's limited mobility during labor.

Expected outcomes
• Patient's self-care needs are met.
• Complications are avoided or minimized.
• Patient or caregiver demonstrates correct use of assistive devices.
• Patient or caregiver carries out bathing and hygiene program daily.

Nursing interventions and rationales
• Advise the patient to take a warm shower. If the patent can't walk, perform a sponge or bed bath, with meticulous perineal care. *This promotes patient comfort and general body cleanliness.*
• Change the patient's gown and sheets whenever they become saturated. Also change the disposable underpad, especially after a vaginal examination. Frequently wipe the patient's face and neck with a cool washcloth, especially during transition. *These measures increase patient comfort and reduce risk of infection.*
• Advise the patient to use her own toiletries, if available. Powder her skin and comb her hair. *These measures increase the patient's comfort.*
• Provide mouth care during labor, and encourage the patient to brush her teeth or use mouthwash *to moisten the mouth and throat.*
• Offer frequent sips of water or allow the patient to suck on some ice, hard candy, or a washcloth saturated with ice water. *These measures maintain throat moisture.*
• Advise the patient to apply lip balm, petroleum jelly, or lemon and glycerin swabs *to heal dry, cracked lips.*

Pain

Pain is associated with the abdominal discomfort and back pain of labor.

Expected outcomes
- Patient describes level and characteristics of pain.
- Patient rates pain using a scale of 1 to 10.
- Patient tries nonpharmacologic methods for pain relief.
- Patient expresses a feeling of comfort and relief from pain.

Nursing interventions and rationales
- Teach the patient about the possible causes of back labor and about coping strategies that she can use. *This gives the patient a sense of control, which decreases her anxiety.*
- Assess fetal position. *An occiput posterior fetal position may cause back labor and indicate the need for interventions.*
- Teach the patient to use relaxation techniques and slow, paced breathing between contractions. *These techniques help the patient relax during labor, reducing her pain.*
- Advise the patient to increase her respiratory rate and to modify her breathing pattern during contractions. *Proper breathing helps maintain relaxation during the later part of labor.*
- Show the patient's partner how to apply firm counterpressures with the heel of one hand to the sacral area. *Counterpressure massage can reduce the patient's pain.*
- Encourage the patient to let her partner know the amount and location of counterpressure that relieves the most pain. *Feedback allows the partner to relieve pain effectively.*
- Help the patient assume a side-lying, upright forward-leaning, or hands-and-knees position. *These positions allow the pressure of the fetus to fall away from the patient's back and relieve pain.*
- If the fetus is in the occiput posterior position, help the patient change positions at least every 30 minutes. *Frequent position changes foster anterior rotation of the fetus.*
- Apply a warm, moist towel to the client's lower back. *Applying heat may help reduce back discomfort.*
- Apply an ice bag or rubber glove filled with ice chips to the patient's lower back. *Applying cold may help decrease back discomfort.*

DISORDERS

This section discusses common maternal and neonatal disorders. For each disorder, you'll find information on causes, assessment findings, diagnostic tests, treatment, nursing interventions, patient education, and evaluation criteria.

Maternal disorders

This section discusses the most common maternal disorders, including ectopic pregnancy, spontaneous abortion, placenta previa, abruptio placentae, premature rupture of the membranes, premature labor, and mastitis and breast engorgement.

Ectopic pregnancy

Ectopic pregnancy is the implantation of the fertilized ovum outside the uterine cavity. More than 90% of ectopic implantations occur in the fallopian tube's fimbria, ampulla, or isthmus, but other sites may include the interstitium, tubo-ovarian ligament, ovary, abdominal viscera, and internal cervical os. (See *Where ectopic pregnancies occur.*) Prognosis is good with prompt diagnosis, appropriate surgical intervention, and control of bleeding. Usually, subsequent intrauterine pregnancy is achieved.

Causes. Conditions that prevent or retard the passage of the fertilized ovum through the fallopian tube and into the uterine cavity include endosalpingitis, diverticula, tubal abnormalities, tumors pressing against the tube, and previous surgery (tubal ligation or resection, or adhesions from previous abdominal or pelvic surgery).

Ectopic pregnancy may result from congenital defects in the reproductive tract or ectopic endometrial implants in the tubal mucosa. Use of an intrauterine device (IUD) may increase the risk of ectopic pregnancy.

Assessment findings. Ectopic pregnancy sometimes produces symptoms of normal pregnancy or no symptoms other than mild abdominal pain (the latter is especially likely in abdominal pregnancy), making diagnosis difficult. Characteristic clinical effects after fallopian tube implantation include amenorrhea or abnormal menses, followed by slight vaginal bleeding, and unilateral pelvic pain over the mass.

Rupture of the tube causes life-threatening complications, including hemorrhage, shock, and peritonitis. The patient experiences sharp lower abdominal pain, possibly radiating to the shoulders and neck, commonly precipitated by activities that increase abdominal pressure such as a bowel movement; she feels extreme pain upon motion of the cervix and palpation of the adnexa during a pelvic examination. She has a tender, boggy uterus.

Diagnostic tests. The following tests confirm ectopic pregnancy.
• *Serum pregnancy test.* Positive results show presence of human chorionic gonadotropin (HCG).
• *Real-time ultrasonography.* This test reveals intrauterine pregnancy or ovarian cyst. It's performed if serum pregnancy test is positive.
• *Culdocentesis.* In this test, fluid is aspirated from the vaginal cul-de-sac to detect free blood in the peritoneum. Culdocentesis is performed if ultrasonography detects the absence of a gestational sac in the uterus.
• *Exploratory laparotomy.* This test confirms ectopic pregnancy and treats it by removing the affected fallopian tube (salpingectomy) and controlling bleeding.

Decreased hemoglobin level and hematocrit from blood loss support the diagnosis. Differential diagnosis must rule out abortion, appendicitis, ruptured corpus luteum cyst, salpingitis, and torsion of the ovary.

Treatment. A positive culdocentesis for blood in the peritoneum indi-

Where ectopic pregnancies occur

In 90% of patients with ectopic pregnancy, the ovum implants in the fallopian tube, either in the fimbria, ampulla, or isthmus. Other possible sites of implantation include the interstitium, tubo-ovarian ligament, ovary, abdominal viscera, and internal cervical os.

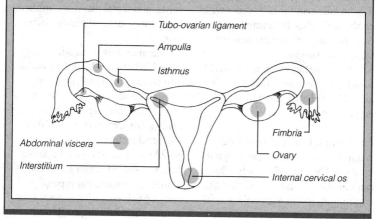

cates laparotomy and salpingectomy possibly preceded by laparoscopy. Patients who wish to have children can undergo microsurgical repair of the fallopian tube. The ovary is saved, if possible. However, ovarian pregnancy necessitates oophorectomy. Interstitial pregnancy may require hysterectomy; abdominal pregnancy requires a laparotomy to remove the fetus, except in rare cases when the fetus survives to term or calcifies undetected in the abdominal cavity. Methotrexate may be given to induce dissolution of the ectopic pregnancy prior to tubal rupture. This avoids surgery and provides improved tubal healing, promoting continued fertility.

Nursing interventions. Patient care measures include careful monitor-ing and assessment of vital signs and vaginal bleeding, preparing the patient with excessive blood loss for emergency surgery, and providing blood replacement and emotional support and reassurance.

Record the location and character of the pain, and administer analgesics as ordered. (Remember, however, that analgesics may mask the symptoms of intraperitoneal rupture of the ectopic pregnancy.)

Check the amount, color, and odor of vaginal bleeding. Determine if the patient is Rh-negative. If she is, administer $Rh_o(D)$ immune globulin (RhoGAM), as ordered. Ask the patient the date of her last menstrual period and to describe the character of this period. Observe for signs of pregnancy (enlarged breasts, soft cervix). Provide a quiet, relaxing environment, and encourage the patient to freely express her feelings of fear, loss, and grief.

Patient education. Inform patients who have undergone surgery involving the fallopian tubes or those with confirmed pelvic inflammatory disease that they are at increased risk for ectopic pregnancy.

Tell the patient who is vulnerable to ectopic pregnancy to delay using an IUD until after she has completed her family.

Evaluation. In a successful treatment, the patient's ectopic pregnancy should be identified early. The patient should understand that she can remain fertile with only one fallopian tube, and she should receive appropriate counseling to deal with her loss.

Abortion

Abortion is the spontaneous or induced (therapeutic) expulsion of the products of conception from the uterus before fetal viability (fetal weight of less than 17^1/2 oz [496 g] and gestation of less than 20 weeks). At least 75% of miscarriages occur during the first trimester. (See *Types of spontaneous abortion.*)

Causes. Spontaneous abortion may result from fetal, placental, or maternal factors. Fetal factors usually cause such abortions at 6 to 10 weeks of gestation and include defective embryologic development from abnormal chromosome division (the most common cause of fetal death), faulty implantation of fertilized ovum, and failure of the endometrium to accept the ovum.

Placental factors usually cause abortion around the 14th week. Factors include premature separation of the normally implanted placenta, abnormal placental implantation, and abnormal platelet function.

Maternal factors usually cause abortion between 11 and 19 weeks and include maternal infection, severe malnutrition, and abnormalities of the reproductive organs (especially incompetent cervix). Other maternal factors include endocrine problems, such as thyroid dysfunction or lowered estriol secretion; trauma, including any type of surgery that necessitates manipulation of the pelvic organs; blood group incompatibility and possibly Rh isoimmunization; and drug ingestion.

The goal of therapeutic abortion is to preserve the mother's health in cases of rape, unplanned pregnancy, or medical conditions such as cardiac dysfunction.

Assessment findings. Prodromal symptoms of spontaneous abortion may include a pink discharge for several days or a scant brown discharge for several weeks before onset of cramps and increased vaginal bleeding. For a few hours the cramps intensify and occur more frequently; then, the cervix dilates for expulsion of uterine contents. If the entire contents are expelled, cramps and bleeding subside. However, if any contents remain, cramps and bleeding continue.

Types of spontaneous abortion

Spontaneous abortions take place without medical intervention. They occur in many ways, as listed below.

• *Threatened abortion:* Bloody vaginal discharge occurs during the first half of pregnancy. Approximately 20% of pregnant women have vaginal spotting or actual bleeding early in pregnancy; of these, about 50% abort.

• *Inevitable abortion:* Membranes rupture and the cervix dilates. As labor continues, the uterus expels the products of conception.

• *Incomplete abortion:* Uterus retains part or all of the placenta. Before the 10th week of gestation, the fetus and placenta usually are expelled together; after the 10th week they're expelled separately. Because part of the placenta may adhere to the uterine wall, bleeding continues. Hemorrhage is possible because the uterus doesn't contract and seal the large vessels that fed the placenta.

• *Complete abortion:* Uterus passes all the products of conception. Minimal bleeding usually accompanies complete abortion because the uterus contracts and compresses the maternal blood vessels that fed the placenta.

• *Missed abortion:* Uterus retains the products of conception for 2 months or more after the death of the fetus. Uterine growth ceases; uterine size may even seem to decrease. Prolonged retention of the dead products of conception may cause coagulation defects such as disseminated intravascular coagulation.

• *Habitual abortion:* Spontaneous loss of three or more consecutive pregnancies constitutes habitual abortion.

• *Septic abortion:* Infection accompanies abortion. This may occur with spontaneous abortion but usually results from a lapse in aseptic technique during therapeutic abortion.

Diagnostic tests. Diagnosis of spontaneous abortion is based on clinical evidence of expulsion of uterine contents, pelvic examination, and laboratory studies. HCG in the blood or urine confirms pregnancy; decreased HCG levels suggest spontaneous abortion. Pelvic examination determines the size of the uterus and whether this size is consistent with the length of the pregnancy. Tissue cytology indicates evidence of products of conception. Laboratory tests reflect decreased hemoglobin level and hematocrit from blood loss. Ultrasonography confirms absence of fetal heartbeats or an empty amniotic sac.

Treatment. An accurate evaluation of uterine contents is necessary before planning treatment. Spontaneous abortion can't be stopped, except in those cases attributed to an incompetent cervix. Control of severe hemorrhage requires hospitalization. Severe bleeding requires transfusion with packed red blood cells (RBCs) or whole blood. Initially, I.V. oxytocin stimulates uterine contractions. If remnants remain in the uterus, dilatation and evacuation (D & E) should be performed.

D & E is also used in first-trimester therapeutic abortions. In second-trimester therapeutic abortions, an injection of hypertonic saline solution or prostaglandin into the amniotic sac or insertion of a prostaglandin vaginal suppository induces labor and expulsion of uterine contents.

After an abortion, spontaneous or induced, an Rh-negative female with a negative indirect Coombs' test should receive $Rh_o(D)$ immune globulin (human) to prevent future Rh isoimmunization.

In a habitual aborter, spontaneous abortion can result from an incompetent cervix. Treatment, therefore, involves surgical reinforcement of the cervix (also known as Shirodkar-Barter procedure, McDonald's procedure, or cerclage) about 14 to 16 weeks after the last menstrual period. A few weeks before the estimated delivery date, the sutures are removed and the patient awaits the onset of labor.

Nursing interventions. Before possible abortion the patient should not have bathroom privileges, because she may expel uterine contents without knowing it. After she uses the bedpan, inspect the contents for intrauterine material.

After spontaneous or elective abortion, note the amount, color, and odor of vaginal bleeding. Save all the pads the patient uses, for evaluation. Administer analgesics and oxytocin, as ordered. Obtain vital signs every 4 hours for 24 hours. Monitor urine output.

Care for the patient who has had a spontaneous abortion includes emotional support and counseling during the grieving process. Encourage the patient and her partner to express their feelings. Some couples may want to talk to a member of the clergy or, depending on their religion, may wish to have the fetus baptized.

The patient who has had a therapeutic abortion also benefits from support. Encourage her to verbalize her feelings. She may feel ambivalent; intellectual acceptance and emotional acceptance of abortion are not the same thing. Refer her for counseling, if necessary.

Patient education. Explain all procedures thoroughly. Tell the patient to expect vaginal bleeding or spotting, but to report excessive, bright-red blood immediately. Also advise her to report bleeding that lasts longer than 8 to 10 days.

Advise the patient to watch for signs of infection, such as a temperature higher than 100° F (37.8° C) and foul-smelling vaginal discharge.

Encourage the gradual increase of daily activities to include whatever tasks the patient feels comfortable doing, as long as these activities don't increase vaginal bleeding or cause fatigue. Most patients return to work within 1 week.

Urge 2 to 3 weeks' abstinence from intercourse, and encourage use of a contraceptive when intercourse is resumed. Instruct the patient to avoid using tampons for 2 to 4 weeks.

Be sure to inform the patient who desires an elective abortion of all the available alternatives. She needs to know what the procedure involves, what the risks are, and what to expect during and after the procedure, both emotionally and physically. Ascertain whether she is comfortable with her decision to have an elective abortion. Encourage her to verbalize her thoughts both when the procedure is performed and at a follow-up visit, usually 2 weeks later. If you identify an inappropriate coping response, refer the patient for professional counseling.

To minimize the risk of future spontaneous abortions, emphasize to the pregnant woman the importance of good nutrition and the need to avoid alcohol, cigarettes, and drugs. Most doctors recommend that the couple wait two or three normal menstrual cycles after a spontaneous abortion has occurred before attempting conception. If the patient has a history of spontaneous abortions, suggest that she and her partner have thorough examinations. For the woman, this includes premenstrual endometrial biopsy, a hormone assessment (estrogen, progesterone, thyroid, follicle-stimulating, and luteinizing hormones), and hysterosalpingography and laparoscopy to detect anatomic abnormalities. Genetic counseling may also be indicated.

Evaluation. After treatment, the patient's mental state should improve. Cervical competence should be restored, the uterus should be healed, and the patient should receive appropriate counseling and support.

Placenta previa

In placenta previa, the placenta implants in the lower uterine segment, where it encroaches on the internal cervical os. Individuals with a low marginal implantation may find that the previa resolves during the course of pregnancy as the placenta migrates upward with uterine growth.

The placenta may cover all or part of the internal cervical os, or it may gradually overlap the os as the cervix dilates. Obstruction may be either complete or partial (incomplete). Obstruction that occurs as the cervix dilates is caused by marginal implantation or a low-lying placenta. The apparent degree of placenta previa may depend largely on the extent of cervical dilation at the time of examination.

Maternal prognosis is good if hemorrhage can be controlled; fetal prognosis depends on gestational age and amount of blood lost. (See *Three types of placenta previa*, page 826.)

Causes. Although the cause of placenta previa is unknown, factors that may affect the site of the placenta's attachment to the uterine wall include early or late fertilization, receptivity and adequacy of the uterine lining, multiple pregnancy (the placenta requires a larger surface for attachment), previous uterine surgery, multiparity, and advanced maternal age.

Three types of placenta previa

In placenta previa, the lower segment of the uterus fails to provide as much nourishment as the fundus. The placenta tends to spread out, seeking the blood supply it needs, and becomes larger and thinner than normal. Eccentric insertion of the umbilical cord often develops, for unknown reasons. Hemorrhage occurs as the internal cervical os effaces and dilates, tearing the uterine vessels. Clinicians distinguish three basic types of the disorder.

Low marginal implantation

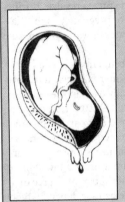

A small placental edge can be felt through the internal os.

Partial placenta previa

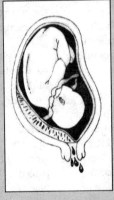

Placenta partially caps the internal os.

Total placenta previa

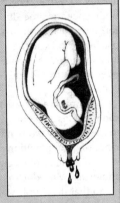

Placenta completely covers the internal os

Assessment findings. Placenta previa usually produces painless third trimester bleeding (in many cases the first complaint). Various malpresentations occur because of the placenta's location and interfere with proper descent of the fetal head. (The fetus remains active, however, with good heart tones.) Complications of placenta previa include shock; the disorder may also lead to death of the mother and fetus.

Diagnostic tests. Diagnostic measures that confirm placenta previa include ultrasound scanning for placental position and pelvic examination (under a double setup because of the likelihood of hemorrhage), performed only immediately before delivery to confirm diagnosis. In most cases, only the cervix is visualized.

Supportive findings include minimal descent of the fetal presenting part and decreased hemoglobin level (from blood loss).

Treatment. Therapy aims to assess, control, and restore blood lost. It can include delivery of a viable neonate and can also prevent coagulation disorders. Immediate therapy includes starting an I.V. using a large-bore catheter; drawing blood for hemoglobin levels and hematocrit as well as typing and crossmatching; initiating external electronic fetal monitoring; monitoring maternal blood pressure, pulse rate, and respirations; and assessing the amount of vaginal bleeding.

If the fetus is premature, treatment consists of observation. If clinical evaluation confirms complete placenta previa, the increased risk of hemorrhage usually requires hospitalization. When the fetus is sufficiently mature, or if severe hemorrhage occurs, immediate delivery by cesarean section may be necessary. Vaginal delivery is considered only when the bleeding is minimal and the placenta previa is marginal, or when the labor is rapid. Because of the possibility of fetal blood loss through the placenta, a pediatric team should be on hand during such a delivery to immediately assess and treat neonatal shock, blood loss, and hypoxia.

Complications of placenta previa require immediate intervention.

Nursing interventions. If the patient shows active bleeding because of placenta previa, continuously monitor maternal blood pressure, pulse rate, respirations, central venous pressure (CVP), intake and output, amount of vaginal bleeding, and fetal heart tones (FHTs). Electronic FHR monitoring is recommended.

Provide emotional support during labor. Because of the infant's prematurity, the patient may not be given analgesics, so labor pain may be intense. However, a regional anesthetic such as an epidural is usually given. Reassure her of her progress throughout labor, and keep her informed of the condition of the fetus. Continued monitoring and prompt management reduce the likelihood of neonatal death.

Patient education. Prepare the patient and her family for a possible cesarean section and the birth of a premature infant. Thoroughly explain postpartum care so they know what measures to expect.

Evaluation. In successful treatment, the patient maintains bed rest. The pregnancy continues until the fetus's lungs mature, and the neonate is delivered without complication. Patient has adequate fluid volume.

Abruptio placentae

In abruptio placentae, the placenta separates from the uterine wall prematurely (usually after the 20th week of gestation), producing hemorrhage. It's a common cause of bleeding during the second half of pregnancy. Firm diagnosis, in the presence of heavy maternal bleeding, usually necessitates termination of pregnancy. Fetal prognosis depends on gestational age and amount of blood lost; maternal prognosis is good if hemorrhage can be controlled.

Causes. The cause of abruptio placentae is unknown. Predisposing factors include traumatic injury such as a direct blow to the uterus, placental site bleeding from a needle puncture during amniocentesis, chronic or pregnancy-induced hypertension, multiparity greater than 5, short umbilical cord, dietary deficiency, smoking, and pressure on the vena cava from an enlarged uterus.

Assessment findings. Abruptio placentae produces a wide range of clinical effects, depending on the extent of placental separation and the amount of blood lost from maternal circulation. (See *Degrees of placental separation in abruptio placentae*.) Mild abruptio placentae (marginal separation) develops gradually and produces mild to moderate bleeding, vague lower abdominal discomfort, mild to moderate abdominal tenderness, and uterine irritability. FHTs remain strong and regular.

Moderate abruptio placentae (about 50% placental separation) may develop gradually or abruptly and produces continuous abdominal pain, moderate dark red vaginal bleeding, a tender uterus that remains firm between contractions, barely audible or irregular and bradycardic FHTs, and possibly signs of shock. Labor usually starts within 2 hours and in many cases proceeds rapidly.

Severe abruptio placentae (70% placental separation) develops abruptly and causes agonizing, unremitting uterine pain (described as tearing or knifelike); a boardlike, tender uterus; moderate vaginal bleeding; rapidly progressive shock; and absence of FHTs.

In addition to hemorrhage and shock, complications may include renal failure, disseminated intravascular coagulation (DIC), and maternal and fetal death.

Diagnostic tests. Diagnostic measures for abruptio placentae include observation of clinical features, pelvic examination (under double setup), and ultrasonography to rule out placenta previa. Decreased hemoglobin level and platelet counts support the diagnosis. Periodic assays for fibrin split products aid in monitoring the progression of abruptio placentae and detect the development of DIC.

Treatment. Treatment of abruptio placentae seeks to assess, control, and restore the amount of blood lost; to deliver a viable infant; and to prevent coagulation disorders. Immediate measures include starting I.V. infusion (via large-bore catheter) of appropriate fluids (lactated Ringer's solution) to combat hypovolemia; placing a CVP line and urinary catheter to monitor fluid status; drawing blood for hemoglobin level and hematocrit determination and coagulation studies as well as for typing and crossmatching; external electronic fetal monitoring; and monitoring of maternal vital signs and vaginal bleeding.

After determination of the severity of abruption and appropriate

Degrees of placental separation in abruptio placentae

Mild separation	Moderate separation	Severe separation

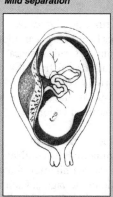

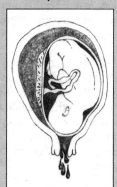

This condition begins with small areas of separation and internal bleeding (concealed hemorrhage) between the placenta and the uterine wall.

The condition may develop abruptly or progress from mild to extensive separation, with external hemorrhage.

In this condition, external hemorrhage occurs, along with shock and possible fetal cardiac distress.

fluid and blood replacement, prompt delivery by cesarean section is necessary with fetal distress. Otherwise, monitoring continues, and delivery is usually performed at the first sign of fetal distress. Because of possible fetal blood loss through the placenta, a pediatric team should be at delivery to assess and treat the newborn for shock, blood loss, and hypoxia. If placental separation is severe and there are no signs of fetal life, vaginal delivery may be performed unless contraindicated.

Complications of abruptio placentae require appropriate treatment. For example, DIC requires immediate intervention with fibrinogen, packed RBCs, and whole blood to prevent exsanguination.

Nursing interventions. Check maternal blood pressure, pulse rate, respirations, CVP, intake and output, and amount of vaginal bleeding every 10 to 15 minutes. Monitor FHTs electronically.

In vaginal delivery, provide emotional support during labor. Because of the infant's prematurity, the mother may not receive analgesics during labor and may experience intense pain. Reassure the patient through labor and keep her informed of the fetus's condition.

Patient education. Prepare the patient and family for cesarean section. Explain postpartum care, so the patient and family know what to expect. Tactfully explore the possibility of neonatal death. Tell the mother the neonate's survival depends primarily on gestational age, blood loss, and associated hypertensive disorders. Assure her that monitoring and prompt management greatly reduce risk of fatality.

Evaluation. Monitoring should identify fetal jeopardy at an early stage. Prompt intervention should prevent further complications. The patient should maintain an adequate fluid volume and satisfactory renal function, and the fetus should survive.

Premature rupture of the membranes

Premature rupture of the membranes (PROM) is a spontaneous break or tear in the amniotic sac before onset of regular contractions, resulting in progressive cervical dilation. PROM occurs in nearly 10% of all pregnancies over 20 weeks' gestation, and labor usually starts within 24 hours; more than 80% of these infants are mature. When the infant is premature, the latent period (between membrane rupture and onset of labor) is prolonged, which increases the risk of mortality from maternal infection, fetal infection, and prematurity.

Causes. Although the cause of PROM is unknown, malpresentation and contracted pelvis commonly accompany the rupture. Predisposing factors may include poor nutrition and hygiene and lack of proper prenatal care; incompetent cervix; increased intrauterine ten-

sion from hydramnios or multiple pregnancies; reduced amniotic membrane tensile strength; and uterine infection.

Assessment findings. Typically, PROM causes blood-tinged amniotic fluid containing vernix caseosa particles to gush or leak from the vagina. Maternal fever, fetal tachycardia, and foul-smelling vaginal discharge indicate infection.

Diagnostic tests. Characteristic passage of amniotic fluid confirms PROM. Physical examination shows amniotic fluid in the vagina. Examination of this fluid helps determine appropriate management. Aerobic and anaerobic cultures and a Gram stain from the cervix reveal pathogenic organisms and indicate uterine or systemic infection.

Alkaline pH of fluid collected from the posterior fornix turns nitrazine paper deep blue. (The presence of blood can give a false-positive result.) If a smear of fluid is placed on a slide and allowed to dry, it takes on a fernlike pattern from the high sodium and protein content of amniotic fluid.

Physical examination also determines multiparity. Fetal presentation and size should be assessed by abdominal palpation (Leopold's maneuvers). Historical, physical, and chemical data determine the fetus's gestational age.

Treatment. Treatment for PROM depends on fetal age and the risk of infection. In a term pregnancy, if spontaneous labor and vaginal delivery don't result within 24 hours after the membranes rupture, induction of labor with oxytocin may follow. However, careful assessment may permit watchful waiting instead of induction of labor. Cesarean hysterectomy may be needed with gross uterine infection.

With advances in technology, a conservative approach to PROM has now been proven effective. With a preterm pregnancy of 28 to 34 weeks, treatment includes hospitalization and observation for signs of infection (maternal leukocytosis or fever, and fetal tachycardia) while awaiting fetal maturation. If clinical status suggests infection, baseline cultures and sensitivity tests are appropriate. If these tests confirm infection, labor must be induced, followed by I.V. administration of antibiotics. You should also make a culture of gastric aspirate or a swabbing from the neonate's ear because he may need antibiotic therapy as well. At delivery, have resuscitative equipment available.

Nursing interventions. After the examination, provide proper perineal care. Send fluid samples to the laboratory promptly. If labor starts, observe the mother's contractions and monitor vital signs every 2 hours. Watch for signs and symptoms of maternal infection (fever, abdominal tenderness, and changes in amniotic fluid, such as foul odor or purulence) and fetal tachycardia. Report such signs and symptoms immediately.

Patient education. Teach the patient in the early stages of pregnancy how to recognize PROM. Make sure she understands that amniotic fluid doesn't always gush; it sometimes leaks slowly.

Stress that she must report PROM immediately, as prompt treatment may prevent dangerous infection. Warn her not to engage in sexual intercourse or to douche after the membranes rupture.

Before physical examination in suspected PROM, explain all diagnostic tests and clarify any misunderstandings. During the examination, stay with the patient and provide reassurance. Such examination requires sterile gloves. Don't use iodophor antiseptic solution or lubricating jelly as it discolors nitrazine paper and makes pH determination impossible.

Evaluation. The patient should avoid infection or other complications. Her pregnancy should continue to at least 34 weeks' gestation.

Premature labor

In premature labor, rhythmic uterine contractions produce cervical change after fetal viability but before fetal maturity. It usually occurs between the 20th and 37th weeks of gestation. Fetal prognosis depends on birth weight and length of gestation.

Causes. The many causes of premature labor include PROM, pregnancy-induced hypertension, chronic hypertensive vascular disease, hydramnios, multiple pregnancy, placenta previa, abruptio placentae, incompetent cervix, abdominal surgery, trauma, structural anomalies of the uterus, infections, and fetal death.

Assessment findings. Premature labor produces rhythmic uterine contractions, cervical dilation and effacement, possible rupture of the membranes, expulsion of the cervical mucus plug, and a bloody discharge.

Diagnostic tests. Premature labor is confirmed by the combined results of prenatal history, physical examination, electronic monitoring, presenting signs and symptoms, and ultrasonography (if available) showing the position of the fetus in relation to the mother's pelvis. Vaginal examination confirms progressive cervical effacement and dilation.

Treatment. Treatment is designed to suppress premature labor when tests show immature fetal pulmonary development, cervical dilation of less than 4 cm, and the absence of contraindications. Such treatment consists of bed rest and, when necessary, drug therapy.

Drugs can suppress premature labor. *Beta-adrenergic stimulants* (terbutaline, isoxsuprine, or ritodrine) stimulate the beta$_2$ receptors, inhibiting contractility of uterine smooth muscle. *Magnesium sulfate* relaxes the myometrium.

Maternal factors that jeopardize the fetus, making premature delivery the lesser risk, include intrauterine infection, abruptio placentae, placental insufficiency, and severe preeclampsia. Fetal problems, particularly isoimmunization and congenital anomalies, can become more perilous as pregnancy nears term.

Treatment and delivery require intensive team effort. The fetus's health requires continuous assessment through fetal monitoring. Sedatives and narcotics that might harm the fetus can't be used. Morphine or meperidine may minimize pain; these drugs have little effect on uterine contractions but depress central nervous system (CNS) function and may cause fetal respiratory depression. These agents should be given in the smallest dose possible and only when absolutely necessary.

Avoid amniotomy, if possible, to prevent cord prolapse or damage to the fetus's tender skull. Maintain hydration through I.V. fluids.

Prevention of premature labor requires good prenatal care, adequate nutrition, and proper rest. Insertion of a purse-string suture (cerclage) to reinforce an incompetent cervix at 14 to 18 weeks' gestation may prevent premature labor in patients with histories of this disorder. Also, some patients have prevented premature labor by receiving terbutaline at home through an I.V. infusion pump. Women at risk can be treated at home and have their contractions monitored via telephone hookup.

Nursing interventions. During attempts to suppress premature labor, maintain bed rest and administer medications, as ordered. Give sedatives and analgesics sparingly.

Minimize the need for these drugs by providing comfort measures, such as frequent repositioning and good perineal and back care.

When administering beta-adrenergic stimulants, sedatives, and narcotics, monitor blood pressure, pulse rate, respirations, FHR, and uterine contraction pattern. Keep the patient in a lateral-recumbent position as much as possible. Provide adequate hydration.

When giving magnesium sulfate, monitor neurologic reflexes. Watch the neonate for signs of magnesium toxicity, including neuromuscular and respiratory depression.

Remember that the premature neonate has a lower tolerance for the stress of labor and is much more likely to become hypoxic than the term neonate. If necessary, administer oxygen to the patient through a nasal cannula. Encourage the patient to lie on her left side or sit up during labor to prevent fetal hypoxia. Observe fetal response to labor through continuous monitoring. Prevent maternal hyperventilation; a rebreathing bag may be necessary. Continually reassure the patient throughout labor to help reduce her anxiety.

Help the patient get through labor with as little analgesic and anesthetic as possible. Explain the option of epidural anesthesia. To minimize fetal CNS depression, avoid administering analgesics when delivery seems imminent. Monitor fetal and maternal response to local and regional anesthetics.

Patient education. Offer emotional support to the patient and family. Encourage the parents to express their fears for the infant's survival.

Explain all procedures. Throughout labor, keep the patient informed of her progress and the condition of the fetus. If the father is present, allow the parents time together to share their feelings.

During delivery, instruct the patient to push only during contractions and only as long as she is told. Pushing between contractions can damage the premature neonate's soft skull. A resuscitation team, consisting of a doctor, nurse, respiratory therapist, and an anesthesiologist or anesthetist, should be in attendance. Have resuscitative equipment available.

After delivery, inform the parents of their baby's condition. Describe his appearance and explain the purpose of any supportive equipment. Help parents gain confidence in their ability to care for their baby. Provide privacy and encourage them to hold and feed the baby, when possible. As necessary, refer them to a home health nurse who can help them adjust to caring for a premature infant.

Evaluation. The neonate should avoid complications.

Mastitis and breast engorgement

Mastitis (parenchymatous inflammation of the mammary glands) and breast engorgement (congestion) are disorders that may affect lactating females. All breast-feeding mothers develop some degree of engorgement, but it's especially likely to be severe in primiparas.

Causes. Mastitis develops when a pathogen that typically originates in the nursing infant's nose or pharynx invades breast tissue through a fissured or cracked nipple and disrupts normal lactation. The most common pathogen of this type is *Staphylococcus aureus;* less commonly, it's *Staphylococcus epidermidis* or beta-hemolytic streptococcus. Predisposing factors include a fissure or abrasion on the nipple; blocked milk ducts; and an incomplete let-down reflex, usually from emotional trauma. Blocked milk ducts can result from a tight bra or prolonged intervals between breastfeedings.

Causes of breast engorgement include venous and lymphatic stasis, and alveolar milk accumulation.

Assessment findings. Mastitis may develop any time during lactation but usually begins 3 to 4 weeks postpartum, with fever (101° F [38.3° C], or higher in acute mastitis), malaise, and flulike symptoms. The breasts (or, occasionally, one breast) become tender, hard, swollen, and warm. Unless mastitis is treated adequately, it may progress to breast abscess.

Breast engorgement generally starts with onset of lactation (day 2 to day 5 postpartum). The breasts undergo changes similar to those in mastitis, and body temperature may be elevated. Engorgement may be mild or severe. A severely engorged breast can interfere with the neonate's capacity to feed because of his inability to position his mouth properly on the swollen, rigid breast.

Diagnostic tests. In a lactating female with breast discomfort or other signs of inflammation, cultures of expressed milk confirm generalized mastitis; cultures of breast skin surface confirm localized mastitis. Cultures also guide appropriate antibiotic treatment. Obvious swelling of lactating breasts confirms engorgement.

Treatment. Antibiotic therapy, the primary treatment for mastitis, generally consists of penicillin G to combat staphylococci; erythromycin or kanamycin is used for penicillin-resistant strains. Although symptoms usually subside 2 to 3 days after treatment begins, antibiotic therapy should continue for 10 days. Other appropriate measures include analgesics for pain and, rarely, when antibiotics fail to control the infection and mastitis progresses to breast abscess, incision and drainage of the abscess.

The goal of treatment of breast engorgement is to relieve discomfort and control swelling and may include analgesics to alleviate pain, and ice packs and an uplift supportive bra to minimize edema.

Nursing interventions. If the patient has mastitis, isolate her and her neonate to prevent the spread of infection to other nursing mothers. Obtain a complete patient history, including a drug history (especially allergy to penicillin). Assess and record the cause and amount of discomfort. Give analgesics, as needed.

Reassure the mother that breast-feeding during mastitis won't harm her neonate. Tell her to offer the neonate the affected breast first. However, if an open abscess develops, she must stop breast-feeding with this breast and use a breast pump until the abscess heals. She should continue to breast-feed on the unaffected side. Suggest applying a warm, wet towel to the affected breast or taking a warm shower to relax and improve her ability to breast-feed.

If the patient has breast engorgement, assess and record the level of discomfort. Give analgesics and apply ice packs and a compression binder, as needed. Ensure that the mother wears a well-fitted nursing bra, usually a size larger than she normally wears.

Patient education. Explain mastitis to the patient and tell her why isolation is necessary. To prevent mastitis and relieve its symptoms, teach the patient good health care, breast care, and breast-feeding habits. Advise her to wash her hands before touching her breasts. Instruct her to combat fever by getting plenty of rest, drinking sufficient fluids, and following prescribed antibiotic therapy.

For breast engorgement, teach the patient how to express excess breast milk manually. She should do this just before nursing to enable the infant to get the swollen areola into his mouth. Caution against excessive expression of milk between feedings, as this stimulates milk production and prolongs engorgement. Explain that because breast engorgement is the result of the physiologic processes of lactation, breast-feeding is the best remedy for engorgement. Suggest breast-feeding every 2 to 3 hours and at least once during the night.

Evaluation. After prompt identification of the infecting organism, the patient should respond to antibiotic therapy and avoid further complications. Free from discomfort, she should understand how to avoid breast engorgement.

Neonatal disorders

This section reviews two conditions which may affect the fetus, neonate, or both: hyperbilirubinemia and erythroblastosis fetalis.

Hyperbilirubinemia

Also known as neonatal jaundice, hyperbilirubinemia is the result of hemolytic processes in the neonate and brings elevated serum bilirubin levels and mild jaundice. It can be physiologic (with jaundice the only symptom) or pathologic (resulting from an underlying disease). Physiologic jaundice is very common. Physiologic jaundice is self-limiting; prognosis for pathologic jaundice varies, depending on the cause. Untreated, severe hyperbilirubinemia may result in kernicterus, a neurologic syndrome resulting from deposition of unconjugated bilirubin in the brain cells and characterized by severe neural symptoms.

Survivors may develop cerebral palsy, epilepsy, or mental retardation, or may have only minor sequelae, such as perceptual-motor disabilities and learning disorders.

Causes. As erythrocytes break down at the end of their neonatal life cycle, hemoglobin separates into globin (protein) and heme (iron) fragments. Heme fragments form unconjugated (indirect) bilirubin, which binds with albumin for transport to liver cells to conjugate with glucuronide, forming direct bilirubin. Because unconjugated bilirubin is fat-soluble and can't be excreted in the urine or bile, it may escape to extravascular tissue, especially fatty tissue and the brain, resulting in hyperbilirubinemia.

This pathophysiologic process may develop several ways. Factors that disrupt conjugation and usurp albumin-binding sites include such drugs as aspirin, tranquilizers, and sulfonamides and such conditions as hypothermia, anoxia, hypoglycemia, and hypoalbuminemia. Other causes include decreased hepatic function, hemolytic disorders, Rh or ABO incompatibility, biliary obstruction, or hepatitis.

Assessment findings. The predominant sign of hyperbilirubinemia is jaundice, which doesn't become clinically apparent until serum bilirubin levels reach about 7 mg/100 ml. Physiologic jaundice develops 24 hours after delivery in 50% of term neonates (usually between days 2 and 3) and 48 hours after delivery in 80% of premature neonates (usually between days 3 and 5). It generally disappears by day 7 in term neonates and by day 9 or 10 in premature neonates. Throughout physiologic jaundice, serum unconjugated bilirubin does not exceed 12 mg/100 ml. Pathologic jaundice may appear anytime after the first day of life and persists beyond 7 days with serum bilirubin levels greater than 12 mg/100 ml in a term neonate, 15 mg/100 ml in a premature neonate, or increasing more than 5 mg/100 ml in 24 hours.

Diagnostic tests. Jaundice and elevated levels of serum bilirubin confirm hyperbilirubinemia. Inspection of the neonate in a well-lit room (without yellow or gold lighting) reveals a yellowish skin coloration, particularly in the sclerae. To verify jaundice, press the skin on the cheek or abdomen lightly with one finger, then release pressure and observe skin color immediately. Signs of jaundice necessitate measuring and charting serum bilirubin levels every 4 hours. Testing may include direct and indirect bilirubin levels, particularly for pathologic jaundice. Bilirubin levels that are excessively elevated or vary daily suggest a pathologic process.

Identifying the underlying cause of hyperbilirubinemia requires a detailed patient history (including prenatal history), family history (paternal Rh factor, inherited RBC defects), present neonate status (immaturity, infection), and blood testing of the neonate and mother (blood group incompatibilities, hemoglobin level, direct Coombs' test, hematocrit).

Treatment. Treatment may include phototherapy, exchange transfusions, albumin infusion, and possibly drug therapy. Phototherapy is the treatment of choice for physiologic jaundice and pathologic jaundice from erythroblastosis fetalis (after the initial exchange transfusion). Phototherapy uses fluorescent light to decompose bilirubin in the skin by oxidation and is usually discontinued after bilirubin levels fall below 10 mg/100 ml and continue to decrease for 24 hours. However, phototherapy is rarely the only treatment for jaundice due to a pathologic cause.

An exchange transfusion replaces the neonate's blood with fresh blood (less than 48 hours old). Possible indications for exchange transfusions include hydrops fetalis, polycythemia, erythroblastosis fetalis, marked reticulocytosis, drug toxicity, and jaundice that develops within the first 6 hours after birth.

Other therapy for excessive bilirubin levels may include albumin administration (1 g/kg of 25% salt-poor albumin), which provides additional albumin for binding unconjugated bilirubin. This may be done 1 to 2 hours before exchange or as a substitute for a portion of the plasma in the transfused blood.

Nursing interventions. Assess and record the neonate's jaundice, and note the time it began. Report the jaundice and serum bilirubin levels immediately. To prevent hyperbilirubinemia, maintain oral intake. Don't skip any feedings because fasting stimulates the conversion of heme to bilirubin. Offer extra water to promote bilirubin excretion.

Patient education. Reassure parents that most neonates experience some degree of jaundice. Explain hyperbilirubinemia, its causes, diagnostic tests, and treatment. Also, explain that the neonate's stool contains some bile and may be greenish.

Evaluation. The neonate's jaundice resolves during the first week of life when the cause is identified and therapy initiated. When phototherapy is successful, the neonate's bilirubin level decreases and kernicterus is avoided.

Erythroblastosis fetalis

A hemolytic disease of the fetus and newborn, erythroblastosis fetalis stems from an incompatibility of fetal and maternal blood, resulting in maternal antibody activity against fetal RBCs. Intrauterine transfusions can save 40% of fetuses with erythroblastosis. However, in severe, untreated erythroblastosis fetalis, prognosis is poor, especially if kernicterus develops. About 70% of these neonates die, usually within the first week of life. Survivors inevitably develop pronounced neurologic damage (sensory impairment, mental deficiencies, cerebral palsy). Severely affected fetuses who develop hydrops fetalis are commonly stillborn; even if delivered live, they rarely survive longer than a few hours.

Causes. Although more than 60 RBC antigens can stimulate antibody formation, erythroblastosis fetalis usually results from Rh isoimmunization

During her first pregnancy, an Rh-negative female becomes sensitized through exposure to Rh-positive fetal blood antigens inherited from the father. A female may also become sensitized from receiving blood transfusions with alien Rh antigens, causing agglutinins to develop; from inadequate doses of $Rh_o(D)$; or from failure to receive $Rh_o(D)$ after significant fetal-maternal leakage from abruptio placentae, amniocentesis or CVS, or previous abortion. Subsequent pregnancy with an Rh-positive fetus provokes increasing amounts of maternal agglutinating antibodies to cross the placental barrier, attach to Rh-positive cells in the fetus, and cause hemolysis and anemia. To compensate for this, the fetus steps up the production of RBCs, and erythroblasts (immature RBCs) appear in the fetal circulation. Extensive hemolysis results in the release of large amounts of unconjugated bilirubin, which the liver is unable to conjugate and excrete, causing hyperbilirubinemia and hemolytic anemia. (See *Pathogenesis of Rh isoimmunization.*)

Assessment findings. Jaundice usually isn't present at birth but may appear as soon as 30 minutes later or within 24 hours. The mildly affected neonate shows mild to moderate hepatosplenomegaly and pallor. In severely affected neonates who survive birth, erythroblastosis fetalis usually produces pallor, edema, petechiae, hepatosplenomegaly, grunting respirations, crackles, poor muscle tone, neurologic unresponsiveness, possible heart murmurs, a bile-stained umbilical cord, and yellow or meconium-stained amniotic fluid. Approximately 10% of untreated neonates develop kernicterus from hemolytic disease and show such signs and symptoms as anemia, lethargy, poor sucking ability, retracted head, stiff extremities, squinting, a high-pitched cry, and convulsions.

Hydrops fetalis causes extreme hemolysis, fetal hypoxia, heart failure, edema, peritoneal and pleural effusions (with dyspnea and crackles), and green- or brown-tinged amniotic fluid.

Other distinctive characteristics of the neonate with hydrops fetalis include marked pallor, hepatosplenomegaly, cardiomegaly, and ascites. Petechiae and widespread ecchymoses are present in severe cases, indicating concurrent DIC. This disorder retards intrauterine growth, so the lungs, kidneys, brain, and thymus are small, and despite edema, his body size is smaller than that of neonates of comparable gestational age.

Diagnostic tests. Diagnostic evaluation uses both prenatal and neonatal findings. It includes maternal history (for erythroblastotic stillbirths, abortions, previously affect-

Pathogenesis of Rh isoimmunization

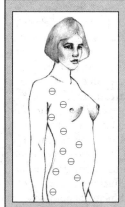

Rh-negative woman prepregnancy.

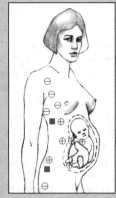

Pregnancy with Rh-positive fetus. Normal antibodies appear.

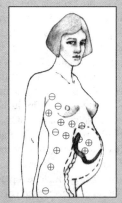

Placental separation.

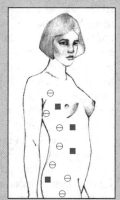

Postdelivery, mother develops anti-Rh-positive antibodies (darkened squares).

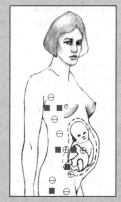

With the next Rh-positive fetus, antibodies enter fetal circulation, causing hemolysis.

ed children, previous anti-Rh titers), blood-typing and screening (titers should be taken frequently to determine changes in the degree of maternal immunization), a paternal blood test (for Rh, blood group, and Rh zygosity), and a history of blood transfusion.

Amniotic fluid analysis may show an increase in bilirubin (indicating possible hemolysis) and elevations in anti-Rh titers. Radiologic studies may show edema and, in hydrops fetalis, enlarged placenta, the halo sign (edematous, elevated, subcutaneous fat layers) and the Buddha position (fetus's legs are crossed).

Neonatal findings indicating erythroblastosis fetalis include direct Coombs' test of umbilical cord blood to measure RBC (Rh-positive) antibodies in the neonate (positive only when the mother is Rh-negative and the fetus is Rh-positive), many nucleated peripheral RBCs, and decreased cord hemoglobin level (less than 10 g), signaling severe disease.

Treatment. Treatment depends on the degree of maternal sensitization and the effects of hemolytic disease on the fetus or neonate.

Intrauterine-intraperitoneal transfusion is performed when amniotic fluid analysis suggests that the fetus is severely affected, and delivery is inappropriate because of fetal immaturity. A transabdominal puncture under fluoroscopy into the fetal peritoneal cavity or in a percutaneous umbilical blood sampling (also known as PUBS) as early as 18 weeks gestation allows infusion of group O, Rh-negative blood. This may be repeated every 2 weeks until the fetus is mature.

Planned delivery, usually 2 to 4 weeks before term date, depends on maternal history, serologic tests, and amniocentesis; labor may be induced from the 34th to 38th week of gestation. During labor, the fetus should be monitored electronically; capillary blood scalp sampling determines acid-base balance. Any indication of fetal distress necessitates immediate cesarean delivery.

Phenobarbital administered during the last 5 to 6 weeks of pregnancy may lower serum bilirubin levels in the neonate. An exchange transfusion removes antibody-coated RBCs and prevents hyperbilirubinemia through removal of the neonate's blood and replacement with fresh group O, Rh-negative blood. Albumin infusion helps to bind bilirubin, reducing the chances of hyperbilirubinemia. Phototherapy by exposure to ultraviolet light also reduces bilirubin levels.

Neonatal therapy for hydrops fetalis consists of maintaining ventilation by intubation, oxygenation, and mechanical assistance, when necessary, and removing excess fluid to relieve severe ascites and respiratory distress. Other appropriate measures include an exchange transfusion and maintenance of the neonate's body temperature.

Gamma globulin that contains anti-Rh-positive antibody ($Rh_o[D]$) can provide passive immunization, which prevents maternal Rh isoimmunization in Rh-negative females. However, it is ineffective if sensitization has already resulted. (See *Preventing Rh isoimmunization*.)

Nursing interventions. Provide explanations of diagnostic tests and therapeutic measures, and emotional support.

Before intrauterine transfusion, obtain a baseline FHR through electronic monitoring. Afterward, carefully observe the mother for uterine contractions and fluid leakage from the puncture site. Monitor FHR for tachycardia or bradycardia.

During exchange transfusion, maintain the neonate's body temperature by placing him under a heat lamp or overhead radiant warmer. Keep resuscitative equipment handy, and warm blood before transfusion. Apply cardiac monitor during exchange transfusion. Watch for complications of transfusion, such as lethargy, muscular twitching, convulsions, dark urine, edema, and change in vital signs. Watch for postexchange serum bilirubin levels that are usually 50% of preexchange levels. Within 30 minutes of transfusion, bilirubin may rebound, requiring repeat exchange transfusions. Measure intake and output. Observe for cord bleeding and complications, such as hemorrhage, hypocalcemia, sepsis, and shock. Report serum bilirubin and hemoglobin levels. Encourage parents to visit and to help care for the neonate as often as possible.

To prevent hemolytic disease in the neonate, evaluate all pregnant females for possible Rh incompatibility. Administer $Rh_o(D)$ I.M., as ordered, to all Rh-negative, antibody-negative females following transfusion reaction, ectopic pregnancy, and spontaneous or therapeutic abortion, or during the second and third trimesters to patients with abruptio placentae, placenta previa, amniocentesis, or PUBS.

Patient education. Reassure the parents that they're not at fault in

Preventing Rh isoimmunization

Administration of $Rh_o(D)$ immune globulin (human) to an unsensitized Rh-negative mother as soon as possible after the birth of an Rh-positive neonate, or after a spontaneous or elective abortion, prevents complications in subsequent pregnancies.

The following patients should be screened for Rh isoimmunization or irregular antibodies:
• all Rh-negative mothers during their first prenatal visit, and at 24, 28, 32, and 36 weeks' gestation
• all Rh-positive mothers with histories of transfusion, a jaundiced infant, stillbirth, cesarean birth, induced abortion, placenta previa, or abruptio placentae.

having a child with erythroblastosis fetalis. Encourage them to express their fears concerning possible complications of treatment. Before intrauterine transfusion, explain the procedure and its purpose.

Evaluation. The Rh-negative mother should be identified early and should prevent complications by receiving Rh-positive antibody prenatally, at 28 weeks' gestation, and after delivery of an Rh-positive neonate.

TREATMENTS

Drug therapy and surgery may be used to assist with labor and delivery and to assure the well-being of the mother and fetus. After birth, treatment seeks to assure the neonate's survival, assist his adjustment to the extrauterine environment and, if necessary, to help him overcome such hazards as respiratory distress, jaundice, or complications from prematurity.

Maternal drug therapy

Drugs may be used to stimulate, augment, or arrest uterine contractions.

Oxytocic drugs

The endogenous hormone oxytocin stimulates uterine contraction. It also exerts a vasopressive, an antidiuretic, and a transient relaxing effect on vascular smooth muscle. Uterine sensitivity to this hormone increases gradually during gestation, then increases sharply before parturition.

Oxytocic agents are primarily given by I.V. infusion to induce or stimulate labor. Prostaglandin gel may be inserted into the cervical area prior to oxytocic induction to soften the cervix. These agents are also used to control postpartum bleeding and may be given I.V., I.M., or by mouth at this time. The nasal form of oxytocin can be given to stimulate lactation and thus relieve breast engorgement.

Adverse maternal reactions to oxytocin include fluid overload, hypertension or hypotension, postpartum hemorrhage, arrhythmias, premature ventricular contractions, afibrinogenemia, nausea and vomiting, and pelvic hematoma. An overdose or a hypersensitivity to the drug may lead to uterine hyper-

tonicity, tetanic contractions, or uterine rupture. In the fetus, the drug may cause bradycardia, neonatal jaundice, and anaphylaxis.

Oxytocin is contraindicated in significant cephalopelvic disproportion, unfavorable fetal position or presentation, obstetric emergencies requiring intervention, fetal distress when delivery isn't imminent, prolonged uterine inertia, severe toxemia, or hypertonic uterine patterns. It shouldn't be given to a patient who has received a sympathomimetic, such as epinephrine or phenylephrine, because severe hypertension or intracranial hemorrhage could occur. (See *Oxytocin administration.*)

Oxytocin must be used cautiously if the patient has a history of cervical or uterine surgery, grand multiparity, uterine sepsis, or traumatic delivery; if the uterus is overdistended; or if the patient is over age 35 and in her first pregnancy. The drug must be used with extreme caution during the first and second stages of labor because cervical laceration, uterine rupture, and maternal and fetal death can occur.

Monitoring and aftercare. Monitor the patient continuously during oxytocin infusion. Oxytocin for induction of labor must be administered via volumetric pump and piggyback setup. Check her blood pressure and pulse every 15 minutes; high doses may cause an initial drop in blood pressure followed by a sustained elevation. Monitor uterine contractions and watch closely for signs of fluid overload. (See

Complications of oxytocin administration, page 844.)

Uterine relaxants

The beta agonists ritodrine, terbutaline, and isoxsuprine relax uterine muscles to suppress premature labor. These relaxants are used when diagnosis of premature labor is certain, gestation is less than 34 weeks, the cervix is dilated less than 4 cm, and no contraindications exist for their use.

Beta agonists usually are administered by I.V. infusion or subcutaneous injection until contractions stop. Then, after discharge, the patient may continue with oral doses until the delivery of a mature infant is assured. Alternatively, some doctors prescribe a 5-day treatment course, which they believe is equally effective and avoids prolonged maternal and fetal exposure. Subcutaneous injections or I.V. infusion may be repeated if premature labor recurs. Some doctors have successfully prescribed terbutaline for use at home with an I.V. pump.

Monitoring and aftercare. Careful monitoring is essential throughout therapy. If a uterine relaxant will be given I.V. or subcutaneously, perform a baseline electrocardiogram (ECG) and connect the patient to a fetal monitor. Also collect serum samples for a CBC and electrolyte and glucose studies, as ordered. During therapy, monitor these laboratory studies, usually at 6-hour intervals, to detect hypokalemia, hypoglycemia, or decreased hemat-

CHARTING TIPS

Oxytocin administration

When administering an oxytocic drug for induction of labor, be certain to document thoroughly. Documentation should include the type and amount of the main I.V. solution; the location, time, and drip rate when it was started; as well as the method used to start the infusion (jelco catheter, butterfly).

Then be sure to document the same information for the oxytocin infusion. State that the oxytocin was started as a piggyback infusion via volumetric (IMED) pump and specify the rate that was ordered. Also be sure to document this information on the fetal monitor strip. Remember to chart the mother's response to the infusion and the procedure.

ocrit. Report abnormal findings to the doctor.

Monitor the patient's cardiac status continuously and report any arrhythmias. Check blood pressure and pulse every 10 to 15 minutes initially, then every 30 minutes or as ordered. Notify the doctor if her pulse rate exceeds 140 beats/minute or if her blood pressure falls 15 mm Hg or more. Tachycardia and hypotension signal the need for a dosage adjustment. Be sure the patient remains in the left-lateral position to provide increased blood flow to the uterus.

If the patient complains of palpitations or chest pain or tightness, decrease the drug dosage and notify

Complications of oxytocin administration

Oxytocin infusion can cause excessive uterine stimulation and fluid overload. To help you forestall these complications, follow these guidelines.

Excessive uterine stimulation

Drug overdose or hypersensitivity may cause excessive uterine stimulation, leading to hypertonicity, tetany, rupture, cervical and perineal lacerations, premature placental separation, fetal hypoxia, or rapid forceful delivery.

To prevent these complications, administer oxytocin with a volumetric pump and use piggyback infusion, so that the drug may be discontinued, if necessary, without interrupting the main I.V. line. Every 15 minutes, monitor uterine contractions, intrauterine pressure, fetal heart rate, and the character of blood loss.

If contractions occur less than 2 minutes apart, last 90 seconds or longer, or exceed 50 mm Hg, stop the infusion, turn the patient onto her side (preferably the left), and notify the doctor. Contractions should occur every 2½ to 3 minutes, followed by a period of relaxation.

Keep magnesium sulfate (20% solution) available to relax the myometrium.

Fluid overload

Oxytocin's antidiuretic effect increases renal reabsorption of water. This can cause fluid overload, leading to seizures and coma.

To identify this complication, monitor the patient's intake and output, especially in prolonged infusion of doses above 20 milliunits/minute. The risk of fluid overload also increases when oxytocin is given after abortion in hypertonic saline solution.

---

the doctor immediately. Keep emergency resuscitation equipment nearby. Assess pulmonary status every hour during I.V. therapy, and monitor intake and output. Fluid overload may lead to pulmonary edema, especially if the patient is receiving corticosteroids along with ritodrine. Auscultate her lungs and report any crackles or increased respirations. Notify the doctor if urine output drops below 50 ml/hour. If signs of pulmonary edema develop, place her in a high Fowler's position, administer oxygen, as ordered, and notify the doctor.

Check the patient's temperature every 4 hours during I.V. infusion.

Report any fever to the doctor. Note the frequency and duration of the contractions. Check the FHR on the monitor every 10 to 15 minutes initially and then every 30 minutes, or as ordered. Immediately notify the doctor if FHR exceeds 180 or falls below 120 beats/minute.

For 1 to 2 hours after I.V. therapy, monitor the patient's vital signs, intake and output, and fetal heart sounds. Perform serial ECGs, as ordered, and assess for uterine contractions. Immediately report tachycardia, hypotension, decreased urine output, or diminished or absent fetal heart sounds.

Patient education. Reassure the patient that drug effects on her neonate should be minimal.

Tell the patient to notify the doctor immediately if she experiences sweating, chest pain, or increased pulse rate. Teach her to check her pulse before oral administration. If her pulse exceeds 130 beats/minute, she shouldn't take the drug and should notify the doctor. Also emphasize the importance of immediately reporting any contractions, low back pain, cramping, or increased vaginal discharge. Instruct her to report other adverse reactions, such as headache, nervousness, tremors, restlessness, nausea, or vomiting to the doctor; he'll probably reduce the drug dosage. Also have her notify the doctor if her urine output decreases or if she gains more than 5 lb (2.2 kg) in a week. Tell her to take her temperature every day and to report any fever to the doctor.

Advise her to take oral doses of the drug with food (to avoid GI upset) and to take the last dose several hours before bedtime (to avoid insomnia). Instruct her to remain in bed as much as possible and not to prepare her breasts for nursing until about 2 weeks before her due date. Emphasize the importance of keeping follow-up appointments.

Surgery

Common obstetric surgeries include amniotomy and cesarean section.

Amniotomy

Performed by a doctor or a nurse-midwife, amniotomy involves inserting a sterile amniohook through the cervical os to rupture the amniotic membranes. This controversial but commonly used procedure allows amniotic fluid to drain, thereby enhancing the intensity, frequency, and duration of contractions. It may be performed to induce labor if the membranes fail to rupture spontaneously after full cervical dilation, to expedite labor after the onset of dilation, or to allow insertion of an intrauterine catheter and a spiral electrode for direct fetal monitoring. Oxytocin infusion may precede amniotomy or follow it by 6 to 8 hours if labor fails to progress.

Factors that influence the decision to perform amniotomy include the presentation, position, and station of the fetus; the degree of cervical dilation and effacement; the gestational age; the presence of complications; the frequency and intensity of contractions; and maternal and fetal vital signs. A high-risk pregnancy may contraindicate this procedure. Amniotomy is contraindicated if the fetal presenting part is not engaged because of the risk of transverse lie and because amniotomy may cause umbilical cord prolapse. Cord prolapse is an obstetric emergency requiring immediate cesarean delivery.

Patient preparation. Reinforce the doctor's or nurse-midwife's explanation of the procedure, and answer the patient's questions. Then, wash your hands.

Monitoring and aftercare. Observe the amniotic fluid for meconium or blood. Note its color and measure the amount of fluid. Take the patient's temperature every 2 hours to detect possible infection. If her temperature rises, begin hourly checks. Continue to monitor uterine contractions and the progress of labor. When performing a vaginal examination after amniotomy, maintain strict aseptic technique to prevent uterine infection. Minimize the number of examinations.

Cesarean section

Cesarean section involves delivering a neonate through an incision of the abdomen and uterus. It's indicated when labor or vaginal delivery carries unacceptable risk for the mother or fetus, as in cephalopelvic disproportion, placenta previa or abruptio placentae, and transverse lie or other malpresentations. Repeat cesarean sections are no longer mandatory. Depending on the type of cesarean incision, a patient may be able to deliver vaginally after having had a previous cesarean birth. In *classic cesarean*, a vertical incision extends from the uterine fundus through the body, stopping above the level of the bladder. In *lower-segment cesarean*, the preferred method, a transverse incision is made across the lower anterior wall behind the bladder. This avoids incision of the peritoneum, reducing the risk of peritonitis.

Vaginal births after cesarean have become increasingly successful.

Patient preparation. Obtain baseline maternal vital signs and FHR. Assess maternal and fetal status frequently until delivery, as policy directs. If ordered, make sure that an ultrasound has been completed to determine fetal position.

For a scheduled cesarean section, you'll be able to discuss the procedure with both parents and provide preoperative teaching. If the procedure is an emergency or the patient is exhausted from a long, inefficient labor, briefly stress the essential points about the procedure. Also, observe the mother for signs of imminent delivery.

Explore the patient's feelings about cesarean section. Reassure her that cesarean birth provides her neonate with the safest, easiest delivery. Describe the equipment in the delivery room or, if possible, show her the room beforehand. Tell her that delivery usually takes about 5 to 10 minutes, although suturing commonly takes up to 40 minutes.

Restrict food and fluids after midnight, if a general anesthetic is ordered. To prepare the patient for surgery, scrub and shave the abdomen and the symphysis pubis, as ordered. Insert an indwelling urinary catheter, as ordered. Tell the mother that the catheter will remain in place for 24 hours or longer. Notify the pediatrician of the anticipated delivery time, and be sure the nursery is alerted.

Administer any ordered preoperative medication. Also give the mother an antacid to help neutralize stomach acid, if ordered. Start an I.V. infusion. Use an 18G or larger catheter to allow blood administration through the I.V., if needed. Make sure the doctor has ordered typing and crossmatching of the mother's blood and that 2 U of blood are available.

Be sure the preoperative checklist is complete. Obtain assistance to transfer the patient to the delivery room or operating room.

Monitoring and aftercare. As soon as possible, allow the mother to see, touch, and hold her neonate, either in the delivery room or after she recovers from the general anesthetic. Contact with the neonate promotes bonding.

Assess the mother for hemorrhage. Check the perineal pad and abdominal dressing on the incision every 15 minutes for 1 hour, then every half hour for 4 hours, every hour for 4 hours, and finally every 4 hours for 24 hours. Perform fundal checks at the same intervals. Monitor vital signs every 5 minutes until stable. Then check vital signs when you evaluate drainage.

Also, monitor intake and output as ordered. Expect the mother to receive I.V. fluids for 24 to 48 hours. In many cases, the doctor will order oxytocin mixed in the first 1 to 2 L of I.V. fluids infused to promote uterine contraction and decrease the risk of hemorrhage.

Assist the mother to turn from side to side every 1 to 2 hours. Encourage her to cough and deep-breathe, and use the incentive spirometer to promote adequate respiratory function. Also apply ice to the incision, as ordered, to reduce pain and swelling. If available, instruct the patient in patient-controlled anesthesia technique.

Anticipate questions about breast-feeding. (See *Breast-feeding after a cesarean section*, page 848.)

Patient education. Instruct the patient to immediately report hemorrhage, chest or leg pain (possible thrombosis), dyspnea, or separation of the wound's edges. She should also report signs and symptoms of infection, such as fever, difficult urination, or flank pain. Note measures to relieve abdominal distention from gas—plenty of fluids and early ambulation. Show her how to move from a lying to a leg-dangling position.

Remind the patient to keep her follow-up appointment. At that time, she can talk to the doctor about using contraception and resuming intercourse.

Neonatal treatments

Following are the most common treatments and surgical procedures for neonatal care. These include Credé's method, thermoregulation, oxygen administration, phototherapy, gavage feeding, and circumcision.

Neonatal eye treatment

Erythromycin ointment is instilled into the neonate's conjunctival sac to prevent gonorrheal conjunctivitis and chlamydial infection.

CRITICAL THINKING

Breast-feeding after a cesarean section

Mrs. Young had just had a cesarean section for cephalopelvic disproportion. She expresses the desire to breast-feed her newborn but is extremely uncomfortable. She knows that breast-feeding is beneficial to her newborn but isn't aware of any benefits to herself. What else could you tell her about the benefits for her? And what could you tell her about positioning of the newborn to promote successful breast-feeding?

Suggested response
Explain that breast-feeding helps her body recover from pregnancy. Reassure her that you can help her find a comfortable way to breast-feed her newborn. Correct positioning can make feeding time much easier.

Usually the antibiotic is placed in the conjunctival sac and spread by closing the eye. Although it may be done in the delivery room, treatment can be delayed for up to an hour to allow parent-child bonding. Antibiotic prophylaxis may not be effective if the infection was acquired in utero from PROM.

Patient preparation. If the neonate's parents are present, explain that the procedure is required by state law. Tell them that it may temporarily irritate the neonate's eyes and make him cry but that the effects are transient.

Thermoregulation

The neonate is very susceptible to hypothermia. Without careful external thermoregulation, the neonate may become chilled, which can result in hypoxia, acidosis, hypoglycemia, pulmonary vasoconstriction, and even death. The object of thermoregulation is to provide a neutral thermal environment that helps the neonate maintain a normal core temperature with minimal oxygen consumption and caloric expenditure. The core temperature varies with the neonate but is about 97.7° F (36.5° C).

Patient preparation. Place a radiant warmer or, if necessary, an isolette in the delivery room and set it at the desired temperature before delivery. Place blankets under a heat source to warm.

Procedure. To avoid heat loss, place the neonate under a radiant warmer during suctioning and initial care in the delivery room. Then, wrap him in a warmed blanket for transport to the nursery. Place him under another radiant warmer until his temperature stabilizes; then, put him in a bassinet.

If the neonate's temperature doesn't stabilize or if he has a condition that affects thermoregulation, place him in a temperature-controlled isolette.

Monitoring and aftercare. Once the neonate's weight is up to about 4 lb,

6 oz (1,985 g), wean him from the incubator by slowly reducing its temperature to that of the nursery. Check him periodically for hypothermia. Never discharge the neonate directly from an isolette.

Always warm oxygen before administering it to a neonate to avoid aggravating heat loss from his head and face. Stimulate the neonate in an isolette by stroking him, talking to him and, if possible, placing a music box in with him.

Patient education. Explain to the mother the importance of maintaining the infant's temperature. Instruct her to keep him wrapped in a blanket and out of drafts when he's not in the bassinet. Explain that keeping the baby dry helps him stay warm.

Oxygen administration
Oxygen relieves neonatal respiratory distress. This distress may be indicated by cyanosis, pallor, tachypnea, nasal flaring, bradycardia, hypothermia, retractions (intercostal, subcostal margin, suprasternal), hypotonia, hyporeflexia, or expiratory grunting.

Oxygen therapy brings hazard to the neonate. When given in high concentrations and for prolonged periods, it can cause blindness in premature neonates, and can contribute to bronchopulmonary dysplasia.

Patient preparation. Because of the neonate's size and special respiratory requirements, oxygen administration generally requires special techniques and equipment. In emergency situations, give oxygen through a manual resuscitation bag and mask of appropriate size until more permanent measures can be initiated. When the neonate merely requires additional oxygen above the ambient concentration, it can be delivered by means of an oxygen hood. When the neonate requires continuous positive airway pressure to prevent alveolar collapse at the end of an expiration, as in respiratory distress syndrome (hyaline membrane disease), administer oxygen through nasal prongs or an endotracheal tube connected to a manometer. If the neonate can't breathe on his own, deliver oxygen through a ventilator. Oxygen must be warmed and humidified.

Procedure. To administer emergency oxygen through a manual resuscitation bag and mask:
• Turn on the oxygen and compressed air flowmeters to the prescribed flow rates. Apply the mask to the neonate's face.
• Provide 40 breaths/minute with enough pressure to cause a visible rise and fall of the neonate's chest. Provide enough oxygen to keep his nail beds and mucous membranes pink.
• Watch his chest movements continuously and check breath sounds. Avoid overventilation.
• Insert a nasogastric tube to keep air out of the stomach.

Monitoring and aftercare. Always take electrical precautions when administering oxygen, to avoid fire or explosion. Explain the situation and the procedures to the parents. Take measures to keep the neonate warm, because hypothermia impedes respiration. Check arterial blood gas (ABG) levels at least every hour if the unstable neonate receives a high concentration of oxygen, and whenever there's a clinical change. If he does not respond to oxygen administration, check for congenital anomalies.

Know how to perform neonatal chest auscultation correctly to pick up subtle respiratory changes. Be able to identify signs of respiratory distress and perform emergency procedures. If required, perform chest physiotherapy and percussion, as ordered, and follow with suctioning to remove secretions. As ordered, discontinue oxygen administration when the neonate's fraction of inspired oxygen is at room air level (20% to 21%) and his arterial oxygen is stable at 60 to 90 mm Hg. Repeat ABG measurements 20 to 30 minutes after discontinuing oxygen, and thereafter as ordered by the doctor or by policy.

Monitor the neonate for any complications of oxygen administration, including signs and symptoms of infection; hypothermia; metabolic or respiratory acidosis; pressure sores on the neonate's head, face, or nose; or signs of pulmonary air leak, including pneumothorax, pneumomediastinum, pneumopericardium, or interstitial emphysema.

Phototherapy

Phototherapy involves exposing the neonate to specific wavelengths of light, which decomposes bilirubin. Neonatal jaundice or hyperbilirubinemia is common.

Phototherapy generally begins while the doctor determines the cause of jaundice. It's usually the only treatment necessary, although some neonates (especially those with hemolytic disease) may require exchange transfusions to reduce excessive bilirubin levels.

Patient preparation. Set up the phototherapy unit over the neonate's crib or isolette, according to the manufacturer's instructions. If using a radiant warmer with a built-in phototherapy unit, position an additional phototherapy unit to the side of the neonate's bed, making sure it's the correct distance from his skin. This additional unit will deliver the required therapeutic energy level because the built-in unit is too far away from the neonate to produce sufficient energy. If a radiometer isn't available, check that the bulbs haven't been used longer than specified by the manufacturer or the institution's policy (usually 400 to 500 hours). Turn on the unit to make sure the bulbs are working properly.

Procedure. Begin by recording the neonate's initial bilirubin level and take his axillary temperature to establish baseline measurements. Then take the following steps.
• Clean the neonate's eyes with cotton balls moistened with normal saline solution. Then instill one drop of methylcellulose in each eye. Place eye pads over the eyes to pre-

vent retinal damage from the phototherapy lights. Make sure his eyes are shut to prevent corneal abrasion. Finally, place the eye mask over the eye pads and secure it with the Velcro strap or paper tape. Make sure the mask isn't too tight to prevent head molding. With a very small premature neonate, consider using a stocking cap over the eye pads instead of a mask.

• Undress the neonate to expose the maximum amount of skin and lay him on the diaper. If required by policy, cover the male neonate's testes with a surgical mask to protect them.

• Turn on the phototherapy lights. Make sure there's nothing between the lights and the neonate to ensure full exposure and to prevent damage to materials such as plastic that could melt under the lights. Always make sure the clear plastic cover is in place on units using fluorescent lights because it removes harmful ultraviolet rays and protects the neonate from bulb breakage.

• If the neonate cries excessively, place a blanket roll to each side of him to calm him.

• Place the radiometer probe in the middle of the crib to measure the amount of radiant energy being emitted by the lights. The measurement should be 4 to 6 μW/cm²/nm.

Monitoring and aftercare. Check bilirubin level at least every 24 hours and more often if the level is rising significantly. Turn off the phototherapy lights before performing the venipuncture to prevent false results. Plot your results on a bilirubin graph to be sure the level isn't rising more than 5 mg/day; a steeper increase indicates the need for additional treatment. Notify the doctor if the bilirubin level exceeds 20 mg/dl in a full-term neonate or 15 mg/dl in a premature one. In addition, do the following.

• Take the neonate's axillary temperature every 1 to 2 hours to prevent hyperthermia and hypothermia. If needed, provide a heat source such as a gooseneck lamp with bulb shield or adjust the temperature of a heated isolette.

• Monitor the neonate's intake and output and bowel movements to help prevent dehydration. Also, monitor specific gravity of urine every 8 hours to help assess hydration.

• Clean the neonate carefully after each bowel movement because the loose, green stools that may result from phototherapy can excoriate the skin. Don't apply an ointment because this can cause burns under the phototherapy lights.

• Reposition the neonate every few hours.

• Feed the neonate every 3 to 4 hours and offer water between feedings; make sure water intake doesn't replace formula or breast milk. If possible, take him out of the crib and remove his eye mask to allow visual stimulation and contact, especially with parents. Check his eyes at this time for signs of irritation or infection.

• Check the neonate's eye mask frequently to prevent slippage, exposure of eyes to the lights, or obstruction of the nostrils. Change the eye pads and the mask daily.

• Finally, watch for signs of infection and metabolic disorders. Check the neonate's hematocrit to detect possible polycythemia. Inspect him for bruising, hematoma, petechiae, and cyanosis. Turn blue lights off during inspection because they may mask cyanosis.

Gavage feeding

Gavage feeding involves passing nutrients directly to the neonate's stomach by a tube passed through the nasopharynx or the oropharynx. The procedure feeds the neonate who is unable to suck because of prematurity, illness, or congenital deformity. It also helps the neonate who risks aspiration because he has gastroesophageal reflux, lacks the gag reflex, or tires easily. In a premature neonate, gavage feeding continues until he can begin bottle-feeding.

Unless the neonate has problems with the feeding tube, you insert it before each feeding, usually through his mouth, and then withdraw it after feeding. This intermittent method stimulates the sucking reflex. If the neonate can't tolerate this, pass the tube through the nostrils and leave it in place for 24 to 72 hours.

Preparation. Determine the length of tubing needed for placement in the stomach. Mark the tube at the appropriate distance.

Procedure. Follow these directions to give a gavage feeding:
• With a tape measure, determine the length of tubing needed to ensure placement in the stomach, according to the institution's policy and the developmental stage of the neonate. Common measurements used are from the bridge of the nose to the xiphoid process, from the tip of the nose to the tip of the earlobe to the midpoint between the xiphoid process and the umbilicus and, for the premature neonate, from the bridge of the nose to the umbilicus. Mark the tube at the appropriate distance with a piece of tape, measuring from the bottom.
• If possible, support the neonate on your lap in a sitting position to provide a feeling of security. Otherwise, place the neonate in a supine position or tilted slightly to the right, with head and chest slightly elevated.
• Stabilize the neonate's head with one hand and lubricate the feeding tube with sterile water with the other hand.
• Insert the tube smoothly and quickly up to the premeasured mark. For oral insertion, pass the tube toward the back of the throat. For nasal insertion, pass the tube toward the occiput in a horizontal plane.
• Synchronize tube insertion with throat movement if the neonate swallows, to facilitate its passage into the stomach. During insertion, watch for choking and cyanosis, signs that the tube has entered the trachea. If these occur, remove the tube and reinsert it. Also, watch for bradycardia and apnea resulting from vagal stimulation. If bradycardia occurs, leave the tube in place for 1 minute and check for return to normal heart rate. If bradycardia persists, remove the tube and notify the doctor.

• If the tube is to remain in place, tape it flat to the neonate's cheek. Don't tape the tube to the bridge of his nose.

• Make sure the tube is in the stomach by aspirating residual stomach contents with the syringe. Note the volume obtained, and then reinject it. If ordered, reduce the volume of the feeding by the residual amount, or prolong the interval between feedings.

Alternatively, or in addition to the above procedure, check placement of the feeding tube in the stomach by injecting 1 to 2 cc of air into the tube while listening for air sounds in the stomach with the stethoscope.

If the tube doesn't appear to be in place, insert it several centimeters further and test again. *Don't* begin feeding until you're sure the tube is positioned properly.

• When the tube is in place, fill the feeding reservoir or syringe with the formula or breast milk. Then, inject 1 ml of sterile water into the tube and pinch the top of the tube to establish gravity flow. Connect the feeding reservoir or syringe to the top of the tube, and then release the tube to start the feeding.

• If the neonate is sitting on your lap, hold the container 4″ (10 cm) above his abdomen. If he's lying down, hold it 6″ to 8″ (15 to 20 cm) above his head. When using a commercial feeding reservoir, observe for air bubbles in the container, indicating passage of formula.

• Regulate flow by raising and lowering the container, so that the feeding takes 15 to 20 minutes, the average time for a bottle feeding. To prevent stomach distention, reflux, and vomiting, don't let the feeding proceed too rapidly.

• When the feeding is finished, pinch off the tubing before air enters the neonate's stomach to prevent distention and to avoid leakage of fluid into the pharynx during removal, with possible aspiration. Then, withdraw the tube smoothly and quickly. If the tube is to remain in place, flush it with several milliliters of sterile water, if ordered.

• Burp the neonate. Hold him upright or in a sitting position, with one hand supporting his head and chest, and gently rub or pat his back until he expels the air.

• Place him on his stomach or right side for 1 hour after feeding to facilitate gastric emptying and to prevent aspiration if he regurgitates.

Monitoring and aftercare. Use the nasogastric approach for the neonate who must have the feeding tube left in place because it's more stable than orogastric insertion. Alternate the nostril used at each insertion to prevent irritation.

Observe the premature neonate for indications that he's ready to begin bottle-feeding: strong sucking reflex, coordinated sucking and swallowing, alertness before feeding, and sleep after it.

Provide the neonate with a pacifier during feeding to relax him, to help prevent gagging, and to promote an association between sucking and feeding.

Circumcision

Circumcision removes the foreskin from the neonate's penis. Usually a doctor performs this minor operation at delivery or within 1 to 2 days for hygienic reasons, to make cleaning the glans easier, and to avoid the risk of phimosis (tightening of the foreskin) in later life.

In the Jewish religion, circumcision is a religious ritual called a *Brith Milah* and is performed by a *mohel* on the eighth day after birth, when the neonate is officially given his name. Because most neonates are sent home before this time, the Brith is rarely done in the health care facility.

REFERENCES AND READINGS

Davis, D. C. "The Discomforts of Pregnancy," *JOGNN* 25(1):73-81, January 1996.

Hart, M.A. "Nursing Implications of Self-care in Pregnancy," *MCN* 21(3):137-43, May/June 1996.

Jonaitis, M.A. "Complications During Pregnancy: Diabetes," *RN* 58(10):40-46, October 1995.

Jones, D.P., and Collins, B.A. "The Nursing Management of Women Experiencing Preterm Labor: Clinical Guidelines and Why They Are Needed," *JOGNN* 25(7):569-92, September 1996.

Letko, M.D. "Understanding the Apgar Score," *JOGNN* 25(4):299-303, May 1996.

Lowdermilk, D.L., et al. *Maternity and Women's Health Care,* 6th ed. St. Louis: Mosby–Year Book, Inc., 1997.

McGregor, L.A. "Short, Shorter, Shortest: Improving the Hospital Stay for Mothers and Newborns," *MCN* 19(2):91-96, March/April 1994.

Minnick-Smith, K., and Cook, F. "Current Treatments for Ectopic Pregnancy," *MCN* 22(1): 21-26, January/February 1997.

Miovech, S.M., et al. "Major Concerns of Women after Cesarean Delivery," *JOGNN* 23(1):53-59, January 1994.

Montgomery, K.S. "Caring for the Pregnant Woman with Sickle Cell Disease," *MCN* 21(5):224-28, September/October 1996.

Olds, S.B., et al. *Maternal-Newborn Nursing: A Family-Centered Approach.* Menlo Park, Calif.: Addison-Wesley Publishing Co., 1996.

Penny-Macgillivray, T. "A Newborn's First Bath: When?" *JOGNN* 25(6):481-87, July/August 1996.

Reeder, S.J., and Martin, L.L. *Maternity Nursing: Family, Newborn, and Women's Health Care,* 18th ed. Philadelphia: Lippincott-Raven Pubs., 1997.

Schroeder, C.A. "Women's Experience of Bedrest in High-Risk Pregnancy," *Image* 28(3):253-58, Fall 1996.

Supplee, R.B., and Vezeau, T.M. "Continuous Electronic Fetal Monitoring: Does It Belong in Low-Risk Births?" *MCN* 18(2):86-93, November/December 1996.

Valaitis, R., at al. "Meeting Parent's Postpartal Needs with a Telephone Information Line," *MCN* 21(2):90-95, March/April 1996.

Vomund, S.L., and Witter, S.E. "Advanced Techniques for the Treatment of Severe Isoimmunization," *MCN* 19(1):18-23, January/February 1994.

Yeo, S. "Exercise Guidelines for Pregnant Women," *Image: Journal of Nursing Scholarship* 26(4):265-71, Winter 1994.

Zwelling, E. "Childbirth in the 1990s and Beyond," *JOGNN* 25(5):425-31, June 1996.

16

PEDIATRIC CARE

While health care providers once sought only to cure disease, practitioners today use a holistic approach, which takes into account the emotional, social, and environmental factors that influence a child's well-being. This chapter will help prepare you for this challenge. It includes instructions on how to perform a complete assessment, body system by body system. In addition, you'll find guidance for formulating nursing diagnoses and putting them into practice. In the treatments section, you'll learn about pediatric cardiopulmonary resuscitation (CPR), and other procedures vital to child health care. Throughout you'll find information on communicating effectively with youngsters and their parents, a vital, if sometimes difficult, part of providing care.

ASSESSMENT

Your health assessment may include a discussion of growth patterns and nutrition as well as an examination of body systems.

Growth patterns and nutrition

This assessment is especially important for any child at nutritional risk, especially one who has failed to thrive or has undergone surgery. Use the same techniques you would in assessing an adult. In addition, plot the child's development on a growth grid and measure head circumference if the child is an infant.

Growth grids

Growth grids allow you to screen for early signs of nutritional deficiencies. Include them in each young patient's chart.

Measure the child's height and weight. Plot your findings on a grid to compare by age and sex. The National Center for Health Statistics has developed growth grids for children up to age 18.

These grids use percentiles rather than ideal weight for height. Consider findings below the 5th percentile or above the 95th percentile abnormal.

Diet history

Obtain a child's diet history from his parents or, if possible, from the child himself. For all pediatric age-groups, assess daily nutritional plan such as the types of meals and number as well as any snacks, any special or modified diet, behavioral peculiarities associated with mealtimes, and any feeding problems.

Examination of body systems

This portion of your assessment may cover the skin, the eyes and vision, the ears and hearing as well as the respiratory, cardiovascular, GI, urinary, nervous, musculoskeletal, hematologic, immune, and endocrine systems.

When taking the patient history, ask the parents about birth history and early development. Also ask about childhood diseases and injuries and any known congenital abnormalities. More specific questions will depend upon which body system is being assessed. (See *Documenting suspicious trauma.*)

Skin

Integumentary problems may occur throughout childhood.

Neonates and infants. Common skin problems include diaper rash, cradle cap, newborn rash (erythema neonatorum toxicum), acne, impetigo, and roseola.

Preschool and school-age children. Younger children are susceptible to common disorders, such as allergic contact dermatitis (from poison ivy, oak, or sumac, or clothing), atopic dermatitis, warts (especially on the hands), viral exanthemas, impetigo, ringworm, scabies, and skin reactions to food allergies.

Adolescents. At puberty, hormonal changes affect the child's skin and hair. Common dermatoses occurring during adolescence include acne, warts, sunburn, scabies, atopic dermatitis, and pityriasis rosea. Allergic contact dermatitis and fungal infections also commonly occur.

Eyes and vision

Often a school nurse or teacher will first notice a child's vision problems and refer him for further evaluation. Behavior problems may relate to difficulty seeing the chalkboard.

When taking the patient history, be alert for clues to familial eye disorders, such as refractive errors or retinoblastoma. Refer a child with a family history of glaucoma to an ophthalmologist, even if he has no obvious symptoms.

Physical examination includes tests for visual acuity and inspection for strabismus. (See *Characteristics of the infant's eye,* page 858.)

Visual acuity. Because 20/20 visual acuity and depth perception develop fully by age 7, you can test vision in school-age children as you would for adults. Test a child age 4 or older with the E chart. No accurate method measures visual acuity in children under age 4. (Testing with Allen cards may provide useful data.)

Strabismus. Strabismus results from the misalignment of each eye's optic axis. As a result, one or both of the child's eyes turn in (crossed eyes), up, down, or out. A child with a deviating eye usually develops double vision (diplopia). Continued disuse of the deviating eye leads to amblyopia, an irreversible loss of visual acuity in the suppressed eye. If the infant or toddler appears to have a deviating eye, refer him to an ophthalmologist. In older children, you can perform the cover-uncover test. The *light reflection test* (Hirschberg's test) also helps to detect strabismus.

Ears and hearing

An infant can localize the direction of sound by age 6 months, and a child's hearing is fully developed by age 5. Investigate the child's speech development by listening to him carefully. Speech development reflects hearing acuity during childhood. (See *Looking at the child's ear,* page 859.)

Prenatal causes of congenital hearing defects include maternal infection (especially rubella during the first trimester) and maternal use of ototoxic drugs. Events at birth that may cause hearing loss include hypoxia (or anoxia), jaundice, and trauma. If the patient has a craniofacial deformity such as a cleft

CHARTING TIPS

Documenting suspicious trauma

Always document your observations accurately when caring for a child. This is especially important when the child is a suspected victim of nonaccidental trauma. Follow these guidelines.
• Be sure to document all physical observations.
• Always document all bruises and their location, size, and color. Color is important as an indication of the age of the bruises.
• Be sure to document other marks observed on the child's body. Be specific about their location, size, and distinguishing characteristics.
• Document parent-child interaction. All observations must be about the observed interaction and not the interpretation of the interaction. Include specific details.

palate he has an increased risk of developing otitis media.

With an infant, make a sudden loud noise, such as clapping your hands, about 12″ (30.5 cm) from his ear. He should respond with the startle reflex or with blinking. To evaluate hearing in a child between ages 2 and 5, use play techniques such as asking him to put a peg in a board when he hears a sound transmitted through earphones. For an older child, try the whisper test, but be sure to use words he knows, and take care to prevent him from lipreading. The child should hear a

Characteristics of the infant's eye

When examining an infant's eye, you'll notice several distinguishing characteristics:
• The eye structure is larger in relation to the body than the adult's eye structure.
• The cornea is thinner and has a greater curvature.
• The cornea's exaggerated curve causes the lens to be more refractive, compensating for the eye's shortness.
• Initially, the iris appears blue. However, the blue coloring is actually from the posterior pigment layer showing through a light or transparent anterior layer. Pigment, deposited in the anterior layer within the first 2 years, determines the adult iris color. Small deposits of pigment make the iris appear blue or green. Large deposits make the iris appear brown.
• The pupil, situated slightly on the nasal side of the cornea, appears larger on examination because of the high refractive power of the cornea. Despite this, the pupils are hard to dilate and small, widening at age 1 and reaching the greatest diameter during adolescence.
• For the first 3 or 4 months, foveal light reflection is not present. Instead, the macula appears bright white and elevated; the peripheral fundus, gray. The fundus may also have a mottled appearance, which is normal in an infant.
• The sclera has a blue tinge because of its thinness and translucence. It turns white as it thickens and becomes hydrated.

whispered question or simple command at 8′ (2.4 m).

Respiratory system

Upper respiratory tract infections commonly occur in children because the respiratory tract is immature and the mucous membranes can't produce enough mucous to warm and humidify inhaled air. A child's respiratory rate may double in response to exercise, illness, or emotion. If the child is quiet, auscultate his lungs first. If you hear fluid, place the stethoscope's diaphragm over his nose to see if the fluid is in the lungs or upper respiratory tract. (See *Assessing a crying child,* page 860.)

Use a flashlight and tongue blade to examine the child's mouth and throat. You can also use the tongue blade to elicit the gag reflex in infants. *Never* test this reflex or examine the pharynx in a child suspected of having epiglottitis; you could cause complete laryngeal obstruction.

While examining the posterior thorax of the older child, be sure to check for scoliosis. (See *Pediatric chest abnormalities,* page 861.)

Laryngotracheobronchitis (croup) is the most common cause of respiratory distress in children over age 3. Its signs include a hacking cough, fever, stridor, and diminished breath sounds with rhonchi. Keep in mind that epiglottitis has similar signs and symptoms.

Intracostal, subcostal, and suprasternal retractions and expiratory grunts are always serious signs in children. Refer an infant or child with any of these signs for treatment

Looking at the child's ear

You'll recognize three major differences between a young child's or infant's ear and an adult's ear.

In a child, the tympanic membrane slants horizontally, rather than vertically. Also, the entire external canal slants upward. These differences require that during the otoscopic examination you hold the child's pinna down and out instead of up and back as you would with an adult.

A child's eustachian tube also slants horizontally. This causes fluid to stagnate and act as a medium for bacteria. These anatomic differences make the infant and young child more susceptible to ear infection.

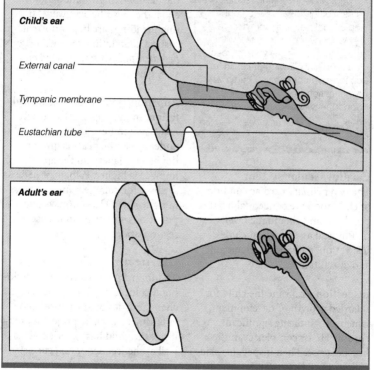

Child's ear

External canal

Tympanic membrane

Eustachian tube

Adult's ear

immediately. He may have pneumonia, respiratory distress syndrome, or left-sided heart failure (HF).

When a child's signs and symptoms include retractions, nasal flaring, cyanosis, restlessness, and apprehension, primarily on inspiration, the trachea or mainstem bronchi may be obstructed. If symptoms occur on expiration, his bronchioles may be obstructed, as occurs in asthma and bronchitis. Foreign body aspiration may cause respiratory distress. (See *Asthma or GI problem?* page 862.)

Cardiovascular system

The two primary cardiac conditions of childhood are congenital heart problems and rheumatic fever.

Physical assessment includes inspection, palpation, percussion, and auscultation.

Inspection. Examine the child for retarded growth or development, which may indicate significant chronic HF or complex cyanotic heart disease. Then inspect his skin. Pallor can indicate a serious cardiac problem in an infant or anemia in an older child. In an infant or child, cyanosis may be an early sign of a cardiac condition.

Check for clubbed fingers, a sign of cardiac dysfunction. (Clubbing doesn't ordinarily occur before age 2.) Also, remember that dependent edema, a late sign of HF in children, appears in the legs only if the child can walk; in infants, it appears in the eyelids.

Blood pressure can help confirm coarctation of the aorta. For children under age 1, the systolic thigh reading should equal the systolic arm reading; for older children, it may be 10 to 40 mm Hg higher, but the diastolic thigh value should equal the diastolic arm value. If thigh readings are below normal, suspect coarctation. (See *Guide to pediatric pulse rate and blood pressure,* page 863.)

Palpation, percussion, and auscultation. In judging cardiac enlargement, remember that in children under age 8, the heart is proportionately smaller and the apical impulse is higher. Palpate or percuss the liver for enlargement, as occurs in right-sided HF, or for systolic pulsations, as occurs in tricuspid regurgitation.

GI system

Abdominal pain is a common childhood complaint. Determine the characteristics of any nausea and vomiting (especially projectile vomiting) the child has experienced as well as the frequency and consistency of bowel movements.

Have a parent hold a young child if possible. Otherwise, position the child so he can see his parent. Abdominal tenseness can impede your examination. To ease tenseness, flex an infant's knees and hips.

Inspection. The contour of a child's abdomen may confirm a GI disorder. An extreme potbelly may result from organomegaly, ascites, neoplasm, defects in the abdominal wall, or starvation; a depressed or concave abdomen may indicate a diaphragmatic hernia. Look for an area of localized swelling. Costal respiratory movements may indicate peritonitis, obstruction, or accumulation of ascitic fluid. When inspecting an infant, stand at the foot of the table and direct a light across his abdomen from the right side. Observe for peristaltic waves. Because peristaltic waves aren't normally visible in a full-term infant, their appearance can indicate obstruction. Reverse peristalsis generally indicates pyloric stenosis; other possible causes include bowel malrotation, duodenal ulcer, GI allergy, or duodenal stenosis.

Inspect for umbilical hernia. The best time to perform this inspection is when the child cries.

Auscultation. Auscultate a child's abdomen as you would an adult's. Significant findings include:
• abdominal murmur, a possible indication of coarctation of the aorta
• high-pitched bowel sounds, a possible indication of intestinal obstruction or gastroenteritis
• venous hum, a possible indication of portal hypertension
• splenic or hepatic friction rubs, a possible sign of inflammation
• double sound, or so-called pistol shot, in the femoral artery, suggesting aortic insufficiency

Pediatric chest abnormalities

When examining a child, note any of the following structural abnormalities of the chest.
• An unusually wide space between the nipples may indicate Turner's syndrome (the distance between the outside areolar edges shouldn't be more than one-fourth of the patient's chest circumference).
• Rachitic beads (bumps at the costochondral junction of the ribs) may indicate rickets.
• Pigeon chest may be a sign of Marfan's or Morquio's syndrome or any chronic upper respiratory tract obstruction; funnel chest may indicate rickets or Marfan's syndrome; barrel chest may indicate chronic respiratory disease, such as cystic fibrosis or asthma. Pigeon chest may also occur as a normal variation.
• Localized bulges may suggest underlying pressures, such as cardiac enlargement or aneurysm.
• Multiple (more than five) café-au-lait spots may be associated with neurofibromatosis. Note that these spots may occur elsewhere on the body.

• absence of bowel sounds, a possible indication of paralytic ileus and peritonitis.

Palpation. Children tend to guard their abdomens when pain is present. Palpate the painful quadrant last. Palpation should reveal a soft, nontender abdomen. Tenderness in

Asthma or GI problem?

Sarah is a three-year-old child brought to the Emergency Department because she is having trouble breathing. Her mother reports that she has had breathing problems intermittently this winter. She also has abdominal pain and has had one vomiting episode this morning.

As you observe Sarah sitting upright in a chair, you see that she is pale and has an anxious expression on her face. Her respirations are shallow at 45 breaths per minute. She has a tight, nonproductive cough and is alert and answers your questions with single words.

Is Sarah having a respiratory or GI problem?

Suggested response

Abdominal pain is a frequent complaint of children. You place a pulse oximeter on Sarah and her oxygen saturation is 91%. When you listen to Sarah"s lungs, you hear inspiratory and expiratory wheezing; you note that she's using accessory muscles for breathing. She has 10 mm Hg pulsus paradoxus and isn't able to use a peak flow meter because of her age.

At this point, you decide that Sarah has had an exacerbation of asthma. You begin oxygen per nasal cannula to maintain oxygen saturation greater than 95% and continuous monitoring by pulse oximetry. You make arrangements for nebulized albuterol treatment. After the first nebulized albuterol, Sarah's respiratory rate is 40, she continues to have inspiratory and expiratory wheezes and her use of accessory muscles is decreased. Her oxygen saturation is 93%. You request another nebulized albuterol treatment. At the completion of this treatment, her respiratory rate is 38, her oxygen saturation is 95%, and she has decreased use of her accessory muscles to breath and only expiratory wheezes.

She receives one more nebulized albuterol treatment for a total of three treatments in the first hour. Her respiratory rate is 32, her oxygen saturation is 98%, she is no longer using her accessory muscles to breathe, and she has no audible wheezes on auscultation. At this time, the supplemental oxygen is discontinued. She will be observed for at least another hour and then sent home.

the right lower quadrant may indicate an inflamed appendix.

Next, ask the child to cough. A reduced or withheld cough may confirm peritoneal irritation, contraindicating checking for rebound tenderness—a potentially painful procedure.

Check for a hernia as you would an adult. Umbilical hernias are commonly present at birth but may not always be visible.

Percussion. Minimal tympany with abdominal distention may result from fluid accumulation or solid

Guide to pediatric pulse rate and blood pressure

Pulse rate		
Age	**Normal range**	**Average**
Neonate	70 to 170	120
1 month to 11 months	80 to 160	120
2 years	80 to 130	110
4 years	80 to 120	100
6 years	75 to 115	100
8 years	70 to 110	90
10 years	70 to 110	90
12 years (female)	70 to 110	90
12 years (male)	65 to 105	85
14 years (female)	65 to 105	85
14 years (male)	60 to 100	80
16 years (female)	60 to 100	80
16 years (male)	55 to 95	75
18 years (female)	55 to 95	75
18 years (male)	50 to 90	70

Blood pressure		
Age	**Female**	**Male**
4 years	98/60	98/55
6 years	105/65	105/60
8 years	108/67	105/60
10 years	112/64	110/65
12 years	115/65	110/65
14 years	112/65	114/65

masses. To screen for abdominal fluid, use the test for shifting dullness, instead of the test for a fluid wave.

In a neonate, ascites usually results from GI or urinary perforation; in an older child, the cause may be HF, cirrhosis, or nephrosis.

Urinary system

Explore any history of colic associated with voiding and persistent enuresis after age 5. Bladder or urethral irritation or emotional difficulties can cause bed-wetting.

Inspect the patient's skin for anemic pallor, which may indicate a congenital renal disorder such as medullary cystic disease. Also inspect for undescended testes and inguinal hernia, anomalies associated with congenital urinary tract malformations.

Palpate the child's abdomen carefully for bladder distention and kidney enlargement. Bladder distention in an older child may indicate urethral dysfunction. In a preschool child, a firm, smooth, and palpable mass adjacent to the vertebral column—but not crossing the midline—suggests Wilms' tumor.

Next, inspect the patient's external genitalia closely for abnormalities associated with congenital anomalies of the urinary tract. Note the location and size of a boy's urethral meatus, the size of his testes, and any local irritation, inflammation, or swelling. The meatus should be in the center of the shaft; you may note epispadias (urethral opening on the dorsum of the shaft) or hypospadias (urethral opening on the underside of the penis or on the perineum).

Note the location of a girl's clitoris, urethral meatus, and vaginal orifice. Check for irritation, swelling, and abnormal discharge—possible signs and symptoms of urethritis.

Nervous system

When taking the patient history, find out if the child has experienced any head or nerve injuries, headaches, tremors, convulsions, dizziness, fainting spells, or muscle weakness. Ask the parents if he's overly active.

During the physical examination, expect to assess the head and neck, cerebral function, cranial nerves (CN), motor function, sensory function, and reflexes.

Head and neck. To examine cranial bones, gently run your fingers over the child's head, checking the sutures and fontanel. Fullness, bulging, or swelling may indicate an intracranial mass or hydrocephalus. Note the shape and symmetry of his head. Abnormal shape accompanied by prominent bony ridges may indicate craniosynostosis (premature suture closure).

A snapping sensation when you press the child's scalp firmly behind and above the ears (similar to the way a table-tennis ball feels when you press it in) may indicate craniotabes, a thinning of the outer layer of the skull. Although bone thinning is normal at the suture lines, premature infants are susceptible to craniotabes. Such thinning can also be a sign of rickets, hypervitaminosis A, syphilis, or hydrocephalus. A resonant, cracked pot sound

(Macewen's sign), heard when you percuss the parietal bone with your finger, is normal in an infant with open sutures. But if the sutures have closed, this can signal increased intracranial pressure.

Assess the child's head and neck muscles. Neck mobility is an important indicator of neurologic diseases such as meningitis. With the child supine, test for nuchal rigidity by cradling his head in your hands. Supporting the weight of his head, move his neck in all directions to assess ease of movement.

Cerebral function. To assess level of consciousness in a young child, use motor cues. Assess his orientation to person and place.

To test attention span and concentration, ask the child to repeat a series of numbers after you. To test a child's recent memory, show him a familiar object and tell him that you'll ask him later what it was. Five minutes later, ask him to recall it.

Cranial nerves. This assessment can be difficult in a child under age 2, but by simple observation you can check for symmetry of muscle movement, gaze, sucking strength, and hearing. In a child over age 2, assess the CNs as you would an adult's, making the following alterations:

• *CN I (olfactory).* Ask the child to identify familiar odors, such as peanut butter and chocolate or peppermint candy. For a very young child who may not be able to identify a smell, try a same-different game

to determine whether he can distinguish one smell from another.

• *CN II (optic).* For visual field testing, follow the procedure for an adult, with one variation: Hold a bright object near the end of your nose to help the young child keep his eyes focused.

• *CN V (trigeminal).* Test the sensory division of this nerve as you would for an adult, but make a game out of it by telling the child that a gremlin's going to brush his cheeks, pinch his forehead, and so on. Test the motor division by having the child bite down hard on a tongue blade as you try to pull it away. At the same time, palpate his jaw muscles for symmetry and contraction strength.

• *CN VII (facial).* Test the muscles controlled by this nerve as you would for an adult, but have him mimic your facial expressions. Test the sensory division of the facial nerve with salt and sugar, as for an adult.

• *CN VIII (acoustic).* Test the cochlear division of the acoustic nerve in a child by checking his hearing acuity and sound conduction.

• *CN IX, X, XI, and XII (glossopharyngeal, vagus, spinal accessory, and hypoglossal).* Test these nerves as you would for an adult, using games when necessary.

Motor function. Assess balance and coordination in a child by watching motor skills such as dressing. You can also have him stack blocks, put a bead in a bottle, or draw.

Left- or right-handedness is well established by the school-age years. A child age 4 should be able to stand on one foot for about 5 seconds, and a child age 6 should be able to do it for 5 seconds with his arms folded across his chest. By age 7, he should be able to do it for 5 seconds with his eyes closed.

Sensory function. Test the sensations of pain, touch, vibration, and temperature in an older child as you would for an adult. (Most of these tests don't apply to younger children.)

Reflexes. Make a special effort to relax a child when assessing his reflexes. Many children and some adults will tighten their muscle, making reflex testing almost impossible. A positive Babinski's sign may normally be present up to age 2.

Musculoskeletal system

Between birth and adulthood the skeleton triples in size. A child's bones are porous and flexible.

Be alert to the possibility of physical abuse. An abused child usually will have multiple bone injuries, in different stages of repair, and may have other serious injuries such as a subdural hematoma. (See *Child abuse: Seeing the reality.*)

Your patient history should include the ages when the child reached major motor-development milestones, such as rolling over (for an infant) or pedaling a tricycle (for an older child).

During the physical examination, expect to assess range of motion (ROM), muscle strength, spine, gait, and hips and legs.

Range of motion and muscle strength. Part of your assessment may involve playing with the child. In infants and toddlers, you'll obviously assess only passive movements for ROM testing. Observe the child's muscles for size, symmetry, strength, tone, and abnormal movements.

Test muscle strength in a preschool or school-age child as you would test it in an adult. To check muscle strength in a toddler or infant, observe his sucking as well as his general motor activity.

Spine and gait. Keep in mind that although accentuated lumbar curvature in adults is abnormal, it occurs normally in children up to age 4. (See *Identifying common spine abnormalities,* page 868.)

To check a child's gait, balance, and stance, ask him to walk, run, and skip away from you and then return. Keep developmental changes in a child's gait in mind, so you don't mistake them for abnormal conditions.

Hips and legs. Inspect the child's gluteal folds for asymmetry, which may indicate a dislocated hip. If hip dislocation is a possibility, test for Ortolani's sign.

Observe the child's legs for shape, length, symmetry, and alignment. Genu varum (bowlegs) is common in children between ages 1½ and 2½; genu valgum (knock-knees) is common in preschoolers. To test for bowlegs, have the child stand straight with his ankles touching. In this position, the knees shouldn't be more than 1″ (2.5 cm) apart. To test a child for knock-knees, have him stand straight with his knees touching. The ankles shouldn't be more than 1″ apart in this position.

Next, observe the child's feet for clubfoot (talipes equinovarus); outward-turned toes (toeing out, or pes valgus), and pigeon toes (toeing in, or pes varus).

Finally, test for tibial torsion. In external tibial torsion, the foot points out while the knee remains straight (toeing out). In internal tibial torsion, the foot points in while the knee remains straight.

Endocrine system

In a neonate or infant, endocrine disorders may cause feeding problems, constipation, jaundice, hypothermia, or somnolence.

In a child, endocrine problems usually cause growth and developmental abnormalities. Height in relation to age and weight in relation to stature and age provide important indices of growth. Poor weight gain with little or no increase in height may indicate a lack of growth hormone. Hyperthyroidism can cause weight loss. Some endocrine disorders selectively affect trunk or extremity growth.

Obtain a thorough family history from one or both parents because many endocrine disorders, such as diabetes mellitus and thyroid problems, can be hereditary. Others, such as delayed or precocious puberty, sometimes show a familial tendency. An older child or adoles-

Child abuse: Seeing the reality

Many people believe child abuse only occurs in poorly educated, disadvantaged families. Don't be blinded by this stereotype. Child abuse exists at every socioeconomic level among seemingly well-adjusted parents and children. The abusive parent may:
• feel intensely anxious about the child's behavior
• feel guilty and angry about the inability to provide for the child
• have also been a victim of child abuse
• believe physical punishment is the best discipline
• lack a strong emotional attachment to the child
• misuse alcohol or other drugs.
   Characteristics of the abused child may include:
• a history of behavior problems
• unusual bruises, welts, burns, fractures, or bite marks
• long sleeves or other concealing clothing, worn to hide injuries
• unusual shyness, toward both adults and children
• a tendency to avoid physical contact with adults
• fearful attitude around parents.

cent can probably give you a more accurate history of his physical growth and sexual development than his parents can, so interview the child when possible.

Determine if the child's facial appearance correlates with his age. When inspecting his mouth, check the number of teeth. Delayed eruption of teeth occurs in hypothyroid-

Identifying common spine abnormalities

When examining the spine of the pediatric or adolescent patient, look for kyphosis and scoliosis. In kyphosis, the patient develops rounded shoulders and exaggerated posterior chest convexity. In scoliosis, the thoracic or lumbar spine curves laterally to the left or right in an S shape. This abnormality is particularly evident when the patient bends over.

Kyphosis

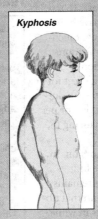

Scoliosis

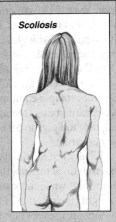

ism and hypopituitarism. Normally, you'll examine a young child's thyroid gland by placing him in the supine position. Endocrine dysfunction can cause both precocious and delayed puberty. Throughout the physical examination, and especially when you're examining the child's breasts, abdomen, and genitalia, inspect for the developmental signs of precocious puberty. Suspect delayed puberty if a child who's reached midadolescence has none of the physical changes associated with puberty. Further diagnostic tests to confirm endocrine dysfunction are just as essential in a child as in an adult.

NURSING DIAGNOSES

When caring for pediatric patients, you'll find that several nursing diagnoses are commonly used. These diagnoses appear below, along with appropriate nursing interventions and rationales. (Rationales appear in italic type.)

Parental role conflict

Related to the child's hospitalization, parental role conflict describes a situation where one or both parents experience role confusion when their child becomes ill. You may notice a change in the way parents interact with the child, or the relationship between the parents may break down. They may seem unwilling to participate in their child's physical or emotional care.

Expected outcomes
• Parents express their feelings and concerns about their child's illness.
• Parents identify and use adaptive coping strategies.
• Parents provide daily physical and emotional care for their child.

- Parents show improved knowledge of their child's illness, prognosis, and developmental needs.
- Parents report feeling less threatened by their child's illness.
- Parents develop an effective support system.

Nursing interventions and rationales

- Orient parents and visitors to the health care facility, visiting procedures, apparatus, and staff. *This helps allay anxiety.*
- Involve parents in caring for their child and encourage questions about the child's status *to decrease feelings of helplessness.*
- Educate parents in normal childhood development. *This knowledge can prepare parents for changes.*
- Encourage parental involvement in appropriate support groups or agencies when necessary. *Such groups can provide emotional support.*
- Facilitate open communication between parents *to help reduce anxiety and tension.*
- Review effective coping techniques *to further reduce anxiety.*

Diarrhea

Related to viral illness, this nursing diagnosis may be associated with infection, malabsorption syndrome, anatomic defects, or allergy. In children, diarrhea can be life-threatening. Monitor all episodes of diarrhea and replace fluids immediately.

Expected outcomes

- Patient regains and retains fluid and electrolyte balance.

- Diarrhea episodes decline or disappear.
- Patient's skin remains clean and free from irritation or ulcerations.

Nursing interventions and rationales

- Maintain accurate records of intake and output. *Fluid losses should be replaced.*
- Weigh the patient daily on the same scale. *Accurate information about weight changes will guide fluid replacement efforts.*
- Monitor the child's hydration status by assessing his mucous membranes and skin turgor. *The child with hypovolemia will have tacky mucous membranes and tenting of the skin.*
- Monitor the perianal skin for breakdown. *Diarrhea stools can be irritating to the child's skin.*

Altered nutrition: Less than body requirements

Altered nutrition, less than body requirements, is related to poor interaction between mother and child. If not treated, this condition may result in a child's failure to thrive.

Expected outcomes

- Patient consumes adequate calories daily.
- Patient gains adequate weight weekly.
- Patient eats independently without being prodded.

Nursing interventions and rationales

• Weigh the child daily on the same scale *to document weight accurately.*
• Maintain an accurate record of intake and output *to calculate nutritional requirements. Intake and output should be balanced.*
• Establish and maintain a feeding schedule for the child. *Both the child and the mother may be unaccustomed to a regular feeding schedule.*
• Observe the feeding methods of the mother and the child's feeding patterns. *This will help diagnose failure to thrive.*

Fear

Related to unfamiliarity, fear has broad applications. When a child enters a health care facility, he's separated from his parents—perhaps for the first time—and he may have to undergo painful procedures. The child may believe he's being punished for some misbehavior.

Expected outcomes

• Patient identifies fear and other feelings related to the possibility of future disability or incapacitation.
• Physical signs and symptoms of fear are decreased.
• Patient uses available support systems to aid coping.

Nursing interventions and rationales

• Encourage the child to identify sources of fear. *This will help you identify the child's misperceptions.*
• Ask the child why he thinks he's in the facility. *His response will help you*

plan patient education and assess need for special emotional support.
• Explain all treatments and procedures and answer any questions. Present information at the child's level of understanding. Avoid becoming too specific. Tell him about painful aspects of treatment last. *This will help reduce anxiety.*
• Orient the child to his surroundings. Make any adaptations to compensate for sensory deficits. *This enhances orientation.*
• Assign the same nurse to care for the child whenever possible *to provide consistency of care and enhance trust.*
• Spend time with the child on each shift *to allow time for expression of feelings.*
• Involve the child by offering realistic choices *to give the child some control over the situation.*
• Orient the family to the child's specific needs, allowing them to participate in giving care. *This helps them provide effective support.*
• Request that the family bring pictures and other small, personal objects to the child. *This helps familiarize the environment.*
• Arrange for a family member to stay with the child *to help him cope.*
• If a language barrier is the source of fear, use family and other resources (such as an interpreter) *to calm him and facilitate communication.*

TREATMENTS

Pediatric patients commonly require different procedures and equipment than adults. Understanding the special needs of these patients can expedite effective treatment or even save a life.

Drug therapy

The physiologic differences between children and adults, including variances in vital organ maturity and body composition, have a strong influence on drug effectiveness.

Drug administration routes are essentially the same for children and adults, but injection sites, administration techniques, and dosages differ greatly in many cases. As a child grows, he undergoes physiologic changes that affect drug absorption, distribution, metabolism, and excretion. These changes in turn affect the choice of drug and effective dosages. And because drug effects are less predictable in children than in adults, careful monitoring after administration is vital.

Providing emergency therapy

Effective management of a pediatric emergency requiring drug therapy calls for quick, accurate dosage calculations and proper administration techniques. (See *Cardiac drugs for common pediatric emergencies,* pages 872 to 874.)

Procedures

This section covers CPR, mist tents, apnea monitoring, and transcutaneous partial pressure of oxygen (Po_2) monitoring.

Pediatric CPR

Cardiac arrest in children usually results from hypoxemia caused by respiratory difficulty or respiratory arrest. Respiratory emergencies may result from obstructions in the airway (such as small toys), injuries (motor vehicle accidents, drowning, or burns), smoke inhalation, apneic episodes, and infections.

Before performing CPR on a child with an airway obstruction, try to determine the cause. In epiglottitis and croup, CPR won't be effective and the child may require an artificial airway.

Although CPR technique for children is basically the same as for adults, important differences do exist. For CPR purposes, consider victims between ages 1 and 8 as children. Depending on the child's size, two-person rescue may be inappropriate. For a child, you'll deliver 20 ventilations per minute instead of 12 (as for an adult), using the heel of one hand, not two. Compress at a depth of 1″ to 1½″ (2.5 to 4 cm). The compression-ventilation ratio is 5:1 in a one- or two-person rescue.

Opening the airway. Follow these steps:
1. Assess the seriousness of the injury. To find out if the child is unconscious, gently shake her shoulder and shout at her. If she's conscious and having trouble breathing, get her to an emergency department immediately. Sometimes, a child will find the position that allows her to breathe most easily. Help her maintain this position. If she's unconscious or in acute distress and you're alone with her, call out for help or dial the appropriate emergency phone number.

(Text continues on page 874.)

Cardiac drugs for common pediatric emergencies

The following drugs and dosages are recommended for pediatric advanced cardiac life support by the American Heart Association.

Drug, route, and dosage	Nursing considerations
adenosine ***To treat supraventricular tachycardia*** *I.V. push:* 0.1 mg/kg given as rapid bolus. Increase to 0.2 mg/kg if initial dose is not effective. Maximum single dose is 12 mg.	• Effective. • Minimal adverse effects. Most adverse effects resolve spontaneously within 1 to 2 min.
atropine sulfate ***To treat symptomatic bradycardia with atrioventricular (AV) block, vagally mediated bradycardia during intubation attempts, and bradycardia accompanied by poor perfusion or hypotension*** *I.V. push:* 0.02 mg/kg per dose. Minimum dose is 0.1 mg. Maximum single dose is 0.5 mg in a child and 1 mg in an adolescent. May be repeated in 5 minutes to a maximum dose of 1 mg in child, 2 mg in adolescent. *Endotracheal:* Same as I.V. dose but absorption may be unreliable.	• Used to treat bradycardia only after ensuring adequate oxygenation and ventilation. • Tachycardia may follow use of atropine in children but drug is usually well tolerated. • Do not give I.V. push in doses less than 0.1 mg because paradoxical bradycardia may occur.
bretylium ***To correct ventricular fibrillation (VF) or pulseless ventricular tachycardia (VT) if defibrillation and lidocaine are ineffective*** *I.V. push:* 5 mg/kg rapidly; may be increased to 10 mg/kg if VF persists after second defibrillation attempt.	• Has been effective in adults with VF unresponsive to electrical defibrillation. No published data available on effectiveness on children.
dobutamine hydrochloride ***To treat low cardiac output and poor myocardial function following resuscitation*** *I.V. infusion:* 2 to 20 mcg/kg/min titrated to patient response.	• Response to drug varies widely. • Higher-than-recommended infusion rates may produce tachycardia or ventricular ectopy.
dopamine hydrochloride ***To treat circulatory shock after resuscitation or when shock is unresponsive to fluid administration*** *I.V. infusion:* 2 to 20 mcg/kg/min, titrated to desired effect. Begin at 2 to 5 mcg/kg/min and titrate upward to 10 to 20 mcg/kg/min as needed to improve blood pessure, urine	• Infuse through a well-established I.V. line. • Infiltration into tissues can produce local necrosis. • If still ineffective when dose is 20 mcg/kg/min, administer epinephrine or dobutamine rather than increase dopamine dose

Cardiac drugs for common pediatric emergencies *(continued)*

Drug, route, and dosage	Nursing considerations
dopamine hydrochloride *(continued)* output, and perfusion.	above 20 mcg/kg/min. • Administer via an infusion pump.
epinephrine *For symptomatic bradycardia* *I.V. push or intraosseous:* 0.01 mg/kg (1:10,000). *Endotracheal:* 0.1 mg/kg of 1:1,000 solution (0.1 ml/kg).	• When using different concentrations of epinephrine in the same patient, take care to avoid errors.
For asystolic or pulseless arrest First dose *I.V. push or intraosseous:* 0.01 mg/kg of 1:10,000 solution (0.1 ml/kg). *Endotracheal:* 0.1 mg/kg of 1:1,000 solution (0.1 ml/kg). Subsequent doses *I.V. push, intraosseous, or endotracheal:* 0.1 mg/kg of 1:1,000 solution. I.V. and intraosseous doses up to 0.2 mg/kg of 1:1,000 solution may be effective. Administer second dose within 3 to 5 min after initial dose. Repeat doses q 3 to 5 min during resuscitation. For persistent asystolic or pulseless arrest, continuous infusion of 20 mcg/kg/min until cardiac activity resumes.	• Be aware that epinephrine's actions are depressed by acidosis; adequate ventilation, circulation, and correction of metabolic acidosis are important.
To treat shock with diminished systemic perfusion from any cause unresponsive to fluid resuscitation and to treat poor perfusion after restoration of a stable rhythm *I.V. infusion:* Begin at 0.1 mcg/kg/min; then titrate to desired effect (0.1 mcg/kg/min). In cases of asystole, may infuse a higher dose.	• Infuse only through a well-established I.V. line and preferably through a central line. • Monitor infusion site closely for infiltration. • Inactivated in alkaline solutions; never mix epinephrine with sodium bicarbonate. • High doses may produce excessive vasoconstriction, resulting in compromised mesenteric, renal, and extremity blood flow.
lidocaine *To treat pulseless VT or VF that persists after defibrillation and epinephrine administration and to treat VT with a pulse* *I.V. push:* 1 mg/kg per dose. Give over 1 to 2	• If possible, administer before synchronized cardioversion of VT that occurs with a pulse. *(continued)*

Cardiac drugs for common pediatric emergencies *(continued)*

Drug, route, and dosage	Nursing considerations
lidocaine *(continued)* minutes to patient with a pulse. Repeat in 5 to 10 minutes if necessary. *I.V. infusion:* 20 to 50 mcg/kg/min. *Endotracheal:* Same as I.V. push dose but absorption may be unreliable.	• Lidocaine infusion rate should not exceed 20 mcg/kg/min in patients with reduced drug clearance ability (shock, HF, or cardiac arrest).
sodium bicarbonate ***To treat metabolic acidosis accompanying prolonged cardiac arrest*** *I.V. push or intraosseous:* 1 mEq/kg per dose (1 ml/kg of 8.4% solution) or 0.3 × kg × base deficit.	• Infuse slowly and only if patient has adequate ventilation. • In cardiac arrest, administer after effective ventilation is established and epinephrine plus chest compressions provide maximum circulation. • Subsequent doses should be based on arterial blood gas (ABG) analysis but may be considered after every 10 minutes of cardiac arrest if ABG analysis is unavailable. • A dilute solution (0.5 mEq/ml) may be used in neonates. • Irrigate the I.V. tubing carefully between infusion of catecholamines or calcium and sodium bicarbonate.

2. Place her in a supine position on a hard, flat surface. When moving her, support her head and neck and roll her head and torso as a unit. If you suspect a head or neck injury, take special care to support her head and neck during this maneuver.

3. A child's small airway can easily be blocked by her tongue. You may be able to clear the obstruction simply by opening the airway, which moves the tongue out of the way and allows the child to breathe.

If the child doesn't have a neck injury, use the *head-tilt, chin-lift maneuver* to open the airway. Kneel next to her at shoulder level. Then place your hand that's closer to her head on her forehead. As you gently tilt the head back, put the fingers of your other hand on her lower jaw and lift the chin up, as shown at the top of the next page.

Two precautions here: Don't place your fingers on the soft tissue of the neck because you may block the airway. Make sure the child's mouth doesn't close completely.

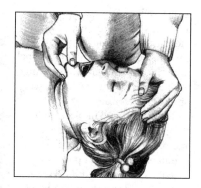

If you suspect a neck injury, use the *jaw-thrust maneuver* to open the airway. Kneel behind the child's head with your elbows resting on the ground. Place two or three fingers of each hand under the angle of her lower jaw, and rest your thumbs on the corners of her mouth. Then lift the jaw.

Checking for breathing. Follow these steps:

1. After opening the airway, check to see if the child is breathing. Place your ear over her mouth so you can listen for and feel air being exhaled. Look for movement of the chest and abdomen. If she's breathing, keep the airway open and monitor her respirations.

2. If she isn't breathing, pinch her nostrils closed with your thumb and forefinger. Take a breath and place your mouth over her mouth to form a tight seal, as shown top right. Give a slow breath for 1 to $1\frac{1}{2}$ seconds, pause to take a breath yourself, then give another slow breath for 1 to $1\frac{1}{2}$ seconds. Air entering a clear airway will make her chest rise.

If the first ventilation isn't successful, reposition her head and try again. If you're still unsuccessful, her airway may be obstructed by a foreign body (see "Clearing an airway obstruction," page 876).

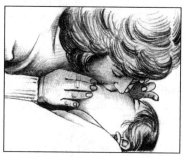

Always begin rescue breathing on a child as soon as possible. In children, cardiopulmonary arrest typically results from a respiratory—not a cardiac—problem. Cardiac arrest develops later, as a result of prolonged hypoxemia. So if you start rescue breathing quickly, your chances of resuscitating a child are very good. Once cardiac arrest develops, your chances of a successful rescue decrease.

Assessing circulation. Follow these steps:

1. Maintain the head tilt with one hand as you assess circulation with the other hand. Locate the carotid artery on the side of the neck, in the groove between the trachea and the sternocleidomastoid muscle. Palpate the carotid artery for 5 to 10 seconds. If the child has a pulse, continue rescue breathing by giving 1 breath every 3 seconds (or 20 breaths per minute).

2. If the child has no pulse, kneel next to her chest so you can start giving chest compressions. Using the hand closer to her feet, locate the lower border of the rib cage on the side nearer to you.

Then hold your middle and index fingers together and move them up the rib cage to the notch where the ribs and sternum join.

3. Put your middle finger on the notch and your index finger next to it. Note the position of your index finger.

4. Lift your hand and place the heel just above the spot where the index finger was. The heel of your hand should be aligned with the long axis of the sternum.

5. Using the heel of one hand only, compress the chest 1″ to 1½″ (2.5 to

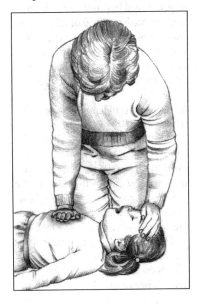

4 cm). Deliver five compressions at a rate of 100 per minute, allowing the chest wall to relax after each compression. To prevent an internal injury, keep your hand in place on the sternum and keep your fingers off the child's ribs.

Leave one hand in place on the sternum to deliver compressions and the other on the forehead to maintain the head-tilt position.

For a child, each CPR cycle consists of five compressions and one ventilation. Count "one and two and three and four and five" as you perform the chest compressions. Pause after your fifth compression and give one ventilation. Give CPR for 10 cycles or 1 minute, then check again for breathing and a pulse. If she isn't breathing or has no pulse, continue CPR. If someone has gone for help, check for breathing and a pulse every few minutes. If you're alone with the child, go for help after you have performed one minute of CPR. Return as quickly as possible and resume CPR.

Clearing an airway obstruction. If the victim is conscious, take the following steps:

1. When a parent is at the scene, ask if the child has had a fever or upper respiratory tract infection recently. If she has, suspect epiglottitis. Don't manipulate the airway; just let the child assume a comfortable position. Then call for help, say that you suspect epiglottitis, and ask for immediate attention. Monitor the child until help arrives, providing rescue breathing as necessary. If she hasn't had a fever or infection or if a parent isn't present, take the following steps to clear her airway.

To make certain her airway is obstructed, ask, "Are you choking?" If she's unable to speak, she has a complete obstruction. If she makes crowing sounds, she has a partial obstruction, and you should encourage her to cough. The cough may clear the partial obstruction or make it complete. If the airway becomes completely obstructed, proceed as follows.

2. Tell the child that you can help her. Stand behind her, then wrap your arms around her waist and make a fist with one hand. Place the top of your fist against her abdomen just above the navel. To avoid injuring her, keep your fist well below the xiphoid process. Grasp your fist with your other hand.

3. Using quick inward and upward thrusts, squeeze her abdomen 6 to 10 times in rapid succession. Deliver each thrust as though it will be

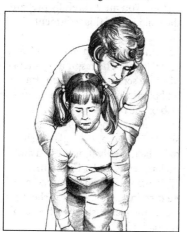

forceful enough to dislodge the obstruction.

These abdominal thrusts will create an artificial cough, using air in the lungs. Because she may lose consciousness during the rescue, you should be aware of any objects in the area that could harm her when she's lowered to the floor.

4. If the child does lose consciousness, lower her to the floor carefully to prevent an injury.

5. Support her head and neck as you place her in a supine position. Then continue your efforts by following Steps 2 through 5 for the unconscious victim of an airway obstruction.

For an unconscious victim. Take the following steps:
1. Ask any bystanders what happened. Begin CPR. If you're unable to ventilate the child, reposition her head and try again. If you're still unable to ventilate, follow Steps 2 through 5.

2. Kneel beside the child. Or, if she's big, you may kneel astride her thighs as you would for an adult. Place the heel of one hand on top of the other. Then place your hands between the umbilicus and the tip of the xiphoid process at the midline of the body. Push inward and upward 6 to 10 times, as though each thrust will be sufficient to remove the obstruction, as shown at the top of the next page.

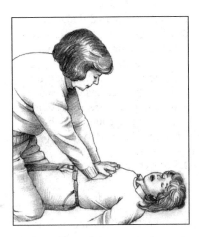

3. After administering 6 to 10 abdominal thrusts, open her mouth by grasping the tongue and lower jaw between your thumb and fingers. This will open the airway.

4. If you see the object, insert the index finger of your other hand deep into the throat at the base of the tongue. Using a hooking motion, remove the obstruction. Don't try to remove an object you can't see.

Attempt to ventilate again. If unsuccessful, reposition the head and attempt to ventilate again. If

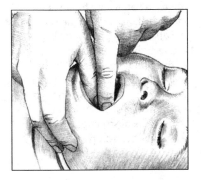

you haven't removed the object and are unable to ventilate, give another 6 to 10 abdominal thrusts, look for the object again, and try to remove it. Continue this process until you can ventilate the child.

5. After you have removed the foreign body or are able to ventilate the child, check for breathing and a pulse. Then proceed with CPR if necessary. Once your rescue has been successful, make sure the child is examined by a doctor.

Mist tents

Also called a Croupette or cool humidity tent, a mist tent contains a nebulizer that creates a cool, moist environment for the child with an upper respiratory tract infection or inflammation. If ordered, pure oxygen may also be supplied. The constant cool humidity helps the patient breathe by decreasing respiratory tract edema, liquefying mucous secretions, and reducing fever. To avoid extreme anxiety and distress, you must carefully prepare the child before this treatment.

Patient preparation. *For the Universal model:* The respiratory therapist may set up the mist-tent frame and plastic tent at the head of the crib or the bed. Cover the mattress as usual with one of the two bed sheets. Then drape the plastic sheet over the upper half of the bed and tuck the ends under the mattress. (For infants, a linen-saver pad may be used instead of a plastic sheet.) Cover the plastic sheet with one of the bath blankets.

Fill the humidity jar three-quarters full with the sterile distilled water. Make sure the filter is clean and in place on the jar, and then screw it in place on the underside of the ice chamber. If ordered, connect the tent to the oxygen flowmeter or air compressor. Fill the ice chamber with crushed ice, and shut the water outlet valve on the chamber.

Turn on the oxygen flowmeter to the ordered setting, or turn on the air compressor. (The exact percentage of oxygen must be measured by an oxygen analyzer.) Allow the mist to fill the tent for about 2 minutes before the patient enters it. Elevate the head of the bed to a position that's comfortable for the patient.

Procedure. Wash your hands and position the patient in the tent. A child is usually put in semi-Fowler's position; an infant seat can be used for a baby. Prop up an older infant or a toddler with a pillow, but don't obstruct the air outlet.

Cover the patient with a light blanket and supply a small towel or cap for his head, to protect him from chills.

Stay with the patient until he's quiet, or have his parents stay with him. Close the zippers on the openings of the tent and tuck the sides of the tent under the mattress. Smooth out all creases or wrinkles.

Because the tent alone won't stop an infant or small child from falling out of bed, raise the side rails all the way. Check on the patient frequently; if possible, place him near the nurses' station.

Monitoring and aftercare. Refill the humidity jar, as necessary. Use only sterile distilled water. Clean the humidity jar at least daily. If this isn't done by the respiratory therapist in your institution, remove the filter screw and tube and clean them with a toothbrush. Drain water from the ice chamber into a large bucket and replace the ice, as necessary. Clean the inside of the tent with soap and water.

Give the child toys to play with while he's in the tent. For the infant, you can string toys across the top bar of the tent. (Avoid allergenic or electrical toys.)

Newer mist therapy units have self-contained cooling units and don't require ice. Change the patient's linen and clothing often because they will quickly become wet from the mist. A nebulizer can supply additional mist, if needed. If you use a nebulizer, watch the patient closely, especially if he has copious mucous secretions that may loosen quickly, creating the risk of aspiration. Chest percussion, postural drainage, and suctioning may be necessary.

Monitor the child's temperature regularly, particularly a small infant's, to prevent hypothermia. If oxygen is required, the percentage used should be monitored by an oxygen analyzer at least twice a shift.

Caregiver education. If the mist tent is to be used at home, teach the parents how to use it, emphasizing the need to clean it correctly.

Apnea monitoring

Infantile apnea is a warning sign of sudden infant death syndrome (SIDS). Apnea monitors sound an alarm when the infant's breathing rate falls below a preset level. Detecting and treating apneic episodes at their onset increases the chances for resuscitation.

Doctors may prescribe apnea monitors for use in premature infants and those with such neurologic disorders as hydrocephalus, neonatal respiratory distress syndrome (hyaline membrane disease), seizure disorders, congenital heart disease with HF, a personal history of sleep-induced apnea, and a family history of SIDS.

A thoracic impedance monitor uses chest electrodes to detect conduction changes caused by respirations. Some monitors of this type have an alarm for bradycardia.

Procedure. All monitors require you to test the alarm system, position the sensor properly, and set the selector knobs appropriately for the patient. Use the following procedure when operating the thoracic impedance monitor:
• Explain the procedure to the parents, if appropriate, and wash your hands.
• Plug in the power cord, attach the leadwires to the electrodes, and then attach the electrodes to the belt. If necessary, apply gel to the electrodes. Or, place the electrodes directly on the infant's chest after applying electrode gel and attach the leadwires.

• Wrap the belt snugly but not restrictively around the infant's chest at the point of greatest movement, optimally at the right and left midaxillary line approximately 3/4″ (2 cm) below the maxilla. Make sure the leadwires are in the appropriate position, according to the manufacturer's instructions.
• Connect the leadwires to the patient cable according to the color code, and then connect the patient cable to the proper jack at the rear of the unit.
• Turn the sensitivity knobs to maximum to allow adjustment of the system.
• Set the alarm delay to the recommended time.
• Turn on the monitor. The alarms will ring until both sensitivity knobs are adjusted. Reset the apnea and bradycardia alarms according to the manufacturer's instructions. Then, adjust the sensitivity controls so the indicator lights blink with each breath and heartbeat.
• If either alarm sounds during monitoring, immediately check the infant's respirations and skin color but don't touch or disturb him until confirming apnea.
• If the infant is still breathing and his skin color is good, readjust sensitivity controls or reposition the electrodes, if necessary.
• If the infant isn't breathing but his skin is pink, wait 10 seconds to see if he starts breathing spontaneously. If he doesn't, try to stimulate breathing by using one of the methods given below.
• If he isn't breathing and he's pale, dusky, or blue, try to stimulate him

immediately. Sequentially, attempt to stimulate respirations by placing your hand on the infant's back, giving him a gentle shake, giving him a vigorous shake, or slapping the bottoms of his feet. If he doesn't begin to breathe immediately, start CPR.

Monitoring and aftercare. Don't put the monitor on top of any other electrical device; make sure it's on a level surface and can't be bumped.

Don't use lotions, oils, or powders on the infant's chest. Periodically check the alarm by unplugging the sensor plug; it should sound after the preset time delay.

Be aware that an apneic episode resulting from upper airway obstruction may not trigger the alarm when the infant continues to make respiratory efforts without gas exchange. However, if the monitor has a bradycardia alarm, the decreased heart rate that results from vagal stimulation accompanying airway obstruction may trigger it. Also, with thoracic impedance monitors without bradycardia alarms, bradycardia during apnea can be read as shallow breathing; this type of apnea monitor fails to distinguish between respiratory movement and the large cardiac stroke volume associated with bradycardia. In this case, the alarm won't trigger until the heart rate is less than the apnea limit.

Caregiver education. Monitoring begins in the health care facility and continues at home. Instruct parents on how to operate the monitor, what to do when the alarm sounds, and how to perform infant CPR.

Transcutaneous monitoring

Using an electrode containing a transducer system, heating device, and temperature probe, a transcutaneous Po_2 ($TCPo_2$) monitor measures the amount of oxygen diffusing through the infant's skin from capillaries directly beneath the surface. This measurement correlates closely with the infant's partial pressure of arterial oxygen level and supplements the established methods of observing skin color and taking periodic arterial blood gas (ABG) measurements to detect hypoxemia and hyperoxemia.

When the electrode is heated to a constant temperature higher than that of the skin, usually 111° F (44° C), it significantly increases capillary blood flow and enhances oxygen diffusion through the tissue beneath the electrode. This procedure is being used widely in intensive care nurseries by staff nurses trained to use the monitor.

Patient preparation. Set up the monitor, and calibrate it, if necessary, following manufacturer's instructions. Ensure that the strip chart recorder is working properly.

Procedure. Follow these steps to attach a $TCPo_2$ monitor:
• Wash your hands and select the monitoring site.
• Clean the site, first using a cotton ball with soap and water, then an alcohol sponge. Dry the skin, attach the adhesive ring to the electrode, and moisten the monitor site with a drop of water, according to manufacturer's instructions.

• Place the electrode on the site, making sure that it's on tight.
• Set alarm switches and electrode temperature according to instructions or your facility's policy.
• Make sure that the reading has stabilized in 10 to 20 minutes. The normal range is 50 to 90 mm Hg but may vary.
• To prevent burns, rotate the electrode site every 4 hours. Recalibrate the monitor each time the position of the electrode is changed.

Monitoring and aftercare. Expect the $TCPO_2$ to vary with the infant's movement and treatment, and to drop markedly whenever the infant cries vigorously. Be prepared to start resuscitation if a sudden significant drop in $TCPO_2$ occurs. Remember that $TCPO_2$ monitoring doesn't replace ABG measurements because it doesn't give information about partial pressure of arterial carbon dioxide and pH. Also, in infants with shock or hypoperfusion, results don't accurately reflect ABG values. Be aware of the potential complications of $TCPO_2$ monitoring: burns and blisters from the electrode and skin reactions to the adhesive ring.

REFERENCES AND READINGS

Anderson, J.E. "Helping Parents Cope with Sudden Death," *Contemporary Pediatrics* 13(12):42-57, December 1996.

Behrman, R.E., et al., eds. *Nelson Textbook of Pediatrics,* 15th ed. Philadelphia: W.B. Saunders Co., 1996.

Burns, C.E., et al. *Pediatric Primary Care.* Philadelphia: W.B. Saunders Co., 1996.

Chameides, L., and Hainski, M.F. *Textbook of Pediatric Advances: Life Support.* Dallas: American Heart Association, 1994.

Jackson, P.L., and Vessey, J.A. *Primary Care of the Child with a Chronic Condition,* 2nd ed. St. Louis: Mosby–Year Book, Inc., 1996.

Kropfelder, L., and Winkelstein, M. "A Case Management Approach to Pediatric Asthma," *Pediatric Nursing* 22(4): 291-95, July-August, 1996.

Robinson, B., et al. "Is that Fast Heartbeat Dangerous? (And What Should You Do About It?)," *Contemporary Pediatrics* 13(9):52-85, September 1996.

Rosenstein, B.J., and Fosareli, P.D. *Pediatric Pearls,* 3rd ed. St. Louis: Mosby–Year Book, Inc., 1997.

Scholer, S.J., et al. "Clinical Outcomes of Children with Acute Abdominal Pain," *Pediatrics* 98(4):680-85, October 1996.

Sherry, S.L., and Jellinek, M.S. "The Many Guises of Depression," *Contemporary Pediatrics* 13(5):63-86, May 1996.

Wilkinson, J.M., ed. *Nursing Diagnosis and Intervention Pocket Guide,* 6th ed. Redwood City, Calif.: Addison-Wesley Publishing Co., 1995.

Wilson, B.A., et al. *Nurses Drug Guide.* Stamford, Conn.: Appleton & Lange, 1997.

Wong, D.L. *Whaley & Wong's Nursing Care of Infants and Children,* 5th ed. St. Louis: Mosby–Year Book, Inc., 1995.

Wong, D. *Wong & Whaley's Clinical Manual of Pediatric Nursing,* 4th ed. St. Louis: Mosby–Year Book, Inc., 1996.

17

GERIATRIC CARE

When caring for an elderly patient, you need to take into account the physiologic and biological changes that normally occur during aging. An elderly patient may have one or more chronic diseases that complicate his management and care.

AGING: NORMAL CHANGES

The heart, lungs, kidneys, and other organs will be less efficient at age 60 than they were at age 20, but aging shouldn't be equated with the unavoidable breakdown of body systems. (See *Aging's effects on body systems,* pages 884 to 886.)

Nutrition

A person's protein, vitamin, and mineral requirements usually remain the same as he ages, whereas caloric needs are lessened. Reduced activity may lower energy requirements.

Other physiologic changes that can affect nutrition in an elderly patient include:
• decreased renal function, causing greater susceptibility to dehydration and formation of renal calculi
• loss of calcium and nitrogen (in patients who aren't ambulatory)
• diminished enzyme activity and gastric secretions
• reduced pepsin and hydrochloric acid secretion, which tends to diminish the absorption of calcium and vitamins B_1 and B_2
• decreased salivary flow and diminished sense of taste
• diminished intestinal motility and peristalsis of the large intestine
• thinning of tooth enamel
• decreased biting force
• gingival retractions, causing a potential loss of teeth
• diminished gag reflex
• decreased tone and mobility of the esophagus, increasing the potential for aspiration.

(Text continues on page 887.)

Aging's effects on body systems

As the body ages, gradual changes in function and appearance occur naturally. You'll need to recognize these normal aspects of aging so you can adjust your assessment techniques accordingly.

Skin, hair, and nails
• Facial lines around the eyes, mouth, and nose
• Subcutaneous fat loss, dermal thinning, decreased collagen
• Prominent supraclavicular and axillary regions, knuckles, and hand tendons and vessels
• Prominent fat pads over bony prominences
• Cell replacement is reduced by 50%.
• Mucous membranes become dry.
• Sweat gland output lessens (number of active sweat glands reduce).
• Body temperature more difficult to regulate
• Skin becomes almost transparent (loss of elasticity).
• Localized melanocyte proliferations are common and cause brown spots (senile lentigo).
• Hair pigment decreases; hair thins
• Facial hair increases in postmenopausal women and decreases in aging men.
• Nails may grow at different rates with longitudinal ridges, flaking, brittleness, and malformations.
• Toenails may discolor.
• Senile keratosis, acrochordon, and senile angioma
• Wounds take longer to heal.

Eyes and vision
• Eye structure and visual acuity changes.
• Eyes sit deeper in the bony orbits.
• Eyelids lose their elasticity.
• Increased incidence of ectropion and entropion.
• Conjunctiva becomes thinner and yellow.
• Pingueculae—fat pads that form under the conjunctiva—may develop.
• Quantity of tears decreases.
• Cornea loses its luster and flattens
• Iris fades or develops irregular pigmentation, turning pale.
• Sclerosis of the sphincter muscles
• Pupil becomes smaller, decreasing the amount of light that reaches the retina.
• Diminished night vision and depth perception
• Sclera becomes thick and rigid, and fat deposits cause yellowing
• Senile hyaline plaques may develop.
• Vitreous can degenerate and detach from retina.
• Lens enlarges and loses transparency.
• Accommodation decreases (impaired lens elasticity [presbyopia]).
• Impaired color vision, especially in the blue and green ranges
• Decreased reabsorption of intraocular fluid.

Ears and hearing
• Bilateral, sensorineural hearing loss
• Presbycusis or senile deafness occurs.

Respiratory system
• Nose enlargement from continued cartilage growth

Aging's effects on body systems *(continued)*

- Tracheal deviations
- Anteroposterior chest diameter increases.
- Kyphosis advances with age.
- Pulmonary function decreases.
- Lung's diffusing capacity declines.
- Decrease in inspiratory and expiratory muscle strength
- Decrease in the lungs' elastic recoil capability (elevated residual volume)
- Reduced maximum breathing capacity, forced vital capacity, vital capacity, and inspiratory reserve
- Airway closure leads to decreased surface area for gas exchange and reduced partial pressures of oxygen.

Cardiovascular system
- Heart size becomes slightly smaller.
- Reduced cardiac output at rest
- Fibrotic and sclerotic changes thicken heart valves and reduce their flexibility.
- Heart's ability to respond to physical and emotional stress may decrease.
- Strength and elasticity of blood vessels decrease.
- Myocardium becomes more irritable.
- Increased fibrous tissue infiltrates the sinoatrial node and internodal atrial tracts (resulting in atrial fibrillation and flutter).
- Veins dilate and stretch.
- Coronary artery blood flow decreases.
- Aorta becomes more rigid (causing rise in systolic blood pressure).
- Increased PR, QRS, and QT intervals, decreased amplitude of the QRS complex, and a shift of the QRS axis to the left.

GI system
- Diminished mucosal elasticity and reduced GI secretions
- Decreased liver weight, reduced regenerative capacity, and decreased blood flow to the liver
- GI tract motility, bowel wall and anal sphincter tone, and abdominal muscle strength may also decrease.

Renal system
- Decline in the glomerular filtration rate
- Renal blood flow decreases.
- Tubular reabsorption and renal concentrating ability decline.
- Bladder muscles weaken.
- Diminished kidney size, impaired renal clearance of drugs, reduced bladder size and capacity, and decreased renal ability to respond to variations in sodium intake.
- Blood urea nitrogen levels rise.
- Residual urine, frequency, and nocturia also increase.

Male reproductive system
- Testosterone production is reduced.
- Testes atrophy and soften and decrease sperm production.
- Prostate gland enlarges and secretions diminish.
- Seminal fluid decreases in volume and becomes less viscous.

Female reproductive system
- Declining estrogen and progesterone levels
- Vulva atrophies with age.
- Pubic hair loss; labia majora flattens
- Vulval tissue shrinks.
- Introitus constricts.

(continued)

Aging's effects on body systems (continued)

- Vagina atrophies and vagina shortens, mucous lining becomes thin, dry, less elastic.
- The pH of vaginal secretions increases.
- Uterus atrophies to one-fourth its premenstrual size.
- Cervix shrinks, no longer produces mucus.
- Endometrium and myometrium become thinner.
- Potential for vaginal and uterine prolapse increases.
- Glandular, supporting, and fatty tissues of the breast atrophy.
- Nipples decrease in size and become flat and nonerect.
- Fibrocystic disease (if present at menopause) usually diminishes and disappears.
- Inframammary ridges become more pronounced.
- Pelvic support structures relax.

Neurologic system

- Nerve transmission slows down.
- Hypothalamus becomes less effective at regulating body temperature.
- Cerebral cortex undergoes a 20% neuron loss.
- Corneal reflex becomes slower.
- Pain threshold increases.
- Decrease in stages III and IV sleep
- Rapid-eye-movement sleep is decreased.

Musculoskeletal system

- Decreasing height
- Decreased bone mass, muscle mass
- Muscle weakness

- Loss of resilience and elasticity in joints and supporting structures
- Synovial fluid becomes more viscous.
- Synovial membranes become more fibrotic.

Immune system

- Immune system begins losing its ability to recognize and destroy mutant cells.
- Decreased antibody response
- Tonsillar atrophy and lymphadenopathy
- B cells and total lymphocytes decrease (occasionally), and T cells decrease in number and become less effective.
- Lymph nodes and spleen become slightly smaller.
- Fatty bone marrow replaces some active blood-forming marrow.
- Vitamin B_{12} absorption diminishes.

Endocrine system

- Decreased ability to tolerate stress (blood sugar increases more in concentration and lasts longer than in a younger adult)
- Ovarian senescence (permanent cessation of menstrual activity)
- Estrogen levels diminish and follicle-stimulating hormone production increases.
- In men, testosterone levels and seminal fluid production decreases.
- Reduced progesterone production
- Decline in serum aldosterone levels (50%)
- Decrease in cortisol secretion rate (25%).

Socioeconomic and psychological factors that affect nutritional status include loneliness, decline of the elderly person's importance in the family, susceptibility to nutritional quackery, and lack of money to purchase nutritionally beneficial foods. Additionally, laxative abuse results in the rapid transport of food through the GI tract, decreasing digestion and absorption.

(See *Illness and injury: Why the risks increase with age.*)

ASSESSMENT

An elderly patient may have a distorted perception of his health problems; he may dwell on them excessively or dismiss them as normal signs of aging. A patient may ignore a serious problem because he doesn't want his fears confirmed. If your elderly patient is seriously ill, the subjects of dying and death may come up during the health history interview. Listen carefully to any remarks your patient makes about dying. Be sure to ask about his religious affiliation and spiritual needs; many elderly patients find comfort in their religious beliefs and practices. Also inquire about the matter of advanced directives (a living will and a durable power of attorney for health care).

History

To counteract hearing and vision loss, sit close to him and face him. Speak slowly in a low-pitched voice. Don't shout at a patient who has hearing loss.

If you have any doubts about your patient's ability to communi-

Illness and injury: Why the risks increase with age

The normal aging process places older adults at risk for incurring certain diseases and injuries. Here are some examples:
- Decreased cerebral blood flow increases risk of stroke.
- An elderly person's spinal cord is tightly encased in vertebrae that may be studded with bony spurs or shrunken around the cord. This means that even a minor fall can cause severe cord damage.
- In elderly women, osteoporosis can cause compression fractures even without a history of trauma.
- Brittle bones make an elderly person especially prone to fractures. When an older patient falls on an outstretched arm or hand or suffers a direct blow to his arm or shoulder, he's very likely to fracture his shoulder or humerus.
- Diminished cardiac rate and stroke volume place an older adult at risk for developing heart failure, hypertensive crisis, myocardial infarction, and arterial occlusion.
- Weakened chest musculature reduces an older person's ability to clear secretions and increases his risk of developing pneumonia, tuberculosis, and other respiratory diseases.
- Prostatic hyperplasia is a common cause of urinary tract obstruction and acute urine retention in elderly males.
- A weakened immune system increases an elderly, debilitated patient's risk of acquiring almost any infection to which he's exposed.

cate before the interview begins, ask him if a family member or a close friend can be present. This gives you an opportunity to observe your patient's interaction with another person and provides more data for the history. However, plan to talk with him privately sometime during your assessment.

Patience is the key to communicating with an elderly patient. Take a little extra time to help him see the relevance of your questions.

Previous illnesses

His detailed recall of all major illnesses, surgical procedures, and injuries is necessary for you to complete the history. As you record his past history, try to ascertain the amount of stress he has had recently and the way he has handled previous health problems. Record his age at the time each medical condition occurred.

Pay special attention to your patient's medication history. Find out what medications—over-the-counter and prescription—he's now taking and has taken in the past as well as the dosage for each. Ask him to show you samples, if possible, of all the medications he currently takes.

Psychosocial history

Ask your elderly patient about his family and friends. Find out what significant relationships he has.

If your patient lacks a support network, record this in the psychosocial history for possible later referral of the patient to a social agency.

If your patient is employed, ask if his health problems will interfere with his returning to work.

If your patient expresses financial concerns, explore them further. Ask your elderly patient if he receives any pensions or Social Security payments.

When appropriate, inquire about the patient's sex life.

Activities of daily living

Assessment of independence in activities of daily living (ADLs) and instrumental ADLs are essential to ensure that adequate services are available. Knowing the patient's functional status helps you set appropriate discharge goals and clarify the need for specific services, such as physical and occupational therapy. To assess ADLs you'll need to evaluate the functional independence or dependence in bathing, dressing, toileting, transferring, continence, and feeding. To assess instrumental ADLs you'll evaluate activities, such as preparing food, doing laundry, using transportation, administering medication, and maintaining finances.

Review of systems

When doing a review of systems for an elderly patient remember normal physiologic changes, and ask pertinent questions.

Skin, hair, and nails. Your patient may report that his skin seems thinner and less elastic than before, that he perspires less, and that his scalp feels dry. Fingernails may thicken and change color slightly. Find out if the patient can take care of his own nails. (See *Disease or signs of aging?*)

Eyes and vision. Has he noticed any increased tearing, or presbyopia? Ask if he's experienced changes in his vision, especially night vision. Does he need more light than usual when reading? Does he have any difficulty driving?

Ears and hearing. Has his hearing been affected by gradual, irreversible hearing loss?

Respiratory system. The elderly patient may be confused or his mental function may be slow, especially if he has hypoventilation and hypoperfusion from respiratory disease. An elderly patient has reduced sensations, therefore he may describe his chest pain as heavy or dull. Check for possible exposure to harmful substances by asking about his former occupation.

Does your patient have trouble breathing? Ask whether he coughs excessively, has a lot of sputum, or coughs up blood. Does he get an annual influenza immunization or a pneumococcal vaccination?

Cardiovascular system. Ask your patient whether he's gained weight recently and if his belts or rings feel tight. Does he tire more easily now than previously? Ask if he has trouble breathing or becomes dizzy when he rises from a chair or bed.

Assess your patient's level of consciousness, noting confusion or slowed mental status—occasionally,

CRITICAL THINKING

Disease or signs of aging?

While assessing the skin turgor of your 90-year-old patient, you note significant tenting of the skin on the back of the hand. You begin to suspect that your patient is showing signs of dehydration. Is this assessment correct?

Suggested response

Your patient isn't showing signs of dehydration. In fact, decreased skin elasticity—especially on areas that have been exposed to the sun—is a normal sign of aging. For more accurate assessment, check skin turgor on the sternum or over the abdomen because these areas have most likely been protected from exposure.

these are early signs of inadequate cardiac output. Ask about chest pain (angina pectoris). His chief complaint may be dyspnea, unexplained behavioral changes, acute signs of cerebral insufficiency, and chronic fatigue rather than chest pain. Also keep in mind that these signs and symptoms in elderly patients may indicate pathology in many systems other than cardiovascular. He may only experience confusion, vomiting, faintness, and dizziness if he's having a myocardial infarction.

Ask your patient about his ADLs, any signs or symptoms associated with these activities, and his response to exertion.

Inquire about a history of smoking, frequent coughing, wheezing, or dyspnea, which may indicate chronic lung disease.

Ask the patient about any adverse reactions he may be having from prescribed medication. Look for weakness, bradycardia, hypotension, confusion (elevated potassium levels) or weakness, fatigue, muscle cramps, and palpitations (inadequate levels of potassium). Overdoses of digitalis glycosides or antiarrhythmia medications may cause anorexia, nausea, vomiting, diarrhea, headache, rash, vision disturbances, or mental confusion.

GI system. An elderly patient may complain about problems related to his mouth and his sense of taste due to decreased saliva production or periodontitis or gingivitis. Are his dentures comfortable and do they work well?

An elderly patient may also have nonspecific difficulty in swallowing. Question him about weight loss, and elimination habits as well as bloating or constipation or lower GI bleeding.

Urinary system. Explore any incontinence the patient reports.

Neurologic system. Inquire about changes in coordination, strength, or sensory perception. Does the patient have headaches or seizures, any temporary losses of consciousness, memory loss, or forgetfulness? Has he had any difficulty controlling his bowels or his bladder?

Musculoskeletal system. If your patient's *chief complaint* is pain associated with a fall, determine if the pain preceded the fall, possibly indicating a pathologic fracture.

Hematologic and immune systems. Ask if your patient experiences joint pain, weakness, or fatigue. Does he have any difficulty using his hands?

Determine your patient's typical daily diet. Also ask if he lives alone and cooks for himself.

Psychological status

When you assess the psychological status of an elderly patient, remember that the most important factors related to promoting mental health include physical health, humor, and physical, mental, and social activity. Adjust your care to the patient's level of functioning. (See *Respecting your patient's level of competency*.)

Common psychological problems among elderly patients include dementia, delirium, depression, grieving, substance abuse, paranoia, and anxiety.

Dementia

Dementia is an irreversible mental state characterized by a decrease in cognitive function, memory impairment, personality change, impaired judgment, and a change in affect. Alzheimer's disease is the most common cause of dementia. Other causes of dementia include multi-infarct dementia, Pick's disease, Creutzfeldt-Jakob disease, Binswanger's disease, and acquired immunodeficiency syndrome.

Delirium

Delirium, or acute confusion, is caused by an underlying illness, a toxic reaction, or occurs as a prelude to death. Delirium produces intellectual deficits, incoherent speech, misinterpretation of reality, disorientation, and memory impairment. The patient is also likely to experience hallucinations, illusions, and changes in motor activity levels. Delirium may result from malnutrition, drug toxicity, fluid and electrolyte imbalances, infection, a decrease supply of oxygen to the brain, depression, restraints, or environmental changes. Because delirium may be reversible when properly treated, early assessment and treatment are essential.

Depression

Although depression is common among older adults, in many cases it's misdiagnosed or overlooked entirely. Consider it as a possibility in any elderly patient. Depression may appear as changes in behavior (apathy, self-deprecation, inertia), changes in thought processes (confusion, disorientation, poor judgment), or somatic complaints (appetite loss, constipation, insomnia). In elderly people, depression frequently mimics Alzheimer's disease.

If you observe any of these signs, question your patient in detail about recent losses, and find out how he's coping with them. Assess his feelings carefully.

Adjusting to loss

Your patient may have to cope with losing his job, income, friends, fam-

FOCUS ON CARING

Respecting your patient's level of competency

Caring for an elderly patient can be a nursing challenge, especially when establishing level of competency. While a particular patient may not be competent to handle complex financial issues, he may be able to make basic decisions regarding daily activities.

To provide optimum care, it's important that you listen carefully to the patient's wishes. Whenever possible, respect your patient's personal decisions such as choice of hairstyles, the timing of personal care, and food preferences.

ily, health, or even his home. These losses can cause stress, which has physiologic and psychological consequences. Unresolved grief can cause a pathologic grief reaction, which may take the form of physical or mental illness. Risk factors for suicide among the elderly include alcohol abuse, bereavement, living alone, retirement, family history of depression or suicide, and loss of health and mobility.

Substance abuse

Your patient may turn to substance abuse or even suicide in response to major life changes and severe stress. Suspect substance abuse or suicidal thoughts if your patient takes an unusual amount of medication or if you note signs of alcohol abuse, such as jaundice and tremor.

Paranoia

If you suspect paranoia, try to determine whether it's a result of sensory-loss problems (which may be corrected by glasses or a hearing aid), psychological problems, or a realistic fear of attack or robbery.

Signs and symptoms of paranoia include expressions of feeling alone and afraid; unpredictable behavior, affect, and thinking; difficulty relating to others; and feelings of being watched or threatened.

Anxiety

In an elderly patient, the need to adjust to physical, emotional, and socioeconomic changes can cause acute anxiety reactions. These changes may raise his anxiety level to the point of temporary confusion and disorientation. Don't dismiss an elderly person's symptom or assume it's the result of dementia. Proper assessment can help diagnose a treatable psychogenic disorder.

Nutritional status

Disabilities, chronic diseases, and surgical procedures such as gastrectomy commonly affect an elderly patient's nutritional status. Be sure to record them in your patient history. Drugs may also affect his nutritional requirements. And mineral oil, which many elderly people use to correct constipation, may impair GI absorption of vitamins.

Assessment measures include common sense, consideration of nutritional risk factors, the dietary history, monitoring of the patient's intake if he's hospitalized, and your objective data. Remember, protein-calorie malnutrition is a major nutritional problem in patients over age 75.

Physiologic status

Your assessment should include a thorough review of the patient's physiologic condition. Keeping in mind the chief complaint, plan to assess skin, hair, and nails; eyes and vision; ears and hearing; as well as each body system, in turn.

Skin, hair, and nails

As a person ages, susceptibility to certain skin disorders increases. For example, actinic keratoses and basal cell epitheliomas from past sun exposure commonly occur in older people. Xerosis, capillary hemangiomas, pedunculated fibromas, and seborrheic keratoses are extremely common. Other characteristic geriatric skin conditions include xanthelasma, plantar keratosis, seborrheic dermatitis, and pigmented nevi. If your elderly patient's mobility has decreased and his circulation is impaired, he may develop stasis dermatitis and possibly stasis ulcers.

Check the patient's skin for pruritus, decubitus ulcers, and skin tears. Also check his toenails for signs of yellowing, a possible indication of a fungal nail infection.

Eyes and vision

When you examine an older patient's eyes, keep in mind that ocular manifestations of aging can affect the entire eye. As you begin your inspection, you may note that his eyes sit deeper in the bony orbits. Look for excess skin on the upper eyelid, which results from normal loss of tissue elasticity. Entropion and ectropion are common in elderly people. You may note drooping of the upper eyelids (blepharochalasis). When it results from normal aging changes, blepharochalasis usually occurs gradually and bilaterally. It may be so severe that it obscures vision. If sudden or unilateral, it may indicate a more serious problem.

When you inspect the conjunctiva, be aware that its luster may appear dimmed, and it may be drier and thinner than in younger patients and may trigger frequent episodes of conjunctivitis. Aging can also affect the lacrimal apparatus. Assess for keratitis sicca—burning, dry, or irritated eyes from decreased tearing.

When you inspect the patient's corneas, you may note lipid deposits on the periphery, known as arcus senilis. The cornea also flattens with age, sometimes causing astigmatism. You may see bilateral irregular iris pigmentation, with the normal pigment replaced by a pale brown color. If your patient had an iridectomy to treat glaucoma, the iris may have an irregular shape.

An elderly patient's pupils may be abnormally small if he's taking medication to treat glaucoma. If an intraocular lens was implanted in the pupillary space after cataract removal, the pupil may be irregularly shaped. Finally, when you examine the patient's macula with an ophthalmoscope, you may note that the foveal light reflex is not as bright as in younger patients.

Be alert for signs and symptoms of vision disorders, such as presbyopia and cataracts.

Medication effects. Remember that certain drugs used to treat such conditions as hypertension and heart failure (HF) may have ocular sequelae. Make sure you've questioned your patient thoroughly about such medications. Steroids, for example, may cause cataracts.

Certain ocular medications (for example, scopolamine hydrobromide) can cause systemic adverse effects (such as disorientation).

Ears and hearing

Periodically assess each elderly patient for hearing loss to rule out conditions that can be treated.

Observe him for behavioral patterns such as anxiety and sleep disturbances. They may be manifestations of the feelings of loss and depression commonly experienced by an elderly person whose hearing is impaired. He may also be disorganized or unreasonable because of his inability to understand what is being said to him.

Suspect presbycusis if your patient complains of gradual hearing loss over many years but has no history of ear disorders or severe generalized disease. In most patients, the physical examination shows no abnormalities of the ear canal or eardrum. If your patient has a history of vertigo, ear pain, or nausea, suspect some pathology other than presbycusis.

Inspection and palpation of the auricles and surrounding areas should yield the same findings as in the younger adult. Examination with the otoscope yields similar results. Remember that the eardrum in some elderly patients may normally appear dull and retracted instead of pearl gray, but this can also be a clinically significant sign.

For early detection of hearing loss in an elderly patient, always perform tuning fork tests. Also evaluate the patient's ability to hear and understand speech, and the need for rehabilitative therapy.

If your patient wears a hearing aid, inspect it carefully for proper functioning and fit. If he reports that what he hears through it sounds fluttery or garbled, it may be broken.

Respiratory system

As you inspect an elderly patient's thorax, be especially alert for degenerative skeletal changes such as kyphosis.

When you percuss his chest, remember that loss of elastic recoil capability in an elderly person stretches the alveoli and bronchioles, producing hyperresonance. During auscultation, carefully observe how well your patient tolerates the examination. He may tire easily because of low tolerance to oxygen debt. Also, taking deep breaths during auscultation may quickly produce light-headedness or syncope. You may hear diminished sounds at the lung bases because some of his airways are closed. Inspiration will be significantly more audible than expiration on auscultation of the lungs.

Keep in mind that older adults are at risk for developing respiratory disorders, but their same signs and symptoms may differ. For example, a patient with pneumonia may exhibit confusion and a slightly increased respiratory rate with no fever.

Cardiovascular system

In an elderly patient who may have chronic lung disease, check for evidence of cor pulmonale and advanced HF: large, distended neck veins; hepatomegaly with tenderness; hepatojugular reflux; and peripheral dependent edema. Check, too, for evidence of chronic obstructive pulmonary disease.

Carefully assess your elderly patient for signs and symptoms associated with cerebral hypoperfusion—such as dizziness, syncope, confusion, unilateral weakness or numbness, aphasia, and occasionally slight clonic, jerking movements.

Record baseline blood pressures bilaterally and use them carefully to determine if pressures are consistently above 160 mm Hg systolic. Because aging causes a person's arterial walls to thicken and lose elasticity, readings—especially systolic readings—may be higher than normal. (See *How prolonged hypertension affects the body.*)

Assess the older adult for postural blood pressure changes in sitting, lying, and standing positions. Orthostatic hypotension commonly occurs in elderly people.

Measure the patient's heart rate for 60 seconds, apically and radially. If the apical rate is below 50

How prolonged hypertension affects the body

Effect	Associated signs and symptoms
Cardiorespiratory system	
Early left-sided heart failure (HF)	Cough
Coronary artery insufficiency	Chest pain
Left-sided HF	Dyspnea, paroxysmal nocturnal dyspnea, and orthopnea
HF, asthma, and chronic obstructive pulmonary disease with bronchospasm	Wheezing
HF, renal disease, or cirrhosis	Edema
Central nervous system	
Transient ischemic attack	Visual disturbances, numbness, tingling, and dizziness
Cerebrovascular accident	Weakness, paralysis, and incontinence
Genitourinary system	
Renal involvement	Hematuria
May be associated with edema, chronic renal insufficiency, or a partial obstruction; may also be an early sign of HF	Nocturia

beats/minute in a hospitalized patient, monitor his vital signs frequently. Determine if the patient has palpitations or symptoms of inadequate cardiac output. When palpating the carotid pulse, be alert for hyperkinetic pulses and bruits over the carotids, which are common in older patients with advanced arteriosclerosis.

Kyphosis and scoliosis distort the chest walls and may displace the heart slightly. Thus, your patient's apical impulse and heart sounds may be slightly displaced. Diastolic murmurs indicate a pathologic condition; soft, early systolic murmurs may be associated with normal aortic lengthening, tortuosity, or sclerotic changes and may not indicate serious pathologic condition. Check for signs of peripheral arterial insufficiency.

GI system

Assessing an older patient's GI system is similar to examining a younger adult's, except the elderly patient's abdominal wall is thinner, and his muscle tone is usually more relaxed. Abdominal distention is more common.

Mouth. Inspect carefully for limited movement of the temporomandibular joint, and be alert for complaints of pain. These signs and symptoms may indicate degenerative arthritis.

Pay particular attention to the elderly patient's teeth. Commonly, you'll find loose teeth (from bone resorption that occurs in periodontal disease) or missing or replaced teeth. (See *Identifying dental appliances,* pages 898 and 899.) Common problems in this age-group include keratosis of the ridge, irritation, fibromas, malocclusion, and mouth disease.

Pathologic changes include oral carcinoma, dysplasia, atrophic glossitis, xerostomia (dry mouth), and denture-related fibrous hyperplasia. Assess for leukoplakia—a flat, white, painless, precancerous lesion that appears on the mucous membranes of the mouth.

Esophagus. Esophageal peristalsis may decrease leading to delayed emptying, irritation, and dilation. It may produce symptoms of gastric reflux, such as a burning sensation

after meals and substernal chest pain (mild to severe stabbing sensation). Pain is centered around food intake and may be accentuated when the patient stoops or lies down. The pain from gastric reflux is difficult to differentiate from cardiac or hiatal hernia pain and necessitates medical consultation.

Refer any elderly patient with dysphagia to a doctor to rule out esophageal cancer.

Hiatal hernia is the most common upper GI problem. Signs and symptoms, including substernal pain, usually appear after periods of intra-abdominal pressure. Ask the patient if his problems seem to occur following bending, straining, vomiting, or coughing. Also assess for ascites and obesity, which also can increase intra-abdominal pressure. Ask the patient if changing his body position relieves the symptoms.

Stomach. Hunter's gastritis, a common geriatric stomach disorder, is chronic inflammation of the stomach. This disorder leads to calcium and iron malabsorption and vitamin B_{12} malabsorption, which can cause pernicious anemia.

The incidence of complications from peptic ulcers and of associated mortality is higher in elderly patients.

Small intestine. Diminished enzyme secretion can cause problems in elderly people because of decreased nutrient absorption and delayed fat absorption. Diminished GI motility and impaired blood flow to the small intestine can also impair nutrient absorption. An inadequate diet commonly causes vitamin and other nutritional deficiencies.

Large intestine. Assess for dehydration in an elderly patient with inadequate water intake, excessive salt intake, or a GI disorder that disturbs water absorption in the large intestine.

Diverticulosis may progress to diverticulitis, causing left lower or middle abdominal pain, changed bowel habits, flatulence, fever, and a palpable mass.

The elderly population has the highest incidence of colorectal cancer. Although some signs and symptoms such as rectal bleeding usually receive prompt attention, others—such as constipation, diarrhea, and changes in bowel habits—are typically vague and may be minimized by the patient. Rectal polyps are difficult to palpate because they're soft.

Constipation may result from several factors, so be sure to ask the patient about use of laxatives, anorectal lesions, low dietary fiber, habitual disregard of the urge to defecate, emotional upset or stress, lack of exercise, insufficient fluid intake, and use of drugs (such as some tranquilizers, antacids, and iron preparations). Percussion of the abdomen will reveal dullness over impacted areas.

Rule out fecal impaction and rectal anomalies such as painful fissures as causes of fecal incontinence. Assess presence and character of bowel sounds as well as presence of fecal impaction and number and consistency of stools. Fecal incontinence is *not* a normal change of aging and indicates pathology.

Liver and biliary system. Always assess an elderly patient for jaundice, which may indicate such causes of common bile duct obstruction as cancer of the head of the pancreas or cholelithiasis. In cholelithiasis, a common condition, midepigastric pain occurs 3 to 6 hours after a heavy or fatty meal.

Genitourinary system

Susceptibility to infection increases with age, and kidney infection from obstruction is a common cause of hospitalization among older patients. An immobilized elderly patient is especially vulnerable to infection from urine stasis or poor personal hygiene. A urinary tract infection (UTI) in an older adult is frequently asymptomatic, or the symptoms are vague and ill defined. If untreated, a UTI in an older adult may progress to renal failure.

Altered cardiac output (such as in HF) lowers renal perfusion and may result in azotemia. The kidneys compensate by retaining sodium and increasing edema. Medications to improve a patient's myocardial contractility and therapy with diuretics may increase his renal function temporarily, but prerenal azotemia commonly results.

Poor musculature from childbearing and from aging may predispose elderly women to cystocele.

Bladder cancer, common after age 50, is more prevalent in men

Identifying dental appliances

Although patients of any age may require tooth replacement, this problem is most common in elderly people. During your examination, you may encounter any of the following dental appliances.

Removable bridge

A removable bridge is designed to replace a missing tooth or teeth. Usually one tooth on either side is crowned (capped) to support the replacement teeth that are fitted to them. The strength of a removable bridge depends on the health of the supporting tooth or teeth. Because bridges are commonly made of gold and porcelain, handle them carefully; they're brittle.

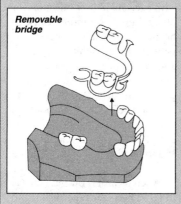

Removable bridge

Partial denture

A partial denture is designed to replace long spans of missing teeth or teeth missing on both sides of the mouth. In many cases, maxillary partial dentures cover the palate partially or fully; mandibular partial dentures cross the midline by way of a connector lingual to the mandible. Most partial dentures are attached mechanically, usually with clasps to supporting teeth. Partial dentures usually consist of porcelain or plastic teeth on an acrylic and metal framework. These appliances can be removed or dislodged; their clasps can be easily bent.

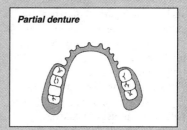

Partial denture

---

than in women. Symptoms of bladder cancer include frequency, dysuria, and hematuria.

Almost all men over age 50 have some degree of prostatic enlargement. In men with benign prostatic hyperplasia or advanced prostate cancer, however, the gland becomes large enough to compress the urethra and sometimes the bladder, obstructing urine flow. If not treat-

ed, benign prostatic hyperplasia can impair renal function.

If your patient does have benign prostatic hyperplasia, you'll probably note nontender and enlarged lateral lobes. These lobes may feel like the thenar eminence of a clenched fist. You may not be able to detect an enlarged median lobe because most of it rests anteriorly. Abdominal palpation and percus-

Complete dentures

Complete dentures are upper and lower appliances that replace all natural teeth. They're commonly made of porcelain and acrylic and can be easily broken. An upper denture usually covers the palate and is held in place by a partial vacuum. A lower denture fits on the mandibular ridge and is designed to permit movement of the tongue. The lower denture is easier to dislodge, break, or aspirate than the upper denture.

Note the type and location of any of these appliances, and check for deterioration. Pathologic lesions commonly associated with dental appliances include periodontitis, gingivitis, candidiasis, fibrous hyperplasia, and chronic irritative ulcers.

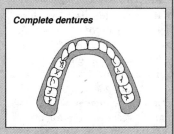

Complete dentures

Female reproductive system

Be alert for signs of gynecologic disorders, such as dyspareunia, senile and atrophic vaginitis, monilia infections resulting in superficial vaginal ulcers that bleed when touched, superficial uterine ulcerations with spotting or bleeding. Bleeding that occurs at least 1 year after menopause may indicate a malignant endometrial tumor.

Diminishing estrogen levels can contribute to osteoporosis.

Ovarian cancer is most common in women between ages 65 and 69.

Neurologic system

You'll usually detect an alteration in one or more senses. Cranial nerves may be affected by aging and produce the following alterations:
• *Olfactory nerve*—progressive loss of smell
• *Optic nerve*—decreased visual acuity, presbyopia, limited peripheral vision
• *Facial nerve*—decreased perception of taste, drooping or relaxation of the muscles in the forehead and around the eyes and mouth
• *Auditory nerve*—presbycusis or loss of high tones, later generalized to all frequencies
• *Glossopharyngeal nerve*—sluggish or absent gag reflex
• *Hypoglossal nerve*—unilateral tongue weakness.

The patient may also exhibit akinesia (a slowing of fine finger movements). Deep tendon reflexes may be diminished or absent and position sense may be impaired. Gait disturbances are also common. In addition, you may encounter

sion may reveal a midline mass, representing a distended bladder.

Keep in mind that normal geriatric laboratory values may differ from those established for younger adults. Also, decreased renal function may make some diagnostic tests hazardous for older patients. (See *How aging kidneys affect diagnostic tests,* page 900.)

How aging kidneys affect diagnostic tests

For elderly patients, normal values for some laboratory tests are different from those established for younger adults because of diminished renal function. An elderly patient's level of blood urea nitrogen, for example, is normally higher by 5 mg/dl.

Because an elderly patient's kidneys have diminished concentrating ability, some diagnostic tests are more hazardous to him than to a younger patient. For instance, dehydration induced in preparation for radiologic studies or as a result of the osmotic diuresis produced by contrast agents may predispose an elderly patient to intravascular volume contraction and further renal deterioration.

decreased ability to differentiate between warm and cold, and sharp and deep pain; or slowed fine motor movements.

Musculoskeletal system

Be alert for signs and symptoms of motor and sensory dysfunction: weakness, spasticity, tremors, rigidity, and various types of sensory disturbances. Difficulty in maintaining equilibrium and uncertain gait may cause damaging falls. Differentiate gait changes caused by joint disability, pain, or stiffness from those caused by neurologic impairment.

Bone softening from demineralization (senile osteoporosis) causes abnormal susceptibility to major fractures. Most patients over age 60

have some degree of degenerative joint disease.

Assess for decreased range of motion (ROM), swelling, tenderness, crepitation, and subcutaneous nodules—common findings in osteoarthritis. Also assess the patient's feet for common musculoskeletal deformation, such as hallux valgus with inflamed bursa and hammertoes with corns.

Hematologic and immune systems

Assessing hematologic and immune function is the same as for a younger adult. However, remember that the elderly patient will have a diminished febrile response to infection.

Endocrine system

Many endocrine disorders cause signs and symptoms in elderly people that resemble changes that normally occur with aging. For this reason, these disorders are easily overlooked during assessment. For example, the mental status changes and physical deterioration of hypothyroidism also characterize normal aging.

Other endocrine abnormalities may complicate your assessment because their signs and symptoms are different in elderly people than they are in other age-groups. Hyperthyroidism, for example, usually causes anxiety, but some elderly patients may instead experience depression or apathy (a condition known as *apathetic hyperthyroidism of the elderly*). What's more, an elderly hyperthyroid patient may initially have signs and symptoms of HF or atrial fibrillation, rather than the classic manifestations associated with this disorder.

NURSING DIAGNOSES

When caring for elderly patients, you'll find that several nursing diagnoses are commonly used. These diagnoses appear below, along with appropriate nursing interventions and rationales. (Rationales appear in italic type.)

Perceived constipation

Perceived constipation is related to diminished GI motility, low roughage diet, decreased activity, lack of privacy, neuromuscular impairment, abuse of enemas and laxatives, and weak abdominal muscles.

Expected outcomes
• Patient states an understanding of normal bowel function.
• Patient states factors causing or contributing to constipation.
• Patient decreases use of laxatives, enemas, and suppositories.
• Patient participates in regular exercise.
• Elimination pattern returns to normal.

Nursing interventions and rationales
Encourage the patient to take these steps *to prevent constipation*:
• Drink 8 oz (237 ml) of water with each meal and drink water or juice frequently between meals, unless contraindicated by cardiovascular or renal disease.

• Increase dietary fiber by adding fresh fruits, fresh vegetables, whole grain breads, cereals, pasta products, and dried fruits.
• Increase exercise to include a brisk walk on a daily basis.

Your interventions should also include the following:
• Teach the patient not to ignore the stimulus to defecate. Allow the patient privacy during defecation, and establish a regular time for elimination, usually 30 to 60 minutes after a meal.
• Avoid medications that further decrease bowel motility or cause constipation, such as narcotic analgesics, tranquilizers, diphenoxylate hydrochloride and atropine (Lomotil), iron, aluminum, or barium products.
• Avoid chronic laxative abuse *to prevent constipation.*
• Inform the patient that bowel movements that occur 3 days apart can be normal, depending on diet and activity level.
• Provide a cup of hot water before meals, *to stimulate defecation.*
• For severe constipation, insert glycerine suppository and have patient attempt to evacuate bowels. Repeat procedure the second day, if necessary. If not effective, give a bisacodyl (Dulcolax) suppository on the third day. Follow with an enema a few hours after giving the suppository if it wasn't effective.
• Monitor for the presence of fecal impaction. An oozing of liquid stool around the impaction is commonly mistaken for diarrhea.

Risk for injury

Risk for injury is related to altered cerebral function, altered mobility, impaired sensory function, and environmental hazards.

Expected outcomes
• Patient identifies factors that increase potential for injury.
• Patient assists in identifying and applying safety measures.
• Patient and family or friend develop strategy to maintain safety.
• Patient performs ADLs to the degree possible within limitations.

Nursing interventions and rationales
• Assess the patient for risk factors that could precipitate injury: poor vision or hearing, altered mental states, unsafe ambulation, unsafe shoes or clothing, drug therapy, depression, environmental hazards, orthostatic hypotension, and hypoglycemia.
• Orient the patient frequently and assess his ability to use the call bell system and ambulate safely.
• Use a night-light and keep bed in lowest position.
• Assess gait stability and provide ambulatory aids, *to increase stability and safety.* Check rubber tips of canes and walkers frequently, *to make sure they're in good repair.* Shoes should have nonskid soles. Older adults with a shuffling gait should wear leather-soled shoes.
• Eliminate environmental hazards, including wet floors, poor lighting, obstacles, broken stairs, throw rugs, exposed electric cords, or cluttered environment. Install handrails.

• Teach the patient to change positions slowly *to avoid orthostatic blood pressure drops.* Use elastic thigh-high hose.

Altered thought processes

Altered thought processes can be related to progressive dementia, depression, alteration in biochemical compounds, isolation, environmental challenge, sensory-perceptual alteration, or drug toxicity.

Expected outcomes
• Patient maintains orientation to time, place, and person.
• Patient's environment is enhanced to compensate for memory deficits.
• Patient voices feelings about memory loss.
• Patient sustains no harm or injury.
• Family members demonstrate techniques for caring for patient, such as reorienting him as needed.

Nursing interventions and rationales
• Assess for drug toxicity, sleep deprivation, sensory deprivation, sensory overload, relocation trauma, fluid and electrolyte imbalance, malnutrition, infection, vision or hearing loss, and decreased respiratory, renal, or circulatory function.
• Reduce and eliminate factors that may contribute to confusion in the older adult. Carefully monitor fluid and electrolyte status and replace as necessary. Promote 2 qt (2 L) of fluid per day unless contraindicated. Provide a nutrient-dense diet. Promote normal sleep-rest activities. Avoid giving sedative or hypnotic drugs when possible. Avoid late

afternoon naps if the patient is unable to sleep through the night. Encourage light exercise 2 to 3 hours before sleep time.

Also, frequently assess the need for medications, appropriateness of dosage, adverse effects, and drug interactions. Promote optimal vision and hearing by keeping rooms well lit, ordering frequent eye and ear examinations, cleaning cerumen out of ears, and ensuring that hearing aids are in good working order and are positioned properly in the ear. Reduce unnecessary stimuli in the environment. Avoid changing rooms and moving furniture or possessions around. Avoid the use of physical restraints whenever possible.

• Provide frequent meaningful sensory input and reorientation. Provide a large clock and calendar in every room. Provide outdoor activities or a bed by the window. Frequently tell the patient your name and what you are planning to do. Encourage family to bring in familiar objects, such as quilts and pictures. Encourage the participation in therapeutic groups, such as those centered on reality orientation, motivation, reminiscing, recreational therapy, pet therapy, music therapy, and sensory training.
• Check the patient frequently *because he may be prone to self-poisoning, wandering, and falls.*
• Monitor water temperature for baths and food temperatures, *to avoid accidental burns.*
• Have the patient wear a medical identification bracelet with a name and address on it and provide a wal-

let identification card. Have a picture taken of all confused patients who might wander. A piece of used clothing can help search dogs locate a wandering patient.

Sensory/perceptual alteration

Related to sensory deprivation, sensory/perceptual alteration is commonly seen in elderly patients who are hospitalized or institutionalized, and in patients who are on isolation precautions. It may be associated with bipolar disease (depression phase), blindness, cerebrovascular accident (CVA), deafness, depression, head injury, hemianopia, or dementia.

Expected outcomes
• Patient's environment is enhanced to ensure safety.
• Patient openly expresses feelings about vision loss.
• Patient regains visual functioning to extent possible.
• Patient maintains orientation to time, place, and person.
• Patient compensates for vision loss by use of adaptive devices.

Nursing interventions and rationales
• Encourage patient to use glasses, hearing aid, or other adaptive devices, *to help reduce sensory deprivation.*
• Reorient the patient to reality. Call him by proper name, using his preferred form. Introduce yourself. Give background information (time, place, date) throughout the

day. Orient him to the environment, including sights and sounds. Use large signs as visual cues. Post the patient's own photo on the door if he is ambulatory and disoriented. Provide for visual contrast in environment. *These measures help reduce sensory deprivation.*

• Arrange the environment to offset the deficit. Place the patient by a window. Encourage family to bring in personal articles, such as photos. Keep articles in the same place. Use safety precautions such as a nightlight when needed. *These measures stimulate the senses.*

• Communicate the patient's response level to family and to staff; record on plan of care and update as needed. *Sensory deprivation level can be evaluated by response to stimuli.*

• Talk to the patient while providing care; encourage the family or significant other to discuss past and present events with patient. Spend time with him to prevent isolation. *Verbal stimuli can improve the patient's reality orientation.*

• Hold the patient's hand when talking. Discuss interests with patient and family or significant other. Obtain needed items such as talking books. *Sensory stimuli help reduce patient's sensory deprivation.*

• Assist the patient and family in planning short trips outside. Educate about mobility, toileting, feeding, suctioning, and so forth. *Trips help reduce patient's sensory deprivation.*

• Avoid the use of physical restraints whenever possible. They cause disorientation from sensory deprivation. (See *Documenting the use of restraints.*)

Risk for altered body temperature

Related to aging, thermoreceptors in an elderly patient may be impaired by any disease, injury, or degenerative change.

Expected outcomes

• Patient's body temperature remains normal.
• Patient exhibits warm, dry skin.
• Patient doesn't exhibit signs of hypothermia or hyperthermia.
• Patient or family members express understanding of factors that cause hypothermia or hyperthermia.
• Patient or family members describe ways to prevent hypothermia or hyperthermia.

Nursing interventions and rationales

• Monitor body temperature every 8 hours or more frequently, as indicated, *to ensure that temperature doesn't vary more than 1° F from average normal (96.8° F [36° C] oral).* If it does, monitor more frequently.

• Instruct the elderly patient in hypothermia precautions. Maintain specific room temperature (70° to 72° F [21.1° to 22.2° C], or as ordered). Dress warmly, even when indoors (particularly in bed). Layer clothing. Keep the patient's hands and feet well covered. Ensure adequate food and fluid intake. Remain as active as possible. Encourage walking or active movement every hour to increase circulation and basal metabolic rate. Have a friend or neighbor check on the patient every day.

• Instruct patient in hyperthermia precautions. Stay out of direct sunlight. Avoid strenuous activity in hot weather. Dress in lightweight, loose-fitting clothing that permits perspiration to evaporate. Select pale colors, if possible. Drink enough fluids. Avoid alcoholic beverages and tobacco. *Precautions aim to maintain optimal health by modifying the environment.*

• Instruct patient about warning signs of hypothermia and hyperthermia, such as lethargy, shivering, nausea, and dizziness, *to prevent complications.*

• Identify patients at risk for hypothermia. Risk factors include inadequate housing, living alone, chronic illness, and drugs such as sedatives, hypnotics, alcohol, and phenothiazines, which can affect the body's thermoregulating system. Other risk factors include dementia, hyperproteinemia, and surgery.

• Assess for signs and symptoms of hypothermia, including cool skin; absence of shivering; pale, waxy skin; bradycardia; arrhythmias; drowsiness; slurred speech; and decrease in blood pressure.

• Assess for signs and symptoms of hyperthermia, including body temperature greater than 100° F (37.8° C) in the absence of infection, weakness, faintness, headache, tachycardia, tachypnea, hallucinations, and confusion.

Functional incontinence

Functional incontinence is the involuntary loss of urine, regardless

CHARTING TIPS

Documenting the use of restraints

If it becomes necessary to apply restraints on your older adult patient, remember to document this important information in the medical record:
• fall assessment and risk analysis
• alternatives used before restraints and their effectiveness
• type of restraint used
• verbal or written order for restraints
• time and date restraints were applied
• times when patient and restraints were monitored
• patient's response to restraints
• care given when released from restraints
• specific patient behavior that creates risk (overlooked documentation in 50% of patients)
• release of liability statement.

of the amount. Types include stress, urge, and reflex incontinence. Alterations in urinary elimination can be caused by a number of factors, including alcohol abuse, obesity, diminished bladder capacity, nocturia, cognitive decline, impaired mobility, and estrogen decline.

Expected outcomes

• Patient maintains a fluid balance.
• Patient achieves urinary continence.
• Patient understands causes of stress incontinence.

• Patient maintains continence with the aid of pads or frequent toileting.
• Patient resumes normal activities.

Nursing interventions and rationales

• Monitor the patient's voiding pattern; document and report intake and output *to ensure correct fluid replacement therapy.*
• Assist with specific bladder elimination procedure, such as:
—habit training, by setting up regular toileting on an individual basis, based on patient's own voiding pattern.
—bladder training, by placing the patient on the toilet every 2 hours while he's awake and once during the night. *Successful bladder training requires adequate fluid intake, muscle-strengthening exercises, and carefully scheduled voiding times.*
—rigid toilet regimen, by placing the patient on the toilet at specific intervals (every 2 hours or after meals). Note whether patient was wet or dry and whether voiding occurred at each interval. *This helps patient adapt to routine physiologic function.*
—external catheter. Apply according to established procedure and maintain patency. Observe condition of perineal skin and clean with soap and water at least twice daily. *This prevents infection and skin breakdown.*
—protective pads and garments. Use only after incontinence management procedures have failed, *to prevent infection and skin breakdown and promote social acceptance.* Allow at least 4 to 6 weeks for trial period.

Establishing continence requires prolonged effort.
• Maintain continence based on patient's voiding patterns and limitations. Use reminders. Orient the patient to toileting environment, time, and place of activity. *A structured environment offers security and helps the patient with elimination problems.*
• Stimulate voiding reflexes. Give patient a drink of water while on the toilet; stroke the area over the bladder; pour water over the perineum. *External stimulation triggers bladder's spastic reflex.*
• For hyperactive patients, provide a distraction such as a magazine to occupy attention while on the toilet. *This reduces anxiety and eases voiding.*
• Provide privacy and adequate time to void *to allow patient to void.*
• Praise successful performance *to encourage compliance.*
• Change wet clothes *to prevent skin breakdown.*
• Teach family members and support personnel to assist, *thus increasing chances for successful treatment.*
• Respond quickly to patient's call light *to avoid delays in routine.*
• Choose the patient's clothing to promote ease in dressing and undressing. (For example, use Velcro fasteners and gowns instead of pajamas.) *This reduces his frustration with voiding routine.*
• Schedule the patient's fluid intake to encourage voiding at convenient times. Maintain adequate hydration up to 3 qt (3 L) daily, unless contraindicated. *Optimal time interval*

between voiding is based on reasonable distention of bladder. Limit fluid intake to 5 oz (150 ml) after supper *to reduce need to void at night.*

• Decrease the patient's use of alcohol.

• Instruct the patient and family on continence techniques to be used at home. Have patient and family demonstrate them.

• Encourage the patient and family to share feelings related to incontinence. *This allows specific problems to be identified and resolved. Attentive listening conveys respect.*

• Refer the patient and family to psychiatric liaison nurse, home health nurse, support group, and similar resources when appropriate *to provide access to additional community resources.*

• Keep skin as clean and dry as possible. Use mild soap and water *to prevent skin breakdown.*

• Assess for UTI, which can cause frequency, urgency, and periods of incontinence if patient can't get to a toilet quickly enough.

• Assess for urine retention, which can lead to overflow incontinence.

• Assess for the presence of stress incontinence. If present, teach elderly women Kegel exercises to strengthen the pelvic floor muscles.

• Assess for drugs, such as sedatives, hypnotics, anticholinergics, and diuretics, which can alter urinary elimination in the older adult.

SPECIAL CONSIDERATIONS

Older adults have a variety of special health needs that require your skilled, knowledgeable care. You need to understand how drugs affect the elderly, in order to improve compliance and avoid adverse reactions.

You also may need to help an older adult patient learn to deal with other age-related concerns, such as managing incontinence and preventing falls. Finally, when your patient can no longer be cared for at home by himself or his family, you may need to help them sort out the available options in long-term care facilities.

Drug therapy

People age 65 or older reportedly purchase 400 million prescriptions per year. Increased medication consumption reflects the increased incidence of chronic disorders.

In elderly patients with chronic disorders, drug therapy may help extend life and may enhance quality of life as well. Treatment obviously requires careful planning and special monitoring to avoid serious adverse reactions and drug interactions. (See *Excessive drug use among older patients,* page 908.)

Pharmacokinetic changes in aging

Age-related changes in body functions may influence the action of drugs—that is, how they are absorbed into the bloodstream, distributed throughout the body, metabolized, and eliminated. (See *Age-related pharmacokinetic changes,* page 909.)

Excessive drug use among older patients

Older patients who have multiple physical dysfunctions may need to consult several doctors and may take several drugs concurrently. However, they may fail to inform each doctor of the various drugs they're already taking. Furthermore, such patients may also take various nonprescription drugs to relieve stomachache, dizziness, or constipation (to name just a few typical complaints).

This excessive use of drugs is called polypharmacy or polymedicine. The patient may obtain prescriptions from three or four doctors and three or four pharmacies. Inherent in this overuse of drugs is the potential for increased adverse drug reactions and interactions (to say nothing of the expense involved).

Identifying excessive use of drugs

Because of your close contact with patients, you're the member of the health care team who is best able to recognize inappropriate use of drugs. Suspect excessive use of drugs if the patient uses:
• several drugs (usually 10 or more)
• drugs for no logical reason—for example, laxatives that aren't needed
• duplicate drugs, such as sleep sedatives and tranquilizers
• an inappropriate dosage
• contraindicated drugs
• drugs to treat adverse reactions.

Pharmacodynamic changes in elderly patients

Age-related changes may increase sensitivity to barbiturates such as pentobarbital, benzodiazepines such as diazepam, and alcohol. Also, age-related changes in the number or function of tissue and organ receptors may alter a drug's effect, for example, drugs that stimulate or block beta-receptors. And, changes in cholinergic and dopaminergic receptors in the nervous system may influence the effect of drugs resulting in extrapyramidal adverse effects and tardive dyskinesia. To compensate, elderly patients commonly require lower dosages of many drugs.

Adverse drug reactions

The older adult is at greater risk for severe adverse drug reactions because they consume more medications, including more toxic medications. Don't overlook or mistake adverse reactions for normal signs of aging. Careful nursing assessment can help identify drug-related adverse effects. (See *Recognizing common adverse drug reactions,* page 910.)

Drug interactions

To help prevent harmful drug interactions, you must be aware of all the medications your patients are taking and keep in mind that your patients may be taking several drugs prescribed independently by different doctors.

Age-related pharmacokinetic changes

Further complicating drug therapy in older people, age-related changes in body functions may influence the action of drugs—that is, how they're absorbed into the bloodstream, distributed throughout the body, metabolized, and eliminated.

Absorption
Absorption may slow or speed up depending on pH levels. For example, absorption from raised pH levels aids absorption of such drugs as oral anticoagulants, iron preparations, digoxin, and tetracycline. Factors that decrease absorption include:
• diminished hydrochloric acid production, which raises gastric pH levels
• decreased blood flow to the intestines and changes in the villi lining of the small intestine's surface
• slowing of stomach emptying and movement of intestinal contents through the GI tract.

Distribution
These factors affect distribution:
• changes in body composition, such as increased body fat and a decrease in lean muscle mass and total body water
• small, frail elderly patients who may require a lower drug dosage.

Metabolism
Factors that slow the rate of metabolism include:
• decrease in liver function
• diminished blood flow to liver
• diminished activity of some enzyme systems
• hepatotoxicity from years of alcohol abuse.

Elimination
Drugs may be eliminated more slowly because of these factors:
• decline in renal function (may slow elimination)
• diminished renal perfusion. As the kidneys excrete drugs more slowly, their half-life and risk of toxicity are prolonged.

Compliance
An elderly patient can have many reasons for noncompliance, such as poor vision or hearing or a physical disability. He may be unable to pay for costly medications; he may be confused about medications and dosage schedules; he may have physical limitations; or he may be socially isolated. When noncompliance is misinterpreted as a lack of therapeutic response, the doctor can mistakenly increase the dosage or prescribe a second drug, further compounding the problem.

Helping to overcome noncompliance in elderly patients is an important nursing responsibility. Ensure that patients know the purpose for all their medications and how to take them correctly.

Urinary incontinence
Incontinence, the uncontrollable passage of urine, results from bladder abnormalities or neurologic dis-

Recognizing common adverse drug reactions

Common signs and symptoms of adverse reactions to medication include hives, impotence, stomach upset, and rashes. Older adult patients are especially susceptible and may experience such serious adverse reactions as orthostatic hypotension, altered mental status, anorexia, dehydration, blood disorders, and tardive dyskinesia.

Keep in mind that such adverse reactions as anxiety, confusion, and forgetfulness may be dismissed as typical elderly behaviors, rather than recognized as adverse effects of a drug.

Orthostatic hypotension

Marked by light-headedness or faintness and unsteady footing, orthostatic hypotension occurs as a common adverse response to antidepressant, antihypertensive, antipsychotic, and sedative medications.

Altered mental status

Agitation or confusion may follow ingestion of alcohol or anticholinergic, antidiuretic, antihypertensive, and antidepressant medications. Paradoxically, depression is a common effect of antidepressant medications.

Anorexia

Anorexia is a warning sign of toxicity—especially from digitalis glycosides such as digoxin. That's why the doctor usually prescribes a low initial dose.

Dehydration

If the patient is taking diuretics such as hydrochlorothiazide be alert for dehydration and electrolyte imbalance. Monitor blood levels and provide potassium supplements, as ordered.

Oral dryness results from many medications. If anticholinergic medications cause dryness, suggest sucking on sugarless candy for relief.

Blood disorders

If the patient takes an anticoagulant such as warfarin, watch for signs of easy bruising or bleeding (such as excessive bleeding after tooth brushing). Easy bruising or bleeding may be signs of other problems, such as blood dyscrasias or thrombocytopenia. Drugs that may cause these reactions include several antineoplastic agents such as methotrexate, antibiotics such as nitrofurantoin, and anticonvulsants such as valproic acid and phenytoin.

Tardive dyskinesia

Characterized by abnormal tongue movements, lip pursing, grimacing, blinking, and gyrating motions of the face and extremities, tardive dyskinesia may be triggered by psychotropic drugs such as haloperidol or chlorpromazine.

---

orders. It may be transient or permanent and may involve large volumes of urine or scant dribbling.

Stress incontinence refers to intermittent leakage resulting from a sudden physical strain leading to increased abdominal pressure.

Overflow incontinence is a dribble resulting from urine retention, which fills the bladder and prevents it from contracting with sufficient force to expel a urine stream. *Urge incontinence* refers to the inability to suppress a sudden urge to urinate. *Total incontinence* is continuous leakage resulting from the bladder's inability to retain any urine due to factors outside the lower urinary tract, such as immobility or dementia.

Urinary incontinence may result from benign prostatic hyperplasia, bladder calculus, bladder cancer, CVA, diabetic neuropathy, Guillain-Barré syndrome, multiple sclerosis, prostatic cancer, chronic prostatitis, spinal cord injury, and urethral stricture. It may also occur after prostatectomy as a result of urethral sphincter damage. Diuretics, sedatives, hypnotics, antipsychotics, anticholinergics, and alpha antagonists are also associated with urinary incontinence.

Assessment

Ask the patient when he first noticed the problem and whether it began suddenly or gradually. Have him describe his typical urinary pattern. Determine his normal fluid intake. Ask about other urinary problems, such as hesitancy, frequency, urgency, nocturia, and decreased force or interruption of the urine stream.

Obtain a medical history. Ask whether the patient is taking any medications, particularly sedatives, hypnotics, anticholinergics, and diuretics.

Have the patient empty his bladder. Inspect the urethral meatus for obvious inflammation or anatomic defect. Have female patients bear down; note any urine leakage. Gently palpate the abdomen for bladder distention. Perform a complete neurologic assessment, noting motor and sensory function and muscle atrophy.

Nursing interventions

Prepare the patient for diagnostic tests, such as cystoscopy, cystometry, and a complete neurologic workup, and implement a bladder retraining program.

Make sure the patient receives adequate fluid intake. Have him void regularly. If appropriate, teach the patient self-catheterization techniques. A patient with permanent urinary incontinence may require surgical creation of a urinary diversion. (See *Biofeedback and incontinence,* page 912.)

Falls

In people age 75 or older, falls account for three times as many accidental deaths as motor vehicle accidents. Lengthy convalescence, the risk of incomplete recovery, and the inability to cope physiologically make falls ominous for the elderly. Injuries that occur because of falls may be psychologically devastating.

Falls can be accidental or may result from temporary muscle paralysis, vertigo, postural hypotension, or central nervous system (CNS) lesions. Many accidental falls are caused by a hazardous environment. They can also result from

Biofeedback and incontinence

Biofeedback is a proven relaxation therapy that allows a patient to control the body's response to stress. Stress-related conditions, such as incontinence (which involves muscle tone) have been treated successfully with biofeedback.

Biofeedback uses electronic feedback devices to teach the patient to be aware of and consciously control involuntary body functions such as heart rate and pulse, blood temperature, digestion, and muscle behavior. For example, by helping the patient to recognize the way that he tenses various muscles when under stress, biofeedback assists the patient to practice relaxing those muscles. Biofeedback can treat incontinence by helping the patient identify and tone muscles that need strengthening.

physiologic factors, such as decreased visual acuity, loss of muscle strength, and decreased coordination.

Assessment

If the patient is found on the floor or reports falling, don't move him until his status is evaluated. Rapidly assess his vital signs, mental status, and functional capacity. Note any signs and symptoms, such as confusion, tremors, weakness, pain, or dizziness. Take steps to control

bleeding, if indicated, and obtain an X-ray if a fracture is suspected. Monitor the patient's status for the next 24 hours.

After the patient is stabilized, review the events that preceded the fall to help avoid future episodes. Review his use of medications, such as tranquilizers and narcotics. Also assess other contributing factors, such as gait disturbances, poor vision, improper use of assistive devices, and environmental hazards.

Nursing interventions

Perform necessary measures to relieve the patient's pain and discomfort. Give analgesics, as ordered. Apply cold compresses for the first 24 hours, and warm compresses thereafter, to reduce the pain and swelling of bruises. If the patient is bedridden, encourage him to remain active, to prevent immobility. Provide appropriate care for a fracture. If indicated, arrange for a home health nurse for the recovery period.

Teach the patient how to reduce the risk of accidental falls by wearing well-fitting shoes with nonskid soles, avoiding use of long robes, and wearing glasses, if he needs them. Advise him to sit on the edge of the bed for a few minutes before rising and to use a walking stick, cane, or walker if he feels even slightly unsteady on his feet.

Suggest ways for the patient to adapt his home to guard against accidental falls, for instance, by applying nonskid treads to stairs and handrails to walls around the bathtub, shower, and toilet.

Teach the patient how to fall safely, for instance, by protecting his hands and face. If the patient uses a walker or a wheelchair, make sure he knows how to cope with a fall, should one occur. Then review with the patient the proper procedure for lifting himself off the floor and either standing up with the walker or getting into the wheelchair.

Long-term care

Most older adults in North America are cared for at home by themselves or by their families. However, as many as 25% will need long-term care (LTC) assistance in their later years.

Several types of LTC facilities are available. A *personal care facility* provides meals, sheltered living, and some medical monitoring. This type of facility is appropriate for someone who doesn't need continuous medical attention.

An *intermediate care facility* provides custodial care for individuals unable to care for themselves due to mental or physical infirmities. They provide room and board and regular nursing care. Physical, social, and recreational activities are provided, and some have rehabilitation programs. A *skilled nursing facility* provides medical supervision, rehabilitation services, and 24-hour nursing care by registered nurses, licensed practical nurses, and nurses' aides to those who have the potential to regain function.

Unfortunately, many older adults dread moving into a nursing home. Some fear being abandoned by their friends and family. Others feel anxious about adjusting to a new setting and routine. Still others are saddened by the loss of their home, possessions, privacy, and independence. The stress of entering an institution threatens an older adult's mental well-being when he's most vulnerable.

Setting the stage for success

Entering an LTC facility can be a positive experience when the following criteria are met:
• The patient selects the facility and enters it voluntarily.
• The facility is located near friends and family.
• The patient is accustomed to being with people, and some of the residents share similar activity and alertness levels.
• The patient recognizes that he needs assistance with physical care or supervision in activities.
• Quality interaction is maintained with at least one staff member and family member or friend.
• Social interaction among residents is encouraged.
• The facility provides adequate environmental stimuli and space.

Helping patient and family

Encourage family members to involve the elderly person in selecting an LTC facility, if possible. This allows the person some control over the situation.

Help the patient and his family sort through the options in LTC facilities. Recommend that they schedule both planned and unannounced visits at several facilities, to compare features, services, environment, and atmosphere. Suggest ways they can determine the quality of care a facility delivers.

Arrange for a social worker to meet with the patient and his family to discuss various options and to help them make the necessary financial arrangements.

REFERENCES AND READINGS

Anderson, K., and Dimond, M. "The Experience of Bereavement in Older Adults," *Journal of Advanced Nursing* 22(2): 308-15, August 1995.

Burrows, A., et al. "Depression in a Long Term Care Facility: Clinical Features and Discordance between Nursing Assessment and Patient Interviews," *Journal of American Geriatrics Society* 43(10):1118-22, October 1995.

DeMaagd, G. "High-Risk Drugs in the Elderly Population," *Geriatric Nursing* 16(5):198-206, September-October 1995.

Johnson, B.K. "Older Adults and Sexuality," *Journal of Gerontologic Nursing* 22(2): 6-15, February 1996.

Mindnich, D., and Hart, B. "Linking Hospital and Community," *Journal of Psychosocial Nursing* 33(1):25-28, 1995.

Teaching Aids for Home Care Nurses. Springhouse, Pa.: Springhouse Corp., 1996.

18

PSYCHIATRIC CARE

Providing care for psychiatric patients requires that you develop a practical, orderly method for dealing with problems as diverse and complex as humanity itself. Your responsibilities include not only planning, implementing, and evaluating care but also establishing a meaningful therapeutic relationship with the patient. But when you encounter intractable psychiatric problems, you'll need to develop a keen awareness of your own attitudes and feelings to prevent frustration from hobbling your efforts.

You'll need to be familiar with the revised fourth edition of the American Psychiatric Association's *Diagnostic and Statistical Manual of Mental Disorders (DSM-IV)*. (See *Understanding the* DSM-IV, page 916.)

ASSESSMENT

Psychiatric assessment refers to the scientific process of identifying a patient's psychosocial problems, strengths, concerns, and treatment goals, and evaluating therapeutic interventions. Recognizing psychosocial problems and how they affect health is important in any clinical setting.

Mental status examination

The mental status examination (MSE) is a tool for assessing psychological dysfunction and for identifying the causes of psychopathology. Your nursing responsibilities may include conducting all or a portion of the MSE. The MSE examines the patient's level of consciousness (LOC), general appearance, behavior, speech, mood and affect, intellectual performance, judgment, insight, perception, and thought content.

Level of consciousness. Begin by assessing the patient's LOC, a basic brain function. Identify the intensity of stimulation needed to arouse the patient.

Describe the patient's response to stimulation, including the degree and quality of movement, content

Understanding the *DSM-IV*

The revised fourth edition of the American Psychiatric Association's *Diagnostic and Statistical Manual of Mental Disorders (DSM-IV)* defines a mental disorder as a clinically significant behavioral or psychological syndrome or pattern that is associated with current distress (a painful symptom) or disability (impairment in one or more important areas of functioning) or with a significantly greater risk of suffering, death, pain, disability, or an important loss of freedom. This syndrome or pattern mustn't be merely an expected, culturally sanctioned response such as grief over the death of a loved one. Whatever its original cause, it must currently be considered a sign of behavioral, psychological, or biological dysfunction.

To add diagnostic detail, the *DSM-IV* uses a multiaxial approach. This flexible approach specifies that every patient must be evaluated on each of five axes, as follows.

Axis I

Clinical disorders—the diagnosis (or diagnoses) that best describes the presenting complaint

Axis II

Personality disorders; mental retardation

Axis III

General medical conditions—a description of any concurrent medical conditions or disorders

Axis IV

Psychosocial and environmental problems that may affect the diagnosis, treatment, and prognosis of the mental disorder

Axis V

Global assessment of functioning (GAF), based on a scale of 1 to 100. The GAF scale allows evaluation of the patient's overall psychological, social, and occupational function. For example, a patient's diagnosis might read as follows:

Axis I: adjustment disorder with anxiety

Axis II: obsessive-compulsive personality disorder

Axis III: Crohn's disease, acute bleeding episode

Axis IV: death of a father and homelessness

Axis V: GAF—53 (current).

and coherence of speech, and level of eye opening and eye contact. Finally, describe the patient's actions once the stimulus is removed.

An impaired LOC may indicate the presence of a medical disorder. If you discover an alteration in consciousness, refer the patient for a more complete medical examination.

General appearance. Appearance helps to indicate the patient's overall mental status. Answer the following questions:
• Is the patient's appearance appropriate to his age, sex, and situation?
• Are skin, hair, nails, and teeth clean?
• Is his manner of dress appropriate?
• If the patient wears cosmetics, are they appropriately applied?

• Does the patient maintain direct eye contact?

Behavior. Describe the patient's demeanor and way of relating to others. Does the patient appear sad, joyful, or expressionless? Does he use appropriate gestures? Does he keep an appropriate distance between himself and others? Does he have distinctive mannerisms, such as tics or tremors?

Is the patient cooperative, mistrustful, embarrassed, hostile, or overly revealing? Describe the patient's level of activity. Is the patient tense, rigid, restless, or calm?

Note any extraordinary behavior. Disconnected gestures may indicate that the patient is hallucinating. Pressured, rapid speech and a heightened level of activity may indicate the manic phase of a bipolar disorder.

Speech. Observe the content and quality of the patient's speech, taking notice of illogical choice of topics, irrelevant or illogical replies to questions, any speech defects such as stuttering, excessively fast or slow speech, sudden interruptions, excessive volume, and barely audible speech. Note slurred speech, an excessive number of words, or minimal, monosyllabic responses.

Mood and affect. *Mood* refers to a person's pervading feeling or state of mind. Usually, the patient will project a prevailing mood, though this mood may change in the course of a day. *Affect* refers to a person's expression of his mood. Variations in affect are referred to as *range of emotion.*

To assess mood and affect, begin by asking the patient about his current feelings. Also look for indications of mood in facial expression and posture.

Does the patient seem able to keep mood changes under control? Mood swings may indicate a physiologic disorder. Medications, recreational drug or alcohol use, stress, dehydration, electrolyte imbalance, or disease may all induce mood changes. After childbirth and during menopause, many women experience profound depression.

Other symptoms of mood disorders include:
• lability of affect—rapid, dramatic changes in the range of emotion
• flat affect—unresponsive range of emotion
• inappropriate affect—inconsistency between expression (affect) and mood.

Intellectual performance. To develop a picture of the patient's intellectual abilities, test the patient's orientation, immediate and delayed recall, recent and remote memory, attention level, comprehension, concept formation, and general knowledge.

Judgment. Assess the patient's ability to evaluate choices and to draw appropriate conclusions. Defects in judgment may also become apparent while the patient tells his history. Pay attention to how the patient handles interpersonal relationships and occupational and economic responsibilities.

Insight. To assess insight, ask "What do you think has caused your anxiety?" or "Have you noticed a recent change in yourself?" Expect patients to show varying degrees of insight. Severe lack of insight may indicate a psychotic state.

Perception. Perception refers to interpretation of reality as well as use of the senses. Proponents of the cognitive theory of depression have suggested that depression arises from distorted perception.

Sensory perception disorders. The patient may experience *hallucinations,* in which he perceives nonexistent external stimuli, or *illusions,* in which he misinterprets external stimuli. Tactile, olfactory, and gustatory hallucinations usually indicate organic disorders.

Not all visual and auditory hallucinations are associated with psychological disorders. Patients may also experience mild and transitory hallucinations. Constant visual and auditory hallucinations may, however, give rise to strange or bizarre behavior. Disorders associated with hallucinations include schizophrenia and acute organic brain syndrome after withdrawal from alcohol or barbiturate addiction.

Thought content. Assess the patient's thought patterns. Are the patient's thoughts well connected to reality? Are the patient's ideas clear, and do they progress in a logical sequence? Observe for indications of morbid thoughts and preoccupations, or abnormal beliefs.

Delusions. Usually associated with schizophrenia, delusions are grandiose or persecutory false beliefs. Delusions may be obvious or may have a slight basis in reality.

Obsessions. Some patients suffer intense preoccupations that interfere with daily living. Patients may constantly think about hygiene, for example. A *compulsion* is a preoccupation that's acted out such as constantly washing one's hands.

Observe also for suicidal, self-destructive, violent, or superstitious thoughts; recurring dreams; distorted perceptions of reality; and feelings of worthlessness.

Sexual drive. Changes in sexual drive provide valuable information in psychological assessment. Prepare yourself for patients who are uncomfortable discussing their sexuality. Avoid language that implies a heterosexual orientation. Introduce the subject tactfully but directly.

Follow-up questions might include:
• Are you currently sexually active?
• Have you noticed any recent changes in your interest in sex?
• Do you have the same pleasure from sex now as before?

Competence. Can the patient understand reality and the consequences of his actions? Does the patient understand the implications of his illness, its treatment, and the consequences of avoiding treatment? Use extreme caution when assessing changes in competence.

Unless behavior strongly indicates otherwise, assume that the patient is competent. Remember that legally, only a judge has the power or right to declare a person incompetent.

Assessing self-destructive behavior

Suicide—intentional, self-inflicted death—may be carried out with guns, drugs, poisons, rope, automobiles, or razor blades, or by drowning, jumping, or refusing food, fluid, or medications. In a *subintentional suicide,* a person has no conscious intention of dying but nevertheless engages in self-destructive acts.

Not all self-destructive behavior is suicidal in intent. A patient who has lost touch with reality may cut or mutilate body parts to focus on physical pain. Such behavior may indicate a borderline personality disorder.

Assess depressed patients for suicidal tendencies. A higher percentage of depressed patients commit suicide than patients with other diagnoses. Chemically dependent and schizophrenic patients also present a high suicide risk.

Suicidal schizophrenics may be agitated instead of depressed. Voices may tell them to kill themselves. Alarmingly, some schizophrenics provide only vague behavioral clues before taking their lives.

On perceiving signals of hopelessness, perform a direct suicide assessment. (See *Recognizing and responding to suicidal patients,* page 920.) Protect patients from self-harm during a suicidal crisis. After treatment, the patient should think more clearly and find reasons for living.

Physical examination

Because psychiatric problems may stem from organic causes or medical treatment, the doctor may order a physical examination for psychiatric patients. Observe for key signs and symptoms and examine the patient by using inspection, palpation, percussion, and auscultation.

DIAGNOSTIC TESTS

Diagnostic studies performed on psychiatric patients include laboratory tests, noninvasive studies, brain imaging studies, and psychological tests. (See *Diagnostic tests for psychiatric disorders,* pages 921 and 922.)

In addition to these diagnostic tests, your patient may undergo a chest X-ray and electrocardiogram (ECG) to screen for heart and pulmonary abnormalities and an electroencephalogram (EEG) to screen for brain abnormalities, especially if he's taking psychotropic medications.

NURSING DIAGNOSES

When caring for patients with psychiatric disorders, you will find that several nursing diagnoses are commonly used. These diagnoses appear below with the appropriate interventions and rationales. (Rationales appear in italic type.)

Impaired social interaction

Related to altered thought processes, impaired social interaction may be associated with such conditions

Recognizing and responding to suicidal patients

Be alert for these warning signs of impending suicide:
• withdrawal
• social isolation
• signs of depression, which may include constipation, crying, fatigue, helplessness, hopelessness, poor concentration, reduced interest in sex and other activities, sadness, and weight loss
• farewells to friends and family
• putting affairs in order
• giving away prized possessions
• expression of covert suicide messages and death wishes
• obvious suicide messages, such as "I'd be better off dead."

Answering a threat
If a patient shows signs of impending suicide, assess the seriousness of the intent and the immediacy of the risk. Consider a patient with a chosen method who plans to commit suicide in the next 48 to 72 hours a high risk.

Tell the patient that you're concerned. Then urge the patient to avoid self-destructive behavior until the staff has an opportunity to help him. You may specify a time for the patient to seek help.

Next, consult with the treatment team about arranging for psychiatric hospitalization or a safe equivalent, such as having someone watch the patient at home. Initiate safety pre-

cautions for those with high suicide risk, including the following:
• Provide a safe environment. Check and correct conditions that could be dangerous for the patient. Look for exposed pipes, windows without safety glass, and access to the roof or open balconies.
• Remove dangerous objects, such as belts, razors, suspenders, light cords, glass, knives, nail files, and clippers.
• Make the patient's specific restrictions clear to staff members, plan for observation of the patient, and clarify day- and night-staff responsibilities.

Patients may ask you to keep their suicidal thoughts confidential. Remember such requests are ambivalent; suicidal patients want to escape the pain of life, but they also want to live. A part of them wants you to tell other staff so they can be kept alive. Tell patients that you can't keep secrets that endanger their lives or conflict with their treatment. You have a duty to keep them safe and to ensure the best care.

Be alert when the patient is shaving, taking medication, or using the bathroom. In addition to observing the patient, maintain personal contact with him. Encourage continuity of care and consistency of primary nurses. Helping the patient build emotional ties to others is the ultimate technique for preventing suicide.

as drug or alcohol withdrawal, delusional disorders, anxiety states, schizophrenia, depression, paranoia, and posttraumatic stress disorder.

Expected outcomes
• Patient understands connection between behavior and safety.
• Patient channels uncontrollable feelings into constructive outlets.

Diagnostic tests for psychiatric disorders

Test	Purpose	Nursing considerations
Dexamethasone suppression test	To serve as an indirect measurement of cortisol hyperactivity that may help to diagnose depression	• Explain the procedure. • Restrict food and fluids for 10 to 12 hours before the test. • Give the patient 1 mg of dexamethasone at 11 p.m. On the following day, collect blood samples at 4 p.m. and 11 p.m. • After the test, observe venipuncture site for bleeding.
Urine glucose	To help identify borderline glycosuria induced by psychotropic drugs	• Explain the procedure. • Obtain a second-voided urine sample in a container. • Dip the reagent strip in the specimen for 2 seconds. Remove from container and begin timing. • Hold the strip in the air and compare to the color chart in exactly 30 seconds. Record the results.
Thyroid function tests (including triiodothyronine [T3], thyroxine [T4], and free thyroxine index)	To rule out a thyroid disorder as a cause of mental distress	• Explain the procedure. • Withhold such medications as steroids, propranolol, and cholestyramine. If such medications must be continued, record this on the laboratory request. • After the test, observe venipuncture site for bleeding.
Computed tomography scan	To help diagnose intracranial lesions and abnormalities	• Explain the procedure. • If contrast enhancement is scheduled, instruct the patient to fast for 4 hours before the test. • Check history for hypersensitivity to iodine, shellfish, or I.V. contrast medium. • Tell him his head will be immobilized. • After the test, watch for residual adverse reactions from the contrast medium. The patient may resume his usual diet.

(continued)

Diagnostic tests for psychiatric disorders *(continued)*

Test	Purpose	Nursing considerations
Magnetic resonance imaging	To detect intracranial structural and biochemical abnormalities	• Explain the procedure. • Emphasize that the opening for the patient's head and body on the scanner is quite small and deep. He'll hear the scanner clicking and thumping, so he may receive ear plugs. • Reassure him he'll be able to communicate with the technician. • Ask if claustrophobia has been a problem. If so, he may need sedation. • Instruct the patient to remove all metal objects. • After the test, the patient may resume normal activity.

• Patient participates in group activities.
• Patient expresses feelings verbally.
• Patient doesn't hurt self or others, or damage his environment.

Nursing interventions and rationales

• Take precautions to ensure a safe and protected environment (provide side rails, assistance with out-of-bed activities, physical restraints, as necessary). *This reduces the potential for patient injury.*
• Assess neurologic function and mental status every shift and reorient patient as often as necessary. *These actions monitor changes in the patient's status.*
• If delusions and hallucinations occur, don't focus on them; provide patient with reality-based information and reassure him of safety. *This increases the patient's ability to grasp reality.*

• Provide specific, non–care-related time with the patient each shift to encourage social interaction. Begin with one-on-one interaction and increase to group interaction as patient's skills indicate. *Gradually increasing social interaction reduces patient's feeling of being overwhelmed.*
• Give positive reinforcement for appropriate and effective interaction behaviors (verbal and nonverbal). *This helps the patient recognize progress and enhances self-esteem.*
• Assist the patient and his family or close friends in progressive participation in care and therapies. *This enhances the patient's feeling of control and independence.*
• Initiate or participate in multidisciplinary patient-centered conferences to evaluate progress and plan discharge. *These conferences involve the patient and family in the plan of care.*

Anxiety

Related to unmet expectations or threats to safety or security, anxiety may be associated with such conditions as anorexia nervosa, phobic disorders, and schizophrenia.

Expected outcomes

• Patient states feelings of anxiety.
• Patient identifies factors that elicit anxious behaviors.
• Patient maintains normal sleep and nutritional patterns.
• Patient discusses activities that tend to decrease anxious behaviors.

Nursing interventions and rationales

• Explore factors that precipitate phobic reactions and anxiety, and explore how the patient typically seeks relief from anxiety. *This is important for understanding the patient's dynamics.*
• Support a phobic patient with desensitization techniques. *Encouraging the patient to expose himself to fears gradually in a safe setting helps overcome problems.*
• Give the patient a chance to express feelings. *Bottled-up feelings continue to affect behavior even though the patient may be unaware of them.*
• Teach relaxation techniques (such as breathing exercises, progressive muscle relaxation, guided imagery, and meditation). *Such measures counteract fight-or-flight response.*
• Help the patient set limits and compromises on behavior when ready. Allow the patient to be afraid. *Fear is a feeling, neither right nor wrong.*

• Help the patient develop his own techniques for dealing with fears. *This establishes alternatives to escape or avoidance behaviors.*

Ineffective individual coping

Related to situational or maturational crisis, ineffective individual coping may be associated with a normal response to stress or with such conditions as alcoholism, bipolar disorder, posttraumatic stress disorder, depression, drug addiction or overdose, drug withdrawal, personality disorder, or self-inflicted injuries.

Expected outcomes

• Patient communicates feelings about the present crisis.
• Patient practices assertive behaviors.
• Patient begins to discuss underlying causes of his feelings.
• Patient identifies at least two new coping tenchiques.

Nursing interventions and rationales

• If possible, assign a primary nurse to patient *to provide continuity of care.*
• Arrange to spend uninterrupted periods of time with patient. Encourage expression of feelings. Try to identify factors that cause, exacerbate, or reduce the patient's inability to cope. *Devoting time for listening helps patient express emotions, grasp situation, and cope effectively.*
• Identify and reduce unnecessary stimuli in environment *to avoid sensory or perceptual overload.*

• Initially, allow patient to depend partly on you for self-care. *Patient may regress to a lower developmental level during initial crisis phase.*

• Explain all treatments and procedures and answer patient's questions *to allay fear.*

• Encourage patient to make decisions about care *to increase sense of self-worth.*

• Praise patient for making decisions and performing activities *to reinforce coping behaviors.*

• Encourage patient to use support systems to assist with coping, *thereby helping restore equilibrium.*

• Help patient look at current situation and evaluate various coping behaviors *to encourage a realistic view of crisis.*

• Encourage patient to try coping behaviors. *A patient in crisis is more likely to accept interventions and develop new coping behaviors.*

• Request feedback from patient about behaviors that seem to work *to encourage him to evaluate them.*

• Refer patient for professional psychological counseling. *Formal counseling increases objectivity and fosters collaborative approach to patient's care.*

Ineffective denial

Related to fear or anxiety, ineffective denial may be associated with such conditions as alcoholism, anxiety, bipolar disorder, and depression. It also may be associated with anorexia nervosa, bulimia, drug addiction, and other self-destructive behaviors.

Expected outcomes

• Patient describes understanding of the present health problem.

• Patient expresses knowledge of the stages of grief.

• Patient demonstrates behavior associated with grief process.

• Patient discusses present health problem with doctors, nurses, and family members.

• Patient shows by conversation or behavior an increased awareness of reality.

Nursing interventions and rationales

• Provide for a specific amount of uninterrupted non-care-related time with patient each day. *This allows patient to express knowledge, feelings, and concerns.*

• Encourage patient to express feelings related to current problem, its severity, and its potential impact on life pattern. *This helps patient resolve concerns.*

• Maintain frequent communication with doctor. *This fosters consistent, collaborative approach to patient's care.*

• Listen to patient with nonjudgmental acceptance *to demonstrate positive regard for patient.*

• Encourage patient to communicate with others. *Patient fixated in denial may withdraw from others.*

• Visit more frequently as patient begins to accept reality; alleviate fears when necessary. *This helps reduce patient's fear of living alone.*

Social isolation

Related to inadequate social skills, fear, or depression, social isolation occurs among elderly patients, patients with present or past history of depression and other psychiatric disorders, and any patient who has no family or friends.

Expected outcomes
• Patient discusses his inadequate social relationships and expresses desire to increase social activity.
• Patient communicates circumstances that may limit social activity.
• Patient and members of the health care team explore ways of reducing barriers to increased social activity.
• Patient reports feeling less socially isolated.

Nursing interventions and rationales
• Assign same caregivers to patient *to promote trusting relationships with staff members.*
• Assign a primary nurse to coordinate patient's care. *This prevents fragmented nursing interventions.*
• Plan a 15-minute period to sit with patient each shift. If patient doesn't want to talk, comment on his behavior or feelings or remain silent. *Active listening communicates concern and encourages patient to initiate interaction.*
• Have patient participate in self-care continuously. *This provides structure and fosters independent action.*
• Discuss patient's living accommodations and lifestyle outside the health care facility. *This increases understanding and helps with discharge planning.*

• Refer to social services for follow-up, if necessary, *to ensure a comprehensive approach to care.*
• Help patient identify social outlets (peer group, participation in group activity). *This promotes goal-directed interaction.*

Impaired verbal communication

Related to psychological barriers, impaired verbal communication may be associated with such conditions as schizophrenia, confusion, alcohol intoxication, Alzheimer's disease, bipolar disease (mania or depression), alcohol withdrawal syndrome, drug overdose, psychosis, or anxiety states.

Expected outcomes
• Patient communicates needs and desires to family, friends, or staff.
• Staff members meet patient's needs.
• Patient incurs no injury or harm.
• Patient begins to make plans to use self-help groups, a speech therapist, or other resources to improve psychological or neurologic status.

Nursing interventions and rationales
• Observe patient closely to anticipate needs; for example, restlessness may indicate need to urinate. *Nonverbal clues give meaning to actions.*
• Maintain a quiet, nonthreatening environment *to reduce anxiety.*
• Introduce yourself and explain procedures in simple terms. *Treating patient as normal may enhance responsiveness.*

• Encourage communication attempts and allow patient time to say or write words in response. *Patient's response time may be slow, thoughts difficult to express.*

• Assess patient's communication status daily, and record. Match communication needs to interventions: for disorientation, use reality orientation techniques; for manic state, reduce environmental stimuli and talk softly and calmly; for alcohol withdrawal syndrome, reassure patient, but don't reinforce presence of hallucinations, and provide quiet environment; for a stutterer, use rhythm or song. *Tailoring communication interventions to the patient improves outcome.*

• Determine patient's past interests and habits from family or close friends and discuss them *to stimulate nonthreatening conversation.*

• Maintain a safe environment for a confused or resistant patient by using side rails, soft restraint or Posey net, and other safety measures according to established policies *to prevent injuries.*

• Refer the patient to psychiatric liaison nurse, social services, community agencies, and such self-help groups as Alcoholics Anonymous (AA). *Exploration and resolution of communication problems may require long-term follow-up.*

Risk for violence: Self-directed or directed at others

Related to organic brain dysfunction, risk for violence, self-directed or directed at others, may be associated with such conditions as delusional disorder, paranoid schizophrenia, posttraumatic stress disorder, mood disorder, senile dementia and psychosis, terminal illness, or use of antipsychotic drugs.

Expected outcomes

• Patient gains control over his anger by verbalizing his feelings, venting his frustration through nondestructive channels, taking time-out periods, and using prescribed medications.

• Patient discusses appropriate ways to handle frustration.

• Patient doesn't harm himself.

• Patient discusses sadness, despair, and other feelings.

• Patient identifies need for continued support groups.

Nursing interventions and rationales

• Provide close supervision and watch for early signs of agitation or increasing anxiety, such as increased motor activity and unreasonable requests or demands. *Early assessment and intervention helps defuse potentially explosive behavior.*

• Use a calm, unhurried approach *to reduce patient's sense of lack of control.* Allow patient to express feelings in nonviolent ways, such as beating a pillow, participating in physical exercise, or working with clay. *This helps patient successfully release tension.*

• Put limits on aggressive behavior *to reinforce expectations that patient act in responsible, controlled manner.*

• Identify and remove from environment stimuli—persons, objects, or situations—that precipitate potentially destructive behavior. *Such stimuli may precipitate aggressive behavior in patients with cognitive and perceptual deficits.*

• Remove from environment anything patient may use to inflict injury on self or others (for example, a belt, razor, or glass objects) *to ensure patient's safety.*

• Administer and monitor effectiveness of medications prescribed to control aggressive behavior. *Medication is the least restrictive intervention and helps reduce patient anxiety and need for physical restraints.*

DISORDERS

This section covers a range of mental and emotional disorders. Patients may come to you seeking help with substance abuse problems, schizophrenic disorders, mood disorders, anxiety disorders, somatoform disorders, personality disorders, and eating disorders, among others.

Substance abuse disorders

Most substance-related disorders arise from substance abuse. Substance abuse refers to the regular use of alcohol or drugs that affect the central nervous system (CNS) and cause behavioral changes. Substance abuse strikes males and females of all ages, cultures, and socioeconomic groups. It follows a pathologic course, impairs social and family relationships or job function, and lasts at least 1 month. Typically, the patient will have abused several drugs or a combination of alcohol and drugs.

Alcoholism

Chronic, uncontrolled intake of alcohol is the nation's largest substance abuse problem. Alcohol abuse may begin as early as elementary school. Alcoholism has no known cure.

Many alcoholics are difficult to identify because they're able to function adequately at work. The homemaker may conceal drinking during the day.

Causes. No definite cause of alcoholism has been clearly identified. However, biologic, psychological, and sociocultural factors contribute to the disorder.

Assessment findings. Characteristically, the alcoholic patient depends on daily or episodic use of alcohol to function adequately. He may experience episodes of anesthesia, amnesia, or violence during intoxication.

In later stages of alcoholism, possible signs and symptoms include unexplained traumatic injuries or mood swings, unresponsiveness to sedatives, poor personal hygiene, and secretive behavior. The patient may attempt to consume alcohol in any form when deprived of his usual supply. If the patient has not yet recognized his drinking problem, he may become hostile or deny its existence.

Diagnostic tests. Laboratory tests can document recent alcohol ingestion. A blood alcohol level of 0.10% weight/volume (200 mg/dl) is accepted as the level of intoxication.

By knowing how recently the patient has been drinking, you can tell when to expect withdrawal symptoms.

A complete serum electrolyte count may be necessary to identify electrolyte abnormalities (in severe hepatic disease, blood urea nitrogen [BUN] level is increased and serum glucose level is decreased). Further testing may show increased serum ammonia levels. Urine toxicology may help to determine if the alcoholic with alcohol withdrawal syndrome or another acute complication abuses other drugs as well.

Liver function studies, revealing increased serum cholesterol value, lactate dehydrogenase, aspartate aminotransferase (AST), alanine aminotransferase (ALT), and creatine kinase levels, may point to liver damage related to alcoholism. Elevated serum amylase and lipase levels point to acute pancreatitis. A hematologic workup can identify anemia, thrombocytopenia, increased prothrombin time, and increased activated partial thromboplastin time.

Echocardiography and ECGs may reveal possible cardiac problems related to alcoholism such as an enlarged heart (cardiomegaly).

Structured, standarized questionnaires are commonly used to assess substance abuse. Well-known scales include the *DSM-IV* structured clinical interview, the addiction severity index, the drinking problems index, the cage questionnaire, and the chemical use, abuse, and dependence scale.

Treatment. Total abstinence is the only effective treatment. Supportive programs that offer detoxification, rehabilitation, and aftercare (including involvement in AA) produce the best long-term results.

Treatment during acute withdrawal may include administration of I.V. glucose for hypoglycemia and forcing fluids containing thiamine and other B-complex vitamins. Other adjunctive therapies include furosemide to reduce overhydration, magnesium sulfate to reduce CNS irritability, chlordiazepoxide or diazepam to prevent alcohol withdrawal syndrome, and phenobarbital for sedation.

Once the alcoholic is sober, treatment aims to help maintain sobriety. Methods include deterrent therapy and supportive counseling. Neither is completely effective.

Deterrent therapy uses a daily oral dose of disulfiram. This drug interferes with alcohol metabolism, producing immediate and potentially fatal distress if the patient drinks alcohol up to 2 weeks after taking it. The reaction includes nausea, vomiting, facial flushing, headache, shortness of breath, red eyes, blurred vision, sweating, tachycardia, hypotension, and fainting. It may last from 30 minutes to 3 hours or longer. The patient needs close medical supervision during this time.

Supportive counseling or individual, group, or family psychotherapy may improve the alcoholic's ability to cope with stress, anxiety, and frustration. If the patient engaged in inappropriate sexual activity while intoxicated, his feelings of guilt and fear of possible exposure to acquired immunodeficiency syndrome must be managed as well.

Some alcoholics may also require job training or help through sheltered workshops, halfway houses, or other supervised facilities.

Nursing interventions. When caring for a patient in alcohol withdrawal, carefully monitor mental status, heart rate, lung sounds, blood pressure, and temperature every 30 minutes to 6 hours, depending on the severity of symptoms. Orient the patient to reality because he may have hallucinations and may try to harm himself or others. You may have to restrain the combative patient temporarily. Take seizure precautions. Administer drugs, as ordered, which may include antianxiety agents, anticonvulsants, or antidiarrheal or antiemetic agents. Participate in the plan of care for medical symptoms and complications. Observe for signs of depression or suicide. Also, encourage adequate nutrition.

Patient education. Educate the patient and his family about the illness. Encourage participation in a rehabilitation program. Warn him that he must abstain from alcohol for the rest of his life.

Warn the patient taking disulfiram that even a small amount of alcohol—including that in cough medicines, mouthwashes, and liquid vitamins—will induce an adverse reaction and that the longer he takes the drug, the greater will be his sensitivity to alcohol. Paraldehyde, a sedative, is chemically similar to

alcohol and may also provoke a disulfiram reaction. These patients should remain under medical supervision.

Tell the patient that AA offers emotional support from others with similar problems. Advise female patients that they may benefit from joining a women's AA group. Offer to arrange a visit from an AA member. Teach the patient's family about Al-Anon and Alateen, two other self-help groups. Explain that involvement in rehabilitation can reduce family tensions.

Evaluation. The patient should recognize that alcoholism is an illness. He should not harm himself or others during withdrawal. He should participate in counseling or self-help groups.

Drug abuse and dependence

Drug abuse involves use of a legal or illegal drug that causes physical, mental, emotional, or social harm. Dependence is marked by physiologic changes, primarily tolerance and withdrawal symptoms.

Abused drugs include cocaine, crack cocaine, opioids (heroin, morphine, and meperidine), barbiturates, nonbarbiturate sedatives, amphetamines, marijuana, hallucinogens, inhalants, and prescribed drugs. The most dangerous form of drug abuse is that in which several drugs are mixed—sometimes with alcohol and various other chemicals.

Causes. The causes of drug abuse are difficult to identify. In young people, drug abuse commonly follows adolescent experimentation with drugs. Abuse sometimes follows the use of drugs for relief of pain or depression.

Assessment findings. Once abuse begins, clinical effects vary according to the substance used, the duration, and the dosage.

Diagnostic tests. Diagnosis depends largely on a history that shows a pattern of pathologic use of a substance with related impairment in social or occupational function for at least 1 month. A urine or blood screen may determine the amount of the substance present.

Treatment. Treatment of acute drug intoxication is symptomatic and depends on the drug ingested. It includes fluid replacement therapy and nutritional and vitamin supplements, if indicated; detoxification with the same drug or a pharmacologically similar drug; sedatives; anticholinergics and antidiarrheal agents; antianxiety drugs for severe agitation, especially in cocaine abusers; and treatment of medical complications.

Treatment of drug dependence commonly involves detoxification, long-term rehabilitation (up to 2 years), and aftercare. The latter means a lifetime of abstinence, usually aided by participation in Narcotics Anonymous or a similar self-help group.

Detoxification is the controlled and gradual withdrawal of an abused drug. Other medications

(such as chlordiazepoxide) may be given to control the effects of withdrawal and reduce the patient's discomfort and the associated risks. Depending on the abused drug, detoxification is managed on an inpatient or an outpatient basis. To minimize severe effects, chronic opiate abusers are commonly detoxified with methadone substitution. Bromocriptine (a dopamine antagonist) is sometimes given to aid cocaine detoxification.

Psychotherapy, exercise, relaxation techniques, and nutritional support may help ease withdrawal from opiates, general depressants, and other drugs. Sedatives and tranquilizers may be administered to help the patient cope with insomnia, anxiety, and depression.

After withdrawal, the patient requires rehabilitation. Inpatient and outpatient programs are available; they usually last 1 month or longer and may include individual, group, and family psychotherapy. Participation in a drug-oriented self-help group (Narcotics Anonymous, Potsmokers Anonymous, Pills Anonymous, and Cocaine Anonymous) may be helpful.

Naltrexone (Trexan) may help outpatient opiate abusers maintain abstinence. Naltrexone is most useful in a comprehensive rehabilitation program.

Nursing interventions. Patient care for drug abusers depends on the drug abused. Expect to observe the patient for signs and symptoms of withdrawal. During the patient's withdrawal from any drug, maintain a quiet, safe environment. Remove harmful objects from the room, and use restraints judiciously. Use side rails for the comatose patient. Reassure the anxious patient that medication will control withdrawal symptoms. Closely monitor visitors who might bring the patient drugs.

Control your reactions to the patient's undesirable behaviors, which commonly include dependency, manipulation, anger, frustration, and alienation. However, be sure to set limits on behavior.

Carefully monitor and promote adequate nutritional intake. Administer medications carefully to prevent hoarding by the patient. Refer the patient for detoxification and rehabilitation, as appropriate.

Patient education. Educate the patient and his family about drug abuse and dependence. Encourage participation in drug treatment programs and self-help groups. Encourage family members to seek help. Suggest private therapy or community mental health clinics.

Evaluation. For treatment to succeed, the patient and his family must be able to identify the importance of participating in counseling or self-help groups. Finally, the patient should do no harm to himself or others.

Schizophrenic disorders

Schizophrenic disorders are marked by withdrawal into self and failure to distinguish reality from fantasy. *DSM-IV* recognizes four types of

schizophrenia: paranoid, disorganized, catatonic, and residual. The different types share these essential features: presence of psychotic features during the acute phase, deterioration from a previous level of functioning, onset before age 45, and presence of symptoms for at least 6 months, with deterioration in occupational functioning, social relations, or self-care.

Schizophrenic disorders produce varying degrees of impairment and usually occur in three phases: prodromal, active, and residual. The *prodromal phase* is insidious, occurring about 1 year before the patient's first hospitalization. During this period, the patient may display signs of a loss of will, inappropriate affect, and impaired job performance. The *active phase* is characterized by psychotic symptoms, such as hallucinations and delusions. The third, *residual phase,* resembles the prodromal phase, although dulling of affect and role impairment may be severer.

As many as one-third of schizophrenic patients have just one psychotic episode and no more. Others experience repeated, acute exacerbations of the active phase. Some patients have no disability between exacerbations; others need continuous institutional care. Prognosis worsens with each acute episode.

Causes. The causes of schizophrenia are unknown, but various theories have been proposed.

Assessment findings. No single symptom or characteristic is present in all schizophrenic disorders. The subtypes differ markedly.

Paranoid schizophrenia. The patient with this disorder characteristically has persecutory or grandiose delusional thought content and auditory hallucinations. Commonly, the patient exhibits stilted formality or intensity during interactions with others. Other clinical features may include unfocused anxiety, anger, argumentativeness, and violence.

Disorganized schizophrenia. Clinical effects of this type of schizophrenia include marked incoherence; regressive, chaotic speech; flat, incongruous, or silly affect; and fragmented hallucinations and delusions. The patient may also exhibit unpredictable laughter, grimaces, mannerisms, hypochondriacal complaints, extreme social withdrawal, and regressive behavior.

Catatonic schizophrenia. These patients exhibit an inability to take care of personal needs, diminished sensitivity to painful stimuli, negativism, rigidity, and posturing. They may have rapid swings between excitement and stupor (the most common sign) or possibly extreme psychomotor agitation with excessive, senseless, or incoherent shouting or talking. This subtype commonly carries an increased potential for destructive, violent behavior.

Residual schizophrenia. While this patient doesn't exhibit prominent psychotic symptoms, he has a previous history of at least one episode of schizophrenia with prominent psychotic symptoms and continues to suffer from two or more characteristic symptoms, such as inappropriate affect, social withdrawal, eccentric behavior, or illogical thinking.

Diagnostic tests. Diagnosis of schizophrenic disorders remains difficult. The following features are important for diagnosing schizophrenic disorders: developmental background, genetic and family history, current environmental stressors, relationship of patient to interviewer, level of patient's premorbid adjustment, course of illness, impaired ability to think abstractly, affect inappropriate to context, and response to treatment.

Psychological tests may help in diagnosis, although none clearly confirms schizophrenia. The dexamethasone suppression test may be used to aid diagnosis, but some psychiatrists question its accuracy. Computed tomography and magnetic resonance imaging scans have shown enlarged ventricles in schizophrenics. The ventricular-brain ratio (VBR) determination may also support diagnosis; some studies have reported an elevated VBR ratio in schizophrenics. Other tests may be performed to rule out drug abuse or other organic disorders. MSE, psychiatric history, and careful clinical observation form the basis for diagnosis.

Treatment. The goals of treatment include equipping patients with the skills they need to live in an unrestrictive environment that offers opportunity for meaningful interpersonal relationships. Another major aim of treatment is control of this illness through continuous administration of carefully selected neuroleptic drugs. Drug treatment aims to manage both the positive and negative symptoms of schizophrenia. (See *Negative and positive symptoms of schizophrenia.*) Drug treatment should be continuous because schizophrenic patients relapse when it's discontinued. Careful monitoring is crucial because patients may develop life-threatening adverse reactions.(See *Neuroleptic malignant syndrome,* page 934.)

Clinicians disagree about the effectiveness of psychotherapy in schizophrenics. Electroconvulsive therapy (ECT) is sometimes used to treat acute schizophrenia and may be helpful when neuroleptic therapy can't be used.

Nursing interventions. Appropriate patient management depends partly on the patient's symptoms and the type of schizophrenia. (See *Spending time,* page 935.) Avoid mutual withdrawal. Express for the patient the message his nonverbal behavior seems to convey; encourage him to do so as well. Emphasize reality in all contacts to reduce distorted perceptions. Give direct, specific, and concise instructions.

Assess the catatonic schizophrenic for physical illness. Remember that the mute patient won't complain of pain or physical symptoms. If he's in a bizarre posture, he is at risk for pressure sores or decreased circulation to a body area. Provide range-of-motion exercises or walk the patient every 2 hours. During periods of

Negative and positive symptoms of schizophrenia

A person with schizophrenia may experience negative symptoms (such as the absence of joy, loss of interest) or positive symptoms (such as grandiosity). Below is a list of typical negative and positive symptoms.

Negative symptoms
- Affect flat and diminished emotional range
- Alogia
- Avolition and apathy, diminished sense of purpose and social drive
- Asocial anhedonia
- Attention impairment

Positive symptoms
- Delusions, thought disorder
- Conceptual disorganization
- Hallucinatory behavior
- Excitement
- Grandiosity
- Suspiciousness or feelings of persecution
- Hostility

hyperactivity, work to prevent physical exhaustion and injury. Your responsibilities may also include meeting the patient's needs for adequate food, fluid, exercise, and elimination. Follow orders with respect to nutrition, urinary catheterization, and enema. Stay alert for violent outbursts, and get help promptly.

Be careful not to crowd the paranoid schizophrenic patient physically or psychologically. He may strike out to protect himself. When he's

Neuroleptic malignant syndrome

Potentially life-threatening, neuroleptic malignant syndrome (NMS) may occur with neuroleptic drug therapy. Once considered rare, NMS strikes 0.5% to 1% of all patients receiving neuroleptic drugs, causing death in 20% to 30% of those affected.

Most neuroleptic drugs block dopamine, a neurotransmitter, at specific receptor sites in the brain. Usually, patients compensate by producing more dopamine. However, patients with fluid and electrolyte imbalances, nutritional deficiencies, and organic brain disorders may be able to overcome the effects of the dopamine blockade and thereby face an increased risk of developing NMS.

Hyperpyrexia constitutes the hallmark sign of NMS. Body temperature may go as high as 108° F (42.2° C). Signs and symptoms of autonomic dysfunction include hypertension, tachycardia, tachypnea, diaphoresis, and incontinence. Severe extrapyramidal symptoms, such as lead-pipe rigidity, opisthotonos, trismus, dysphagia, dyskinetic movement, and flexor-extensor posturing, may also occur. Mental status changes include delirium, mutism, stupor, and coma.

Treatment

Discontinuation of neuroleptics usually leads to recovery in 5 to 7 days. Drug therapy may include amantadine (Symmetrel), an antiviral and antiparkinsonian agent that alleviates extrapyramidal signs and hyperpyrexia, and bromocriptine (Parlodel), a dopamine agonist that counteracts dopamine blockade. Dantrolene (Dantrium), a skeletal muscle relaxant, may be given to decrease muscle contractions.

---

newly admitted, minimize contact with staff.

To help a paranoid schizophrenic patient, you need to be flexible. Allow him some control. Approach him in a calm and unhurried manner. Respond neutrally. Don't take his remarks personally. Don't try to combat his delusions with logic. Build trust; be honest and dependable. Don't threaten or make promises you can't fulfill.

Make sure the patient's nutritional needs are met. If he thinks food is poisoned, let him fix his own food when possible, or offer foods in closed containers he can open. Also monitor the patient carefully for adverse effects of neuroleptic drugs: drug-induced Parkinsonism, acute dystonia, akathisia, tardive dyskinesia, and neuroleptic malignant syndrome. Document and report adverse effects promptly.

If the patient is hallucinating, explore the content of the hallucinations. If he hears voices, find out if he thinks he must do what they command. Tell the patient you don't hear the voices, but you know they are real to him. If the patient is expressing suicidal or homicidal thoughts, institute suicide or homicide precautions. Document his behavior and your precautions. Notify the doctor and the potential victim. Document the patient's comments and who was notified.

Set limits firmly but without anger. Avoid a punitive attitude. Don't touch the patient without telling him first exactly what you're going to do. Consider postponing procedures that require physical contact with staff if the patient becomes suspicious or agitated.

The following guidelines apply to all types of schizophrenics:
• Avoid promoting dependence.
• Evaluate symptoms carefully because institutionalization may produce symptoms and disabilities that are not part of illness.
• Ask the patient to clarify private language, autistic inventions, or neologisms.
• Expect the patient to put you through a rigorous period of testing before he shows evidence of trust.
• Mobilize all resources to provide a support system for the patient to reduce his vulnerability to stress.
• Evaluate positive and negative symptoms, disorganization, and cognitive deficits.

Patient education. Distinguish adult behavior from regressive behavior; reward adult behavior. Increase the patient's sense of his own responsibility in improving his level of functioning.
• Engage the patient in reality-oriented activities, such as inpatient social skills training groups, outpatient day care, and sheltered workshops. Provide reality-based explanations for distorted body images or hypochondriacal complaints.

FOCUS ON CARING

Spending time

When working with a patient who is a catatonic schizophrenic, you'll need to spend some time with him—even if he's mute and unresponsive. The patient is acutely aware of his environment although he seems not to be. Your presence can be reassuring and supportive.

• Encourage the patient to engage in meaningful interpersonal relationships; don't avoid patient. Convey optimism about possible improvement to him.
• Encourage compliance with neuroleptic medication regimen to prevent relapse.
• Involve the patient's family in treatment; teach them symptoms associated with relapse (tension, nervousness, insomnia, decreased concentration ability, and loss of interest), and suggest ways to manage these symptoms.
• Support the patient in learning social skills.
• Active involvement in an effective psychiatric rehabilitation program is important in maintaining the patient's level of functioning.

Evaluation. Note if the patient's hallucinations and delusions have decreased and whether he spends more time focused on reality. Evaluate whether he completes his activities of daily living and takes his

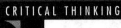

Grief, dementia, or psychosis?

Two days after admission for a serious suicide attempt, Jay Montoc, 63, says he's much better today and promises not to attempt suicide. However, he also states that he doesn't know how to go on living since his wife died 2 months ago. He says he's going crazy and that he sees things that are not there. He tells you that he followed a woman who looked like his deceased wife for several blocks, even though he knew it was unrealistic.

A problem—or not?
Questioning him, you learn that these transient hallucinations followed his wife's death and always involve seeing or hearing her. He says this is crazy because he knows she is dead. He denies and shows no evidence of any symptoms of other thought disorder. His sad mood matches his sense of loss and bereavement. You conduct a Folstein Mini Mental status examination, which is normal.

medications as ordered. (See *Grief, dementia, or psychosis?*)

Mood disorders

When a person's mood becomes so intense and persistent that it interferes with social and psychological function (and the altered mood can't be attributed to another physical or mental problem), he probably suffers from a mood disorder. Major mood disorders include bipolar and depressive disorders.

Bipolar disorder

The patient with this disorder experiences severe pathologic mood swings from euphoria to sadness. Usually, recovery is spontaneous and mood swings tend to recur. The cyclic (bipolar) form consists of separate episodes of mania (elation) and depression; however, manic or depressive episodes can be predominant, or the two moods can be mixed. When depression is the predominant mood, the patient has the unipolar form of the disease. The manic form is more prevalent in young patients, and the depressive form in older ones. Bipolar disorder recurs in 80% of patients; as they grow older, the attacks of illness recur more frequently and last longer. This illness is associated with significant mortality because of the number of depressed patients who commit suicide.

Causes. Causes are not clearly understood but are believed to be multiple and complex, and may involve genetic, biochemical, and other risk factors.

Genetic factors. Increasing evidence supports the role of genetics in transmitting bipolar disorder. Several studies implicate a dominant X-linked gene. Incidence among relatives of affected patients is higher than in the general population and highest among maternal relatives.

Biochemical factors. Just as lowered norepinephrine levels occur during an episode of depression, the opposite appears to be true during a manic episode. An excess of this biogenic amine may cause elation and euphoria. Other biochemical factors associated with mania include altered dopamine and serotonin function.

Risk factors. Although bipolar affective disorder commonly appears without identifiable predisposing factors, events that may precede the onset of illness include early loss of a parent, parental depression, incest, abuse, bereavement, disruption of an important relationship, and severe accidental injury.

Assessment findings. The manic and the depressive phases of bipolar disorder produce characteristic mood swings and other behavioral and physical changes. Before the onset of overt symptoms, many patients with this illness have an energetic and outgoing personality with a history of wide mood swings.

Depressive episode. Clinical features of this phase include loss of self-esteem, overwhelming inertia, hopelessness, withdrawal, sadness, and helplessness. Elderly patients may show poor concentration instead of sadness.

In addition, note if the patient exhibits any of the following:
• increased fatigue, difficulty sleeping
• tiredness on awakening
• anorexia, causing significant weight loss without dieting
• psychomotor retardation with slowed speech and movement and difficulty concentrating. (The patient may offer slow, one-word answers in a monotonic voice.)
• multiple somatic complaints, such as constipation, fatigue, headache, chest pains, or heaviness in the limbs. These physical symptoms may be the only clues to an elderly patient's depression.
• guilt and self-reproach over past events
• feelings of worthlessness and a belief that he's wicked and deserves to be punished.

Acute manic episode. This episode is marked by recurrent, distinct episodes of persistently euphoric, expansive, or irritable mood. It must be associated with three to four of the following symptoms that persist for at least 1 week:
• increase in social, occupational, or sexual activity with restlessness
• unusual talkativeness
• flight of ideas or the subjective experience that thoughts are racing
• inflated self-esteem, grandiosity
• decreased need for sleep
• distractibility
• excessive involvement in potentially destructive activities (gambling, shopping sprees, reckless driving). The manic patient ignores the need to eat, sleep, or relax.

Hypomania. More common than acute mania, hypomania consists of a classic triad of symptoms: elated but unstable mood, pressure of speech, and increased motor activity. Hypomania isn't associated with flight of ideas, delusions, or absence of self-control.

Other signs and symptoms include hyperactivity, easy distractibility, talkativeness, irritability, impatience, and impulsiveness and excessive involvement in pleasurable activities with high risk of painful consequences.

Diagnostic tests. Psychological tests such as rating scales of increased or decreased activity, speech, or sleep may support the diagnosis, which rests primarily on observation and psychiatric history.

Treatment. Treatment for an acute manic or depressive episode may require brief hospitalization to provide drug therapy or ECT. Fluoxetine (Prozac), monoamine oxidase (MAO) inhibitors such as phenelzine (Nardil), and tricyclic antidepressants (TCAs) such as imipramine (Tofranil) relieve depression without causing the amnesia or confusion that commonly follows ECT.

In ECT, an electric current is passed through the temporal lobe to produce a controlled grand mal seizure. An effective treatment for persistent depression, ECT is less effective in the manic phase. It's the treatment of choice for middle-aged, agitated, and suicidal patients.

Lithium therapy can dramatically relieve symptoms of mania and hypomania and may prevent recurrence of depression. Because therapeutic doses of lithium produce adverse effects in many patients, compliance may be a problem. In those who fail to respond to lithium, or to treat acute symptoms before onset of lithium effect, haloperidol (Haldol) or carbamazepine (Tegretol) may be effective. (Onset of lithium effect takes 7 to 10 days.)

Nursing interventions. Be prepared to help the patient get through both manic and depressive episodes.

Depressive episodes. The patient needs continual positive reinforcement to improve his self-esteem. Encourage him to talk or to write down his feelings. Listen attentively and respectfully and allow him time to formulate his thoughts. Provide a structured routine, including activities to promote interaction with others (for instance, group therapy), and keep reassuring him that depression will lift.

Record all observations and conversations with the patient because these records are valuable for evaluating his condition. To prevent possible self-injury or suicide, remove harmful objects from the suicidal patient's environment (glass, belts, rope, bobby pins), observe him closely, and strictly supervise his medications.

If he's too depressed to take care of his physical needs, help him.

Manic episodes. Help the patient during this phase of illness by providing emotional support, maintaining a calm environment, and setting realistic goals for behavior. Encourage short naps during the day and assist with personal hygiene. Provide diversionary activities suited to a short attention span; firmly discourage him if he tries to overextend himself. When necessary, reorient the patient to reality.

Set limits in a calm, clear, and self-confident manner in response to the manic patient's demanding, hyperactive, manipulative, and acting-out behaviors. Avoid leaving an opening for the patient to test or argue. Listen to the patient's requests attentively and with a neutral attitude, but avoid power struggles. Explain that you will consider the request seriously and will respond later. Collaborate with other staff members to provide consistent responses to the patient's acting out.

If the patient's anger escalates from verbal threats to hitting an object, tell him firmly that threats and hitting are unacceptable. Then tell him that staff will help him move to a quiet area so that he will not hurt himself or others. Staff who have practiced as a team can prevent acting-out behavior or remove and confine a patient. Alert the staff team promptly when acting-out behavior escalates. Once the incident ends and the patient regains self-control, discuss his feelings with him and offer suggestions to prevent recurrence. (See *Documenting safety measures*.)

Finally, remember the manic patient's physical needs. Encourage him to eat; he may jump up and walk around the room after every mouthful but will sit down again if you remind him.

Evaluation. Look for the patient to make fewer inappropriate requests and to control manic behavior. Assess whether he consumes adequate amounts of food and fluids.

CHARTING TIPS

Documenting safety measures

When charting about your psychiatric patient, remember to chart information regarding protection of human rights. This includes charting access to informed consent. Be sure to document that you have provided the least amount of restrictive treatment (for agitation) and ensured that patients who are restricted in any way (by restraints, for example) have adequate nourishment, activity, circulation, and bathroom breaks. For your legal protection, always document adequate safety and protection measures for the patient.

Depression

Major depression is characterized by at least one 2-week episode of depressed mood. At some point in their lives, 15% to 30% of adults are diagnosed as having major depression. Incidence is also high among patients hospitalized with medical illness.

Depression may be difficult to treat, especially in children, adolescents, elderly people, or those with a history of chronic disease, but treatment has become more effective.

Causes. The multiple causes of depression are controversial and not completely understood. Current research suggests possible genetic, familial, biochemical, physical, psychological, and social causes. In many patients, the history identifies a specific personal loss or severe stress that may trigger a person's predisposition to major depression.

Assessment findings. The primary feature of major depression is a persistent and prominent dysphoric mood, with loss of interest in usual activities, which may shift periodically to anger or anxiety.

In addition, look for at least four of the following symptoms of at least 2 weeks' duration:
• appetite disturbance (weight loss of at least 5% of body weight in a month without dieting, or significant appetite or weight increase)
• sleep disturbance (insomnia or hypersomnia)
• energy loss and fatigue
• psychomotor agitation or retardation
• feelings of worthlessness, self-reproach, excessive guilt
• difficulty in concentration, decision making, or thinking
• recurrent suicidal thoughts, suicide attempts, or death wishes.

Diagnostic tests. To support a diagnosis of depression, the doctor may use the Beck Depression Inventory and other psychological tests, the dexamethasone suppression test, and an EEG, which shows evidence of sleep disturbance.

Treatment. Primary treatment methods—psychotherapy, drug and somatic therapy (including ECT)—along with possible adjuvant therapies aim to relieve depressive symptoms. Research confirms the effectiveness of antidepressant drug therapy, which, when combined with psychotherapy, is more effective than either method alone. Drug therapy usually includes seratonin uptake inhibitors such as fluoxetine, TCAs, and less commonly, MAO inhibitors. Drug treatment may include sedatives if the patient suffers insomnia. Monitor the patient carefully to prevent hoarding of doses.

In severely depressed or suicidal patients who don't respond to other treatments, ECT may improve mood dramatically. However, ECT should be prescribed only after a complete evaluation, including history, physical examination, chest X-ray, and ECG. ECT may cause adverse effects—arrhythmias, fractures, confusion, drowsiness, memory loss (usually temporary), sluggish respirations and, occasionally, permanent memory loss or learning difficulties. Consequently, before such treatment, ECT should be discussed thoroughly with the patient and his family.

Nursing interventions. The depressed patient needs a therapeutic relationship to boost self-esteem. Encourage the patient to talk about and write down his feelings. Show him he's important by setting aside uninterrupted time each day to listen attentively, allowing time for sluggish responses. Record all observations of and conversations with the patient because they are valuable for evaluating his response to treatment. Provide a structured routine, including noncompetitive activities, to build the patient's self-confidence and encourage interaction with others.

Watch carefully for signs of suicidal ideation or intent. Ask the patient directly about thoughts of death or suicide. Such thoughts signal an immediate need for consultation and assessment. Failure to detect suicidal thoughts early may result in suicide.

If the patient is too depressed to take care of himself, help him with personal hygiene. Encourage him to eat, or feed him if necessary. Offer warm milk or back rubs at bedtime to improve sleep.

If the patient requires ECT, expect the course of treatment to include two or three treatments per week for 3 to 4 weeks. Before each ECT, give the patient a sedative, and insert a nasal or oral airway. Monitor vital signs. Offer support by talking calmly or by gently touching the patient's arm. Afterward, he may be drowsy and have transient amnesia, but he should be alert, and oriented, within 30 minutes. The period of disorientation lengthens after subsequent treatments.

Patient education. Reassure the patient that he can help ease his depression by expressing his feelings, participating in pleasurable activities, and improving grooming and hygiene. Help him avoid isolation by urging him to join noncompetitive group activities.

Evaluation. Note whether the patient reports any thoughts of death or suicide, or gives suicidal clues—especially as depression lifts.

The patient should participate in activities and improve his personal hygiene and grooming. His self-esteem and self-confidence should improve.

Anxiety disorders

When anxiety and inner conflict become overwhelming, a psychiatric disorder may develop. Types of anxiety disorders include obsessive-compulsive disorder, phobias and posttraumatic stress disorder (PTSD).

Obsessive-compulsive disorder

Obsessive thoughts and compulsive behaviors represent recurring efforts to control overwhelming anxiety, guilt, or unacceptable impulses that persistently and involuntarily enter the consciousness. Obsession refers to a recurrent idea, thought, or image. Compulsion, the action component, refers to a ritualistic, repetitive, and involuntary defensive behavior as an expression of anxiety. Compulsive behaviors are repeated because they reduce the anxiety associated with the obsession. The typical onset of this disorder is in adolescence or early adulthood.

Obsessions and compulsions cause significant distress and may severely impair occupational and social functioning. An obsessive-compulsive disorder is usually chronic, in many cases with remissions and flare-ups. The patient recognizes that his obsessions are a product of his own mind, and the patient's description of his own behavior may offer the best clue to this diagnosis. However, the patient also needs evaluation for other physical or psychiatric disorders. The prognosis is better than average when symptoms are quickly identified, diagnosed, and treated, and when the patient can recognize and adjust environmental stress.

Causes. Researchers have not uncovered a single cause for obsessive-compulsive disorder. Some studies suggest the possibility of brain lesions, but the most useful research and clinical studies point to an explanation based on psychological theories.

Research shows that obsessive-compulsive children are conformist, excessively mature, and try too hard to please adults.

Behaviorists see obsessive-compulsive disorder as a conditioned response to anxiety-provoking events. Associating anxiety with a neutral object or event causes obsessional preoccupation. Compulsive behavior is also learned and reinforced. In the past, such behavior helped control the person's anxiety, so he practices it again, even though it's no longer helpful.

Major depression, organic brain syndrome, and schizophrenia may contribute to the onset of obsessive-compulsive disorder.

Assessment findings. Compulsive actions may be simple, mild, and uncomplicated or dramatic, elaborately complex, and ritualized. Their meanings may be obvious or may reflect inner psychological distortions that are unraveled only through intensive psychotherapy.

The patient's anxiety may be so strong that he will avoid the situation or the object that evokes his compulsion. Common compulsions include the following: repetitive touching, doing and undoing (opening and closing doors, rearranging things), washing (especially hands), and checking (to be sure no tragedy has occurred).

When the obsessive-compulsive phenomena are mental, they may go undetected unless the patient reveals them. The obsessive patient may have repeated thoughts of violence or contamination or constant worry about a tragic event.

Treatment. Treatment of obsessive-compulsive states aims to reduce anxiety, resolve inner conflicts, relieve depression, and teach more effective ways of dealing with stress. Such treatment (especially during an acute episode) typically includes drug therapy using tranquilizing and antidepressant drugs such as fluoxetine and behavorial therapy. Clomipramine (Anafranil) is indicated for the treatment of obsessive-compulsive disorder. Intensive long-term psychotherapy, brief supportive psychotherapy, behavior therapy, and group therapy have also been effective.

Nursing interventions. Patient care should focus on reducing the associated anxiety, fears, and guilt; building self-esteem; and helping him understand how compulsive behavior releases anxiety.

Create an atmosphere for open discussion; don't show shock or criticism of the ritualistic behavior. Approach the patient unhurriedly. Encourage him to express his anxious feelings. Explore the patterns leading to the behavior or recurring problems. Identify disturbing topics of conversation that reflect underlying anxiety or terror. Listen attentively and offer feedback.

Help the patient learn new ways of behaving. Encourage use of appropriate defense mechanisms to relieve loneliness and isolation. Engage the patient in activities that will raise his self-esteem and confidence. Encourage diversionary activities such as listening to music.

Allow the patient time to carry out the ritualistic behavior (unless it is dangerous) until he can be distracted into some other activity. Set limits on unacceptable behavior (for example, limit the number of times per day he may indulge in compulsive behavior). Gradually shorten the time allowed. Help him focus on other feelings or problems for the rest of the time.

Help the patient identify progress and set realistic expectations. Evaluate behavioral changes and encourage the patient to do the same. Keep your demands on him reasonable. Avoid creating situations that increase frustration.

Be flexible; observe which interventions do and don't work. Find ways to deal with the frustration that the patient arouses in you.

Keep the patient's physical health in mind. For example, compulsive hand washing may cause skin breakdown, and rituals or preoccu-

pations may cause inadequate food and fluid intake and exhaustion.

Patient education. Explain how to channel emotional energy to relieve stress (through such activities as sports and creative endeavors).

Evaluation. Assess whether the patient has adequately expressed his feelings and frustrations. Look for compulsive behaviors to decrease and for demonstration of new problem-solving strategies.

Posttraumatic stress disorder

PTSD involves the psychological consequences of a traumatic event. PTSD can be acute, chronic, or delayed and can follow a natural disaster (flood, tornado), a man-made event (war, imprisonment, torture, car accidents, incest, large fires), an assault, or a rape.

Causes. In most people with PTSD, the stressor is a necessary but insufficient cause of the persisting symptoms. Psychological, physical, genetic, and social factors may also contribute to PTSD.

Risk factors. Very young and very old people have more difficulty coping with traumatic events. Pre-existing psychopathology can also predispose a patient to PTSD.

Assessment findings. Characteristic symptoms that persist after unusual trauma confirm this diagnosis. The patient experiences recurrent, intrusive recollections or nightmares, or psychological distress at exposure to events that symbolize trauma. Other

ALTERNATIVE THERAPY

Yoga

Yoga is a form of mind-body medicine that uses exercise (postures and coordinated breathing techniques) and meditation to achieve physical and mental self-discipline. The postures help the person develop strength and flexibility by using all the muscles in the body, increasing circulation, and stretching and aligning the spinal column. Breathing exercises and meditation help reduce stress and anxiety.

symptoms include sleep disturbances, chronic anxiety or panic attacks, memory impairment, guilt, difficulty concentrating, and feelings of detachment that destroy interpersonal relationships.

Assess also for headaches, depression, suicidal thoughts, rage, and use of violence to solve problems, persistent avoidance of stimuli associated with trauma, and diminished general responsiveness. Onset may be delayed, acute, or chronic.

Diagnostic tests. A psychiatric examination should include an MSE and tests for organic impairment and should focus on other syndromes that accompany PTSD, such as depression, generalized anxiety, and phobia.

Treatment. Goals of treatment include reducing the target symptoms, preventing chronic disability, and promoting occupational and social rehabilitation. Specific treatment may emphasize behavioral techniques (relaxation therapy to decrease anxiety and induce sleep, or progressive desensitization); antianxiety and antidepressant drugs; or brief or ongoing psychotherapy to minimize the risks of dependency and chronicity.

Many Veterans Administration centers serve those traumatized by Vietnam and other wars, and crisis clinics run highly effective support groups. In group settings, victims of PTSD can work through their feelings with others who have had similar conflicts. Group settings are appropriate for most degrees of symptoms presented. Some group programs include spouses and families in their treatment process. Rehabilitation in physical, social, and occupational areas is also available for those with chronic PTSD. Many patients need treatment for depression, alcohol and drug abuse, or medical conditions before psychological healing can take place. (For information on one alternative therapy, see *Yoga*.)

Nursing interventions. The goal of intervention is to encourage the victim of PTSD to complete the mourning process so that he can go on with his life. Keep in mind that such a patient tends to sharply test your commitment and interest. First examine your feelings about the event (war or other trauma). Expressing disdain or shock may reinforce the patient's poor self-image and sense of guilt.

Follow these guidelines:
• Know and practice crisis intervention techniques as appropriate.
• Establish trust by accepting the patient's level of functioning and by assuming a positive, consistent, and nonjudgmental attitude.
• Help the patient to regain control by identifying situations in which he lost control and by talking about past and precipitating events (conceptual labeling) to help with later problem-solving skills.
• Praise the patient who commits to working on his problem.
• Deal constructively with anger. Identify how anger escalates, and explore preventive measures that family members can take to help the patient regain control. Provide a safe, staff-monitored room in which the patient can deal with violent urges by displacement (such as pounding and throwing clay.) Encourage him to move from physical to verbal expressions of anger.
• Relieve shame and guilt precipitated by real actions—such as killing and mutilation—through clarification (put behavior into perspective), atonement (help the patient realize that social isolation and self-destructive behavior are not valid methods of repentance), and restitution (have clergy help him conquer guilt, once the patient learns to accept authority and trust others).
• Encourage the patient to express feelings of survivor guilt.

Patient education. Refer the patient to group therapy with other victims and to appropriate community resources. Encourage patients who abuse drugs to participate in chemical dependency programs.

Evaluation. Look for the patient to safely express feelings of shame, guilt, and anger. He should demonstrate an improved ability to relax; assess for evidence of improved memory and sleep as well as attempts to reestablish relationships.

Somatoform disorders

The patient with a somatoform disorder complains of physical symptoms, but the organic basis for these symptoms remains elusive.

Somatization disorder

In somatization disorder, the patient experiences multiple signs and symptoms that suggest a physical disorder, but no verifiable disease or pathophysiologic condition exists to account for them. Commonly, the patient with somatization disorder undergoes repeated medical evaluations, which can be potentially damaging and debilitating. Unlike the hypochondriac, he isn't preoccupied with the belief that he has a specific disease. Exacerbations occur during times of stress.

Causes. This disorder has no specific cause. Its symptoms can begin or worsen after recent unemployment, a disruption in personal relationships, or other loss.

Assessment findings. The essential feature of this disorder is the pattern of recurrent, multiple symptoms and complaints that have no apparent physical basis and that have persisted for at least 6 months. These complaints can involve any body system but most commonly involve the GI tract, the neurologic system, or the cardiopulmonary system. (See *Symptoms of somatization disorder.*)

Diagnostic tests. No specific test or procedure verifies somatization disorder. Diagnostic evaluation should rule out physical causes that may produce vague, confusing symptoms, such as multiple sclerosis, hypothyroidism, systemic lupus erythematosus, or porphyria. Psychological evaluation may rule out depression, schizophrenia with somatic delusions, hypochondriasis, psychogenic pain, and malingering.

Treatment. Rather than eradicate the patient's symptoms, treatment seeks to help him learn to live with them. After diagnostic evaluation has ruled out organic causes, the patient should be told that he has no serious illness but will receive care to ease his symptoms.

Most important, the patient needs a continuing, supportive relationship with a sympathetic health care provider—someone who acknowledges the patient's symptoms. The patient should have regularly scheduled appointments for review of symptoms and basic physical evaluation and, above all else, assessment of his coping skills. Follow-up appointments should last approximately 20 to 30 minutes and should focus on new symptoms or any change in old symptoms to avoid missing a developing physical disease. As many as 30% of patients initially diagnosed with somatization disorder eventually develop an organic disease. Patients with somatization disorder rarely acknowledge any psychological aspect of their illness.

Nursing interventions. Acknowledge the patient's symptoms and support his efforts to function and cope despite distress. Under no circumstances should you tell the patient his symptoms are imaginary. But do tell him the results and meanings of tests. Gently point out the time relation between stress and physical symptoms.

Remember, your job is to help the patient to manage stress, not get rid of symptoms. Often, his interpersonal relationships are linked to his symptoms. Remedying the symptoms can impair his interactions with others.

Patient education. Develop a plan of care with some input from the patient and his family. Encourage and help them to understand his need for troublesome symptoms.

Evaluation. The patient should demonstrate an improved ability to ease stress and relax. He should be able to describe the relation between his symptoms and stress.

Symptoms of somatization disorder

Cardiopulmonary symptoms
• Shortness of breath (without exertion)
• Palpitations
• Chest pain
• Dizziness

GI symptoms
• Abdominal pain (excluding menstruation)
• Nausea and vomiting (excluding motion sickness)
• Flatulence
• Diarrhea
• Intolerance to foods

Female reproductive symptoms
• Irregular menses
• Excessive menstrual bleeding
• Vomiting throughout pregnancy

Pseudoneurologic symptoms
• Amnesia

• Dysphagia
• Loss of voice or hearing
• Double or blurred vision
• Blindness
• Fainting or loss of consciousness
• Seizures
• Difficulty walking, weakness, or paralysis
• Urine retention or dysuria

Pain
• In extremities
• In back
• During urination

Sexual symptoms
• Burning sensation in sexual organs or rectum (except during intercourse)
• Sexual indifference
• Dyspareunia or lack of pleasure during sex
• Impotence

Hypochondriasis

The patient with hypochondriasis misinterprets the severity and significance of physical signs or sensations. This leads to a preoccupation with having a serious disease, which persists despite medical reassurance to the contrary. Hypochondriasis meets his needs by allowing him to assume a dependent sick role. He remains unaware of this benefit and isn't consciously causing his symptoms. Hypochondriasis causes severe social and occupational impairment.

Hypochondriasis may lead health care providers to overlook a serious organic disease, given the patient's previously unfounded complaints. Significant complications or disabilities may result from multiple evaluations, tests, and invasive procedures.

Causes. Hypochondriasis isn't linked to any specific cause; however, it commonly develops in people or relatives of those who have experienced an organic disease.

Assessment findings. The dominant feature of hypochondriasis is the misinterpretation of symptoms—usually multiple complaints that involve a single organ system—as signs of serious illness; however, as medical evaluation proceeds, complaints may shift and change. Symptoms can range from specific to general, vague complaints and may reflect a preoccupation with normal body functions.

Diagnostic tests. Projective psychological testing may show a preoccupation with somatic concerns; however, a complete history, including emphasis on current psychological stresses, provides the basis for diagnosis. Diagnostic tests may be performed to rule out underlying organic disease, but invasive procedures should be kept to a minimum.

Treatment. Interventions seek to help the patient lead a productive life despite distressing symptoms and fears. After medical evaluation is complete, inform the patient that he doesn't have a serious disease, but that continued medical follow-up will help control his symptoms. Providing a diagnosis will not make hypochondriasis disappear, but it may ease some anxiety.

Regular outpatient follow-up can help the patient deal with his symptoms and is necessary to detect organic illness. As many as 30% of these patients later develop an organic disease. Unfortunately, because the patient can be quite demanding and irritating, consistent follow-up commonly proves difficult. Usually, these patients resist psychiatric treatment.

Nursing interventions. Create a supportive relationship that helps the patient feel cared for and understood. The patient with hypochondriasis feels real pain and distress; don't deny his symptoms. Instead, help him find new ways to deal with stress other than development of physical symptoms. Recognize that the patient will probably never be symptom-free.

Patient education. If the patient is receiving a tranquilizer, both he and his family should know dosages, expected effects, and possible adverse effects (for example, drowsiness, fatigue, blurred vision, and hypotension). Warn the patient to avoid alcohol or other CNS depressants. Warn him to take the drug only as prescribed to prevent dependence; to avoid hazardous tasks until he has developed a tolerance to the tranquilizer's sedative effects; and to continue the tranquilizer as directed because abrupt withdrawal may be hazardous.

Help the patient learn strategies (such as imagery, relaxation, hypnosis, and massage) to reduce distress.

Evaluation. Look for the patient to reduce his level of stress and to identify possible adverse effects.

Personality disorders

In personality disorders, a patient displays a chronic pattern of inflexible, maladaptive traits that influence his affect, cognition, behavior, and style of interacting with others. These disorders cause severe emotional distress and impair social and occupational function. Usually, patients don't receive treatment;

when they do, it's managed on an outpatient basis. Essential to diagnosis is the patient's history that shows maladaptive personality traits as characteristic of lifelong behavior.

Causes. Only recently have personality disorders been categorized in detail, and research continues to identify their causes. Various theories attempt to explain their origin, including biological, social, and psychodynamic theories.

Assessment findings. Signs and symptoms of personality disorders differ according to the diagnosis: paranoid, schizoid, compulsive, passive-aggressive, borderline, histrionic, and narcissistic. They differ among people and within the same person at different times.

Diagnostic tests. Psychological evaluation must rule out other psychiatric disorders. The major feature of this disorder is the person's long-term pattern of functioning.

Treatment. Measures depend on individual symptoms, but all patients require a trusting relationship with a therapist. Drug therapy is usually ineffective but may help to relieve acute anxiety or depression. Family and group therapy usually proves effective. Inpatient milieu therapy in crisis situations and possibly for long-term treatment of borderline personality disorders may be effective. Inpatient treatment remains controversial, however, because patients with personality disorders tend to be noncompliant.

Nursing interventions. Keep in mind that many of these patients don't respond well to interviewing, whereas others are charming masters of deceit. Offer patient, persistent, consistent, and flexible care. Take a direct, involved approach to ensure the patient's trust.

Nursing goals for the patient with a personality disorder include teaching social skills; reinforcing appropriate behavior; setting limits on inappropriate behavior; encouraging expression of feelings, self-analysis of behavior, and accountability; and helping the patient seek appropriate employment.

Evaluation. Look for the patient to demonstrate improved social skills, increased self-esteem, and respect for reasonable limits on behavior.

Eating disorders

Patients with bulimia and anorexia nervosa—primarily women—need help to overcome psychological obstacles to healthful eating.

Bulimia

Patients with bulimia go on repeated eating binges. Typically, they induce vomiting so that they may eat more. Other clinical features include diuretic or laxative abuse, excessive sleep, vigorous exercise, and strict dieting or fasting. Patients with bulimia are obsessed with body shape and weight. Afraid of losing control, they become depressed after a binge-purge episode.

This disorder primarily begins in adolescence or early adulthood. In men, bulimia usually occurs among those involved in sports or physical training.

Causes. The cause of bulimia remains unknown, but psychosocial factors that probably contribute to its development include family disturbance or conflict, maladaptive learned behavior, struggle for control or self-identity, cultural overemphasis on physical appearance, and weight requirements associated with competitive activities such as gymnastics. Recent psychiatric theory considers bulimia a syndrome of depression.

Assessment findings. Cardinal symptoms include episodic binge eating (as often as several times a day) and purging through vomiting, laxatives, or diuretics. Purging allows the patient to feel in control of food intake and allows eating to continue. Assess for frequent weight fluctuations, although purging and exercise usually keep weight within normal range.

Other characteristic features include an excessive exercise schedule, a distorted body image, bad breath or sweet breath from mouthwash, and feelings of despair, hopelessness and worthlessness, guilt, anxiety, or low self-esteem. Also look for enlarged lymph glands in the neck, gingival or dental problems, and pruritus ani.

Diagnostic tests. Bulimia is seldom confused with any other physical disorder. Laboratory tests may rule out hypokalemia or alkalosis associated with electrolyte imbalances or dehydration.

Treatment. The patient with bulimia knows that her eating pattern is abnormal but can't control it. Therefore, interventions focus on breaking the binge-purge cycle and helping the patient regain control over eating behavior. Usually performed on an outpatient basis, treatment includes behavior modification therapy, possibly in highly structured psychoeducational group meetings. The patient may also undergo individual psychotherapy and family therapy, which address the eating disorder as a symptom of unresolved conflict. The doctor may order antidepressant drugs such as imipramine. The patient may also benefit from self-help groups such as Overeaters Anonymous.

Nursing interventions. Help the patient regain control over eating behavior by encouraging her to keep a daily record of everything she has eaten, to eat only at mealtimes, and only at the table, and to reduce her access to food by limiting choice or quantity. You can also help her develop more adaptive coping skills. Encourage her to express feelings, reinforce her realistic perceptions about weight and appearance, and urge her to participate in therapy.

Patient education. Recommend the American Anorexia/Bulimia Association and Anorexia Nervosa and

Related Eating Disorders, Inc., as sources of additional information and community support.

Evaluation. Assess whether the patient realizes that social and family pressures influence eating disorders. Look for signs of increased control of eating and binge-purge behavior.

Anorexia nervosa

Anorexia nervosa is characterized by self-imposed starvation and consequent emaciation, nutritional deficiencies, and atrophic changes. The patient may gorge, vomit, and purge during starvation or after returning to normal weight. Primarily affecting adolescent and young adult females, anorexia nervosa also affects older women and occasionally affects males. It usually develops in a patient who's of normal weight or only about 5 lb (2.3 kg) overweight.

Mortality ranges from 5% to 15%, the highest mortality associated with a psychological disturbance.

Causes. The cause is unknown. Clearly, however, social attitudes that equate slimness with beauty play a role in this disorder. Other emotional factors may contribute as well.

Assessment findings. Cardinal symptoms include a 25% or greater weight loss coupled with a compulsion to be thin. The patient may engage in ritualistic behavior or restless activity, such as exercising avidly without apparent fatigue. She frequently becomes angry. Despite evidence to the contrary, she believes that she is fat. Note any indications of despair, hopelessness, guilt, anxiety, low self-esteem, or depression.

The patient's systolic blood pressure may fall below 50 mm Hg, signaling circulatory collapse, and she may develop cardiac arrhythmias, possibly leading to cardiac arrest.

Diagnostic tests. Laboratory data are usually normal unless weight loss exceeds 30%. Initial blood tests include complete blood count (CBC), creatinine, BUN, uric acid, total serum cholesterol value, total serum protein, albumin, electrolytes (sodium, potassium, chloride, bicarbonate), calcium, AST and ALT, and fasting blood glucose measurements. The doctor may also order urinalysis and an ECG.

Treatment. Measures aim to promote weight gain and control the patient's compulsive gorging and purging, and to correct starvation symptoms. The patient may require inpatient treatment in a medical or psychiatric health care facility. Inpatient treatment may be as brief as 2 weeks or may stretch from a few months to 2 years or longer. Results are often discouraging. Many clinical centers are now developing inpatient and outpatient programs. However, interventions must wait until the patient has achieved normal weight and hydration, and greater emotional stability.

Treatment approaches may include behavior modification; curtailing activity for physical reasons (such as cardiac arrhythmias); vitamin and mineral supplements; a reasonable diet, with or without liquid supplements; hyperalimentation (subclavian, peripheral, or enteral); and group or family therapy or individual psychotherapy.

To be successful, therapy should address the patient's underlying problems of low self-esteem, guilt, and anxiety; feelings of hopelessness and helplessness; and depression. Most therapists consider task-centered approaches and therapeutic flexibility important requirements for success.

Nursing interventions. During hospitalization, regularly monitor vital signs and intake and output. Weigh the patient weekly, if possible, before she has eaten breakfast or dressed. Check the patient's body orifices before weighing. However, because many patients fear being weighed, be flexible with your routine.

Meet the patient's nutritional needs. Frequently offer small portions of food or drinks, if she wants them. She may accept nutritionally complete liquids more readily.

Reassure her that any edema or bloating is temporary. Express understanding of her anxiety.

Encourage the patient to recognize and assert her feelings freely. She may gradually learn that expressing her true feelings won't result in her losing control or love. Be patient in your dealings with her. Remember, the anorexic patient uses exercise, preoccupation with food, ritualism, manipulation, and lying as mechanisms that preserve the only control she feels she has.

Her family may need therapy to change their behavior. Advise them to avoid discussing food with her. Try to establish an agreement between the patient, her family, and her therapist on who should monitor her weight.

Patient education. If tube feedings become necessary, explain them to the patient. Discuss her need for food matter-of-factly. Point out that improved nutrition can correct abnormal laboratory findings.

Refer the patient and her family to Anorexia Nervosa and Related Eating Disorders, Inc., a national support organization.

Evaluation. The patient should express her feelings with the staff and begin to establish healthier relationships with her family. Her eating patterns and weight should stabilize.

TREATMENTS

The nurse's role in helping emotionally troubled people has grown considerably. Besides carrying out the traditional task of administering drugs and monitoring their effects, nurses may act as primary therapists in milieu therapy or may direct behavior therapies.

This section discusses drug therapy, psychotherapy, detoxification, and ECT.

Drug therapy

Many drugs used to treat psychiatric disorders require changes in dosage and careful monitoring. Antidepressant drugs include tricyclic antidepressants (such as amitriptyline and doxepin), heterocyclics (such as amoxapine and bupropion), MAO inhibitors (such as isocarboxazid and tranylcypromine), and the phenylpropylamine derivative fluoxetine. Other common psychiatric drugs include benzodiazepines such as alprazolam and chlordiazepoxide to treat anxiety and tension as well as acute alcohol withdrawal, antipsychotics (phenothiazines) such as chlorpromazine and mesoridazine to treat psychotic disorders, butyrophenones such as haloperidol and thiothixene to treat psychotic disorders and acute agitation, and selective serotonin reuptake inhibitors such as fluvoxamine maleate to treat obsessive-compulsive or personality disorders.

Counseling

Types of counseling include psychotherapy, behavior therapy, and milieu therapy.

Psychotherapy

The psychological treatment of mental and emotional disorders involves a range of approaches. Regardless of the approach, most types of psychotherapy aim to change a patient's attitudes, feelings, or behavior.

The success of therapy depends largely on the compatibility between patient and therapist, the treatment goals selected, and the patient's commitment.

Individual therapy. This type of therapy requires a series of counseling sessions and may be short- or long-term. It involves mutually agreed-upon goals, with the therapist mediating the patient's disturbed patterns of behavior to promote development.

Cognitive therapy. This therapy aims to identify and change patients' negative generalizations and expectations to reduce depression or distress. Cognitive theory states that depression stems from the patient's belief that the future is bleak and hopeless. Cognitive therapists assign homework that includes making lists of pleasurable activities and reducing automatic negative thoughts and conclusions.

Group therapy. Guided by a psychotherapist, a group of people experiencing similar emotional problems meet to discuss their concerns with one another. Duration varies from a few weeks to several years. Group therapy is especially useful in treating addictions.

Family therapy. The goal here is to alter relationships within the family and to change problematic behavior of one or more members. Useful in treating adjustment disorders of childhood or adolescence, marital discord, and abuse, family therapy may be short- or long-term.

Crisis intervention. This type of therapy seeks to help the patient develop adequate coping skills to resolve an immediate, pressing problem. The crisis can be a developmental one (such as a marriage or death) or a situational one (such as an illness). Therapy seeks to restore the previous level of functioning and may include family members. Therapy may last from 1 session to 6 months.

Patient preparation. Review the patient's psychiatric history, treatment history, and current psychiatric status to help assess his needs. Explain the therapeutic techniques to him and help him establish a treatment goal.

You'll probably share patient information with the treatment team or therapist. Maintain confidentiality unless the patient plans to harm himself or someone else.

Monitoring and aftercare. Observe the patient for signs of increased distress, depression, anxiety, and restlessness. If the patient feels uncomfortable with therapy, he may display loss of appetite, irritability, or insomnia. Reassure the patient that talking about his feelings will help relieve distress. Also explain that he may feel worse during the early stages of treatment because he is facing frustration and conflict. Reinforce any gains that he has made.

Patient education. If appropriate, refer the patient to a self-help group. Instruct him to contact his therapist if symptoms recur.

Behavior therapy

Behavior therapy assumes that problem behaviors are learned and, through special training, can be unlearned. Unlike psychotherapy, it tends to de-emphasize the patient's thoughts and feelings about them.

The behavioral approach relies on a cluster of therapies, rather than on just one, to change a behavioral pattern. Commonly used therapies include desensitization, assertiveness training, flooding, token economy, positive conditioning, and social skills training. Suitable for adults or children, behavior therapies can be used for individuals or for groups.

Behavior therapies may use different techniques, such as positive or negative reinforcement, shaping, modeling, punishment, or extinction. *Positive reinforcement* increases the likelihood of a desirable behavior being repeated by promptly praising or rewarding the patient. In contrast, *negative reinforcement* involves the removal of a negative stimulus only after the patient provides a desirable response. *Shaping* initially rewards any behavior that resembles the desirable one. Then, step by step, the behavior required to gain a reward becomes progressively closer to the desired behavior. *Modeling* provides a reward when the patient imitates the desired behavior. *Punishment* discourages problem behavior by inflicting a penalty such as temporary removal of a privilege. *Extinction* is a technique that simply ignores undesirable behavior—provided, of course, that the behavior isn't dangerous. Depending on his beliefs and training, the therapist selects one or more behavioral therapies for the patient or group.

Patient preparation. Before therapy begins, determine whether the patient is amenable to the behavioral approach. Consider his age, intellectual function, and mental status. Review with the therapist which behavior requires alteration and why.

Counsel the patient about which behaviors need changing, the goals of therapy, and the techniques used to accomplish them. Make clear exactly what's expected of him and what he can expect from the staff.

Monitoring and aftercare. Monitor the patient throughout therapy, reinforcing acceptable behaviors, and discouraging unacceptable ones. If unacceptable behaviors persist, inform the therapist. He may need to try another technique.

Patient education. If appropriate, teach the patient's family the basic techniques used to correct problem behaviors. Recommend an outpatient therapist to reinforce desirable behaviors and to respond to patient or family problems or questions. Remember that family members, friends, coworkers, and community members may tolerate problem behavior or feel reluctant to interfere.

Milieu therapy

Milieu therapy uses the patient's environment as a tool for overcoming mental and emotional disorders. The patient's surroundings become a therapeutic community, with the patient himself involved in planning, implementing, and evaluating his treatment as well as in sharing with staff and other patients the responsibility for establishing group rules and policies. This helps the patient learn to interact appropriately with staff and other patients. Staff usually wear street clothes instead of uniforms, keep units unlocked, and run activities in a community room, which is the center for meetings, recreation, and meals. Staff also provide individual, group, and occupational therapy.

Patient preparation. Explain the purpose of milieu therapy to the patient, stating your expectations and how he can participate in the therapeutic community. Orient him to the community's routines. Introduce him to other patients and staff.

Monitoring and aftercare. Regularly evaluate the patient's symptoms and therapeutic needs. Oversee his activities, encouraging him to keep a schedule typical of life outside the health care facility. Also encourage him to interact with others. Point out the importance of respecting others and his environment.

Patient education. If the patient returns to the outside community, encourage him to keep follow-up appointments with his therapist.

Other therapies

Other important psychiatric treatments include detoxification programs and ECT. (For an introduction to an alternative therapy, see *Chinese therapy,* page 956.)

ALTERNATIVE THERAPY

Chinese therapy

In Chinese medicine, depression is viewed as a disharmony resulting from emotional and physical reactions to outside stimuli, and the treatment involves correcting these imbalances. Recommended approaches include dietary assessment and alterations, exercise and meditation, acupuncture or acupressure, and combination herbal therapy.

For other disharmonies, such as anxiety and stress, the Chinese healer prescribes different recommendations for diet, exercise, and meditation. Similarly, different meridian points are selected for acupuncture and acupressure. Chinese medicine also specifies particular herbs used in herbal therapy to treat anxiety.

Detoxification

Chinese medicine recommends a comprehensive program of detoxification to assist people in breaking free from their dependency on substances, whether that substance is caffeine, food, heroin, or cocaine. The comprehensive program includes three stages of detoxification: acute, short-term, and long-term. The program begins with a careful assessment to determine what damage has occurred to the person and the nature of the imbalance within the body-spiritual-emotional domains of the person. Specific corrective actions are prescribed to help the person reestablish and maintain harmony.

Detoxification

Detoxification programs offer a relatively safe alternative to self-withdrawal after prolonged dependence on alcohol or drugs. Performed in outpatient centers or in special units, these programs provide symptomatic treatment as well as counseling or psychotherapy on an individual, group, or family basis.

Alcohol withdrawal, requiring total abstinence, usually proves severer and potentially deadlier than drug withdrawal. Its symptoms vary from morning hangover in mild alcoholism to alcohol withdrawal syndrome (also known as delirium tremens), a condition of severe distress marked by menacing hallucinations, gross uncontrollable tremors, extreme restlessness, vomiting, profuse diaphoresis, and elevated pulse rate and blood pressure.

To help the patient through withdrawal, the doctor gradually lowers the dosage of the abused drug or substitutes a drug with similar action; for example, he may substitute methadone for heroin or treat cocaine addiction with bromocriptine or naltrexone. If these options aren't available, treatment is supportive and symptomatic.

Treating patients undergoing detoxification requires skill and compassion. Because substance abusers commonly try to manipulate people, you'll need to control your feelings of frustration.

Preparation. If the patient is in acute distress, arrange for immediate treatment. Otherwise, perform a psychosocial evaluation to examine his family and social life. The patient will probably rationalize or minimize his abuse. If possible, substantiate what he tells you with family members or friends. Assess the patient's level of motivation and the support systems available to him.

Next, take a medical history to find out if the patient has a history of any psychiatric disorder, prior drug or alcohol abuse treatment, seizures, or delirium. The doctor will probably order a neurologic workup as well as a urinalysis, CBC, liver function tests, serum electrolyte and glucose levels, and a chest X-ray. Obtain urine and blood samples for alcohol and drug screening to provide information on the most recent ingestion. Medical and psychosocial evaluations help determine appropriate treatment and decide whether it should be provided on an inpatient or outpatient basis.

Procedure. If the patient is in acute distress, provide a quiet, softly lit environment to avoid overstimulation and agitation. Remove any potentially harmful objects.

If the patient is experiencing alcohol withdrawal syndrome, give antianxiety agents, anticonvulsants, and antidiarrheals or antiemetics, as ordered. Monitor his mental status, vital signs, and lung sounds every 30 minutes. Orient him to reality because he may be having hallucinations. If he's combative or disoriented, restrain him. Take seizure and suicide precautions. If ordered, give I.V. glucose for fluid replacement and hypoglycemia, and thi-

amine and other B-complex vitamins for nutritional deficiencies.

If the patient is undergoing opioid withdrawal, detoxify him with methadone, as ordered. To ease withdrawal from opioids, depressants, and other drugs, provide nutritional support, suggest mild exercise, and teach relaxation techniques. If appropriate, temporarily administer sedatives or tranquilizers.

After withdrawal from alcohol or drugs, the patient needs rehabilitation to prevent recurrence of abuse. For the alcoholic, rehabilitation may include aversion therapy, using a daily oral dose of disulfiram, and supportive counseling or individual, group, or family psychotherapy. For the drug abuser, rehabilitation may include psychotherapy.

Monitoring and aftercare. Encourage the patient's participation in rehabilitation programs and self-help groups. Be alert for any continued substance abuse after admission to the detoxification program. Carefully administer any prescribed medications to prevent hoarding by the patient, and closely monitor visitors, who might bring the patient drugs or alcohol. If you suspect any abuse, obtain a blood and urine sample for screening and report any positive findings to the doctor. Obtain urine samples for screening whenever the patient returns to the facility from an off-premises visit.

Observe the patient for signs of infection. Also watch for signs of vitamin deficiency and malnutrition. With the dietitian's help, ensure that the patient maintains an adequate diet. Offer bland foods if he experiences GI distress.

Patient education. To prevent relapse, encourage professional and family support after the patient leaves the detoxification program. Emphasize the benefits of joining an appropriate self-help group, such as AA or Narcotics Anonymous. Recommend that the spouse or mature children accompany the patient to group meetings. Also, refer the family to a support group, if necessary. Stress to the patient that he ultimately must accept responsibility for avoiding abused substances.

Electroconvulsive therapy

Also referred to as electroshock therapy, ECT was first introduced in 1937 as the primary intervention for all types of emotional disorders. Early misuse (because of ignorance or the unavailability of proper anesthesia) resulted in severe memory loss, fractures, and death.

Today, ECT is recognized as a legitimate treatment for major depression when medication is contraindicated or faster onset is warranted. It's also used for acute mania and, less commonly, for acute short-term schizophrenia with affective symptoms when psychotropic drugs are ineffective. The number of treatments varies with the disorder's severity and the patient's response; however, the patient usually receives two or three treatments a week, with an interval of 48 hours between sessions.

In ECT, an electrical stimulus travels through electrodes placed on the patient's temples, causing a generalized tonic-clonic seizure. The resulting seizure reduces hypothalamic stress and stimulates biogenic amine metabolism.

Although, in rare cases, ECT can cause arrhythmias and even death, untreated depression carries a higher mortality risk because of suicide. However, ECT is contraindicated in recent myocardial infarction with cardiac decompensation, CNS tumors, organic brain syndrome, and aortic aneurysm. This treatment should be used cautiously during pregnancy and old age and in patients with glaucoma, confusion, or cardiac disease.

Patient preparation. Explain the treatment to the patient and family, including its risks, its expected effects, and the use of anesthesia. Correct any misconceptions and allow them to voice their fears and hopes. Prepare the patient for a complete physical examination and EEG.

Stop any psychotropic drugs the day before ECT to prevent any interactions. Restrict foods and fluids after midnight to prevent aspiration while under anesthesia. Just before ECT, ask the patient to void. If he wears dentures, ask him to remove them. Make sure that emergency resuscitation equipment is available.

Monitoring and aftercare. After the patient awakens, assist him to get dressed and help orient him. Call him by name, and let him know that the treatment is complete. Reassure him as necessary. Until he becomes oriented, keep the bed's side rails raised. Check the patient's vital signs until they return to normal. Also monitor cardiac rhythm.

Ask the patient if he's experiencing headache or nausea. If he reports discomfort, give analgesics or antinausea drugs, as ordered.

Patient education. If the patient receives ECT as an outpatient, make sure a family member or companion provides transportation home. Inform him that he mustn't drive or operate machinery until confusion and drowsiness completely subside. He may resume his daily activities only when he feels physically able.

Remind the family or companion that temporary anterograde and retrograde amnesia and mild confusion can occur after ECT. These symptoms usually diminish or disappear within 8 weeks. Tell the family or companion not to leave the patient alone until his confusion has subsided. Once home, the patient needs the support of his family. Encourage them to make sure the patient follows the doctor's orders and keeps follow-up appointments.

REFERENCES AND READINGS

Coyne, A.C., et al. "The Relationship Between Dementia and Elder Abuse," *American Journal of Psychiatry* 150(4):643-46, 1993.

Craig, C. "Clinical Recognition and Management of Adult Attention Deficit Hyperactivity Disorder," *The Nurse Practitioner* 21(11):101-11, 1996.

Dannenberg, A.L., et al. "Intentional and Unintentional Injuries in Women," *Annals of Epidemiology* 4(2):133-39, 1994.

Diagnostic and Statistical Manual of Mental Disorders, DSM-IV, 4th ed., rev. Washington, D.C.: American Psychiatric Association, 1994.

Diseases, 2nd ed. Springhouse, Pa.: Springhouse Corp., 1997.

Hollinger, P.C., et al. *Suicide and Homicide Among Adolescents.* New York: Guilford, 1994.

Kapur, S., et al. "Antidepressant Medications and the Relative Risk of Suicide Attempts and Suicide," *Journal of American Medical Association* 268(24): 3441-45.

Leaman, T.L. *Healing the Anxiety Disease.* New York: Plenum Publishing Corp., 1992.

Leon, A.C., et al. "The Social Costs of Anxiety Disorders," *British Journal of Psychiatry* 27(Supp):19-22, 1995.

McIntyre, L., et al. "Depression and Suicide: Assessment and Intervention," *Home Health Care Management and Practice* 9(1):8-18, 1996.

Nursing98 Drug Handbook. Springhouse, Pa: Springhouse Corp., 1998.

Stoudemire, A., et al. "Psychopharmacology in the Medical Patient," in *Psychiatric Care of the Medical Patient.* Edited by Stoudemire, A., and Fogel, B. S. New York: Oxford University Press, 1993.

Stuart, G.W., and Sundeen, S.J. *Principles and Practice of Psychiatric Nursing,* 4th ed. St. Louis: Mosby–Year Book, Inc., 1991.

Stuck, A.E., et al. "A Trial of Annual In-home Comprehensive Geriatric Assessments for Elderly People Living in the Community," *New England Journal of Medicine* 333:1184-89, 1995.

Valente, S.M. "Diagnosis and Management of Panic Disorder and Generalized Anxiety Disorder in Primary Care," *Nurse Practitioner* 21(8):26-47, 1996.

Valente, S.M. "Evaluating Suicide Risk in the Medically Ill Patient," *Nurse Practitioner* 18(9):41-49, 1993.

Valente, S.M., and Frierson, A. "Suicide Risk in Young African Americans," *Glowing Lamp/JOCEPS* 43(1):11-16, 1996.

Wise, M.G., and Griffies, W.S. "A Combined Treatment Approach to Anxiety in the Medically Ill," *Journal of Clinical Psychiatry* 56(2)(Suppl.):14-19, 1995.

APPENDIX

Internet sites for nurses

The Internet is yet another way for you to gain information that will help you in your practice. The World Wide Web (WWW) is the most popular part of the Internet. It contains electronic publications, drawings, and photos.

On the web, you'll find sites for universities offering nursing education. Try the American Assocation of Colleges of Nursing (http://www.aacn.nche.edu). You can also use a search engine to locate individual programs. For example, searching on "nursing education" and "San Antonio" (http://www.uthscsa.edu/nursing/ce.htm) helps you find the University of Texas Health Science Center at San Antonio–School of Nursing.

Most major nursing associations have sites on the web, and some state nursing associations now do too; others are developing them through the American Nurses Association's Nursing World website.

Once you have found your favorite sites for information, your computer may allow you to "bookmark" them, giving you immediate access without re-entering the whole Internet or website address. The following are some of the most popular websites.

Website	Internet address	What it provides
ACLS Algorithms	http://www.cardiac.org/aclsalgr.html#algor	Instructions on advanced cardiac life support, step-by-step through the branches of the algorithm tree
American Diabetes Association	http://www.diabetes.org	Pathophysiology of diabetes, treatment, and information about insulin
Centers for Disease Control and Prevention	http://www.cdc.gov	Guidelines for infection control, hazardous substances, and immunizations
Digital Anatomist	http://www1.biostr.washington.edu/DigitalAnatomist.html	Anatomy atlas, including two- and three-dimensional pictures of various regions of the anatomy with information about the region
Drug Formulary	http://www.intmed.mcw.edu/drug.html	Enter the brand name of a drug and you can get the generic name, how supplied, dosage, and cost

Internet sites for nurses *(continued)*

Website	Internet address	What it provides
Hospital Web	http://neuro-www.mgh.harvard.edu/hospitalweb.nclk	Websites of hospitals and medical organizations in the United States and the world
Joint Commission on Accreditation of Healthcare Organizations (JCAHO)	http://www.jcaho.org	Information on JCAHO products and services; links to data on accreditation for home care, long-term care, and others
Laboratory Values	http:/www.ghsl.nwu.edu/Norm.html	Normal laboratory values for blood, sweat, urine, and CSF in a table format
MedWeb: Nursing	http://www.gen.emory.edu/MEDWEB/keyword/Nursing.html	Upcoming nursing conferences, associations, and electronic publications
National Council of State Boards of Nursing, Inc. (NCSBN)	http://www.ncsbn.org	Publications order form, events calendar, NCLEX examination information, and an online library
National League for Nursing (NLN)	http://www.nln.org	Testing services, publications and products (including videos), calendar of events
National Library of Medicine	http://www.nlm.nih.gov	Vast array of general information about medicine, aural heart sounds, ECG readings, motion pictures of procedures such as angiography, interactive chat rooms
Nursing and Health Care Resources	http://www.bath.ac.uk/~exxrw/nurse.html	Websites lists, news groups, mailing lists on mental health, midwifery, alternative therapy, and related fields
Nursing Index	http://www.lib.umich.edu/tml/nursing.html	Career opportunities, organizations, nursing research, and discussion groups in annotated format

Internet sites for nurses *(continued)*

Website	Internet address	What it provides
NursingNet	http://myspot.com/cgi-bin/nic-cgi/chat2.pl	Chat room for communication between users to ask questions and get quick responses
Nutrition	http://www.fsi.umn.edu/tools.htp	Nutrient components of specific foods
Perioperative Nursing Resources	http://www.aorn.org/nsgtoday/internet/links.htm	General nursing information, OR nursing, nursing organizations, and research
PharmInfoNet	http://pharminfo.com	Alphabetic formulary with links to articles from *Medical Sciences Bulletin*
Physical Exam	http://www.medinfo.ufl.edu/year1/bcs/clist/index.html	Diagrams on how to complete a history and a physical
Psychiatry On-Line	http://www.priory.com/journals/psych.htm	A peer-reviewed, independent journal
RxList	http://www.rxlist.com	Drug interactions for most commonly used agents
Sigma Theta Tau	http://stti-web.iupui.edu	Programs, research, membership and chapters, publications, philanthropy, library, and Online Journal of Knowledge Synthesis for Nursing
Springhouse Corporation	http://www.springnet.com	CE tests (100+ contact hours with immediate online grading), job listings, conference database, product ordering, articles and references on wide range of nursing topics (sponsored by *Nursing97*)
Virtual Hospital	http://vh.radiology.uiowa.edu	Medical specialties, multimedia textbook, guidelines, patient simulators, and teaching files

INDEX

---

i refers to an illustration; t refers to a table; **boldface** refers to a color illustration.

---

i refers to an illustration; t refers to a table; **boldface** refers to a color illustration.

i refers to an illustration; t refers to a table; **boldface** refers to a color illustration.

---

i refers to an illustration; t refers to a table; **boldface** refers to a color illustration.

---

i refers to an illustration; t refers to a table; **boldface** refers to a color illustration.

i refers to an illustration; t refers to a table; **boldface** refers to a color illustration.

i refers to an illustration; t refers to a table; **boldface** refers to a color illustration.

---

i refers to an illustration; t refers to a table; **boldface** refers to a color illustration.